Min Zhuo *Editor*

Molecular Pain

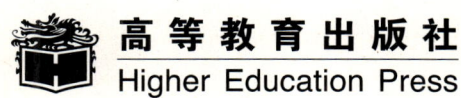
高等教育出版社
Higher Education Press

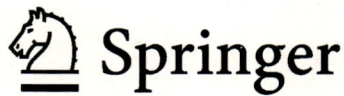
Springer

Min Zhuo
Department of Physiology
University of Toronto
Medical Sciences Bldg, Rm 3342
1 King's College Circle
Toronto, Ontario, Canada M5S 1A8

E-mail: *min.zhuo@utoronto.ca*

图书在版编目（CIP）数据

疼痛的分子机理=Molecular Pain /（美）卓敏主编. 北京：
高等教育出版社，2007.10
　ISBN 978-7-04-018954-4

　Ⅰ. 疼… Ⅱ. 卓… Ⅲ. 疼痛-研究-英文 Ⅳ. R441.1

中国版本图书馆 CIP 数据核字（2006）第 064136 号

图字：01-2007-3413 号

Copyright © 2007 by
Higher Education Press
4 Dewai Dajie, Beijing 100011, P. R. China

Distributed by Springer Science+Business Media, LLC under ISBN 978-0-387-75268-6 worldwide except in mainland China by the arrangement of Higher Education Press.

ISBN 978-7-04-018954-4

Printed in P. R. China

Major Contributors

Lan Bao, MD, PhD

Principal Investigator, Professor

Laboratory of Molecular Cell Biology

Institute of Biochemistry and Cell Biology

Chinese Academy of Sciences

No. 320 Yue Yang Rd

Shanghai 200031, China

Phone: 86-21-54921764

Fax: 86-21-54921762

E-mail: baolan@ion.ac.cn

Haruhiko Bito, MD, PhD

Associate Professor and Head

Department of Neurochemistry

The University of Tokyo, Graduate School of Medicine

7-3-1 Hongo, Bunkyo-ku

Tokyo 113-0033, Japan

Phone: 81-3-5841-3559

Fax: 81-3-3814-8154

E-mail: hbito@m.u-tokyo.ac.jp

Yves De Koninck, PhD

Professor and Director

Department of Psychiatry

Centre de recherche Université Laval Robert-Giffard (CRULRG)

2601, Chemin de la Canardière

Bureau F-5579 Beauport (Quebec) G1J 2G3, Canada

Phone: 418-663-5747 ext. 6885

Fax: 418-663-5873

E-mail: Yves.DeKoninck@crulrg.ulaval.ca

Alaa El-Husseini, PhD

Assistant Professor and Invesitgator

Brain Research Centre

University of British Columbia

Department of Psychiatry

Room 4N2-2255 Wesbrook Mall

Vancouver BC V6T 1Z3, Canada

Phone: 604-822-7526

Fax: 604-822-7981

E-mail: alaa@interchange.ubc.ca

Paul W. Frankland, PhD

Canada Research Chair in Cognitive Neurobiology

Hospital for Sick Children Research Institute

Department of Integrative Biology

555 University Ave.

Toronto ON M5G 1X8, Canada

Phone: 416-813-7654 ext.1823

Fax: 416-813-6846

E-mail: paul.frankland@sickkids.ca

Gerald F. Gebhart, PhD

Professor and Director

Center for Pain Research

University of Pittsburgh

Pittsburgh PA 15213, USA

Phone: 412-383-5911

Fax: 412-383-5466
E-mail: gebhartgf@upmc.edu

Peter A. Goldstein, MD
Assistant Professor
Department of Anesthesiology
Weill Medical College
Cornell University
New York NY 10021, USA
Phone: 212-746-5325
Fax: 212-746-4879
E-mail: pag2014@mail.med.cornell.edu

Jianguo G. Gu, PhD
Associate Professor
Department of Oral & Maxillofacial Surgery & Di-
    agnostic Sciences
College of Dentistry and McKnight Brain Institute
University of Florida
Box 100416
1600 SW Archer Road
Gainesville, Florida 32610, USA
Phone: 352-392-5989
Fax: 352-392-7609
E-mail: jgu@dental.ufl.edu

Sheena Josselyn, PhD
Assistant Professor
Department of Brain & Behavior
Hospital for Sick Children Research Institute
McMaster Bldg Rm 4017B, 555 University Ave
Toronto ON M5G 1X8, Canada
Phone: 416-813-7654 ext.1824
Fax: 416-813-6846
E-mail: sheena.josselyn@sickkids.ca

Bong-Kiun Kaang, PhD
Professor
Neurobiology Laboratory
Department of Biological Sciences
    & Institute of Molecular Biology & Genetics
College of Natural Sciences
Seoul National University

San 56-1 Silim-dong Kwanak-gu
Seoul 151-742, Korea
Phone: 82-2-880-7525
Fax: 82-2-884-9577
E-mail: kaang@snu.ac.kr

Jon H. Kaas, PhD
Distinguished Professor, Department of Psychology
Associate Professor, Department of Cell Biology
Kennedy Center Investigator
Vanderbilt University
Department of Psychology
301 Wilson Hall
Nashville TN 37240, USA
Phone: 615-322-6029
Fax: 615-343-8449
E-mail: jon.h.kaas@vanderbilt.edu

Rohini Kuner, PhD
Principal Investigator
Institute of Pharmacology
University of Heidelberg
Department of Molecular Pharmacology
366 IM Neuenheimer Feld
Heidelberg 69120, Germany
Phone: 49-6221-54-8289
Fax: 49-6221-54-8549
E-mail: rohini.kuner@urz.uni-heidelberg.de

John F. MacDonald, PhD
Ernest B. and Leonard B. Smith Professor and Chair
    Physiology
Department of Physiology
University of Toronto
1 King's College Circle
Toronto ON M5S 1A8, Canada
Phone: 416-978-0711
Fax: 416-978-4940
E-mail: j.macdonald@utoronto.ca

Annika Malmberg, PhD
Principal Scientist, Head of Analgesia Discovery Re-
    search and Head of *in Vivo* Analgesia

Elan Pharmaceuticals
800 Gateway Boulevard
South San Francsico CA 94080, USA
Phone: 650-794-4253
Fax: 650-877-7486
E-mail: annika.malmberg@elan.com

Christophe Mulle, PhD
Professor and Director
Institut Francois Magendie
Université Victor Segalen Bordeaux 2
1 rue C. Saint-Saëns
Bordeaux 33077, France
Phone: 0557574086
Fax : 0557574082
E-mail: mulle@u-bordeaux2.fr

Timothy J. Ness, MD, PhD
Professor and Co-Director
University of Alabama Birmingham
Department of Anesthesiology
619 19th St S ZRB 940
Birmingham AL 35233-6810, USA
Phone: 205-975-9643
Fax: 205-934-7437
E-mail: tim.ness@ccc.uab.edu

Volker E. Neugebauer, MD, PhD
Associate Professor
Department of Anatomy & Neurosciences
The University of Texas Medical Branch
Galveston TX 77555-1069, USA
Phone: 409-772-2124
Fax: 409-772-2789
E-mail: voneugeb@utmb.edu

Zhizhong Z. Pan, PhD
Assistant Professor
The University of Texas-MD Anderson Cancer Center
Department of Anesthesiology and Pain Medicine
Division of Anesthesiology and Critical Care
1515 Holcombe Blvd.
Houston TX 77030, USA

Phone: 713-792-5559
Fax: 713-745-4754
E-mail: zzpan@mdanderson.org

Huixin Qi, PhD
Research Assistant Professor
Department of Psychology
Vanderbilt University
Nashville TN 37203, USA
Phone: 615-322-7491
Fax: 615-343-8449
E-mail: huixin.qi@vanderbilt.edu

Alfredo Riberio-da-Silva, PhD
Professor
McGill University
Department of Pharmacology & Therapeutics
Department of Anatomy & Cell Biology
3655 Prom. Sir William Osler
Montreal, Quebec, H3G 1Y6, Canada
Phone: 514-398-3619
Fax: 514-398-6690
E-mail: alfredo.ribeirodasilva@mcgill.ca

Michael W. Salter, MD, PhD
Canada Research Chair in Neuroplasticity and Pain (Tier I)
Senior Scientist, Programs in Brain and Behaviour and Cell Biology
The Hospital for Sick Children
Professor of Physiology; Director, University of Toronto Centre for the Study of Pain
University of Toronto
Elizabeth McMaster Bldg 555 University Ave, Rm 5018
Toronto ON M5G1X8, Canada
Phone: 416-813-6272
Fax: 416-813-7921
E-mail: mike.salter@utoronto.ca

Kathleen A. Sluka, PT, PhD
Associate Professor
Graduate Program in Physical Therapy & Rehabilita-

tion Science
University of Iowa, Iowa, USA
1-242 Medical Education Building
Iowa City, Iowa 52242-1190, USA
Phone: 319-335-9791 or 9799
Fax: 319-335-9707
E-mail: kathleen-sluka@uiowa.edu

Stefan Strack, PhD

Assistant Professor
Department of Pharmacology
University of Iowa, College of Medicine
2-432 BSB
Iowa City IA 52242, USA
Phone: 319-335-7965
Fax: 319-338-8930
E-mail: stefan-strack@uiowa.edu

Andrew J. Todd, PhD

Professor
Institute of Biomedical and Life Sciences
University of Glasgow
West Medical Building University Avenue
Glasgow G12 8QQ YT, UK
Phone: 441413305868
Fax: 441413302868
E-mail: a.todd@bio.gla.ac.uk

Makoto Tominaga, MD, PhD

Professor
Okazaki Institute of Integrative Bioscience
Section Cell Signaling
Higashiyama 5-1 Myodaiji
Okazaki 444-8787, Japan
Phone: 81-5-6459-5286
Fax: 81-5-6459-5285
E-mail: tominaga@nips.ac.jp

Lu-Yang Wang, PhD

Associate Professor
Department of Physiology, University of Toronto
Canada Research Chair in Brain & Behavior (Tier II)
Senior Scientist, Program in Brain and Behavior Re-

search & Division of Neurology
The Hospital for Sick Children (HSC)
555 University Ave
Toronto ON M5G 1X8, Canada
Phone: 416-813-8711
Fax: 416-813-5086
E-mail: luyang.wang@utoronto.ca

Ling-Gang Wu, PhD

Investigator
National Institute of Neurological Disorders and Stroke
  36 Convent Drive, Bldg 36, Rm. 1C12
Bethesda, MD 20892, USA
Phone: 301-451-3338
Fax: 301-480-1466
E-mail: Wul@ninds.nih.gov

Tian-Le Xu, PhD

Investigator and Chief
Laboratory of Synaptic Physiology
Institute of Neuroscience
Chinese Academy of Sciences
No.320 Yue Yang Rd
Shanghai 200031, China
Phone: 86-21-54921751
Fax: 86-21-54921735
E-mail: tlxu@ion.ac.cn

Megumu Yoshimura, MD, PhD

Professor and Chair
Department of Integrative Physiology
Graduate School of Medical Sciences
Kyushu University
3-1-1 Maidashi, Higashi-ku
Fukuoka 812-8582, Japan
Phone: 81-9-2642-6085
Fax: 81-9-2642-6093
E-mail: yoshimum@physiol.med.kyushu-u.ac.jp

Xu Zhang, MD, PhD

Principal Investigator and Professor
Laboratory Sensory Sys
Institute Neuro Science

Chinese Academy of Sciences
No.320 Yue Yang Rd
Shanghai 200031, China
Phone: 86-21-54921761
Fax: 86-21-64713446
E-mail: xu.zhang@ion.ac.cn

Zhi-Qi Zhao, PhD
Professor
Institute of Neurobiology
Fudan University
Shanghai 200433, China.
Phone: 86-21-55522878
Fax: 86-21-55522876
E-mail: zqzhao@fudan.edu.cn

Min Zhuo, Ph D
Canada Research Chair in Pain and Cognition, Tier I
EJLB-CIHR Michael Smith Chair in Neurosciences
   and Mental Health
Professor
Department of Physiology
University of Toronto
Medical Sciences Bldg, Rm 3342
1 King's College Circle
Toronto, Ontario, M5S 1A8, Canada
Phone: 416-946-0532
Fax: 416-978-4940
E-mail: min.zhuo@utoronto.ca

Preface

The initial idea for this book came from Dr. Li Bingxiang at Higher Education Press during an international symposium in beautiful southern China. Unlike traditional textbooks on pain, she proposed I write a new book that included recent progress in the neurobiology of pain. This idea revived my long-term interest in editing a book on molecular pain.

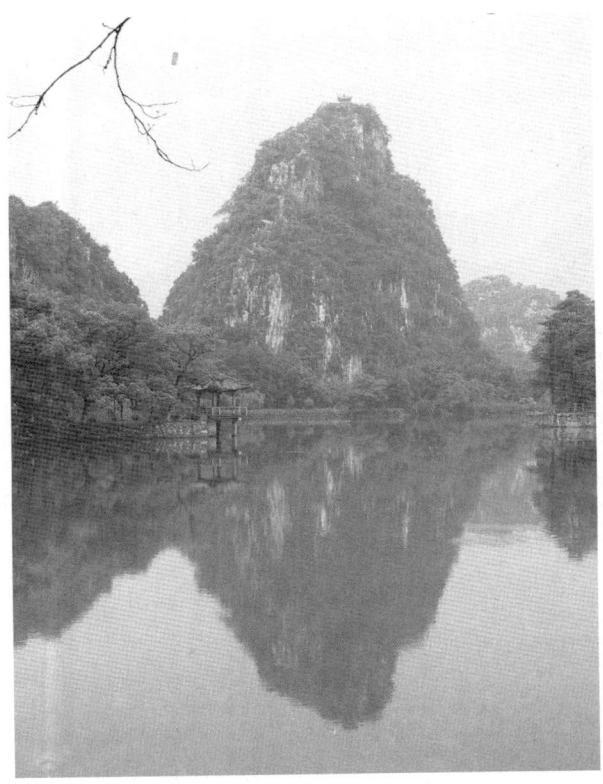

A scenery view of the southern China.

There are at least four major reasons why I felt this book was necessary. First, there are only a few textbooks on pain available, and some of them are outdated.

Second, the existing pain textbooks mainly focus on basic animal research and the clinical treatment of pain. Due to space limitations and the breadth of the topic, coverage of basic neuroscience is not sufficient.

Third, molecular biologists are making rapid progress toward finding molecular and gene involvement in pain. This progress is visible in a number of ways: the gene-chip used in pharmaceutical companies; the increase in molecular biologists interested in pain; and the use of transgenic mice in pain research. These scientists must be brought together with pain scientists.

And finally, an integrative approach is becoming standard in pain research. New investigators in the field need to be trained in multiple aspects of neurobiology.

Support from my friends and fellow scientists was essential to this book. The idea for this book was met with a strong positive response from many scientists, though not all of them could contribute chapters due to personal time constraints. I am confident that many of these excellent scientists will be able to contribute new chapters to future editions.

Help from Michelle and Melissa was essential to

put this book together. Funding from the EJLB-CIHR Michael Smith Chair and the Canada research Chair made it possible for me to work on this book. Additional help from lab members was also appreciated. My wife Kelly and my daughters Morgan and Danielle gave me enough energy and support to take on this rather difficult task.

I look forward to hearing readers' suggestions and comments on the book, though I know that not every pain-related topic is fully covered. In most cases, experts were contacted to write a chapter, but couldn't due to various commitments. This book is not intended to cover every topic related to pain; for instance, I have skipped over discussion of sensory receptors and the genetic background of pain. My goal was to focus on several topics in which neuroscience and pain interact to produce a basic understanding of mechanisms.

I hope that readers will find this book helpful and useful, and I sincerely hope that this book will enable doctors to relieve their patients' pain effectively.

The Guide to Use This Book

Unlike traditional textbooks, this book is edited as a series of topical seminars given by active researchers. The order of chapters is topic related, rather than the traditional layout of the pain textbooks, which is from periphery to the brain, and from basic to clinic. Most of topics are selected based on the recent progress as well as basic discovery at neurobiological levels in terms of our understanding. Many particular areas related to pain and analgesia are not covered, in part due to either the lack of molecular and cellular understanding of the process or the limit space.

Therefore, the readers are encouraged to use this book, together with the classic textbook of Pain (Wall and Melzeck). If necessary, the basic neuroscience textbooks are also recommended including the Principle of Neural Science (Kandel, Schwartz, Jessell).

Clinical studies are usually well covered in other pain-related textbooks. However, due to the limitation of new translational researches, we did not cover the clinical pain researches. Readers are encouraged to use the textbook of pain if needed.

Considering the rapid progress in neuroscience and pain related researches, the readers are highly recommended to use the PubMed in combination with this book.

The book is designed to teach basic principles for pain while introducing the most recent progress in exploring basic pain mechanism. We will aim at undergraduate students (late years), graduate students, post-doc fellows, medical students, nursing students, and clinical pain fellows. Although the book is focused on pain, we would like to also teach the students to use Pain as a model for investigating brain mechanisms.

Contents

Part I Genes, Neurons and Neurotransmission

Genes and Neurons

CHAPTER 1

Bong-Kiun Kaang

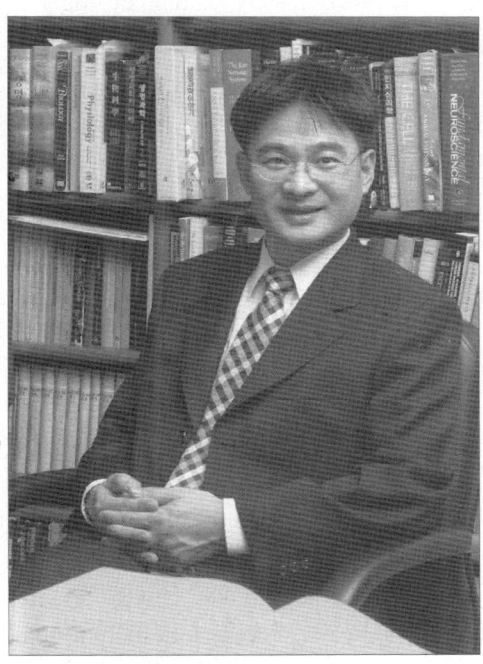

Dr. Kaang is a Professor in the Department of Biological Sciences, Seoul National University, Seoul, Korea. He graduated from Seoul National University. After gaining a Ph.D. in Neuroscience at Columbia University, he continued postdoctoral training in Eric Kandel's Laboratory. Dr. Kaang is interested in the molecular mechanisms of learning and memory.

MAJOR CONTRIBUTIONS

1. Kaang BK, Kandel ER, Grant SG. 1993. Activation of cAMP-responsive genes by stimuli that produce long-term facilitation in *Aplysia* sensory neurons. *Neuron*, 10(3): 427-435.

2. Chang DJ, Li XC, Lee YS, Kim HK, Kim US, Cho NJ, Lo X, Weiss KR, Kandel ER, Kaang BK. 2000. Activation of a heterologously expressed octopamine receptor coupled only to adenylyl cyclase produces all the features of presynaptic facilitation in aplysia sensory neurons. *Proc Natl Acad Sci USA*, 97(4): 1829-1834.

3. Park H, Lee JA, Lee C, Kim MJ, Chang DJ, Kim H, Lee SH, Lee YS, Kaang BK. 2005. An Aplysia type 4 phosphodiesterase homolog localizes at the presynaptic terminals of Aplysia neuron and regulates synaptic facilitation. *J Neurosci*, 25(39): 9037-9045.

4. Jang DH, Han JH, Lee SH, Lee YS, Park H, Lee SH, Kim H, Kaang BK. 2005. Cofilin expression induces cofilin-actin rod formation and disrupts synaptic structure and function in Aplysia synapses. *Proc Natl Acad Sci USA*, 102(44): 16072-16077.

5. Kim H, Lee SH, Han JH, Lee JA, Cheang YH, Chang DJ, Lee YS, Kaang BK. 2006. A Nucleolar Protein ApLLP Induces ApC/EBP Expression Required for Long-Term Synaptic Facilitation in Aplysia Neurons. *Neuron*, 49(5): 707-718.

MAIN TOPICS

Function of neurons
  Shape of neurons
  Types of neurons and glia
  Signaling and information processing in neurons
Genes involved in neural function
  Cytoskeletons
  Growth cone guidance molecules
  Neurotransmitter and neuropeptides
  Receptors & channels
  Plasticity-related genes
  Neurotrophic factors and cell death genes

SUMMARY

Genes encode proteins that are critical for the development and regulation of neural circuits involved in various aspects of brain function such as emotion, thought, learning, and neurological disease. We would like to understand the manner in which proteins responsible for neuronal activities are related to mental processes or brain diseases. Molecular genetics provides the means to determine the genes involved in a particular function of the brain. The human genome project has revealed that a human cell has approximately 30,000-60,000 genes. Neurons differ from other types of cells because they express a set of genes that is specific to them. Neurons are estimated to express ~40% of their total genes, some of which are also expressed in other types of cells. Neuron-specific genes encode neuropeptides, enzymes involved in the synthesis of neurotransmitters (NT), ion channels and receptors, synaptic proteins, and neurotrophic receptors. However, genes expressed in other cell types, such as those encoding protein kinases, cytoskeletal proteins, growth factors, etc., collaborate with neuron-specific genes and are thus involved in neuron-specific behavior such as axon guidance, synaptic plasticity, and neuronal cell death. In this chapter, we examine the basic structure of neurons and discuss genes and proteins that play a key role in neuronal functions. Although complex functions of the brain are determined by the pattern of neuronal connectivity and probably by the number of neurons, it is important to understand the molecular machinery of neurons and synapses given that genetic defects are known to cause many neurological disorders. In addition, remarkable progress has been made to develop drugs that target specific molecules or genes involved in neuronal functions.

INTRODUCTION

Neurons are the basic functional units of the nervous system. The human brain contains ~10^{11} neurons. Each neuron interconnects with thousands of other neurons through a synaptic structure to form precise neural circuits, which enable us to perceive, think, move, and feel. Complexity of behavior depends on the complexity of patterns of neuronal connections. Any pathological, cellular or molecular change in neurons can lead to specific neurological diseases depending on the site where the neurons or circuits are affected. A first step toward understanding the complexity of human behavior and the nature of neurological disorders is to determine the organization of neurons in functional systems and the manner in which they interact with each other during information processing in the nervous system.

In this chapter, we will study the basic structure and function of neurons, and examine various genes that encode proteins involved in neuronal development as well as in basic neuronal functions.

FUNCTION OF NEURONS

Shape of Neurons

A neuron receives neural signals from other neurons through its dendrites and cell body. The nerve impulses are then transmitted along the axon to the axon terminal where NT is released to stimulate other neurons. The cell body or soma contains the nucleus where specific genes are transcriptionally regulated in order to perform the specific function of individual neurons. In many neurons, dendrites have specialized protruding structures termed as spines that receive synaptic inputs from axon terminals.

Generally, in the vertebrate nervous system, axons are wrapped in a myelin sheath. This myelination enables fast, saltatory conduction of the nerve impulses through the axons. The myelin sheath is interrupted by the node of Ranvier, which is highly enriched in ion channels and pumps. The axon terminals contact other neurons to form a connection site termed as the synapse. The presynaptic and postsynaptic cells are separated by a space termed as the synaptic cleft (Fig.1.1).

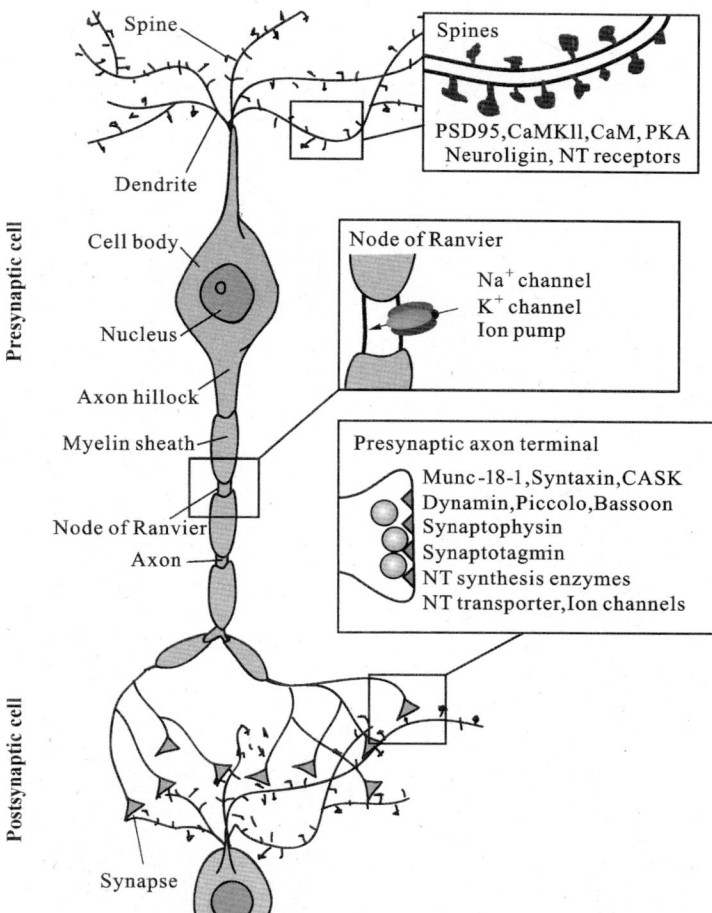

Fig.1.1 Structure of a neuron. The presynaptic cell transmits electrical signals to the postsynaptic cell at a site named the synapse. Some of the key molecules are listed for three different regions in the neuron. Some of these molecules could be expressed in non-neuronal cells.

Types of Neurons and Glia

Although all neurons have the same basic architecture, they can be classified into numerous types on the basis of multiple criteria (Fig.1.2). Based on the number of neurites radiating from the cell body, some neurons are termed as unipolar (single neurite), bipolar (two neurites), or multipolar (many neurites). Based on the dendritic shapes, neurons are differentiated as pyramidal cells or stellate cells. Based on the function, sensory neurons carry the information from the sensory surfaces of the body, whereas motor neurons control muscles. Most neurons are termed as interneurons since they form connections only with other neurons. Depending on the types of NT released, neurons are termed as cholinergic, glutamatergic, serotonergic, dopaminergic, GABAergic neurons, etc.

In fact, neurons are not the major cells in the nervous system. Ninety percent of cells in the nervous system are non-neuronal cells termed as glia or glial cells. Glial cells provide physical and chemical support to the neurons. Astrocytes reabsorb the NT spilled from neurons along with K^+ ions that are accumulated in the extracellular fluid due to excessive neural activity. Oligodendrocytes in the central nervous system and Schwann cells in the peripheral nervous system provide the myelin sheath that insulates axons. Microglia removes dead materials and cells from the nervous system. Ependymal cells contribute to the formation of cerebrospinal fluid and recently, they have been shown to contain neural stem cells [BOX 1.1] that have the potential to produce new neurons and glia.

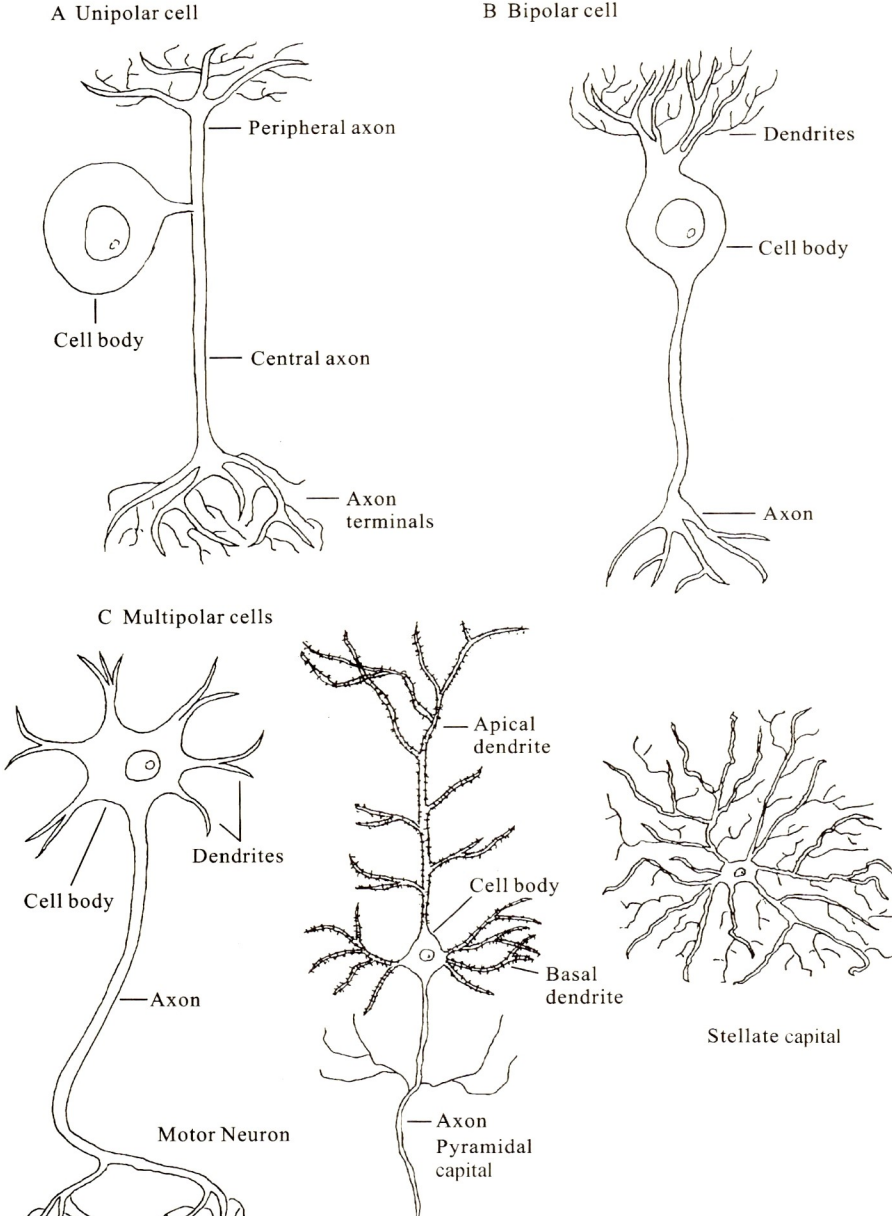

Fig.1.2 Classification of neurons. A. Unipolar cell containing a single process. Dorsal root ganglion cell. B. Bipolar cells containing two processes. Bipolar cells in the retina. C. Multipolar cells containing many processes. Three examples are shown: motor neuron, pyramidal cell, stellate cell (adapted from Kandel *et al.*, Principles of Neural Sciences).

Signaling and Information Processing in Neurons

One of the most important functions of neurons is to generate an electrical signal, carry this signal, and transfer it to another target cell. This neuronal signaling is one of the key features of information processing in the nervous system. Thus, it is important to understand the manner in which this signaling is generated and the nature of the molecular components involved in this signaling function. Neural signaling is initiated from the axon hillock, a specialized trigger zone near the cell body. When the membrane potential is depolarized above the threshold in the axon hillock, it generates an electrical signal termed as the action potential. When a depolarizing stimulus can sufficiently activate the Na^+ channels to cause a trigger, a positive feedback occurs, which allows more Na^+ to enter, ensuring a sudden increase in Na^+ influx. The membrane potential approximates the Na^+ equilibrium potential (E_{Na}). From this point onwards, the sodium channels become desensitized and they close. At the peak of membrane depolarization, delayed rectifying potassium channels start to open because they are also sensitive to voltage change. Finally, the membrane potential almost returns to the resting potential thus completing one round of action potential.

The action potential moves along the axon to the axon terminal (Fig.1.3).

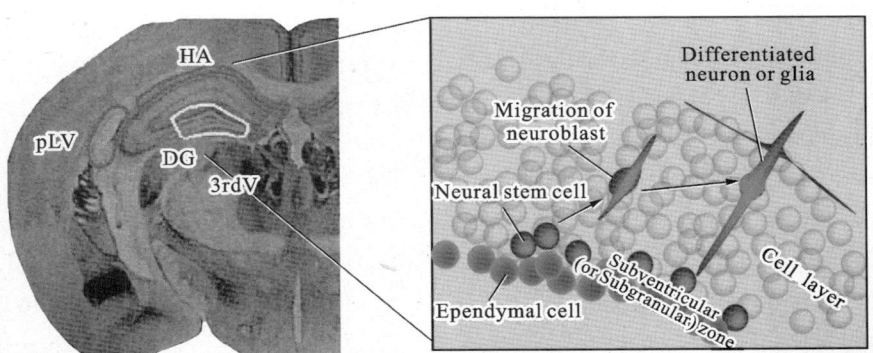

Stem cells are undifferentiated cells that have the potential to differentiate into other cell types. With this potential, it has been used to replace defected cells in patients. Neural stem cells have also been identified in the ependymal cell layers lining the lateral ventricle (pLV), the adjacent subventricular zone (3rd V: third ventricle) and the hippocampus (DG: dentate gyrus, HA: hippocampal arch). Neural stem cells in the ependymal cell layer lining the surface of the subventricular or subgranular zone migrate rostrally to give rise to differentiated neurons or glial cells in the cell layer.

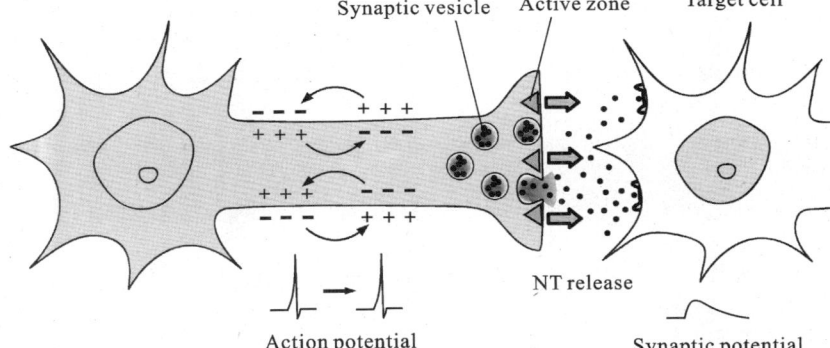

Fig.1.3 Communication between neurons is mediated by action potential propagation and neurotransmitter (NT) release at the synapse. The response of the target is determined by the temporal and spatial patterns of synaptic inputs and the types of NT receptors activated.

The axon terminal makes a synaptic contact with the postsynaptic membrane. When the action potential reaches the presynaptic terminal, voltage-dependent Ca^{2+} channels open to allow the extracellular Ca^{2+} to flow into the presynaptic terminal. Synaptic vesicles containing NT molecules are present at the presynaptic terminal. Ca^{2+}-triggered synaptic vesicle release is one of the most complex mechanisms in which the interaction between v-SNARE and t-SNARE proteins plays a key role in the active zone. Due to membrane fusion between the vesicles and the plasma membrane, NT molecules are released into the synaptic cleft.

Synaptotagmin present at the vesicle membrane is known to act as a Ca^{2+} sensor. Recently, numerous proteins such as piccolo and bassoon have been identified as components of the active zone. Synaptic vesicles are recycled by clathrin-mediated endocytosis and then transported to early endosome where budding of new synaptic vesicles occurs. NTs released from the presynaptic terminals bind to the receptors clustered at the postsynaptic membrane in the dendrites or dendritic spines. These receptors are usually ligand-gated ion channels or ionotropic receptors.

The activation of NT receptors can induce

changes in the membrane potential, i.e., either depolarization by excitatory NT (e.g., glutamate) or hyperpolarization by inhibitory NT (GABA or glycine). NT receptors are clustered by a scaffold complex or by so-called postsynaptic density (PSD), which contains numerous scaffold proteins and signaling components such as PSD 95, CaMKII, etc. The activation of postsynaptic neurons by NT and neural activity can produce synaptic plasticity, a phenomenon involving a plastic change in the synaptic strength or efficacy. Second messengers such as Ca^{2+} and cAMP are transiently increased by synaptic or neural activity. These messengers play a key role in producing synaptic plasticity (e.g., long-term potentiation). Ca^{2+} activates CaM kinases to induce AMPA receptor trafficking to the postsynaptic membrane or to induce local protein synthesis in the dendritic spines. These kinases appear to produce a retrograde signal such as nitric oxide that can cross over the synaptic cleft to enhance the presynaptic release. The cAMP signal can trigger PKA and MAPK to move toward the cell nuclei to induce new gene expression.

Postsynaptic neurons can integrate and process neural signals from different synaptic inputs by spatial summation, or they can integrate repetitive signals from the same synaptic input by temporal summation. Furthermore, the postsynaptic neuron can associate different synaptic inputs or produce a change in synaptic strength depending on the pattern of neural activity in collaboration with the presynaptic neurons.

GENES INVOLVED IN NEURAL FUNCTION

The completion of the genome projects for *Caenorhabditis elegans*, *Drosophila melanogaster*, and humans provides an understanding of the complete gene set of the proteins that function in the nervous system [BOX 1.2]. The genomes of these organisms share a conserved, large repertoire of neuronal proteins, although in the human genome, there is an increase in the number of some members of protein families. In addition, it became possible to screen neuron-specific genes or a set of genes that are induced under a specific neurobiological condition [BOX 1.3]. In this section, I will highlight some selected neuronal proteins that are critical in neuronal functioning.

BOX 1.2   Proteins involved in neural structure, function, and development.

Number of proteins in selected families in human (*H. sapiens*), fly (*D. melanogaster*), and nematode (*C. elegans*).

Protein family	Human	Fly	Nematode
Acetylcholine receptor	17	12	56
Voltage-gated Ca^{2+} channels	38	9	12
Voltage-gated K^+ channels	39	7	14
Voltage-gated Na^+ channels	11	4	4
Myelin-related	10	1	0
Neuropilin	2	0	0
Plexin	9	2	0
Semaphorin	22	6	2
Synaptotagmin	10	3	3
Connexin	14	0	0
Ephrins	7	2	4
Cadherin	100	14	16

The publications of the sequences of genomes enable a comparative analysis of genes expressed in nervous systems. This box shows the representative proteins involved in neural structure, function, and development from worm, fly, and human. Correlating with the unique properties of nervous system such as the generation of action potentials and neurotransmitter release, voltage-gated channels consist large protein families. Other neural protein families are involved in pathway finding by axons and neuronal network formation (cadherins, ephrins, semaphorins, neuropilins, and plexins). Protein families predominantly expressed only in vertebrate genome are myelin-related proteins which provide insulation and increase the speed of propagation of action potentials. Note that there is a marked increase in the number of neural protein families in the human genome. This finding can partially explain that the human nervous system is more complicated than other nervous systems in terms of the number and connectivity of neurons, the number of distinct neural cell types, the increased length of axons, and the increase in glial cell number.

BOX1.3   Microarray analysis for profiling of neural specific or neural activity-induced genes.

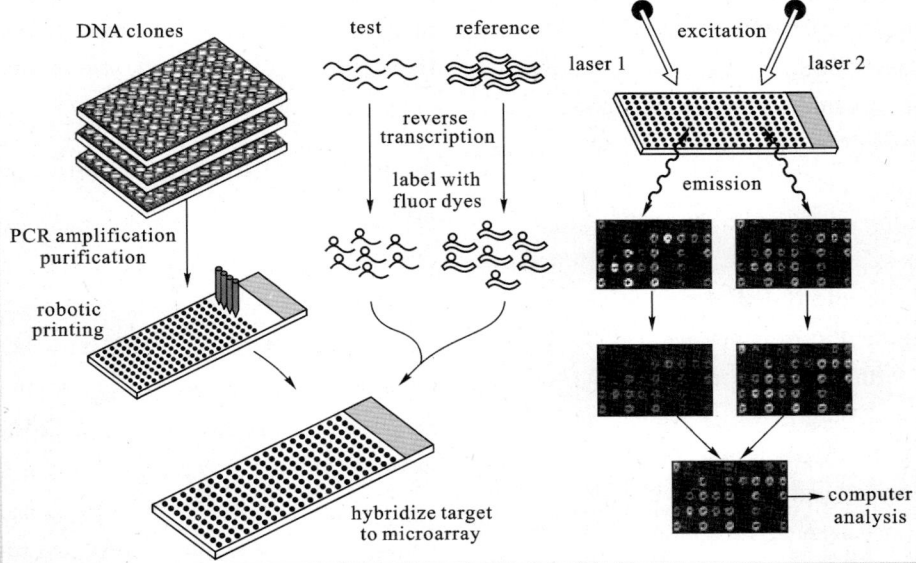

cDNA Microarray overview (adapted from Duggan *et al.*, Nature Genetics, 1999, 21)

Microarrays are defined as immobilized oligonucleotides or cDNA (EST or known genes) at high density. The attached DNAs serve as hybridization target for labeled probes which can be generated by labeling extracted RNA with fluorescence, radioactivity, or chemiluminescence. This technology provides a chance to analyze huge number of genes (>10,000) simultaneously. Recently, molecular biologists adopted this approach to elucidate set of neural specific genes and differentially expressed genes at specific developmental time points, in specific brain area, and certain physiological conditions (seizure, memory consolidation etc.).

There are several specific challenges in adapting this technology to neurobiology: (i) the extreme complexity of nervous system make it difficult to collect homogeneous neuronal population, (ii) the amount of RNA extracted from single neuron or even specific brain tissue is very limited. To enrich differentially expressed genes in specific population of neurons or brain tissues, other techniques such as representational difference analysis (RDA) and suppressive subtractive hybridization (SSH) are combined to enriched transcripts in interest. To overcome the problem of RNA amount, several amplification methods have been developed. If both linearity and uniformity of the amplifications are guaranteed, those techniques will facilitate the use of microarray technology by neurobiologists.

Cytoskeleton

Neuronal morphology is largely determined by the various cytoskeletons present within the neuron. Cytoskeletons contain microtubules, actin filaments, and intermediate filaments (neurofilaments). These cytoskeletons are connected to each other by various cross-linking proteins. Microtubules shape the neuronal structure and play a key role in transporting materials between the cell body and distal neurites and synapses. These materials such as proteins, RNA, and vesicles are transported by motor proteins that move along the microtubule railway. There are many microtubule-associated proteins, of which, MAP2 is well known as a dendrite-specific marker protein.

Actin is highly enriched in the cytoskeleton and is thus involved in shaping the periphery of the cell membrane, dendritic spines, and presynaptic terminals. Dynamic changes in actin polymerization/depolymerization are involved in growth cone guidance and are regulated by various signaling pathways. Intermediate filaments and neuron-specific filaments termed as neurofilaments are known to stabilize the neuronal structure.

Growth Cone Guidance Molecules

The function of the growth cone is to enable a neuron to find the target cell in order to make synaptic contact with it. Growth cones use diffusible molecules or extracellular matrix molecules as guideposts during the long journey to the target cells. Target cells usually secrete diffusible molecules to attract a growth cone. The growth cone finally recognizes the target cell and makes synaptic contact with it. The growth cones and neurites contain a family of integrin molecules, which are the membrane proteins; these integrin molecules can interact with extracellular matrix molecules such as laminin. This interaction determines direction of movement of the growth cone.

Cell-cell interactions are also important in neurite outgrowth. The cadherin superfamily and NCAM, a member of the immunoglobulin (Ig) superfamily of adhesion molecules, are involved in cell-cell interaction and neuritic fascicle (bundle) formation by homophilic or heterophilic interactions between the member proteins within each superfamily. Diffusible factors affect axonal outgrowth as well as neuronal survival. For example, netrin acts as a chemoattractant to attract the growth cone. Netrin receptors include unc-5H and Dcc/neogenin, which are Ig superfamily members.

In contrast, ephrins and semaphorins act as chemorepellants and repel the growth cone. Ephrin activates a receptor tyrosine kinase named as Eph kinase that inhibits axon growth. Semaphorins bind to neuropilin and plexin, which are also Ig superfamily

members, and repress axon growth. When growth cone receptors are activated by guidance molecules, they activate or inactivate small GTP-binding proteins that lead to a change in actin polymerization/depolymerization. Growth cone directions are determined by actin dynamics.

Neurotransmitters and Neuropeptides

NTs are locally synthesized at the presynaptic terminal (Table 1.1). Neurons contain specific enzymes that are involved in NT synthesis. These enzymes are distributed within the cytosol and vesicles present at the axon terminal. NTs are packaged into the vesicles by H^+-dependent transporters. Specific enzymes involved in the first step of NT biosynthesis are usually regulated at the transcriptional or posttranslational level by neural activity and other relevant stimuli. NT released into the synaptic cleft is removed by degradation by a specific enzyme, chelation by a binding protein, or by reuptake into the presynaptic terminal and the nearby surrounding glial cells.

Table 1.1   Neurotransmitters and neuropeptides.

Classic Neurotransmitters (small, rapid-acting molecules)	Key Biosynthetic Enzymes
Acetylcholine	Choline acetyltransferase
Biogenic amines	
Dopamine	Tyrosine hydroxylase
Norepinephrine	Tyrosine hydroxylase and dopamine β-hydroxylase
Epinephrine	Tyrosine hydroxylase and dopamine β-hydroxylase
Serotonin	Tyrosine hydroxylase
Histamine	Histidine decarboxylase
Amino acids	
γ-Aminobutyric acid	Glutamic acid decarboxylase
Glycine	Enzymes operating in general metabolism
Glutamate	Enzymes operating in general metabolism
Neuropeptides (large, slow-acting molecules)	
Adrenocorticotropic hormone (ACTH)	Leucine enkephalin
Angiotensin II	α-melanocyte-stimulating hormone(MSH)
Bombesin	Methionine enkephalin
Bradykinin	Motilin
Carnosine	Neurotensin
Cholecystokinin (CCK)	Oxytocin
β-endorphin	Somatostatin
Gastrin	Substance P
Glucagon	Thyrotropin-releasing hormone (TRH)
Gonadotropin-releasing hormone (GnRH)	Vasoactive intestinal polypeptide (VIP)
Insulin	Vasopressin

Neuropeptides are large, slow-acting molecules and synthesized in the rough endoplasmic reticulum (RER) in the cell body (Table 1.1). Neuropeptide precursors are processed and cleaved by specific enzymes in the Golgi and stored in the vesicles. These vesicles are transported by anterograde motor proteins to the presynaptic terminals along the microtubule. Unlike the small translucent vesicles containing conventional NT, neuropeptide-containing vesicles are large, dense-core vesicles. These vesicles are not released at the active zone, and thus require a large Ca^{2+} influx through bursts of action potential.

Receptors and Channels

Neurons have a variety of receptors on their plasma membrane in order to receive various chemical signals such as NT, neuropeptides, growth factors, and neurohormones from other cells. Ionotropic receptors are ion channels that are specifically activated by NT (Fig.1.4). Other types of receptors are metabotropic receptors that are activated by NT, neuropeptides, and growth factors and mediate the intracellular signal cascades. Steroids can activate another type of receptor, termed as nuclear receptors, which act as transcription factors.

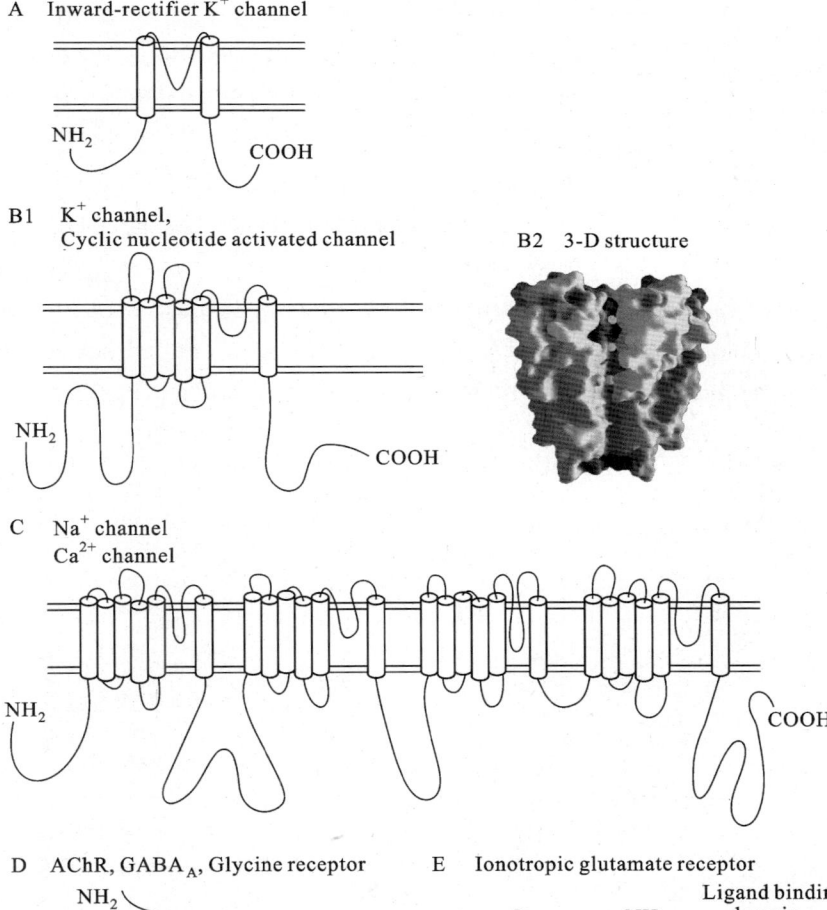

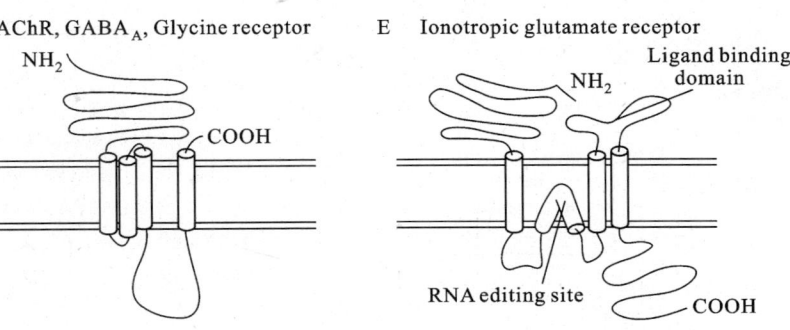

Fig.1.4 General structure of ion channels. A. Inward rectifier K^+ channels have only the pore loop region and two membrane-spanning regions. B1. A typical voltage-gated K^+channel. Cyclic nucleotide activated channels also share this topology. Four channel subunits are assembled to form a functional channel. B2. Three dimensional structure of a K^+channel (adapted from Science, 1998, 280:69) C. The major subunits of voltage-gated Na^+ and Ca^{2+} channels. These α subunits are composed of four repeat units of six transmembrane regions and one pore loop. D. AChR, $GABA_A$, and glycine receptor have the four domains named M1-M4 spanning the plasma membrane. Five subunits are assembled to form a complete channel. E. Ionotropic glutamate receptors include NMDA receptors, AMPA receptors, and kainate receptors (adapted from Kandel *et al.*, Principles of Neural Sciences).

Ion channels play a key role in generating the electrical signal in the nervous system (Fig.1.4). Some channels are leaky channels that are involved in producing the resting membrane potential. Other channels are usually gated by specific stimuli such as voltage change, NT, second messenger, mechanical force, and temperature change. Most of these ion channels are classified into gene families that are considered to have evolved from an ancestral gene by gene duplication and rearrangement (Fig.1.4).

The structure and gating mechanism of ion channels were extensively studied by Rod Mackinnon and his colleagues at Rockefeller University. They revealed the three-dimensional structure of the pore structure and gating mechanism by using a voltage-sensitive K^+ channel. Ion channels are good drug targets because the neural functions involved in the cognition, behaviors, and brain diseases are mostly carried out by ion channels (Fig.1.4).

Plasticity-related Genes

Neural plasticity is one of the most critical functions in the nervous system and is involved not only in learning and memory but also in neurological diseases such as drug addiction and depression.

Long-term potentiation (LTP) is one of the best-studied synaptic plasticities and is found in many brain areas, including hippocampus, amygdala, and cerebral cortex. LTP has been most extensively studied in area CA1 of the hippocampus (Fig.1.5). NMDA receptors play a critical role in initiating LTP by generating Ca^{2+} influx, which can activate αCaMKII and probably other kinases. αCaMKII phosphorylates AMPA receptor and other proteins. This phosphorylation can increase the unitary conductance of AMPA receptors containing GluR1. It is also shown that the phosphorylation of another site of GluR1 by αCaMKII can induce the synaptic translocation of the AMPA receptor to increase the sensitivity of the postsynaptic membrane to glutamate. The PDZ domain-containing proteins SAP97 and syntenin are involved in AMPA receptor trafficking to the synaptic site.

On the other hand, in long-lasting LTP, cAMP production by Ca^{2+}-activated adenylyl cyclase and subsequent PKA activation are critical events that lead to CREB phosphorylation, which in turn induces other transcription factors such as C/EBP and Egr1 (Zif 268).

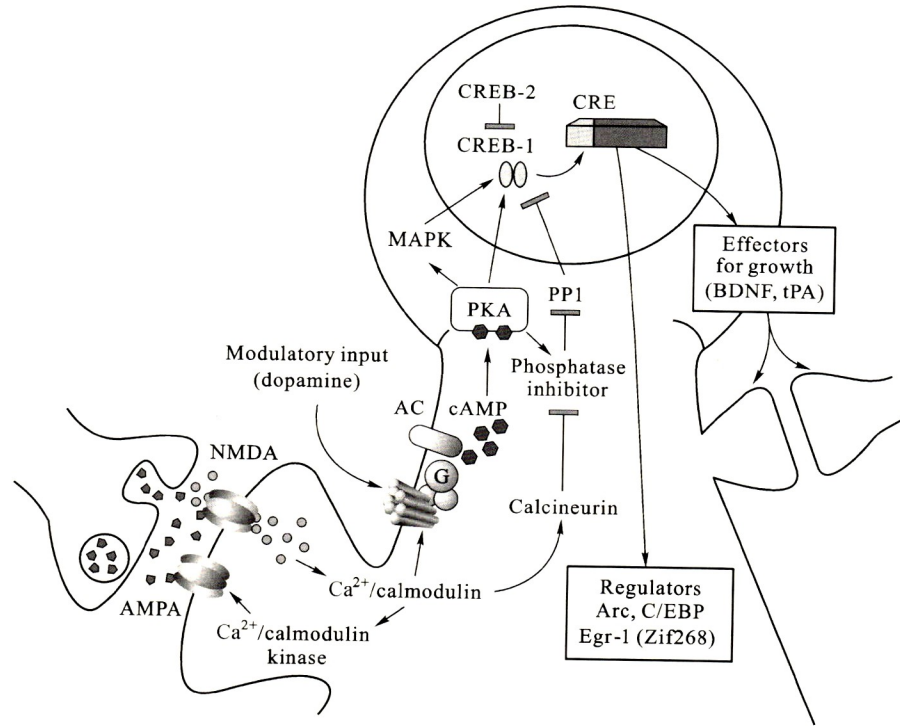

Fig.1.5 Key molecules involved in LTP in the Schaffer collateral pathway (adapted from Kandel, Science, 2001, 294). AC, adenylyl cyclase; PP1, protein phosphatase 1; BDNF, brain-derived neurotrophic factor; tPA, tissue plasminogen activator; Arc, activity-regulated cytoskeletal-related molecule.

These factors are considered to induce proteins that are involved in strengthening the synaptic structure and function(Fig.1.5).

Neurotrophic Factors and Cell Death Genes

Neurotrophic factors are critically involved in neuronal differentiation, growth, synaptogenesis, and synaptic plasticity. NGF, BDNF, and NT-3/4 are well-known neurotrophic factors (Fig.1.6). Non-neu-ronal growth factors such as GDNF, CNTF, LIF, PDGF, and FGF are also critically involved in neuron and glial cell differentiation (Fig.1.6). The neurotrophic factor receptors are TrkA, TrkB, and TrkC, which have a different affinity to each neurotrophic factor. The receptors for their cognate non-neuronal growth factors are GFRα, RET, gp130, LIFR, and CNTFR.

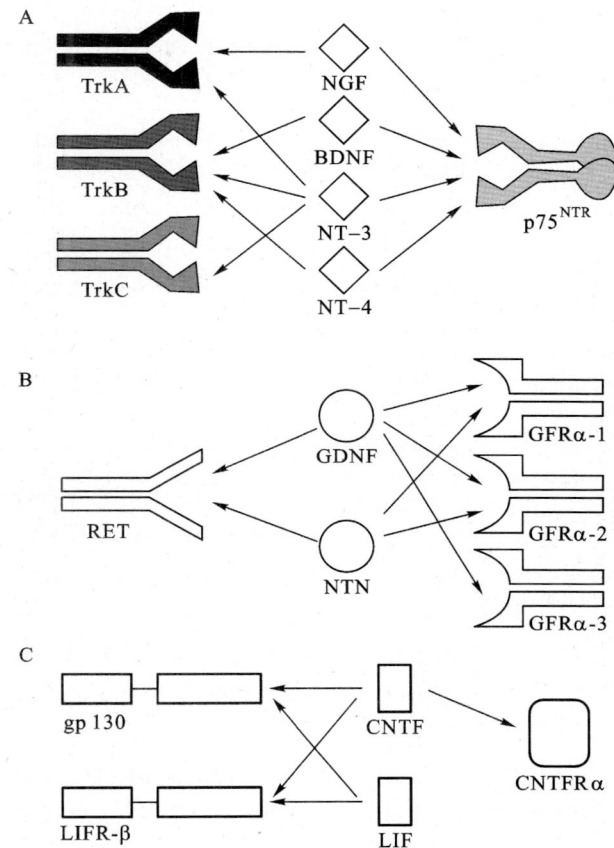

Fig.1.6 Neurotrophic factors and their cognate receptors. A. The neurotrophins, NGF (nerve growth factor), BDNF (brain-derived neurotrophic factor), NT-3(neurotrophin-3), and NT-4 (neurotrophin-4) bind to p75^{NTR} and different members (TrkA, B and C) of the Trk tyrosine kinase family. B. GDNF (glial cell-derived neurotrophic factor) and NTN (neurturin) bind to the same receptor subunit RET. They also bind differentially to GFRα receptors. C. The neurokines, CNTF (ciliary neurotrophic factor) and LIF (leukemia inhibitory factor) use the same receptor subunits, gp130 and LIFR-β. CNTF also activates CNTFRα (adapted from Trends Neurosci, 1998 (21): 438).

Elimination of neurotrophic factors activates a cell death program that results in neuronal death. In fact, the role of neurotrophic factors is to suppress a cell death program instead of stimulating a beneficial metabolism that leads to neuronal survival. Once a cell suicide program is activated, it causes apoptosis, which is characterized by cell shrinkage and nuclear condensation. The cellular debris is eventually phagocytosed by microglia.

In the absence of neurotrophic factors, Bcl-2, an antiapoptotic protein, is inactivated. Inactivation of Bcl-2 leads to the activation of Apaf-1. Apaf-1 shows ATP-dependent hydrolytic activity, which is required to process and activate caspases that cleave substrate proteins and eventually result in cell death.

The tyrosine kinase receptor is considered to phosphorylate protein substrates that promote Bcl-2 activities. Bcl-2 proteins form dimers. Other proteins such as Bax, a proapoptotic protein, can bind to Bcl-2 and inhibit its activity.

$$NT$$
$$\downarrow$$
$$\text{Receptor Tyrosine Kinase}$$
$$\downarrow$$
$$Bax \longrightarrow \dashv Bcl2 \longrightarrow \dashv Apaf\text{-}1 \rightarrow Caspase\ cleavage \rightarrow Cell\ death$$

CONCLUSIONS AND FUTURE DIRECTIONS

Modern genetic approaches, including the genome projects and DNA chip techniques, combined with a basic knowledge of neuroscience obtained during the 20th century have revealed many neuron-specific and other genes that are activated in a specific neurobiological phenomenon. Neuron-specific genes encode neuropeptides, enzymes involved in the synthesis of NTs, ion channels and receptors, synaptic proteins, and neurotrophic receptors. However, the genes expressed in many other cell types, such as those encoding protein kinases, cytoskeletal proteins, growth factors, etc., collaborate with neuron-specific genes and are thus involved in neuron-specific behavior such as axon guidance, synaptic plasticity, and neuronal cell death. All these genes are involved in shaping neuronal morphology, generating neural signaling and synaptic function, and responding to various chemical and electrical signals that act on neurons at every moment during our development and daily life. We are not only interested in finding neuron-specific genes but are also eager to understand the manner in which the expression of these genes and/or the activities of these gene products are regulated under certain conditions such as in neurological and psychiatric diseases. For example, we need to understand the nature of the key molecular components involved in pain mechanism if we want to develop a new drug for analgesia. Similarly, molecular studies on neuronal cell death mechanisms can provide an insight into many neurodegenerative diseases. Notably, neurons are rather heterogeneous in nature in terms of their position and role in different systems. Thus, the future challenge would be to detect molecular genetic changes at the single neuron level. These efforts combined with high throughput screening would help in developing specific drugs for key molecules that are critically involved in certain neurological diseases at the system level. Thus, future molecular biological efforts may shed light on providing solutions for some of the most debilitating psychiatric and neurological diseases such as pain, schizophrenia, manic depression, Alzheimer's disease, and Parkinson's disease.

GENERAL CITATIONS

Cao Y, Dulac C. 2001. Profiling brain transcription: neurons learn a lesson from yeast. *Curr Opin Neurobiol*, 11:615-620.

Cavallaro S, D'Agata V, Manickam P, Dufour F, Alkon DL. 2002. Memory-specific temporal profiles of gene expression in the hippocampus. *Proc Natl Acad Sci USA*, 99: 16279-16284.

Duggan DJ, Bittner M, Chen Y, Meltzer P, Trent JM. 1999. Expression profiling using cDNA microarrays. *Nat Genet*, 21: 10-14.

Eberwine J, Kacharmina JE, Andrews C, Miyashiro K, McIntosh T, Becker K, *et al*. 2001. mRNA expression analysis of tissue sections and single cells. *J Neurosci*, 21: 8310-8314.

Geschwind DH, Ou J, Easterday MC, Dougherty JD, Jackson RL, Chen Z, *et al*. 2001. A genetic analysis of neural progenitor differentiation. *Neuron*, 29: 325-339.

Ibanez CF. 1998. Emerging themes in structural biology of neurotrophic factors. *Trends Neurosci*, 21: 438-444.

Kandel ER. 2001. The molecular biology of memory storage: a dialog between genes and synapses. *Biosci Rep*, 21: 565-611.

Kandel ER, Schwartz JH, Jessell TM. 2000. *Principles of Neural Science*, 4th ed. New York: McGraw-Hill.

Luo L. 2002. Actin cytoskeleton regulation in neuronal morphogenesis and structural plasticity. *Annu Rev Cell Dev Biol*, 18: 601-635.

Malenka RC, Nicoll RA. 1999. Long-term potentiation—a decade of progress? *Science*, 285: 1870-1874.

Sandberg R, Yasuda R, Pankratz DG, Carter TA, Del Rio JA, Wodicka L, *et al*. 2000. Regional and strain-specific gene expression mapping in the adult mouse brain. *Proc Natl Acad Sci USA*, 97: 11038-11043.

Tojima T, Ito E. 2004. Signal transduction cascades underlying de novo protein synthesis required for neuronal morphogenesis in differentiating neurons. *Prog Neurobiol*, 72: 183-193.

DISCOVERY CITATIONS

Cao Y, Dulac C. 2001. Profiling brain transcription: neurons learn a lesson from yeast. *Curr Opin Neurobiol*, 11: 615-620.

Cavallaro S, D'Agata V, Manickam P, Dufour F, Alkon DL. 2002. Memory-specific temporal profiles of gene expression in the hippocampus. *Proc Natl Acad Sci USA*, 99: 16279-16284.

Duggan DJ, Bittner M, Chen Y, Meltzer P, Trent JM. 1999. Expression profiling using cDNA microarrays. *Nat Genet*, 21: 10-14.

Wang HG, Lu FM, Jin I, Udo H, Kandel ER, de Vente J, *et al*. 2005. Presynaptic and postsynaptic roles of NO, cGK, and RhoA in long-lasting potentiation and aggregation of synaptic proteins. *Neuron*, 45: 389-403.

Wu H, Nash JE, Zamorano P, Garner CC. 2002. Interaction of SAP97 with minus-end-directed actin motor myosin VI. Implications for AMPA receptor trafficking. *J Biol Chem*, 277: 30928-30934.

Ying SW, Futter M, Rosenblum K, Webber MJ, Hunt SP, Bliss TV, *et al*. 2002. Brain-derived neurotrophic factor induces long-term potentiation in intact adult hippocampus: requirement for ERK activation coupled to CREB and upregulation of Arc synthesis. *J Neurosci*, 22: 1532-1540.

Zurn AD, Winkel L, Menoud A, Djabali K, Aebischer P. 1996. Combined effects of GDNF, BDNF, and CNTF on motoneuron differentiation in vitro. *J Neurosci Res*, 44: 133-141.

Synapses: Coupling of Presynaptic Voltage-gated Ca^{2+} Channels to Vesicular Release of Neurotransmitter

CHAPTER 2

Lu-Yang Wang

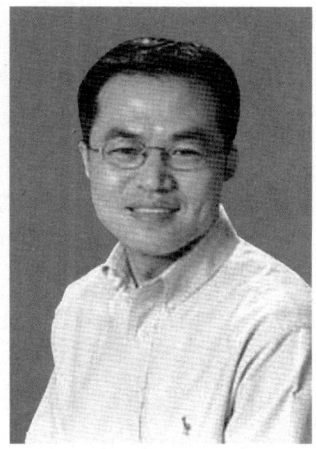

Dr. Wang is a Senior Scientist in The Division of Neurology & The Program for Brain and Behavior Research, The Hospital for Sick Children. He is also an Associate Professor, Department of Physiology, University of Toronto. He graduated from China Pharmaceutical University and continued graduate studies at the University of Toronto, obtaining a M.S. in Cardiac Pharmacology. After gaining a Ph.D. in Neuropharmacology at the University of Toronto, he continued postdoctoral training in Neuroscience at the Yale University School of Medicine.

MAJOR CONTRIBUTIONS

1. Wang LY, Salter MW, MacDonald JF. 1991. Regulation of kainate receptors by cAMP-dependent protein kinase and phosphatases. *Science*, 253:1132-1135.
2. Wang LY, Taverna FA, Huang XP, MacDonald JF, Hampson DR. 1993. Phosphorylation and modulation of a kainate receptor (GluR6) by cAMP-dependent protein kinase. *Science*, 259:1173-1175.
3. Wang LY, Orser BA, Brautigan DL, MacDonald JF. 1994.
Regulation of NMDA receptors in cultured hippocampal neurons by protein phosphatases 1 and 2A. *Nature*, 369: 230-232.
4. Wang LY, Kaczmarek LK. 1998. High Frequency firing helps replenish the readily releasable pool of synaptic vesicles. *Nature*, 394:384-388.
5. Fedchyshyn MJ, Wang LY. 2005. Developmental transformation of the release modality at the calx of Held synapse. *J Neurosci*, 25:4131-4140.

MAIN TOPICS

Ca^{2+} domain and vesicular release of neurotransmitter

Temporal fidelity of synaptic transmission

Physiological roles of modality switch in developmental plasticity of transmitter release

Short-term plasticity: facilitation vs. depression

SUMMARY

Ca^{2+} inflow through voltage-gated calcium channels (VGCCs) at the nerve terminal is an indispensable trigger for fusion of synaptic vesicles (SVs) with active zones (AZs) and neurotransmitter release, but many issues regarding how the magnitude and temporal profile of Ca^{2+} transients influence release efficacy and short-term plasticity remain controversial. One of such issues under intensive debate for the last two and half decades is the coupling modality between VGCCs and SVs. In one view, VGCCs and SVs are physically tethered at release sites and Ca^{2+}

influx can readily reach Ca^{2+} sensors on SVs situated in the immediate vicinity of the inner mouth of the channel, leading to a fusion event ("*nanodomain*" model). In the other view, VGCCs are sufficiently far apart from SVs and release of a single SV requires cooperative actions of several neighbouring channels in order for Ca^{2+} to reach the fusion threshold at the release sensor ("*microdomain*" model). These two conceptual models are mutually exclusive, supported by compelling but irreconcilable experimental evidence. Because coupling modality plays a critical role in controlling the efficiency of quantal release and dynamic gain range at any given synapse, which modality that central synapses use remains to be one of the core questions for understanding the mechanisms of transmitter release. This chapter will attempt to provide some new insights and prospective outlook for understanding how the nerve terminal develops different release modality so as to fine-tune quantal output and temporal fidelity of synaptic transmission.

INTRODUCTION

Since the landmark studies by Bernard Katz *et al.* in the 1960s, it has been widely accepted that presynaptic release of neurotransmitter requires an elevation of intracellular Ca^{2+} ($[Ca^{2+}]_i$). The major route of Ca^{2+} elevation is through voltage-gated Ca^{2+} channels (VGCCs) clustered near the active zones (AZs), where synaptic vesicles (SVs) containing neurotransmitter are usually docked near or at release sites. Upon arrival of an action potential (or spike) at the nerve terminal, openings of VGCCs raise $[Ca^{2+}]_i$ in their vicinity and trigger the engagement of release machinery (i.e., SNAREs) and fusion of SVs with AZs, ultimately leading to unloading of neurotransmitters from SVs. However, a large body of work in the last four decades demonstrates that Ca^{2+} does not merely trigger neurotransmitter release, the spatial and temporal profiles of "Ca^{2+} domain" near the inner mouth of VGCCs play critical roles in regulating the amplitude and time course of transmitter release as well as various forms of short-term presynaptic plasticity.

Ca^{2+} DOMAIN AND VESICULAR RELEASE OF NEUROTRANSMITTER

Early work at the neuromuscular junction demonstrates that the relation between Ca^{2+} and quantal output (Q) is non-linear and can be quantitatively described by equation: $Q \propto [Ca^{2+}]^m$, where the parameter m is defined as Ca^{2+} cooperativity. The classical definition of Ca^{2+} cooperativity usually refers to the cooperative action of Ca^{2+} at the sensor of the release machinery (e.g., synaptotagmins), to which a minimal of 3-4 Ca^{2+} ions must bind before fusion takes place. Depending on the types of synapse, the m values fall usually in the range of 2-4, meaning that 1-fold increase in Ca^{2+} influx through VGCCs will lead to an amplification of quantal output by 4-16-fold. In addition to being a gain factor, m has also been implicated as an inference index for Ca^{2+} domain interactions under appropriate experimental conditions. From extensive work in the frog neuromuscular junction (NMJ), squid giant synapse and chick ciliary ganglion calyx synapse, it has been proposed that VGCCs are tightly coupled to the release sites where SVs are docked. Consequently, release of a single SV requires activation of a small number of VGCCs. In chick calyx synapse, there is direct evidence that opening of a single VGCC is sufficient to trigger a fusion event. These findings lead to the "*nanodomain*" model in which a docked SV is physically associated with one or a couple of VGCCs (Fig.2.1). Release of a single tightly-coupled SV from such synapses exhibits low m values (1-2) because such a modality requires little cooperative actions among Ca^{2+} domains. In contrast, in central synapses such as hippocampal synapses, cerebellar parallel fiber-Purkinjie cell synapses and the immature calyx of Held synapses, not only many VGCCs (up to 60 VGCCs) but also different types of VGCCs typically N-and P/Q-type are involved in triggering release of a single SV. These results form the basis of "*microdomain*" model for central synapses, in which many channels have to act in a cooperative manner (with high m values, 3-5) to induce a

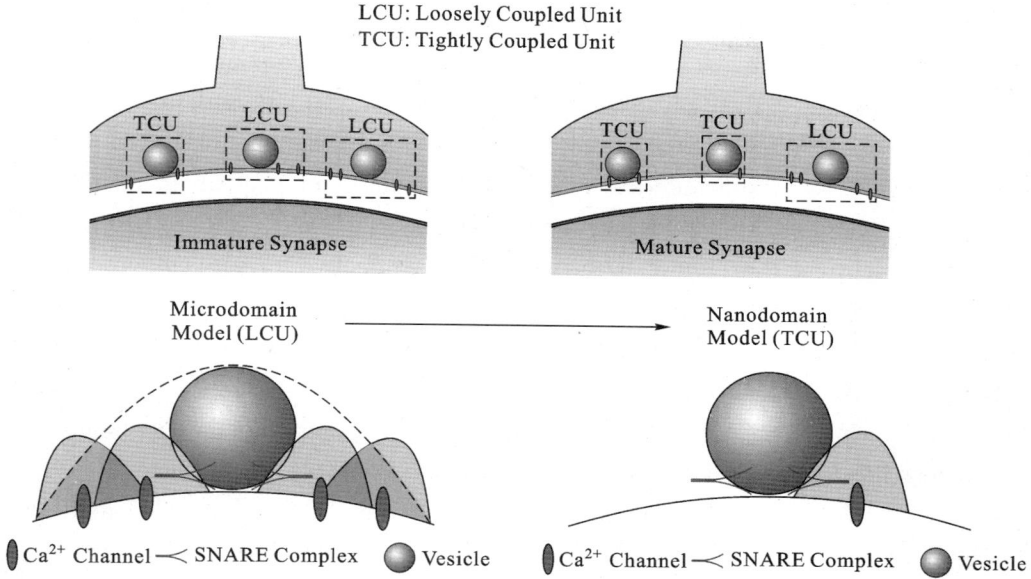

Fig.2.1   Transformation of release modality from microdomain to nanodomain coupling. Diagrams illustrating developmental transformation of mixed populations of loosely- coupled units (LCU, microdomain) and tightly coupled units (TCU, nanodomain).

fusion event (Fig.2.1).   Emerging evidence from the immature calyx of Held synapse and other synapses demonstrate that N-type VGCCs failed to fully compensate for synaptic deficits in P/Q-channel knockout mice, in line with the view that the latter type may likely occupy the preferred "slots" for mediating vesicular fusion in the active zone. However, whether developmental evolution of release modality requires a switch in the subtype of VGCCs, being from N-type in immature synapses to predominantly P/Q-type in mature synapses remain to be an open question. As the *m effect* on synaptic strength is a powerful amplification factor in controlling the dynamic range of any given synapse, understanding which of these two release modalities is preferred for quantal release is of fundamental importance. Evidence to support either model has been generated from synapses of various preparations that are functionally distinct. The size of Ca^{2+} domains and their interactions are dependent on the extracellular concentration of Ca^{2+} ($[Ca^{2+}]_e$), which may also differ by more than ten-fold ($[Ca^{2+}]_e$: 5-10 mM for the frog, squid and chick; 1-2 mM for mammalian central synapses). These differences in experimental condition and preparation made it difficult to resolve this important issue.

The calyx of Held synapse in the rat or mouse auditory pathway has become a prominent preparation for studying fundamental mechanisms underlying synaptic transmission and plasticity. At maturity, this synapse is known for being capable of faithfully relaying synaptic inputs from the contralateral cochlear nucleus (CN) to the ipsilateral medial and lateral superior olives (MSO and LSO), where neurons encode the relative interaural timing and intensity differences of sound stimuli received at each cochlea for sound localization. From the initial onset of synapse formation at postnatal day 4/5 (P4/5) to functional sensory inputs (i.e., hearing) at P11/12 and final maturation at P14, this axosomatic synapse must achieve the capacity of high-fidelity neurotransmission at extraordinarily high rates (up to 600 Hz).   Within such a short time, profound adaptations in biophysical properties of pre- and postsynaptic elements take place in a highly convergent manner to facilitate the development of such a capacity. Clearly defined critical period and rapid development of its functionality make this synapse an ideal model for studying synaptic transmission and developmental plasticity. The large size and compact structure of this giant synapse present additional technical advantages for direct biophysical analysis of synaptic properties.

In our recent attempt to address the core question how the calyx of Held synapse develops its ability to control quantal output, we have taken advantage of the large size of the synapse and compared coupling properties of VGCCs and SVs in immature and mature synapses. By paired voltage-clamp recordings of graded presynaptic Ca^{2+} currents (I_{Ca}) and excitatory postsynaptic currents (EPSCs, as a readout of transmitter release), we discovered that immature terminals required significantly greater threshold I_{Ca} to evoke release, and displayed much higher Ca^{2+} cooperativity value than mature ones [P8-12: m=4.8-5.5 vs. P16-18: m=2.8-3.0; in 1 mM $[Ca^{2+}]_o$], implying that the number of VGCCs involved in triggering release of a single SV decreases as maturation progresses. Raising temperature from 22°C to 35°C or $[Ca^{2+}]_o$ from 1 to 2 mM reduced the difference in m value between two age groups, likely due to the fact that an increase in temperature or the driving force for Ca^{2+} through individual open channels increases the size of Ca^{2+} domains and the likelihood of domain overlapping. This reduces the total number of VGCCs required for a fusion event, hence leading to an apparent decrease in m in immature synapses. However, the m value remained significantly different between two age groups at 35°C or 2 mM $[Ca^{2+}]_o$, and was independent of postsynaptic receptor desensitization, implying that presynaptic coupling modalities in immature and mature synapses are distinct under physiological conditions. Using two Ca^{2+} buffers (EGTA and BAPTA), we further demonstrated that spatial coupling between VGCCs and SVs shortens with maturation. Because of similar equilibrium dissociation constants (K_D) but very different forward-rate constants (k_{on}~160-fold difference) for binding Ca^{2+} ions, it is expected that if VGCCs were tightly coupled to SVs, slow buffers like EGTA should not be able to intercept Ca^{2+} ions before they reach the Ca^{2+} sensors of the release machinery, therefore minimally attenuating transmitter release. However, EGTA would effectively attenuate release if VGCCs were physically distant from SVs, providing sufficient time for EGTA to bind Ca^{2+} ions in transit.

In contrast, fast buffers like BAPTA should be able to intercept Ca^{2+} ions and decrease synaptic strength independent of the coupling tightness. We found that injection of slow Ca^{2+} buffer EGTA (10 mM) potently attenuated transmitter release in immature terminals but produced little effect in mature ones (P16-18), whereas fast Ca^{2+} buffer BAPATA (1 mM) was equally effective for both age groups. In fact, the extent of release attenuation by EGTA was strongly correlated with the postnatal developmental stage. These results suggest that a majority of VGCCs in immature synapses are loosely-coupled to SVs but the coupling tightens during maturation, hence the relative portion of tightly-coupled units (TCUs) versus loosely-coupled units (LCUs) increases with age. Consistent with this, when LCUs were functionally blocked by EGTA (10 mM), immature synapses behaved like mature ones with similar m values. Taking together, these concrete evidences led us to propose a developmental transformation of the release modality from "*microdomain*", involving the cooperative action of many loosely coupled VGCCs, to "*nanodomain*" in which openings of fewer tightly coupled VGCCs effectively induce a fusion event at the calyx of Held synapse. Because these experiments were done in the same preparation and $[Ca^{2+}]_e$, one could imagine that either release modality may operate in different central synapses depending on their functionality or developmental stages. Independent observations made in developing hair cell synapses have also led to the similar conclusions to ours. Although these biophysical studies provide concrete and compelling evidence to validate these two conceptual models, morphological correlates have yet to be identified at the developing presynaptic structures.

TEMPORAL FIDELITY OF SYNAPTIC TRANSMISSION

Armed with biophysical evidence for a developmental transformation of release modality at the calyx of Held synapse, we next consider the question how tightening spatial coupling would influence the development of temporal fidelity of release. The timing of neurotransmitter release is usually inferred from synaptic delay, which refers to the time interval between the arrival of a spike at the nerve terminal and the onset of postsynaptic response. Classical studies at the frog NMJ by Katz and Miledi (1965) and subsequently by Barret and Stevens (1972) indicate that synaptic delay is invariant. This view leaves the assumption that temporal fidelity of secretion is not modifiable. However, recent evidence from the goldfish Mauthner-cell synapse and crayfish NMJ suggests that synaptic delay is not invariant. Paired-pulse depression in the Mauthner-cell synapse is associated with a prolongation in synaptic delay while facilitation at the crayfish NMJ leads to an activity-dependent shortening in synaptic delay. Our own work in this regard not only demonstrates that synaptic delay can be modulated, but also implicates an important role for the release modality in this modulation.

In the developing calyx of Held synapse, synaptic delay shortens with maturation. In light of a developmental transformation in the release modality, we postulate that long synaptic delay in immature synapses where "*microdomain*" modality predominates, is a result of required time for Ca^{2+} ions to transit and for multiple Ca^{2+} domains to overlap so as to initiate a fusion event. In contrast, tight "*nanodomain*" coupling between VGCCs and SVs in mature synapses minimizes the transit time for Ca^{2+} ions to reach the release sensor and the need for cooperative interaction, hence leading to transmitter release with synaptic delays near their lower limits. To test these postulations, we have probed the effects of release modality on synaptic delay with paired recordings of I$_{Ca}$ and EPSCs. Because the width of action potential becomes narrower as maturation progresses, one may argue that the difference in synaptic delay between immature and mature synapses (as previously observed) may be due to the timing difference in Ca^{2+} entry, which usually occurs during the repolarization phase of an action potential. To avoid such a complication, we used an identical command spike waveform for both age groups and found that immature synapses showed significantly longer synaptic delay than mature ones following the alignment of the peak of presynaptic I$_{Ca}$, indicating a genuine difference in synaptic delay. An increase in [Ca^{2+}]$_o$ from 1 to 2 mM reduced synaptic delay in immature synapses, in line with the idea that an expansion in individual Ca^{2+} domain size by high [Ca^{2+}]$_o$ reduces time for Ca^{2+} ions to transit and for overlapping Ca^{2+} domains. By using voltage steps of incremental durations to recruit an increasing number of VGCCs, we found that synaptic delay was inversely correlated with the amplitude of I$_{Ca}$. However, the slope factor derived from linear fits to the data was significantly higher for immature synapses than that for mature ones at both room and near physiological temperatures, indicating that synaptic delay in immature synapses has a stronger Ca^{2+}-dependence than that in mature synapses. These preliminary results demonstrated that synaptic delay, instead of being invariant, is strongly dependent on Ca^{2+} domain interactions and hence release modality. When presynaptic I$_{Ca}$ is small, synaptic delay is long as a result of a low probability of domain overlapping. On the other hand, large I$_{Ca}$, involving a greater number of recruited VGCCs, shortens synaptic delay as domain interactions are facilitated. Thus, synaptic delay in immature synapses shows much steeper dependence on I$_{Ca}$ than that in mature synapses. In contrast, synaptic delay in mature synapses becomes less dependent on Ca^{2+} domain interactions due to tight coupling of VGCCs to SVs, hence showing little changes in response to the same voltage paradigm to recruit VGCCs. Taken together, these lines of evidence implicate the transformation in release modality from "*microdomain*" to "*nanodomain*" as the most likely subsynaptic substrate for developmental shortening of synaptic delay. As temporal fidelity of synaptic response is strongly dependent on timing of unitary quantal release, we suggest that "*nanodomain*" coupling presents the maximal likelihood for synchronized release and ensures high-fidelity synaptic transmission.

PHYSIOLOGICAL ROLES OF MODALITY SWITCH IN DEVELOPMENTAL PLASTICITY OF TRANSMITTER RELEASE

In many central synapses including the calyx of Held synapse, release probability (P_r) estimated by single action potential (AP) declines as maturation progresses. At the first glance, this decrease in P_r appears to be contradictory to our model, in which a developmental transformation in release modality from "microdomain" to "nanodomain" predicts an increase in P_r, as a consequence of shortened diffusion distance for Ca^{2+} ions to reach the release sensor. On the basis of input-output relationship in the form of $I_{EPSC} = a[I_{Ca}]^m$, we postulate that developmental shortening of spike width (*AP effect*) and transformation of the release modality (*m effect*) are two determining factors for the decrease in P_r. Because VGCCs open in a stochastic manner, a broad spike in the immature synapse would recruit a large number of VGCCs (large I_{Ca}), and induce quantal release (large I_{EPSC}) that follows a high power function (i.e., m=4-5), as predicted by "microdomain" modality. On the other hand, in the mature synapse, a narrow spike would activate few VGCCs and hence small Ca^{2+} transients (small I_{Ca}), limiting the number of activated release sites while low m value (2-3) associated with the "nanodomain" release modality would also constrain the amplification effect of incoming Ca^{2+}. Therefore, a combined decrease of the "AP effect" and "m effect" in developing synapses may effectively reduce P_r (*m effect* on synaptic strength) while synaptic delay is also shortened (*m effect* on temporal fidelity). In the meantime, developmental increase in the number of AZs and Ca^{2+}-dependent replenishment of depleted release sites may compensate for the decease in P_r. Together, these parallel changes may help preserve the readily releasable pool of SVs during repetitive activity and reduce the extent of short-term depression as we and other groups have shown, ultimately leading to high-fidelity neurotransmission.

Our recent work suggests that the waveform of action potentials profoundly influences the number and kinetics of presynaptic VGCCs and quantal output at the immature calyx of Held synapse. To specifically test the *AP Effect* and *m Effect* on transmitter release, we have carried out preliminary experiments in which presynaptic terminals were voltage-clamped into a series of pseudo AP waveforms with upstroke and repolarization time course closely mimicking developmental changes in real APs. In immature age group of synapses, we found that quantal outputs evoked by real APs recorded from immature (AP_I) and mature terminals (AP_M) are strongly correlated with the input-output relationship derived from pseudo APs. Within the physiological range of developmental AP shortening (i.e., from AP_I to AP_M), we noted that one-fold reduction in the total Ca^{2+} charge integral produced more than 16-fold decrease in quantal output, in line with the prediction based on "*microdomain*" model for *AP Effect* and *m Effect* on P_r. At near physiological temperature we have made qualitatively similar observations. However, whether such a correlation exists in mature synapses with predominantly "*nanodomain*" modality, and how transformation in release modality influences synaptic delay under physiological conditions remains to be determined.

SHORT-TERM PLASTICITY: FACILITATION VS. DEPRESSION

Like most physiological information in neural circuits, auditory signals often coded in waves of action potential bursts. This presents an important question whether/how different release modalities described above impact on short-term plasticity, more specifically, the amplitude and temporal fidelity of individual synaptic responses within a train. In response to the same pattern of inputs, different synapses may display a variety of behavioural phenotypes such as short-term facilitation (STF) or depression (STD) or a mixture of both interplaying as repetitive activity proceeds. Although multiple theoretical models have been proposed for these phenotypes, the FD simulation model by Dittman *et al.* (2000) captures major features of synaptic responses in a train (Fig.2.2). In this model, synaptic strength at any given time of a train is a product of facilitation (F) and depression (D), where F is proportional to the release probability (P_r),

and D corresponds to the number of release-competent sites that may enter into a refractory state. Residual Ca²⁺ ions are related to both F and D, in that a small increase in F leads to a large decrease in D. In the early phase of a train, F predominates as a result of power function of residual Ca²⁺ from preceding

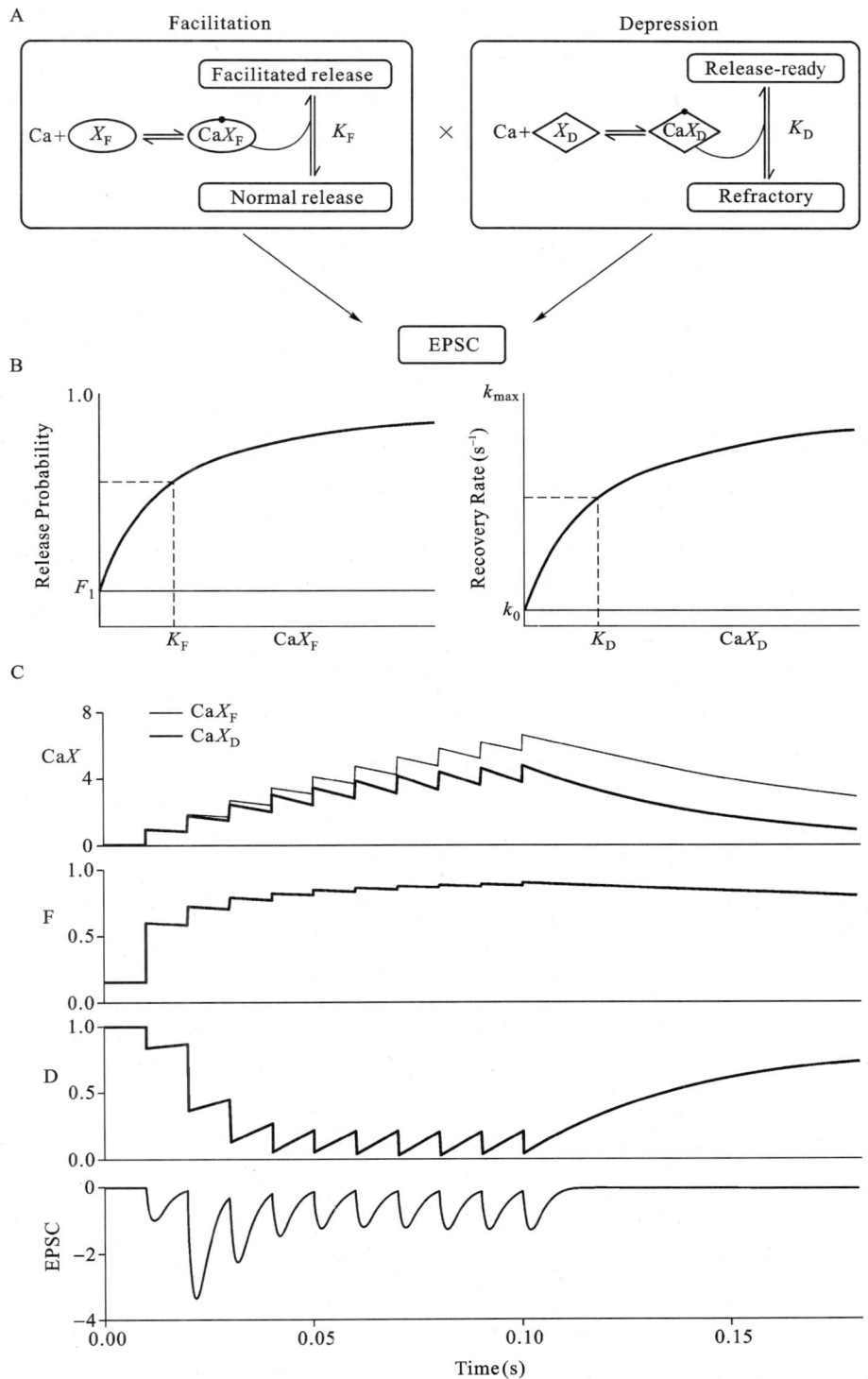

Fig.2.2 FD model for Ca-dependence of short-term plasticity. A. Left, Residual presynaptic calcium binds to site X_F, and the complex CaX_F then binds to the release site causing an enhancement of release probability. Right, Schematic of residual presynaptic calcium binding to site X_D, which then binds with the refractory release site driving a transition back to the release-ready state. B. Left, F plotted as a function of CaX_F ranging from a minimal probability of F_1 (no residual calcium) to a maximum of 1. The dissociation constant for CaX_F is K_F. Right, the recovery rate for depression is plotted as a function of CaX_D with a minimum rate of k_o, a maximum rate of k_{max}, and CaX_D dissociation constant K_D. C. Presynaptic levels of CaX_F (*thin line*) and CaX_D (*thick line*), fraction of available synapses that undergo release (F), fraction of release-ready synapses (D), and normalized EPSC during a train of 10 stimuli at 100 Hz.

event(s), leading to STF. However, F eventually saturates, leaving D to take over the later phase of the train and hence STD. An additional component also driven by activity-dependent build-up of residual Ca^{2+} is Ca^{2+}-dependent recovery (CDR) from STD, which may counteract effect of or compete with D. Although there is substantial evidence to support each component of this model, only synaptic strength but not delay has been simulated.

Previous work from our group and others indicate that in response to a train of stimuli at high-frequencies (100-300 Hz, 2 mM $[Ca^{2+}]_o$), STD in synaptic strength usually dominates in both immature and mature calyx of Held synapse. However, the extent of STD is much more prominent in the former than the latter. Such a difference in STD has been attributed to higher P_r and more pronounced postsynaptic desensitization in immature synapses, both of which decrease as maturation progresses. In addition, STF can also be observed early in the train in immature synapses. Hence, we could view the calyx of Held synapse as a model of short-term synaptic plasticity, where a synapse, during repetitive stimulation, exhibits facilitation, depression or some superposition of the two (as simulated by the FD model), depending on its developmental stage. We would like to propose that developmental shortening of spike width (*AP effect*) and transformation of the release modality (*m effect*) are two determining factors for short-term plasticity. Since VGCCs open in a stochastic manner, a broad spike in the immature synapse would recruit a large number of VGCCs, and induce quantal release that follows a high power function (i.e., m=5-6; $I_{EPSC} = a[I_{Ca}]^m$), as predicted by "*microdomain*" modality. During the early phase of a train, residual Ca^{2+} would boost F by *m effect*. However, a small increase in F would lead to a large decrease in D. Hence, robust facilitation usually precedes profound depression within a train of synaptic response in immature synapses. On the other hand, in the mature synapse, a narrow spike would activate few VGCCs and hence small Ca^{2+} transients, limiting the number of activated

release sites and fusion events. During repetitive activity in a train, low m value (2-3) associated with the "*nanodomain*" release modality would also constrain the amplification effect of residual Ca^{2+} build-up on F and D. Therefore, both facilitation and depression in synaptic strength are less prominent in mature synapses. A developmental increase in the number of AZs and activity-dependent CDR may also contribute to the reduction in STD (as predicted by the FD model). Therefore, by effectively reducing the extent of STD, a combination of "*AP effect*" and "*m effect*" in mature synapses may help the development of high-fidelity neurotransmission.

If STF and STD in synaptic strength were indeed dependent on the release modality as proposed above, one could make another extrapolation that synaptic delay of individual synaptic responses during a train would also be influenced in parallel, particularly for immature synapses where "*microdomain*" dominates. As synaptic delay in immature synapses is strongly dependent on Ca^{2+} and shortens when Ca^{2+} domain interactions are facilitated, it could be predicted that repetitive activity in a train may promote such interaction and progressively shorten synaptic delay along with facilitation in synaptic strength.

CONCLUSION

In the context of aforementioned issues, we have rationalized the central role of release modality in regulating synaptic strength, synaptic delay and short-term plasticity in transmitter release. Perhaps we have raised more questions than we have answered, we believe that synaptic strength and synaptic delay are two parallel but intermingled quantal parameters that are dependent on spatial coupling between VGCCs and SVs. Spatial rearrangement of VGCCs and SVs may underlie developmental transformation of the release modality from "*microdomain*" to "*nanodomain*". This transformation reduces cooperativity m and limits the amount of quantal output {as $I_{EPSC}=a[I_{Ca}]^m$}, hence preventing the terminal from depleting the readily-releasable pool (RRP) of SVs during repetitive activity. Release modality switch may also reduce the jitter in synaptic delay, therefore ensuring temporal fidelity of high-frequency neurotransmission. Understanding the role of the release modality and its developmental transformation may shed light not only on the core question we are addressing at the developing calyx of Held synapse, but also on common mechanisms underlying spatiotemporal aspects of synaptic transmission and short-tem plasticity in other central synapses.

GENERAL CITATIONS

Augustine GJ, Charlton MP, Smith SJ.1987. Calcium action in synaptic transmitter release. *Annu Rev Neurosci*, 10: 633-693.

Lin JW, Faber DS. 2002. Modulation of synaptic delay during synaptic plasticity. *Trends Neurosci*, 25:449-455.

Oertel D. 1999. The role of timing in the brain stem auditory nuclei of vertebrates. *Annu Rev Physiol*, 61: 497-519.

Reid CA, Bekkers JM, Clements JD. 2003. Presynaptic Ca²⁺ channels: a functional patchwork. *Trends Neurosci*, 26: 683-687.

von Gersdorff H, Borst JG. 2002. Short-term plasticity at the calyx of held. *Nat Rev Neurosci*, 3: 53-64.

DISCOVERY CITATIONS

Adler EM, Augustine GJ, Duffy SN, Charlton MP. 1991. Alien intracellular calcium chelators attenuate neurotransmitter release at the squid giant synapse. *J Neurosci*, 11: 1496-1507.

Augustine GJ. 1990. Regulation of transmitter release at the squid giant synapse by presynaptic delayed rectifier potassium current. *J Physiol*, 431: 343-364.

Barrett EF, Stevens CF. 1972. The kinetics of transmitter release at the frog neuromuscular junction. *J Physiol*, 227: 691-708.

Borst JG, Sakmann B. 1996. Calcium influx and transmitter release in a fast CNS synapse. *Nature*, 383: 431-434.

Borst JG, Sakmann B. 1999. Effect of changes in action potential shape on calcium currents and transmitter release in a calyx-type synapse of the rat auditory brainstem. *Philos Trans R Soc Lond B Biol Sci*, 354: 347-355.

Borst JG, Helmchen F, Sakmann B. 1995. Pre- and postsynaptic whole-cell recordings in the medial nucleus of the trapezoid body of the rat. *J Physiol*, 489 (Pt 3): 825-840.

Cao YQ, Piedras-Renteria ES, Smith GB, Chen G, Harata NC, Tsien RW. 2004. Presynaptic Ca²⁺ channels compete for channel type-preferring slots in altered neurotransmission arising from Ca²⁺ channelopathy. *Neuron*, 43: 387-400.

Datyner NB, Gage PW. 1980. Phasic secretion of acetylcholine at a mammalian neuromuscular junction. *J Physiol*, 303: 299-314.

Dittman JS, Regehr WG. 1998. Calcium dependence and recovery kinetics of presynaptic depression at the climbing fiber to Purkinje cell synapse. *J Neurosci*, 18: 6147-6162.

Dittman JS, Kreitzer AC, Regehr WG. 2000. Interplay between facilitation, depression, and residual calcium at three presynaptic terminals. *J Neurosci*, 20: 1374-1385.

Dodge FA, Jr, Rahamimoff R. 1967. Co-operative action a calcium ions in transmitter release at the neuromuscular junction. *J Physiol*, 193: 419-432.

Fedchyshyn MJ, Wang LY. 2005. Developmental transformation of the release modality at the calyx of held synapse. *J Neurosci*, 25: 4131-4140.

Forsythe ID. 1994. Direct patch recording from identified presynaptic terminals mediating glutamatergic EPSCs in the rat CNS, *in vitro*. *J Physiol*, 479 (Pt 3): 381-387.

Gentile L, Stanley EF. 2005. A unified model of presynaptic release site gating by calcium channel domains. *Eur J Neurosci*, 21: 278-282.

Inchauspe CG, Martini FJ, Forsythe ID, Uchitel OD. 2004. Functional compensation of P/Q by N-type channels blocks short-term plasticity at the calyx of held presynaptic terminal. *J Neurosci*, 24: 10379-10383.

Iwasaki S, Takahashi T. 1998. Developmental changes in calcium channel types mediating synaptic transmission in rat auditory brainstem. *J Physiol*, 509 (Pt 2): 419-423.

Iwasaki S, Takahashi T. 2001. Developmental regulation of transmitter release at the calyx of Held in rat auditory brainstem. *J Physiol*, 534: 861-871.

Johnson SL, Marcotti W, Kros CJ. 2005. Increase in efficiency and reduction in Ca²⁺ dependence of exocytosis during development of mouse inner hair cells. *J Physiol*, 563: 177-191.

Joshi I, Wang LY. 2002. Developmental profiles of glutamate receptors and synaptic transmission at a single synapse in the mouse auditory brainstem. *J Physiol*, 540: 861-873.

Joshi I, Shokralla S, Titis P, Wang LY. 2004. The role of AMPA receptor gating in the development of high-fidelity neurotransmission at the calyx of Held synapse. *J Neurosci*, 24: 183-196.

Jun K, Piedras-Renteria ES, Smith SM, Wheeler DB, Lee SB, Lee TG, *et al.* 1999. Ablation of P/Q-type Ca$^{(2+)}$ channel currents, altered synaptic transmission, and progressive ataxia in mice lacking the alpha(1A)-subunit. *Proc Natl Acad Sci USA*, 96: 15245-15250.

Katz B, Miledi R. 1965. The effect of temperature on the synaptic delay at the neuromuscular junction. *J Physiol*, 181: 656-670.

Llinas R, Sugimori M, Simon SM. 1982. Transmission by presynaptic spike-like depolarization in the squid giant synapse. *Proc Natl Acad Sci USA*, 79: 2415-2419.

Luebke JI, Dunlap K, Turner TJ. 1993. Multiple calcium channel types control glutamatergic synaptic transmission in the hippocampus. *Neuron*, 11: 895-902.

Meinrenken CJ, Borst JG, Sakmann B. 2003. Local routes revisited: the space and time dependence of the Ca^{2+} signal for phasic transmitter release at the rat calyx of Held. *J Physiol*, 547: 665-689.

Mintz IM, Sabatini BL, Regehr WG. 1995. Calcium control of transmitter release at a cerebellar synapse. *Neuron*, 15: 675-688.

Naraghi M, Neher E. 1997. Linearized buffered Ca^{2+} diffusion in microdomains and its implications for calculation of [Ca^{2+}] at the mouth of a calcium channel. *J Neurosci*, 17: 6961-6973.

Neher E. 1998. Vesicle pools and Ca^{2+} microdomains: new tools for understanding their roles in neurotransmitter release. *Neuron*, 20: 389-399.

Parnas H, Hovav G, Parnas I. 1989. Effect of Ca^{2+} diffusion on the time course of neurotransmitter release. *Biophys J*, 55: 859-874.

Sabatini BL, Regehr WG. 1997. Control of neurotransmitter release by presynaptic waveform at the granule cell to Purkinje cell synapse. *J Neurosci*, 17: 3425-3435.

Stanley EF. 1993. Single calcium channels and acetylcholine release at a presynaptic nerve terminal. *Neuron*, 11: 1007-1011.

Stanley EF. 1997. The calcium channel and the organization of the presynaptic transmitter release face. *Trends Neurosci*, 20: 404-409.

Stevens CF, Wesseling JF. 1998. Activity-dependent modulation of the rate at which synaptic vesicles become available to undergo exocytosis. *Neuron*, 21: 415-424.

Takahashi T, Momiyama A. 1993. Different types of calcium channels mediate central synaptic transmission. *Nature*, 366: 156-158.

Taschenberger H, von Gersdorff H. 2000. Fine-tuning an auditory synapse for speed and fidelity: developmental changes in presynaptic waveform, EPSC kinetics, and synaptic plasticity. *J Neurosci*, 20: 9162-9173.

Taschenberger H, Leao RM, Rowland KC, Spirou GA, von Gersdorff H. 2002. Optimizing synaptic architecture and efficiency for high-frequency transmission. *Neuron*, 36: 1127-1143.

Trussell LO. 1999. Synaptic mechanisms for coding timing in auditory neurons. *Annu Rev Physiol*, 61: 477-496.

Vyshedskiy A, Allana T, Lin JW. 2000. Analysis of presynaptic Ca^{2+} influx and transmitter release kinetics during facilitation at the inhibitor of the crayfish neuromuscular junction. *J Neurosci*, 20: 6326-6332.

Waldeck RF, Pereda A, Faber DS. 2000. Properties and plasticity of paired-pulse depression at a central synapse. *J Neurosci*, 20: 5312-5320.

Wang LY, Kaczmarek LK. 1998. High-frequency firing helps replenish the readily releasable pool of synaptic vesicles. *Nature*, 394: 384-388.

Wheeler DB, Randall A, Tsien RW. 1994. Roles of N-type and Q-type Ca^{2+} channels in supporting hippocampal synaptic transmission. *Science*, 264: 107-111.

Wu LG, Saggau P. 1994. Pharmacological identification of two types of presynaptic voltage-dependent calcium channels at CA3-CA1 synapses of the hippocampus. *J Neurosci*, 14: 5613-5622.

Wu LG, Westenbroek RE, Borst JG, Catterall WA, Sakmann B. 1999. Calcium channel types with distinct presynaptic localization couple differentially to transmitter release in single calyx-type synapses. *J Neurosci*, 19: 726-736.

Yamada WM, Zucker RS. 1992. Time course of transmitter release calculated from simulations of a calcium diffusion model. *Biophys J*, 61: 671-682.

Yoshikami D, Bagabaldo Z, Olivera BM. 1989. The inhibitory effects of omega-conotoxins on Ca channels and synapses. *Ann N Y Acad Sci*, 560: 230-248.

Synaptic Vesicle Cycle at Nerve Terminals

CHAPTER 3

Ling-Gang Wu, Jianhua Xu

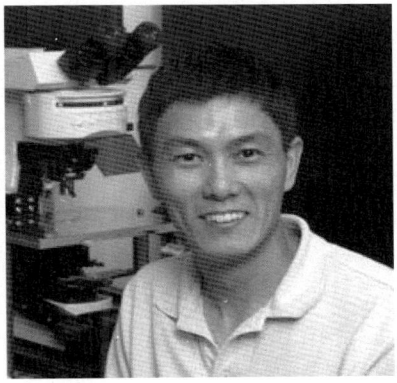

Dr. Wu is an Investigator in the National Institute of Neurological Disorders and Stroke, Bethesda, USA. He graduated from Second Military Medical University, China and obtained a M.S. in Physiology. After gaining a Ph.D. in Neuroscience from Baylor College of Medicine, he pursued postdoctoral training at the same institution, followed by training at the University of Colorado Medical School and the Max Planck Institute.

Dr. Jianhua Xu is a research fellow in Dr. Wu's laboratory.

MAJOR CONTRIBUTIONS

1. Wu LG, Saggau P. 1997. Presynaptic inhibition of elicited neurotransmitter release. *Trends Neurosci*, 20(5): 204-212. (Review)
2. Wu LG, Borst JG, Sakmann B.1998. R-type Ca^{2+} currents evoke transmitter release at a rat central synapse. *Proc Natl Acad Sci USA*, 95(8): 4720-4725.
3. Sun JY, Wu LG. 2001. Fast kinetics of exocytosis revealed by simultaneous measurements of presynaptic capacitance and postsynaptic currents at a central synapse. *Neuron*, 30(1): 171-182.
4. Sun JY, Wu XS, Wu LG. 2002. Single and multiple vesicle fusion induce different rates of endocytosis at a central synapse. *Nature*, 417(6888): 555-559.
5. Xu J, Wu LG. 2005. The decrease in the presynaptic calcium current is a major cause of short-term depression at a calyx-type synapse. *Neuron*, 46(4): 633-645.

MAIN TOPICS

Vesicle pools

Vesicle mobilization, docking, priming and fusion

Three endocytic pathways

The dynamic time course of endocytosis

The time course of endocytosis is regulated by stimulation

Mechanisms that may regulate the time course of endocytosis

Clathrin-dependent versus clathrin-independent endocytosis

Regulation of endocytosis by single rate-limiting factors

The effects of calcium on endocytosis

Hypotheses that may account for calcium-mediated facilitation of endocytosis

The functional significance of regulation of endocytosis

The contribution of slower endocytosis to short-term synaptic depression

The maintenance of transmitter release by retrieving vesicles into the reserve pool and/or the readily releasable pool

Is endocytosis fast enough to limit transmitter release from the fusion pore?

SUMMARY

Synaptic vesicle fusion at the plasma membrane is followed by vesicle retrieval. There are three different pathways for retrieving vesicles: classic clathrin-mediated endocytosis, a "kiss-and-run" form of endocytosis, and bulk endocytosis. These forms of endocytosis may take as long as tens to hundreds of seconds or as short as one second or less. The time course of endocytosis is determined by the neuronal firing frequency and duration. The dynamic time course could be a result of multiple endocytic pathways and/or regulation by a variety of modulators. The newly formed vesicles via various endocytic pathways may join the readily releasable pool or the reserve pool, likely depending on which pathway they are generated. Vesicles in the reserve pool can be mobilized to the readily releasable pool, when the latter is depleted. Vesicle recycling is critical for the maintenance of transmitter release during repetitive stimulation. Regulation of any step in the vesicle cycling process, including endocytosis, could thus provide a mechanism by which synaptic plasticity is achieved.

INTRODUCTION

Synaptic transmission is the fundamental building block for the function of the nervous system. Synaptic transmission is initiated by an action potential, which opens voltage-gated calcium channels at the nerve terminal. Calcium influx through calcium channels triggers vesicle fusion with the plasma membrane and the opening of a fusion pore. Transmitter is released through the fusion pore to act on the postsynaptic receptor, which generates a postsynaptic current. These processes, summarized as synaptic transmission, may be repeated very often because neurons may be subject to various frequencies of action potential trains *in vivo*. A typical nerve terminal in the central nervous system contains a couple of hundred vesicles. These vesicles would eventually be exhausted if there were no further supply of vesicles. Fortunately, synaptic vesicle fusion is followed by vesicle membrane re-

trieval, endocytosis, to form new vesicles. Newly formed vesicles are reused for exocytosis. Such a vesicle cycling process is essential for the maintenance of the vesicle supply during repetitive nerve activity. Here we will review the cellular and the molecular mechanisms underlying the vesicle cycling process. We will introduce different vesicle pools in the nerve terminal, discuss how vesicles become mature for release, and review how vesicle membrane is retrieved after fusion. We will also discuss the significance of modulation of the vesicle cycling process to synaptic transmission and synaptic plasticity. Our main focus is the cellular and the molecular mechanisms mediating various vesicle retrieval pathways.

VESICLE POOLS

Synaptic vesicles are generally assigned into at least two pools, the readily releasable pool (RRP), where vesicles are immediately available for release, and the reserve pool, where vesicles can be mobilized to the RRP. The RRP can be depleted by a number of ways depending on the approaches available for the preparation. These approaches include a train of 10-30 action potentials at a high frequency, a few milliseconds of depolarization at the nerve terminal (Fig.3.1A and 3.1B), 1-3 s of hypertonic shock (Fig.3.1C), and a rapid increase of the cytosolic calcium level by photolysing caged calcium compounds. Although these stimuli are different in their pathways to trigger vesicle release, they have been shown to utilize the same RRP vesicles. The RRP contains about 7-50 vesicles per active zone, which accounts for about 1-5% of the total number of vesicles. The remaining vesicles are in the reserve pool. It should be mentioned that in some studies, the term "reserve pool" is used to represent the vesicles only available during intense stimulation, such as high potassium application or prolonged stimulation with action potentials at a high frequency. A new term "the recycling pool" is created to refer to those vesicles that can be released upon moderate physiological stimulation. Thus, the recycling pool includes the RRP and a fraction of vesicles mobilized from the reserve pool.

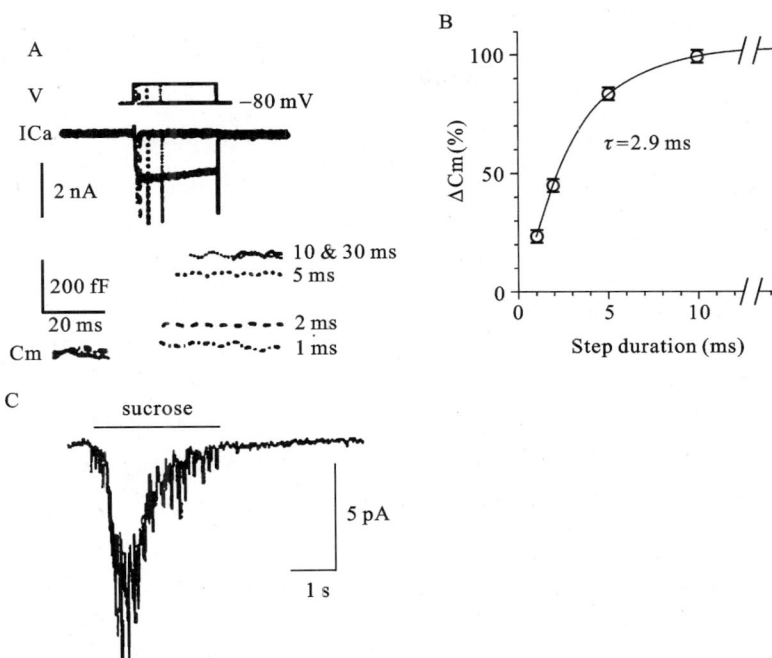

Fig.3.1 Measurements of the size of the readily releasable pool (RRP). A and B. In the rat calyx of Held, the amount of release, measured as the membrane capacitance jump (A, lower; B) induced by various lengths of depolarization (A, upper; B) was saturated by a 10 ms depolarization pulse from −80 to +10 mV. Thus, a 10 ms depolarization is sufficient to deplete a pool of vesicles immediately available for release, defined here as the RRP. C. In cultured hippocampal neuron, hypertonic sucrose solution depletes vesicles in the RRP.

The above pools are defined based on functional measurements. Morphological studies demonstrated that some of the synaptic vesicles are docked at the active zone, whereas most vesicles are not. It is believed that docked vesicles may correspond to the vesicles in the RRP, whereas non-docked vesicles may correspond to vesicles in the reserve pool. However, a recent study in the frog neuromuscular junction challenges this idea. The study suggests that vesicles in the RRP may not necessarily locate close to the active zone, instead a fast track may exist to transport these vesicles for a rapid release. Whether this recent finding applies to other synapses remains to be determined.

VESICLE MOBILIZATION, DOCKING, PRIMING AND FUSION

The RRP can be readily depleted by repetitive nerve activities. In a traditional view, the empty RRP will be replenished with vesicles from the reserve pool. The time constant for replenishment is in the order of a few seconds at resting conditions. At higher frequency firing, however, replenishment is speeded up by the increase of the intracellular calcium concentration. It remains unclear what molecular mechanism

mediates the calcium-induced enhancement of replenishment. The calcium-dependent enhancement of replenishment may help to relieve depletion of the RRP during higher frequency firing. Since depletion of the RRP may be a major cause for short-term depression of synaptic transmission, the calcium-dependent enhancement of replenishment may help to relieve short-term depression, a synaptic plasticity involved in the information processing of the neuronal network. A recent study challenges the idea that the calcium-dependent enhancement of replenishment plays a significant role to relieve short-term depression. This study suggests that calcium-dependent replenishment plays little role during moderate frequency firing (<100 Hz) at a calyx-type synapse, because depletion is not the major mechanism. Instead, inactivation of the presynaptic calcium current is the major mechanism causing short-term depression. It remains unclear whether the finding at the calyx-type synapse applies to other synapses. Some recent studies suggest that newly formed vesicles may replenish the RRP without going through the reserve pool. More detailed discussion on this issue will be presented later.

When a vesicle is mobilized to the RRP, it may dock at the active zone. Acquisition of fusion competence may require multiple steps and may involve both lipid and protein changes, but it is defined collectively as priming (Fig.3.2). According to the widely accepted SNARE hypothesis, the priming reaction includes the formation of protein complex between proteins located on vesicle membrane and plasma membrane. As illustrated in Fig.3.3, synaptobrevin (or VAMP) is a SNARE protein on the vesicle membrane, while syntaxin and SNAP-25 are SNARE proteins on the plasma membrane (Fig.3.3, stage 1). During priming, synaptobrevin interacts with both syntaxin and SNAP-25 to form a loose SNARE complex (Fig.3.3, stage 2). Because the SNARE complex is formed by SNARE proteins on the opposing vesicle membrane and plasma membrane, it is also called

trans-SNARE in order to distinguish from the cis-SNARE complex formed by proteins on the same membrane. Before fusion the loose SNARE complex will proceed into a tight complex by a zippering process (Fig.3.3, stage 3) which is speculated as driving the vesicle membrane to merge with the plasma membrane (Fig.3.3, stage 4). Although many other proteins appear to have critical roles in synaptic vesicle exocytosis, it seems likely that the SNAREs represent the minimal machinery for fusion. The importance of SNARE proteins in release has been well demonstrated by studies that detected failures of exocytosis and/or fusion after treatment with botulinum toxins and tetanus toxin which can cleave critical domains of specific SNARE protein(s).

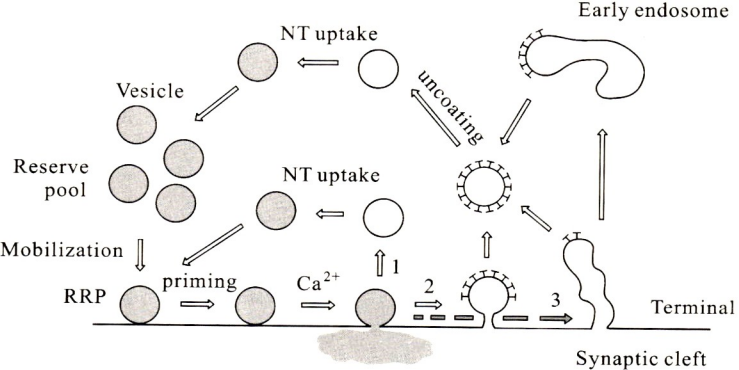

Fig.3.2   An overview of the synaptic vesicle cycle. Vesicles are mobilized from the reserve pool into the readily releasable pool (RRP), primed for fusion competence and, triggered by the Ca^{2+} influx to fuse with plasma membrane and release neurotransmitter (NT). The exocytosed membrane can be internalized by a number of pathways: (1) a reversed step of transient fusion ("kiss-and-run"), (2) clathrin-mediated endocytosis, (3) retrieval of a large piece of membrane, called bulk endocytosis, which may form an endosome, from which clathrin-coated vesicles may be formed. In addition, clathrin-coated vesicles may be formed from the tip of a large piece of membrane which remains at the plasma (3). After reloading of neurotransmitter, newly retrieved vesicles may fill the RRP or the reserve pool for the next round of release.

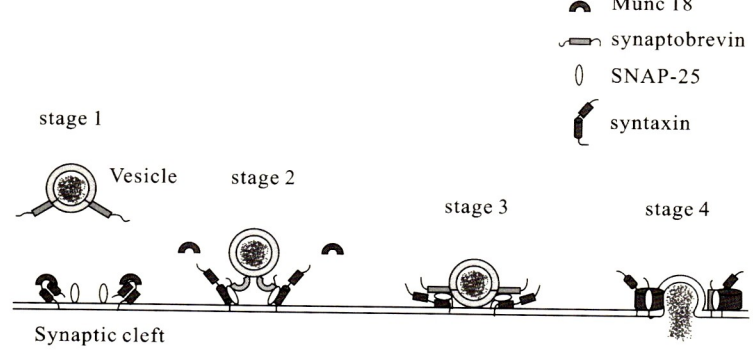

Fig.3.3   The SNARE hypothesis for synaptic vesicle exocytosis. Synaptobrevin/VAMP on vesicle membrane forms a loose trans-SNARE complex with SNAP-25 and syntaxin. Munc 18, which originally interacts with syntaxin, was dissociated from syntaxin. The interaction among SNARE proteins brings the opposing membranes close, and a further zippering process may even provide the driving force for fusion.

High intracellular concentrations of calcium trigger rapid neurotransmitter release and thus are expected to act on late steps of synaptic vesicle fusion. Synaptotagmin, a calcium-binding protein on synaptic vesicle membrane, has been shown to be the primary calcium sensor for triggering fusion. Synaptotagmin is an integral membrane protein with two C2 domains (C2A and C2B) that bind calcium, SNARE proteins and phospholipids. There are several isoforms of synaptotagmin with differential intracellular localization and tissue expression patterns. Synaptotagmin I is selectively enriched in synaptic vesicles, and its absence leads to a severe loss of calcium-dependent synchronous release. Synaptotagmin I is believed to govern the fast, synchronous release of neurotransmitter, while other synptotagmin isoforms are responsible for nonsynchronous release. A current model suggests that calcium binding induces the interaction of one or both C2 domains with proteins and lipids in the plasma membrane, thus helping to catalyze SNARE-mediated membrane fusion.

THREE ENDOCYTIC PATHWAYS

After vesicle fusion, vesicle membrane must be retrieved to form new vesicles (Fig.3.2). In the early 1970s, two groups used electron microscopy to examine how vesicles are retrieved after fusion at the frog neuromuscular unction. Stimulating at 10 Hz for 1 min, Heuser and Reese observed decreased numbers of synaptic vesicles and the appearance of membrane cisternae emanating from the plasma membrane. If a rest period was allowed after stimulation, vesicles reappeared, apparently at the expense of the cisternae. Clathrin-coated pits and vesicles were frequently observed, particularly at sites remote from the active zone. In contrast, Ceccarelli *et al.* observed little change in the ultrastructure of the terminal following stimulation at low frequency (2 Hz). After release, vesicles were recycled fast enough to prevent depletion of vesicles. These two sets of observations have widely been interpreted as indicating that two mechanisms of vesicle release and retrieval exist at the frog

neuromuscular junction: some vesicles collapse fully into the plasma membrane and are then recycled by clathrin-mediated endocytosis (Fig.3.2, 2) while other vesicles release neurotransmitter without full collapse and are then retrieved by a direct and rapid reversal of the fusion process (Fig.3.2, 1). The latter mechanism, termed "kiss-and-run", provides a rapid and economical way of recycling vesicles. A third mechanism of endocytosis, involving the formation of a deep membrane infoldings (Fig.3.2, 3), has also been consistently observed in the frog neuromuscular junction, lamprey, reticulospinal synapses, snake motor nerve terminals, rat hippocampal neurons, goldfish bipolar cells, and the calyx of Held. These large membrane invaginations occur away from the site of fusion and their formation is not thought to directly involve clathrin. The current view is that the cisternae are not formed by the coalescence of internalized clathrin-coated vesicles as originally proposed. Instead, they are formed directly from the plasma membrane, and synaptic vesicles are thought to be formed by clathrin-mediated endocytosis from the infolded membrane connected to (Fig.3.2, 3) or disconnected from the plasma membrane.

Of these three basic mechanisms of retrieval, the best understood one is clathrin-mediated endocytosis. Clathrin-coated vesicles are observed in nerve terminals, generally at the outer margin of the active zone and their number is increased when fixation is performed during a peak of endocytic activity. Under electron microscope, it is able to identify polygonal clathrin lattices that form the outer shell and main scaffold of the coat. Clathrin and the clathrin adaptor complexes (AP-2 and AP-180), which participate in clathrin-mediated budding from the plasma membrane, are enriched in the nervous system, where they are concentrated in nerve terminals. Incubation of lysed synaptosomes in the presence of brain cytosol, ATP and GTPγS (a condition that enhances coat formation and blocks uncoating) results in the massive generation of clathrin-coated endocytic buds. Genetically induced disruption of genes encoding clathrin adaptors in *Drosophila* produces drastic impairment of synaptic vesicle recycling. Microinjections into giant axons of antibodies or peptides that perturb the function of the clathrin coat induce a powerful inhibition of synaptic vesicle membrane endocytosis and synaptic transmission. These observations strongly support a role of the clathrin-mediated pathway in synaptic vesicle endocytosis. The current model for clathrin-mediated endocytosis suggests a pathway of four steps, i.e., nucleation of the coat, invagination of the pit, fission, and uncoating (Fig.3.4, see also the color plate). The heterotetrameric adaptor complex AP-2 and AP-180 may bind to transmembrane proteins at the surface and recruit clathrin triskelions that assemble into the lattice over the membrane surface. Formation of the lattice deforms the membrane to form a coated pit which will develop into the size of a vesicle. Subsequent scission of the vesicle from the surface requires the large GTPase, dynamin. The formation of clathrin-coat and disconnection of coated vesicle from plasma membrane may involve accessory proteins, such as endophilin, amphiphysin, auxilin, synaptojanin, and stoned B. Coated vesicles or invagination fail to pinch off when the function of dynamin is disturbed by mutations in dynamin (e.g., *shibire* mutant of *Drosophila*), by microinjection of antibodies of dynamin or peptide domain interfering with the interaction of dynamin and other accessory proteins, or by blocking GTPase activity of dynamin with GTPγS.

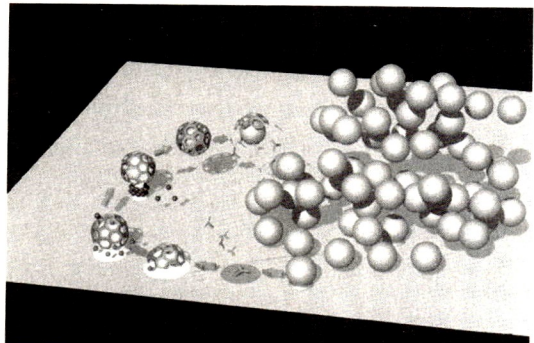

Fig.3.4 The model of clathrin-mediated endocytosis. The clathrin triskelia are recruited to form coat on the cytosolic face of plasma membrane, and this induces the membrane invagination. Around the neck of the coated pit, a complex of fission machinery (red spheres), composed of dynamin and its binding proteins, assembles and pinches off the coated vesicle. The coats are rapidly shed off (reprinted from *Synapses*, p.230, eds. by Cowan, Sudhof and Stevens, with permission of the Johns Hopkins University Press).

The molecular mechanism of "kiss-and-run" mode or rapid form of endocytosis is also under investigation. A couple of studies suggest that it is a clathrin-independent pathway, but requires dynamin.

THE DYNAMIC TIME COURSE OF ENDOCYTOSIS

Electron microscopic studies in 1970s provided some insights to the kinetics of endocytosis. Heuser and Reese found that a clathrin-mediated form of endocytosis is in a time scale of minutes. In contrast, Ceccarelli and his colleagues proposed a "kiss-and-run" of endocytosis in a time scale of seconds. However, quantitative time course measurements are difficult with electron microscopy. To overcome this difficulty, three techniques have been developed in the last decade to study live synapses: (i) imaging of vesicles loaded with FM dyes, (ii) imaging of vesicles expressed with a pH sensitive mutant of GFP, synaptopHluorin, and (iii) membrane capacitance measurement at nerve terminals. Imaging with FM dyes can be applied to the majority of synapses, but the time resolution is limited to seconds. Imaging with synaptopHluorin requires genetic manipulations, but offers a real-time measurement at a resolution of less than one second, provided that the re-acidification of endocytosed vesicles is much faster than endocytosis. The measurement of capacitance offers the fastest time resolution, down to milliseconds, but requires patch-clamping the nerve terminal. Large terminals that can be patch-clamped include (i) ribbon-type synapses, such as the goldfish retinal bipolar nerve terminal and the mouse cochlear inner hair cell, (ii) neurohypophysial nerve terminals containing large dense-core vesicles and unknown microvesicles, and (iii) nerve terminals containing conventional active zones, such as calyces of Held in the auditory brain stem and hippocampal mossy fiber boutons.

With these quantitative techniques, endocytosis on the order of tens to hundreds of seconds was readily observed in early studies at cultured hippocampal synapses, goldfish retinal bipolar nerve terminals, and frog neuromuscular junctions, and subsequently confirmed at other synapses (Fig.3.5A, lower). Rapid endocytosis, on the order of 0.1-2 s, was first observed with capacitance measurements at the goldfish retinal bipolar synapse, and subsequently confirmed in the neurohypophysial nerve terminal, the mouse cochlear inner hair cell, the rat calyx of Held (Fig.3.5A, upper) and the hippocampal mossy fiber bouton. Recent imaging studies also indicate the existence of rapid endocytosis at small conventional boutons. At cultured hippocampal synapses, vesicles loaded with FM2-10, a dye that dissociates from the membrane to the solution faster than FM1-43, are

destained to a larger extent than those loaded with FM1-43. This result implies the existence of rapid endocytosis, which is too fast for FM1-43 to leave from the vesicle membrane to the bath solution. However, FM2-10 may preferentially stain the readily releasable pool of vesicles at frog neuromuscular junctions, which provides an alternative interpretation for why destaining of FM2-10 is faster. Partly to resolve these issues, labeling of single vesicles with FM1-43 or synaptopHluorin has recently been achieved at cultured hippocampal boutons. For most single vesicles labeled with FM1-43, action potentials

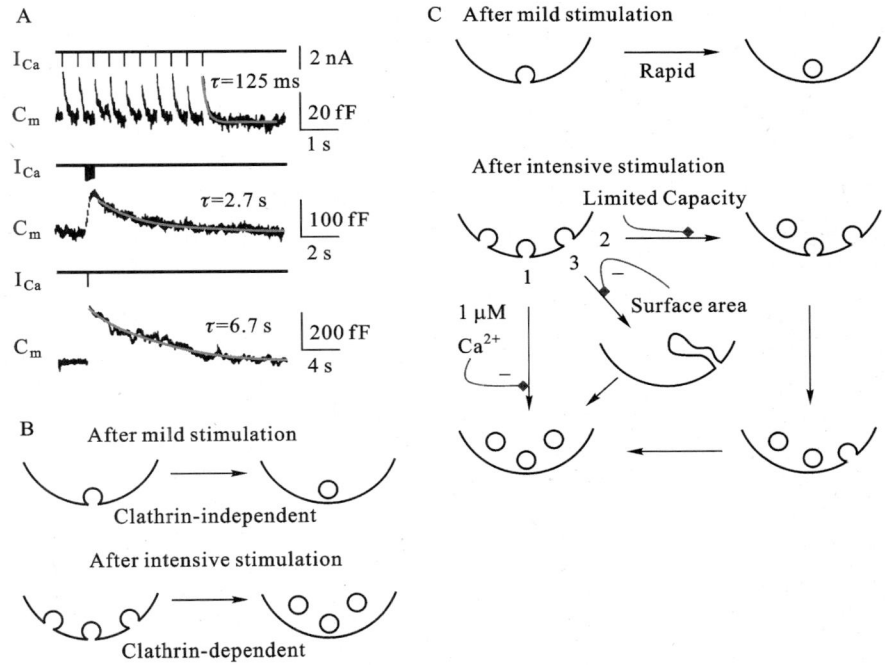

Fig.3.5   Stimulation-dependent slow down of endocytosis and its potential underlying mechanisms. Endocytosis slows down after higher frequencies of stimulation at the calyx of Held. Sampled calcium current (I_{Ca}) and membrane capacitance (C_m) induced by 10 action potential-equivalent stimuli (AP-e) at 2 (upper), 20 (middle), and 333 (lower) Hz. The scale for I_{Ca} applies to all three traces. A model at the molecular level that may account for the stimulation-dependent slow down of endocytosis. Endocytosis is mediated by a rapid (thick arrow), clathrin-independent mechanism and a slow (thin arrow), clathrin-dependent mechanism after mild and intensive stimulation, respectively. Three models at the cellular level that may account for the stimulation-dependent slow down of endocytosis (e.g., panel A). After mild stimulation, all models agree that endocytosis of a vesicle in a nerve terminal is relatively rapid (thick arrow). After intensive stimulation, more vesicles remain fused with the plasma membrane and their retrieval may be prolonged by three different mechanisms. First (thin arrow), the residual calcium in the range of 1 μM or less may inhibit (−) endocytosis, as reported at the goldfish retinal bipolar nerve terminal. Second (thick arrows), as proposed in cultured hippocampal synapses, although retrieval of each vesicle is rapid, the capacity of such rapid endocytosis is limited, resulting in a slow time course of overall retrieval. Third (medium sized arrows), as proposed in the calyx of Held, an increased surface area or tension at the plasma membrane may slow (−) endocytosis, perhaps by slowly forming long infoldings from several fused vesicles, followed by slow regeneration of vesicles. These cartoons do not indicate the exact location of retrieval (applies to Fig.3.2 and 3.3).

trigger only partial dye loss, suggesting that fusion and retrieval, estimated to be less than 1.4 s, is fast enough to prevent full dye loss from the plasma membrane to the solution. Furthermore, imaging studies at cultured hippocampal synapses expressed with synaptopHluorin show that single vesicle fusion and retrieval may take only 400-860 ms and fast endocytosis may occur during repetitive stimulation. In conclusion, the time course of endocytosis ranges from hundreds of milliseconds to hundreds of seconds.

THE TIME COURSE OF ENDOCYTOSIS IS REGULATED BY STIMULATION

At goldfish bipolar nerve terminals, neurohypophysial nerve terminals and calyces, endocytosis after a depolarization pulse of longer duration is prolonged. At frog neuromuscular junction, hippocampal synapses and calyces, endocytosis after a longer train of action potentials is prolonged. At calyces, endocytosis after a higher frequency train of action potential-like stimuli is also prolonged (Fig.3.5A). These consensus findings establish a principle that endocytosis after an increased duration or frequency of stimulation is prolonged.

While endocytosis is prolonged after high frequency stimulation, several lines of indirect evidence suggest fast endocytosis during stimulation, at least at cultured hippocampal synapses. First, destaining of FM1-43 from individual vesicles during a 10 Hz train is much slower than that predicted for complete fusion with departitioning of FM1-43 from the membrane to the aqueous solution. This result implies that endocytosis is too fast for FM1-43 to dissociate from the membrane at hippocampal synapses, which is different from results obtained at goldfish retinal bipolar nerve terminals. Secondly, the decrease of the EPSC is slower than the decrease of the FM2-10 destaining rate during 10-30 Hz nerve stimulation. The onset of this difference may be as short as 1-3 s, implying that recycled vesicles, which have lost FM2-10, are reused

in 1-3 s after fusion. Finally, a recent imaging study at cultured hippocampal nerve terminals expressed with synaptopHluorin suggests that endocytosis during repetitive stimulation is faster than that after stimulation.

MECHANISMS THAT MAY REGULATE THE TIME COURSE OF ENDOCYTOSIS

Clathrin-dependent Versus Clathrin-independent Endocytosis

Two major hypotheses have been proposed to account for the slow down of endocytosis after intensive stimulation. First, at frog neuromuscular junctions, clathrin-dependent endocytosis was observed after intensive high frequency nerve stimulation, whereas the "kiss-and-run" hypothesis was proposed for low frequency stimulation. At adrenal medulla chromaffin cells, prolonged depolarization shifts the mode of endocytosis from clathrin-independent rapid endocytosis to clathrin-dependent slow endocytosis. At *Drosophila* neuromuscular junctions, there are two morphologically and pharmacologically distinct endocytic pathways, which are similar to clathrin-dependent and "kiss-and-run" pathways, respectively. Furthermore, examination of *Drosophila* with a mutant in endophilin, a protein involved in clathrin-mediated endocytosis, suggests both clathrin-dependent and clathrin-independent forms of endocytosis. Clathrin-independent endocytosis may be rapid because it escapes loading by FM1-43. These results led to the first hypothesis that intensive stimulation triggers clathrin-mediated slow endocytosis, whereas mild stimulation triggers clathrin-independent, rapid endocytosis (Fig.3.5B).

Regulation of Endocytosis by Single Rate-limiting Factors

The first hypothesis predicts only two fixed rates of endocytosis. However, endocytosis gradually slows down from less than a second to minutes as the stimulation intensity increases at many synapses (e.g.,

Fig.3.5A). This led to the second major hypothesis that the time course of endocytosis is regulated by a single rate-limiting factor generated by stimulation. Three such factors have been proposed at three different synapses. First, an increase of the intracellular calcium concentration up to 1 μM may inhibit endocytosis at goldfish bipolar cells (Fig.3.5C). Second, the endocytic capacity may be limited to about one vesicle per second per bouton at cultured hippocampal synapses, perhaps owing to a limited resource that mediates endocytosis. Saturation of this capacity may slow down endocytosis (Fig.3.5C). Third, the above two mechanisms could not fully account for the slow down of endocytosis observed at the calyx. Since single and multiple vesicle fusion at an active zone are correlated with rapid and slow endocytosis, respectively, it was proposed that different numbers of fused vesicles may generate different sizes of membrane infoldings, which may be retrieved at different rates (Fig.3.5C).

Recent studies have identified some regulatory mechanisms that may help to explain the dynamic time course of endocytosis. For example, at goldfish bipolar synapses, blocking hydrolysis of ATP but not GTP inhibits both rapid and slow endocytosis, and increasing the osmolarity of the cytosolic solution inhibits slow but not fast endocytosis. At cultured hippocampal synapses, the time course of endocytosis after single vesicle fusion depends on the release probability of the bouton. Rapid endocytosis is predominant at boutons with lower release probability, whereas slow endocytosis is predominant at boutons with higher release probability. These observations offer an explanation for why rapid endocytosis occurs during repetitive stimulation, during which boutons with a lower release probability, and thus a faster endocytosis, may be recruited for release.

The Effects of Calcium on Endocytosis

The reported effects of calcium on endocytosis are apparently controversial. Here we attempt to provide some explanations for this apparent controversy. At the goldfish bipolar nerve terminal, an increase of the intracellular calcium level to about 1 μM blocks endocytosis. However, imaging with FM dyes at goldfish bipolar nerve terminals suggests that endocytosis occurs at the intracellular calcium concentration of 0.8-20 μM. At the calyx, increasing the intracellular calcium concentration to about 1 μM does not slow endocytosis. Furthermore, at the frog neuromuscular junction, the residual calcium level (up to 1 μM) induced by various durations of nerve stimulation is not correlated with the rate of endocytosis. These results suggest that calcium inhibition of endocytosis may be at most a cell-type specific, but not a general mechanism.

In contrast to the inhibitory or lack of effect of low micromolar concentrations of calcium on endocytosis, high micromolar concentrations of calcium seem to speed up endocytosis. At the mouse cochlear inner hair cell, increasing the intracellular calcium level to tens of micromolar triggers rapid endocytosis. At chromaffin cells, an increase of the extracellular calcium concentration to tens of millimolar, which may increase the peak calcium concentration induced by depolarization, shifts the mode of exo- and endocytosis to the rapid "kiss-and-run" mode. At the goldfish retina, calcium buffers like EGTA and BAPTA, which may reduce the calcium concentration in the microdomain created by the opening of calcium channels, reduced the amplitude of rapid endocytosis and increased the amplitude of slow endocytosis. However, imaging of FM dyes at the goldfish retina suggests that endocytosis is inhibited by increasing the intracellular calcium concentration above 20 μM. At cultured hippocampal synapses, elevation of the extracellular calcium concentration seems to speed up both rapid and slow endocytosis. In conclusion, the majority of studies support the hypothesis that higher micromolar ranges of cytosolic calcium speed up endocytosis. Such a mechanism offers an explanation for why endocytosis can be rapid during high frequency stimulation at cultured hippocampal synapses.

The conclusion that high concentrations of calcium speed up endocytosis seems contradictory to the result that endocytosis after intensive stimulation is slower than that after mild stimulation. This discrepancy may be accounted for by the following hypothesis. A single action potential triggers release by increasing the calcium concentration at the release site to tens of micromolar. Thus, the calcium concentration during single or low frequency action potentials may be sufficiently high to trigger rapid endocytosis. If rapid endocytosis is of limited capacity, the capacity may be saturated during higher frequency stimulation. After intensive stimulation, fused vesicles exceeding the capacity of rapid endocytosis may be retrieved by a slower mechanism.

Hypotheses that May Account for Calcium-mediated Facilitation of Endocytosis

The molecular mechanism by which higher concentrations of calcium speed up endocytosis is not clear. Recent studies suggest several possibilities. At PC12 cells, the frequency of the stand-alone foot of amperometric recordings, in which fusion pores open and close without dilating, is increased by transfection with synaptotagmin IV, an important transducer of calcium signals in evoked exocytosis. This result suggests that the amount of synaptotagmin IV at the vesicle may be involved in determining whether the vesicle undergoes "kiss-and-run" or not. At cultured hippocampal synapses, the splice variants of synaptotagmin VII, a calcium binding protein, may differentially regulate the rate of vesicle cycling. At Drosophila neuromuscular junctions, inactivation of synaptotagmin I, which mediates calcium-dependent exocytosis, blocks slow endocytosis. This result suggests that synaptotagmin I may couple exocytosis to slow endocytosis. A study at Drosophila neuromuscular junctions proposed that calcium mediates endocytosis by promoting clathrin assembly at the plasma membrane. At synaptosomes, slow endocytosis induced by extremely prolonged depolarization may be triggered by dephosphorylation of a series of endocytic proteins by calcineurin, a calcium-dependent protein phosphatase.

THE FUNCTIONAL SIGNIFICANCE OF REGULATION OF ENDOCYTOSIS

The Contribution of Slower Endocytosis to Short-term Synaptic Depression

Studies of a temperature-sensitive paralytic Drosophila mutant, shibire[ts], provide direct evidence for the importance of endocytosis in maintaining transmitter release. In wild-type Drosophila neuromuscular junctions, repetitive nerve stimulation leads to a decrease of the synaptic current to a steady-state level (Fig.3.6A, left). This steady-state level is abolished (Fig.3.6A, right) in shibire[ts] mutants at non-permissive temperatures, at which endocytosis is blocked. These results predict that decreasing the rate of endocytosis results in a decreased steady-state level of synaptic transmission, thus a larger extent of short-term synaptic depression during repetitive nerve stimulation. This prediction is confirmed at the frog neuromuscular junction, where it was shown that as the duration of nerve stimulation at 30 Hz increases from 10 to 300 s, the rate of endocytosis slows down, short-term synaptic depression increases, and the time course of recovery from depression increases (Fig.3.6B). These observations lead to a model in which slower endocytosis causes a slower replenishment of the reserve pool of vesicles (Fig.3.6D, k_2), which in turn causes a slower replenishment of the readily releasable pool from the reserve pool (Fig.3.6D, k_3), and thus contributes to the generation of short-term synaptic depression.

The Maintenance of Transmitter Release by Retrieving Vesicles into the Reserve Pool and/or the Readily Releasable Pool

At cultured hippocampal synapses, neuromuscular junctions, and rat calyces, only a small fraction of the total pool of vesicles undergoes vesicle recycling during repetitive stimulation. This feature makes vesicle recycling particularly important to sustain synaptic

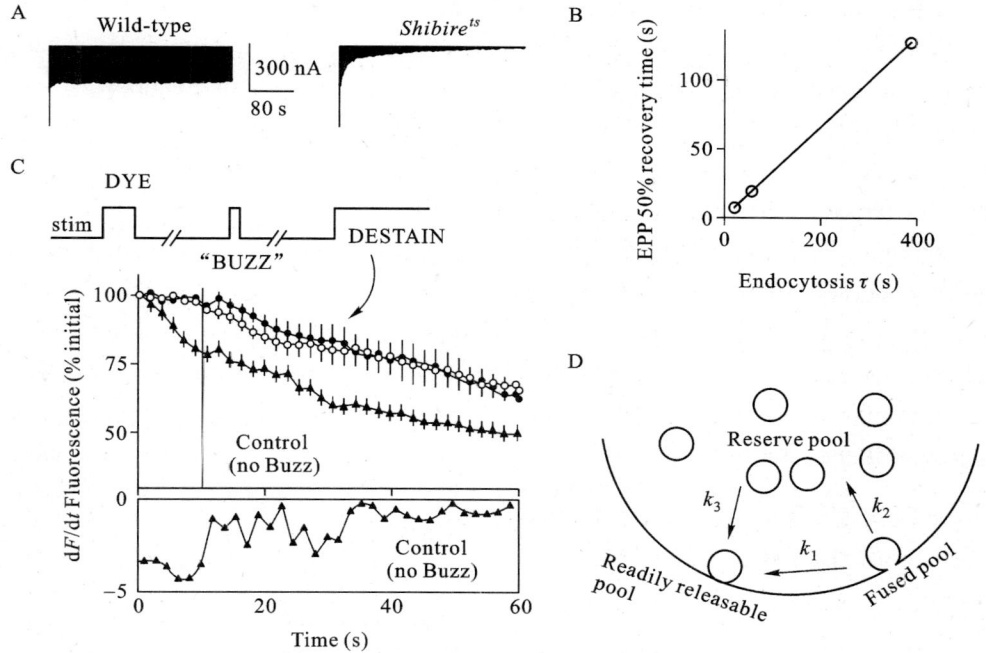

Fig.3.6   Endocytosis is essential for the maintenance of synaptic transmission. Decline of synaptic current amplitude during 400 s 10 Hz tetanic stimulation at 32°C in wild-type (left) and in a *shibire*ᵗˢ mutant (right) *Drosophila* neuromuscular junction. The block of endocytosis in the *shibire*ᵗˢ mutant results in the decline of the synaptic current to zero, suggesting an essential role for endocytosis to maintain synaptic transmission during repetitive stimulation. The relation between the 50% recovery time of the end plate potential (EPP) and the time constant of endocytosis after 10 (lower circle), 60 (middle circle), and 300 s (upper circle) of nerve stimulation at 30 Hz at frog neuromuscular junctions. The data were fit well with a linear regression line, suggesting that slower endocytosis may contribute to slower recovery from short-term synaptic depression. Vesicles in the readily releasable pool recycle selectively to their pool of origin at the frog neuromuscular junction. After dye loading of total recycling pool and washing, terminals were given a weak stimulus ("buzz") (either 30 Hz for 10 s (filled circles) or 5 Hz for 2 min (open circles)) designed to deplete the readily releasable pool; controls (triangles) did not receive this stimulation. After a 20 min rest, the terminals were destained with 30 Hz stimulation. The graph shows the fluorescence of terminals during final destaining, each normalized to the brightness at the beginning of the final destaining. Control terminals destained progressively. Terminals given the prestimulus buzz showed a distinct lag before starting to lose dye, suggesting that release during the lag was sustained by recycled vesicles which have lost their dye during fusion evoked by the prestimulus buzz. The destinations of retrieved vesicles. Vesicles fused at the plasma membrane (fused pool) may be retrieved directly to the readily releasable pool and/or the reserve pool with a rate constant of k_1 and k_2, respectively. It is likely that k_1 is larger than k_2. Vesicles in the reserve pool may also be mobilized to the readily releasable pool with a rate constant of k_3. These cycling routes may be essential for the maintenance of synaptic transmission and regulation of these routes may result in synaptic plasticity.

transmission. Recycled vesicles are generally assumed to enter the reserve vesicle pool before entering the readily releasable pool (Fig.3.6D, k_2, k_3). However, recent studies suggest that they may also directly enter the readily releasable pool (Fig.3.6D, k_1). Following brief stimulation that depletes the readily releasable pool at cultured hippocampal synapses, the ability to release neurotransmitter recovers 10-fold more rapidly than that of FM2-10 destaining. This result suggests that rapidly endocytosed vesicles, which have lost FM2-10, re-enter the readily releasable pool

and are capable of being released. Consistent with this suggestion, the decrease of the EPSC is slower than that of the FM2-10 destaining rate during 10-30 Hz nerve stimulation. The onset of the difference may be as short as 1-3 s during 30 Hz stimulation, suggesting a rapid reuse of vesicles in 1-3 s after exocytosis. At frog neuromuscular junctions, replenishment of the reserve vesicle pool is slow, with a half-time of about 8 min, and transmitter release during low (2-5 Hz) or high (30 Hz) frequency stimulation is at least partly maintained by vesicle recycling to the readily releasable pool without entering the reserve pool (Fig.3.6C). Surprisingly, vesicles in the functionally defined readily releasable pool are found randomly throughout the vesicle cluster at frog neuromuscular junctions. It is unclear whether vesicle recycling at frog neuromuscular junctions is as fast as in the cultured hippocampal synapses. Although it is currently unknown what determines the destination of endocytosed vesicles, it seems reasonable to propose a general hypothesis that rapidly endocytosed vesicles recycle directly to the readily releasable pool, whereas the slowly endocytosed vesicles recycle to the reserve pool.

Is Endocytosis Fast Enough to Limit Transmitter Release from the Fusion Pore?

While rapid endocytosis helps to maintain transmitter output during repetitive stimulation, could it be so fast to permit only partial release of transmitter from the fusion pore and thus limit the quantal size? Studies with patch amperometry and cell-attached capacitance measurements suggest so for dense-core vesicles at endocrine cells. Whether such a mechanism occurs for clear-core vesicles at synapses remains unclear. At cultured neurons of the leech, clear-core vesicles discharge transmitter serotonin with a time constant of 260 μs. Therefore, rapid endocytosis, in the range of 0.1-2 s, is too long to limit diffusion of transmitter from clear core vesicles. A study at cultured hippocampal synapses found that a fraction of vesicles released by a hypertonic shock do not permit FM dyes to enter or escape from them. This observation led to the suggestion that the vesicle interior may be exposed very transiently, likely less than 6 ms, or a special configuration of the fusion pore may prevent dye exchange. However, no significant decrease in the quantal size is observed, implying that the fusion pore opening is still long enough to release all transmitters from the vesicle.

CONCLUSIONS

It is well established that the time course of synaptic vesicle endocytosis after stimulation may range from hundreds of milliseconds to hundreds of seconds, and it increases as the stimulation duration and/or frequency increase. Rapid endocytosis might also occur during repetitive stimulation, and is facilitated by high concentrations of calcium. Endocytosed vesicles may enter the reserve pool and/or the readily releasable pool to sustain synaptic transmission during repetitive stimulation. Regulation of the kinetics of endocytosis may contribute to the generation of certain forms of synaptic plasticity, such as short-term synaptic depression. There are still many unresolved major questions. Some examples are listed in the following. First, the cellular, molecular, and ultra-structural mechanisms that determine and mediate different rates of endocytosis are not well understood. Although many hypotheses have been proposed, future work is needed to determine whether there is a general mechanism that regulates the rate of endocytosis. Secondly, it is unclear whether vesicles formed by rapid and slow endocytosis replenish different pools of vesicles, such as the readily releasable pool and the reserve pool, respectively. Thirdly, it remains unclear whether regulation of endocytosis is a general property by which many forms of synaptic plasticity are achieved. Fourthly, how calcium facilitates endocytosis is not well understood. A likely possibility is the binding to synaptotagmins. Finally, the molecular mechanism involved in vesicle mobilization from the reserve pool to the readily releasable pool is not well understood. Addressing these issues in the future may greatly improve our understanding of the vesicle cycling process.

GENERAL CITATIONS

Cousin MA, Robinson PJ. 2001. The dephosphins: dephosphorylation by calcineurin triggers synaptic vesicle endocytosis. *Trends Neurosci*, 24: 659-665.

Jahn R, Lang T, Sudhof TC. 2003. Membrane fusion. *Cell*, 112: 519-533.

Lindau M, Alvarez de Toledo G. 2003. The fusion pore. *Biochim Biophys Acta*, 1641: 167-173.

Murthy VN, de Camilli P. 2003. Cell biology of the presynaptic terminal. *Annu Rev Neurosci*, 26: 701-728.

Rizzoli SO, Betz WJ. 2004. The structural organization of the readily releasable pool of synaptic vesicles. *Science*, 303: 2037-2039.

Rizzoli SO, Betz WJ. 2005. Synaptic vesicle pools. *Nat Rev Neurosci*, 6: 57-69.

von Gersdorff H, Borst JG. 2002. Short-term plasticity at the calyx of held. *Nat Rev Neurosci*, 3: 53-64.

Wu LG. 2004. Kinetic regulation of vesicle endocytosis at synapses. *Trends Neurosci*, 27: 548-554.

DISCOVERY CITATIONS

Albillos A, Dernick G, Horstmann H, Almers W, Alvarez de Toledo G, Lindau M. 1997. The exocytotic event in chromaffin cells revealed by patch amperometry. *Nature*, 389: 509-512.

Aravanis AM, Pyle JL, Tsien RW. 2003. Single synaptic vesicles fusing transiently and successively without loss of identity. *Nature*, 423: 643-647.

Artalejo CR, Elhamdani A, Palfrey HC. 2002. Sustained stimulation shifts the mechanism of endocytosis from dynamin-1-dependent rapid endocytosis to clathrin- and dynamin-2-mediated slow endocytosis in chromaffin cells. *Proc Natl Acad Sci USA*, 99: 6358-6363.

Beutner D, Voets T, Neher E, Moser T. 2001. Calcium dependence of exocytosis and endocytosis at the cochlear inner hair cell afferent synapse. *Neuron*, 29: 681-690.

Bollmann JH, Sakmann B, Borst JG. 2000. Calcium sensitivity of glutamate release in a calyx-type terminal. *Science*, 289: 953-957.

Ceccarelli B, Hurlbut WP, Mauro A. 1973. Turnover of transmitter and synaptic vesicles at the frog neuromuscular junction. *J Cell Biol*, 57: 499-524.

Delgado R, Maureira C, Oliva C, Kidokoro Y, Labarca P. 2000. Size of vesicle pools, rates of mobilization, and recycling at neuromuscular synapses of a *Drosophila*, mutant, *shibire*. *Neuron*, 28: 941-953.

Gandhi SP, Stevens CF. 2003. Three modes of synaptic vesicular recycling revealed by single-vesicle imaging. *Nature*, 423: 607-613.

Heidelberger R, Heinemann C, Neher E, Matthews G. 1994. Calcium dependence of the rate of exocytosis in a synaptic

terminal. *Nature*, 371: 513-515.

Heuser JE, Reese TS. 1973. Evidence for recycling of synaptic vesicle membrane during transmitter release at the frog neuromuscular junction. *J Cell Biol*, 57: 315-344.

Klyachko VA, Jackson MB. 2002. Capacitance steps and fusion pores of small and large-dense-core vesicles in nerve terminals. *Nature*, 418: 89-92.

Koenig JH, Ikeda K. 1989. Disappearance and reformation of synaptic vesicle membrane upon transmitter release observed under reversible blockage of membrane retrieval. *J Neurosci*, 9: 3844-3860.

Koenig JH, Ikeda K. 1996. Synaptic vesicles have two distinct recycling pathways. *J Cell Biol*, 135: 797-808.

Kuromi H, Kidokoro Y. 1998. Two distinct pools of synaptic vesicles in single presynaptic boutons in a temperature-sensitive *Drosophila* mutant, *shibire*. *Neuron*, 20: 917-925.

Pyle JL, Kavalali ET, Piedras-Renteria ES, Tsien RW. 2000. Rapid reuse of readily releasable pool vesicles at hippocampal synapses. *Neuron*, 28: 221-231.

Richards DA, Guatimosim C, Betz WJ. 2000. Two endocytic recycling routes selectively fill two vesicle pools in frog motor nerve terminals. *Neuron*, 27: 551-559.

Richards DA, Guatimosim C, Rizzoli SO, Betz WJ. 2003. Synaptic vesicle pools at the frog neuromuscular junction. *Neuron*, 39: 529-541.

Rizzoli SO, Betz WJ. 2004. The structural organization of the readily releasable pool of synaptic vesicles. *Science*, 303: 2037-2039.

Sankaranarayanan S, Ryan TA. 2000. Real-time measurements of vesicle-SNARE recycling in synapses of the central nervous system. *Nat Cell Biol*, 2: 197-204.

Schneggenburger R, Neher E. 2000. Intracellular calcium dependence of transmitter release rates at a fast central synapse. *Nature*, 406: 889-893.

Shupliakov O, Low P, Grabs D, Gad H, Chen H, David C, *et al.* 1997. Synaptic vesicle endocytosis impaired by disruption of dynamin-SH3 domain interactions. *Science*, 276: 259-263.

Sun JY, Wu LG. 2001. Fast kinetics of exocytosis revealed by simultaneous measurements of presynaptic capacitance and postsynaptic currents at a central synapse. *Neuron*, 30: 171-182.

Sun JY, Wu XS, Wu LG. 2002. Single and multiple vesicle fusion induce different rates of endocytosis at a central synapse. *Nature*, 417: 555-559.

Takei K, McPherson PS, Schmid SL, de Camilli P. 1995. Tubular membrane invaginations coated by dynamin rings are induced by GTP-gamma S in nerve terminals. *Nature*, 374: 186-190.

Takei K, Mundigl O, Daniell L, de Camilli P. 1996. The synaptic vesicle cycle: a single vesicle budding step involving clathrin and dynamin. *J Cell Biol*, 133: 1237-1250.

Verstreken P, Kjaerulff O, Lloyd TE, Atkinson R, Zhou Y, Meinertzhagen IA, *et al.* 2002. Endophilin mutations block clathrin-mediated endocytosis but not neurotransmitter release. *Cell*, 109: 101-112.

von Gersdorff H, Matthews G. 1994. Dynamics of synaptic vesicle fusion and membrane retrieval in synaptic terminals. *Nature*, 367: 735-739.

von Gersdorff H, Matthews G. 1994. Inhibition of endocytosis by elevated internal calcium in a synaptic terminal. *Nature*, 370: 652-655.

Wang CT, Lu JC, Bai J, Chang PY, Martin TF, Chapman ER, *et al.* 2003. Different domains of synaptotagmin control the choice between kiss-and-run and full fusion. *Nature*, 424: 943-947.

Wu LG, Betz WJ. 1996. Nerve activity but not intracellular calcium determines the time course of endocytosis at the frog neuromuscular junction. *Neuron*, 17: 769-779.

Wu LG, Betz WJ. 1998. Kinetics of synaptic depression and vesicle recycling after tetanic stimulation of frog motor nerve terminals. *Biophys J*, 74: 3003-3009.

Xu J, Wu LG. 2005. The decrease in the presynaptic calcium current is a major cause of short-term depression at a calyx-type synapse. *Neuron*, 46: 633-645.

Part II Glutamate, Excitatory Transmission and Pain

Postsynaptic Excitatory Transmission

CHAPTER 4

John F. MacDonald, Suhas Kotecha, Michael F. Jackson, Michael Beazely

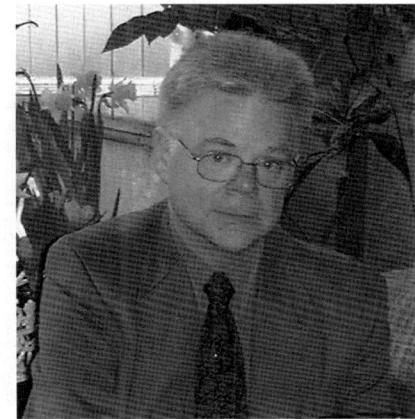

Dr. MacDonald is a Professor and Chair in the Department of Physiology, University of Toronto. He graduated from The University of British Columbia and obtained a Ph.D. in Physiology. He pursued postdoctoral training at St. Andrews University, McGill University, and NINCDS.

Suhas Kotecha, Michael F. Jackson and Michael Beazely are members of Dr. MacDonald's laboratory.

MAJOR CONTRIBUTIONS

1. Lu W, Man, Ju W, Trimble WS, MacDonald JF, Wang YT. 2001. Activation of synaptic NMDA receptors induces membrane insertion of new AMPA receptors and LTP in cultured hippocampal neurons. *Neuron*, 29: 243-254.

2. Huang Y, Lu W, Ali DW, Pelkey KA, Pitcher GM, Lu YM, Aoto H, Roder JC, Sasaki T, Salter MW, MacDonald JF. 2001. CAKbeta/Pyk2 kinase is a signaling link for induction of long-term potentiation in CA1 hippocampus. *Neuron*, 29: 485-496.

3. Kotecha SA, Oak JN, Jackson MF, Perez Y, Orser BA, Van Tol H, MacDonald JF. 2002. A D2 class dopamine receptor transactivates a receptor tyrosine kinase to inhibit NMDA receptor transmission. *Neuron*, 35: 1111-1122.

4. Aarts M, Iihara K, Wei W-Y, Xiong Z, Arundine M, Mac-

mitter systems (e.g., cholinergic and dopaminergic systems). We have shown that long-distance cross-talk between receptors for "long" transmitters and glutamate receptors occurs through the sharing of overlapping signal transduction pathways and may also make use of the signal relay mechanism of growth factor receptor "transactivation".

INTRODUCTION

Glutamate is without a doubt the most ubiquitous, and therefore, arguably the most significant transmitter in the mammalian central nervous system. Glutamate is also a major excitatory transmitter in the nervous systems of most invertebrates and has been extensively studied for its role as the transmitter at the neuromuscular junction of crustaceans. Interestingly, through evolution the neuromuscular junction role of glutamate has been superceded in vertebrate skeletal muscle by acetylcholine (ACh). This "centralization" of the transmitter glutamate seems mirrored by a similar internalization of γ-amino-butyric acid (GABA) to form the primary inhibitory transmitter. Although many other transmitter systems, including ACh, are found in the mammalian central nervous system, they are most often organized into discrete pathways to form so called "long transmitter systems". This contrasts with local or "short transmitter" networks of inhibitory interneurons where transmission is primarily GABAergic. The relatively small number of presynaptic neurons for many cholinergic (ACh), catecolaminergic (e.g., noradrenalin) and indolaminergic (e.g., serotonin) pathways are sequestered in discrete nuclei, whose axons project diffusely to remote postsynaptic target regions of the brain. The shear ubiquity of glutamate as an excitatory transmitter dictates that presynaptic glutamatergic neurons are both close as well as far from their postsynaptic targets ("short" and "long" transmitter).

More recent genetic approaches have begun to unravel the transmitter role of glutamate in the central nervous system of simple animals such a *Caenorhabditis elegans* and *Drosophila melanogaster*. Such

findings are of considerable potential value in anticipating how glutamatergic transmission in mammals has evolved to form the repertoire of complex cellular behaviours underlying the integration of sensory information into the perceptions of pain. Our understanding of invertebrate giant axons and synapses has contributed so much to our fundamental understanding of neuronal transmission in the mammalian nervous system and the analogies of invertebrate central glutamatergic transmission and those of the mammal are just beginning to be exploited using genetic approaches.

EXCITATORY SYNAPTIC POTENTIALS

Using voltage-clamp techniques one can observe the underlying currents responsible for generating epsps as excitatory synaptic currents (epscs). Glutamatergic epscs are the result of inward currents generated by the influx of cations (and K^+ efflux) into the postsynaptic neuron. A unitary epsp (response to transmitter released from a single terminal) is exceedingly small (usually just a few millivolts in amplitude) relative to the endplate potential generated at the neuromuscular junction (from 20 to 70 mV). Transmission at the neuromuscular junction is almost all or none as a very high "safety factor of transmission" is required between motoneurons and muscle. Clearly it is advantageous that every command signal from a skeletal motoneuron pool leads to a guaranteed muscular action potential and hence contraction. In contrast, excitatory signals on most principle cells of the central nervous system employ extremely large numbers of small epsps whose spatial and temporal summation is essential to reach threshold for the generation of an action potential (the output signal of the neuron). Indeed, most excitatory synapses found on the dendrites of central neurons are both topographically and "electrically" remote from potential trigger zones responsible for generation of the action potential. The cellular integration of these excitatory signals is considerably more complicated because a variety of physical factors (e.g., membrane capacitance, dendritic spine structure, dendrite diameter, dendritic branching, etc.) as well as the presence of active conductances (voltage-dependent ion channels) in the dendrites and cell body serve to filtre, amplify and integrate these excitatory signals. Furthermore, the attenuating actions of inhibitory synaptic inputs, largely located at the cell body, also contribute through counter acting membrane hyperpolarization and membrane shunting.

The transience of postsynaptic glutamatergic responses means that these receptors would appear best adapted for very rapid excitatory signaling. Indeed this is the case; however, rapid and short-lasing excitatory signaling is only one aspect of postsynaptic glutamatergic responsiveness. The degenerative lack of signaling capacity provided by the unanimity of employing glutamate at so many synapses, has been counteracted through a diversity in the number of postsynaptic glutamate receptor subtypes and via the coupling of receptors to signal transduction pathways capable of regulating a myriad of protein posttranslational processes, protein translation itself and ultimately gene expression. So the simple excitatory signal is transduced into major and long-lasting events whose consequences far out last the transient electrical signals.

GENERATING GLUTAMATERGIC ESPS

Each glutamatergic epsp is mediated by ionotropic postsynaptic glutamate receptors of the α-amino-3-hydroxy-5-methyl-4-isoxazole propionic acid (AMPA) and the N-methyl-D-aspartate (NMDA) receptor classes (Fig.4.1). Unitary glutamatergic epsps invariably are mediated by AMPA receptors (AMPAR) with little contribution by NMDA receptors (NMDAR) due to their depression by extracellular Mg^{2+} which blocks the open channels. There is also good evidence that a further class of ionotropic kainate receptors occupies synapses in some specialized pathways and it is possible that other more exotic ionotropic synaptic receptors, perhaps related to the GluRδ may yet be

detected. Beyond this a broad spectrum of subtypes of AMPA or NMDA receptors arises because of their tetrameric subunit composition (see Chapter 7). AMPA and NMDA receptors are non-selective cation channels whose ion permeabilities depend upon the given composition of receptor subunits. Both receptors are thought to be tetrameric combinations a) GluR1,2,3,4 subunits for AMPARs and for NMDARs, two of 11 splice variants of NR1 combined with one NR2B or NR2A (or NR3A or B) or pairs of NR2A or 2B subunits. The relative high Ca^{2+} permeability of NMDA receptors, as well as a subpopulation of GluR2 lacking AMPA receptors, endows a much greater intracellular signaling role for NMDA versus AMPA receptors. Subsynaptically, high densities AMPA and NMDA receptors are found immediately beneath the glutamate release sites by virtue of their anchoring, through protein-protein interactions, to proteins of the postsynaptic density (PSD). The postsynaptic density is a highly diverse protein signaling complex which includes many scaffolding proteins, signaling enzymes, as well as interacting protein bridges or links to the cytoskeleton and endoplasmic reticulum (and intracellular Ca^{2+} stores). Somewhat more peripheral, or perisynaptic to the immediate post and subsynaptic region, are metabotropic receptors for glutamate (mGluRs). These are heptahelical or G-protein

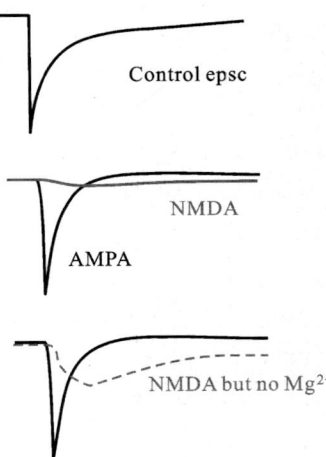

Fig.4.1 Epscs consist of a large, rapid AMPAR and a smaller, slower NMDAR component. A voltage-dependent block by Mg^{2+} greatly reduces the NMDA component at resting membrane potential.

coupled receptors (GPCRs). Coupling of these receptors is via, but is not restricted to G-proteins signaling, and these receptors provide mechanisms to target intracellular signal transduction pathways, calcium release machinery, as well as ionotropic glutamate receptors.

EXTRASYNAPTIC VERSUS SYNAPTIC RECEPTORS

It is assumed that primary signaling at excitatory synapses is mediated by PSD anchored glutamate receptors ("synaptic receptors") (Fig.4.2). However, it is clear that there are populations of ionotropic glutamate receptors that exist well beyond the physical restrictions provided by the PSD, and that synaptically released glutamate can "spill-over" to activate these receptors. The definition of "extrasynaptic" receptors on central neurons has always been some what nebulous. One reasonable definition would be that non-PSD anchored receptor proteins can be defined as "extrasynaptic" glutamate receptors. Such a definition is not meant to imply that extracellular receptors are devoid of protein-protein interactions with potential intracellular scaffolding proteins. Indeed, extrasynaptic receptors may have their own compliment of connected signaling proteins much in the way integrin and other adhesion receptors form seeding structures for intracellular protein signaling complexes. The large carboxy-terminals of NMDARs suggest that this is a very likely scenario. Another possibility is that extrasynaptic NMDA receptors, with their very high affinity for glutamate, could be tonically activated by ambient concentrations of glutamate (and glycine or D-serine required co-agonists for these receptors). By analogy tonically activated $GABA_A$ receptors, of specific subunit composition, appear to play important functional roles in the modulation of neuronal activity in the central nervous system.

Evidence suggests that the anchored synaptic pool of receptors can be supplemented by receptors entering from the extrasynaptic pool perhaps by through intramembrane transport mechanisms such as that provided by lipid rafts. Therefore, there is reason to believe that synaptic and extrasynaptic receptor pools are dynamically related. Of perhaps even greater importance has been the dramatic increase in our understanding of the trafficking of glutamate receptors from intracellular pools into synaptic pools. This trafficking reflects subunit specific mechanisms of receptor insertion and endocytosis as well regulation of receptor protein synthesis and degradation (see Chapter 8). One should note the striking discovery that the internalization of NMDA receptors is governed by the binding of the receptors co-agonist glycine. This finding by provides a clear tie between co-agonist regulation and functional modulation of NMDARs in central neurons.

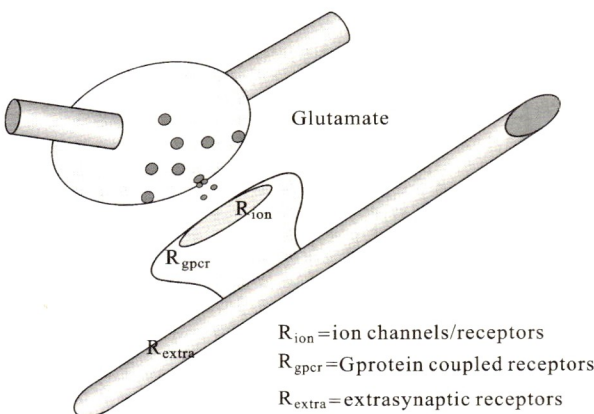

Fig.4.2 Synaptic receptors associate with the PSD in the spine whilst extrasynaptic receptors form a separate domain. NMDARs likely form the bulk of extrasynaptic receptors as they have a much higher affinity for glutamate than do AMPARs.

LOCAL CROSS-TALK BETWEEN RECEPTORS

A key difference between AMPARs and NMDARs is the permeability of the later for Ca^{2+}; and, the remarkable repertoire of regulatory mechanisms associated with modulation of NMDAR activity. The requirement of a glycine or D-serine co-agonist in order for functional gating of these channels is still, in many ways perplexing. Why require binding of two different molecules in order to achieve gating? The simply answer would seem to be that by regulating extracellular concentrations of these two amino acids it is possible to modulate the gain of NMDAR transmission at synapses. Although an equally valid alternative is that the co-agonists may be employed to change the gain of tonic currents associated with activation of extracellular NMDARs. The Salter's group demonstration that NMDAR internalization is tied to the binding of the co-agonist immediately suggests

that glycine and D-serine are not only permissive to gating but are also tied to the surface expression of receptors. Increases in extracellular co-agonists would potentially act as a positive feedback to enhance the activity of NMDARs. This would act in concert with the well characterized positive feedback on NMDAR receptors provided by membrane depolarization and the relief of Mg^{2+} channel blockade.

BOX 4.1

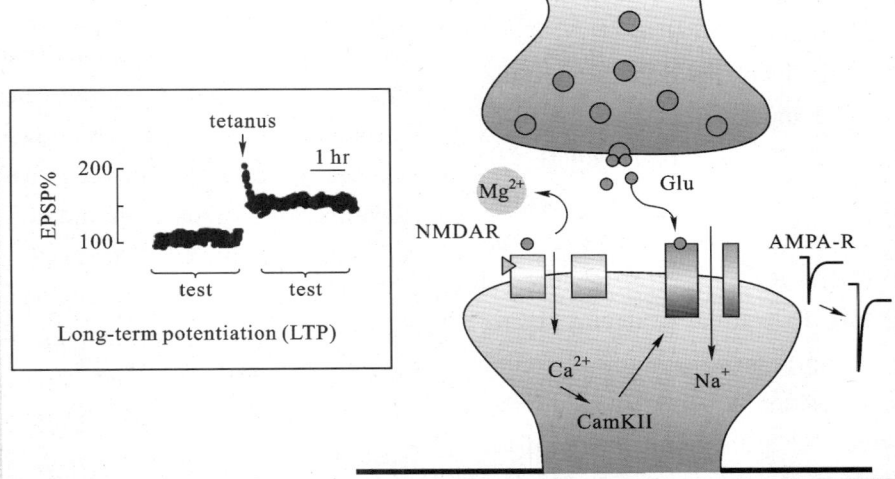

At CA1 synapses in the hippocampus afferent excitatory synapses evoke epsps in postsynaptic CA1 neurons. These epsps are primarily mediated by AMPARs. If a strong or tetanic stimulation is imposed, epsps are subsequently enhanced for periods lasting many hours (Long-term potentiation). At these synapses entry of Ca^{2+} through NMDARs is required to induce LTP; although, once it is activated NMDARs are no longer required to maintain LTP. The strong stimulation causes enough depolarization that the voltage-dependent block of NMDARs by extracellular Mg^{2+} is relieved allowing Ca^{2+} and Na^+ influx and further depolarizing the cell to cause even more relief of the Mg^{2+} block. Therefore, this positive

feedback between depolarization and the relief of the Mg^{2+} block sets off a strong activation of NMDARs postsynaptically and provides the Ca^{2+} entry signal responsible for setting off the events responsible for inducing LTP. One of these events is the activation of CaMKII which leads to an enhancement of AMPAR activity and also facilitates the incorporation of additional AMPARs into the synapses helping to contribute to he potentiation of LTP. The relief of the Mg^{2+} block is not the only means of amplifying the NMDAR Ca^{2+} signal (see Fig.4.3). Longer lasting components of LTP require changes in gene expression, new proteins and remodeling of synaptic spines.

This positive feed back provided by the voltage-dependent blockade by extracellular Mg^{2+} is often sited as providing the amplification required at many synapses to induce the NMDAR-mediated Ca^{2+} influx

required for the induction of LTP. However, there are additional biochemical components of the positive feedback responsible for NMDAR-dependent LTP.

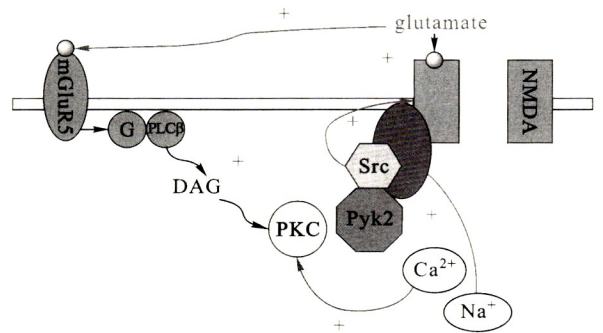

Fig.4.3 Biochemical positive feedback pathways act to amplify NMDAR activity during strong stimulation such as during induction of LTP.

These include a Na^+-dependent activation of the tyrosine kinase, Src, resulting in enhanced NMDAR activity and indirect Src and/or Fyn activation resulting from Ca^{2+} influx through NMDARs as well as activation of mGluRs, PKC and Pyk2 (Fig.4.3). The potential cross talk between glutamate receptors themselves is also substantial. In some cases the influx of Ca^{2+} via NMDARs alters the function of mGluRs and AMPARs. Indeed the structural organization of the PSD complex has the serine/threonine kinase, CaMKII, in a position of being bound directly to the NMDAR. Presumably, the combination of the high concentration of Ca^{2+} in the internal microdomain of the channel and the physical proximity of the kinase provides an ideal mechanism for localized biochemical signaling which then leads to phosphorylation of AMPAR subunits and increases in AMPAR expression in the synapses. Also, activation of mGluRs will modulate NMDARs via signal transduction pathways which require PKC and the release of intracellular Ca^{2+}. Therefore, glutamate receptors, as a part of the PSD signaling complex, play a major role in modulating and regulating their own activity and expression.

There are also several fundamental questions that have not yet been adequately addressed. Could the coupling of receptors to scaffolding proteins have functional consequences as a result of the physical properties of protein-protein interactions? For example, NMDARs are coupled via α-actinin2 to actin in the dendritic spines and this interaction is regulated by Ca^{2+} influx via the channels. Given that NMDAR activity is altered by membrane stretch one can question whether or not mechanical changes in the tension provided by alterations in such protein interactions might be a mechanism of modulating NMDAR channel activity. Indeed, NMDAR activity is under the influence of myosin light chain kinase acting by a mechanism involving actin-myosin interactions and requiring an intact cytoskeleton.

With the understanding that there are so many excitatory glutamatergic pathways it would seem reasonable to anticipate that some or many of the "long transmitter systems" would themselves target excitatory transmission. In spite of the many studies that show "long transmitter" systems modulate glutamate receptors surprisingly little is known about the topographical relationships between these and glutamate receptors. Very fundamental questions have yet to be definitively answered. The large pyramidal hippocampal neurons of the CA1 region serve as an example of this lack of understanding. Cholinergic pathways are believed to impinge upon these neurons, and muscarinic AChRs (also GPCRs) when activated, cause a marked enhancement of NMDAR activity. Are the muscarinic receptors located in the subsynaptic region of the excitatory synapse? If so, does this mean that presynaptic cholinergic synapses co-localize to single dendritic spines? This seems unlikely so perhaps the presynaptic cholinergic synapses (perhaps of an enpassant type synapse) are located somewhere else such as at non-spine locations? Are the muscarinic receptors bound directly to NMDARs? Are the muscarinic receptors within the excitatory PSD complex or are the muscarinic receptors located in a region essentially "extrasynaptic" with respect to glutamate receptors? Theoretically answering these simple questions should be rather straight forward. Employing immuno-histochemical approaches in concert with a highly selective labeled antibody it should be a simple matter to physically locate the position of muscarinic receptors in relationship to glutamate receptors. To some extent this has been accomplished with the suggestion that these receptors are found in the puncta associated with glutamate receptors and dendritic spines. Nevertheless, this evidence still falls far short of demonstrating the co-localization or lack thereof, of muscarinic and glutamate receptors within the PSD. Having receptors for two entirely different transmitters located at the same synapse presents some conceptual challenges. By definition a synapse has usually been considered to be a specialization to accommodate the release of a given presynaptic transmitter or co-transmitter. Recent evidence reviewed subsequently (see Part Ⅱ, Chapter 11) points out that direct binding between different types of receptors proteins not only occurs but that such protein-protein interactions can modify the functional properties of either partner receptor. Whether or not these direct inter-receptor interactions actually occur in synapses and include glutamate receptors has yet to be firmly established. For that matter this kind of heterologous receptor interaction could be occurring with extrasynaptic glutamate receptors.

Considering that "long" transmitters have both ionotropic and metabotropic receptors (GPCRs) one might anticipate that their ionotropic receptors will also be found in higher density within postsynaptic specializations associated with release sites for the "long" transmitter. However, if the release of the "long" transmitter results in a significant and generalized diffusion away from its release sites then its receptors might be located just about anywhere on the postsynaptic cell. Of course the 2nd messenger and signal transduction systems activated by these receptors need not be in close proximity to glutamate receptors and the PSD complex. Indeed, these signaling cascades could be some distance from the synaptic spine. Ultimately the signaling cascades employed by one receptor to alter another receptor may be extensive and complex.

REMOTE CROSS-TALK BETWEEN RECEPTORS

The more conventional view of synaptic transmission would state that synapses for different transmitters are topographically organized on the postsynaptic cell (Fig.4.4). For example, excitatory glutamatergic synapses are usually dendritic and inhibitory GABAergic synapses are most often located on the soma. There may actually be a considerable degree of physical overlap of synaptic domains on central neurons. Nevertheless, it seems reasonable to suppose that glutamatergic synapses are located some distance from those for "long" transmitters. This brings up the question as to how remotely located transmitter synapses of the same cell can communicate with each other? Many "long" transmitter receptors are GPCRs that could communicate to excitatory synapses via second messengers etc. However, we have identified a highly unique mechanism whereby "long" transmitter systems can communicate with excitatory glutamatergic synapses. In addition to transmitter receptors there are many other kinds of plasma membrane receptors on neurons. Receptors and ligands for cell adhesion complexes and growth factor receptors are prime examples. These receptors can themselves form the functional scaffolding of distinct intracellular signaling complexes. Signaling by such complexes often regulates the development, differentiation and proliferation of neurons and their pre-cursor cells. Much of the information about these signaling systems comes from cancer research where both GPCRs and growth factor receptors have been implicated very strongly in oncogensis. In adulthood at least some of these signaling complexes are presumably critical for maintenance of neurons, but there is evidence that some may also be important for synaptic plasticity and the re-modeling of synaptic structures.

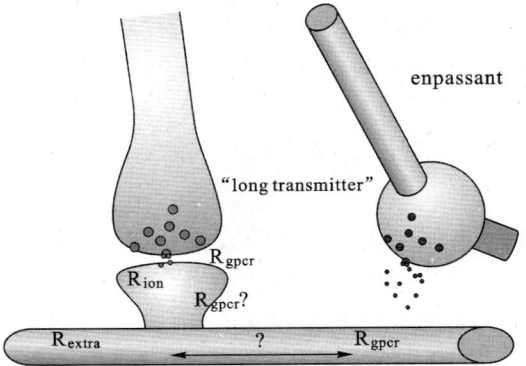

Fig.4.4   How can remotely located receptors for a "long" transmitter communicate with glutamate receptors?

TRANSACTIVATION: SIGNALING BETWEEN TRANSMITTER SYSTEMS

We have recently found that at least one growth factor receptor can serve as a pivotal "signal and integration relay" for communication between a major "long transmitter" (dopaminergic) and regulation of excitatory glutamatergic transmission in the hippocampus. The origin of our hypothesis comes directly from cancer research and studies of GPCRs and growth factors in model cell lines. For some time it has been known that genes for GPCRs can be oncogenic and lead to uncontrolled proliferation and cell growth. Surprisingly it was appreciated that the primary means of oncogensis for these receptors is "piggy- backed" upon growth factor receptor tyrosine kinases such as the epithelial growth factor and platelet-derived growth factor (PDGF) receptors. When activated by their cognate ligands, receptor dimerization ensues leading to autophosphorylation at a series of tyrosine residues thus presenting a series of SH2 binding domains for interacting target signaling proteins. These receptors function to regulate growth, differentiation, and proliferation of many cell types but they are well known to be oncogenic themselves. A variety of GPCRs can "transactivate" (not to be confused with transactivation of genes) one or more of these growth factors through mechanisms that are not entirely understood. In brief "transactivation" refers to the capacity of a GPCR to activate a growth factor receptor in the apparent absence of the growth factor ligand. There are a variety of potential mechanisms to account for "transactivation" ranging from direct interactions between G-protein subunits and the growth factor receptor to GPCR activation of Src which then stimulates dimerization, to a GPCR activation of an ectoplasmic metalloproteinase which cleaves a precursor growth factor ligand to release the endogenous ligand itself. Much further work will have to be done to understand how GPCRs transactivate growth factor receptors and to determine if there is one common or a variety of specific mechanisms employed for particular receptor interactions.

Some time ago, we examined the hypothesis that the Platelet-derived Growth Factor Receptor (PDGFR) in hippocampal neurons have a role to play in regulating excitatory synaptic transmission. PDGFRs are dimers which form multiple receptor subtypes of which the PDGFα and PDGFRβ are the best studied in the central nervous system. PDGF is perhaps misnamed because its receptors and its ligands are also wide spread through out the central nervous system. For example, the PDGFβ receptor is highly expressed in CA1 pyramidal neurons as are the ligands PDGFAA and PDGFBB.

Applications of PDGFBB to both cultured and isolated hippocampal neurons causes a long-lasting depression of NMDAR mediated currents (Fig.4.5) and NMDAR mediated synaptic transmission at CA1 synapses. The PDGFR actions on NMDARs required

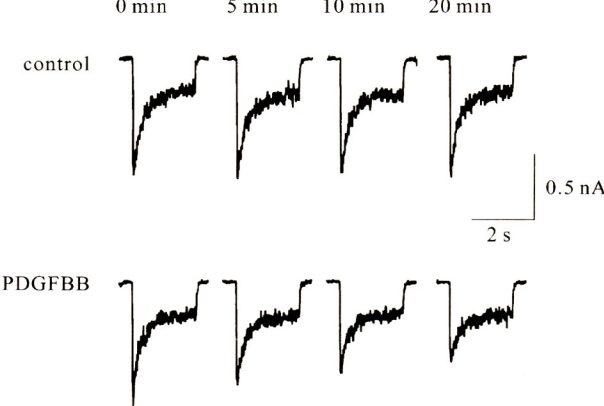

Fig.4.5 Applications of PDGFBB inhibit peak currents evoked by repeated applications of NMDA in a hippocampal neuron.

tyrosine phosphorylation of Y1021 (Fig.4.6), stimulation of phospholipase Cγ, a rise in intracellular Ca^{2+} and a Ca^{2+}/calmodulin-dependent inhibition of NMDAR activity. In preliminary experiments with applications of quinpirole, a D2 dopamine receptor agonist, we observed a remarkably similar long-lasting depression of NMDARs (Fig.4.7). We then made a conceptual jump to the hypothesis that dopamine receptors of the D2 class might be "transactivating" the PDGFR leading to down regulation of NMDAR channels in CA1 hippocampal neurons. Indeed, the long-lasting inhibition of NMDARs as a result of D4 receptor (a member of the D2 class) stimulation was blocked by relatively selective inhibitors of auto-phosphorylation of the PDGFR (Fig.4.8) as well as by inhibitors of PLCγ, inhibitors of intracellular Ca^{2+} release and by strong intracellular buffering of Ca^{2+}. Furthermore, we could demonstrate that D4 receptor activation leads to autophosphorylation of the PDGFR which is indicative of transactivation of this receptor. Transactivation also led to stimulation of other important signaling pathways in these neurons including the mitogen activated protein kinase or MAPK pathway. Our results are of some conceptual interest because they provide a highly novel mechanism whereby a "long" transmitter can signal to excitatory synapses simply by "piggy-backing" upon the presence of a growth factor receptors signaling complex.

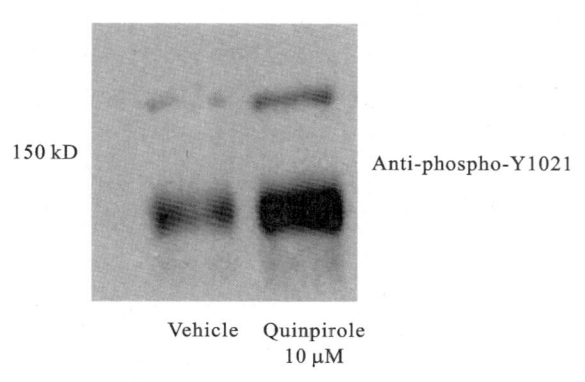

Fig.4.6 Western blot probed with a phosphosite specific antibody for tyrosine phosphorylation of residue 1021 on the PDGFR. Phosphorylation of this site is indicative of transactivation of the receptor and formation of a stimulatory site for PLCγ.

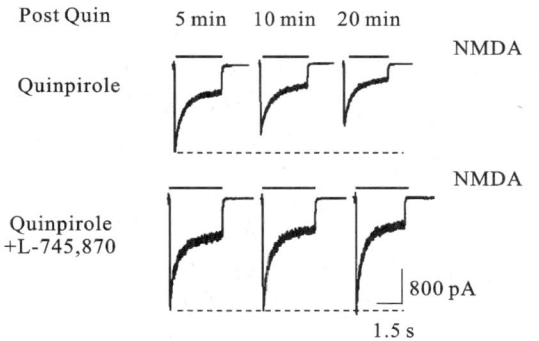

Fig.4.7 Quinpirole applications also cause a long-lasting inhibition of peak NMDA currents. A selective D4 antagonist, L-745,870, blocked this inhibition.

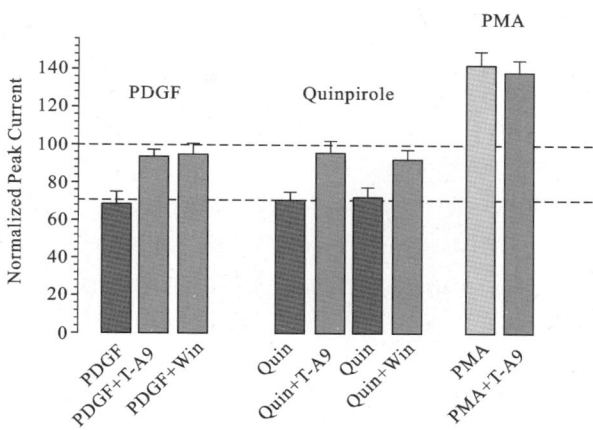

Fig.4.8 Summary data shows that the inhibition of peak currents by PDGFBB and quinpirole is blocked by two different PDGFR inhibitors (TA-9 and Win). These inhibitors did not change the enhancement of peak currents induced by applications of a PKC stimulator PMA.

Although we still do not have a clear picture of the direct physical relationship between D4, PDGF and NMDA receptors transactivation is appealing because there is no intrinsic requirement that the receptors be in close proximity to one another (Fig.4.9). It presents an ideal way for GPCRs and growth factor receptors to both target the genes responsible for re-modeling synapses and couple these signals with critical NMDARs located in the synapses.

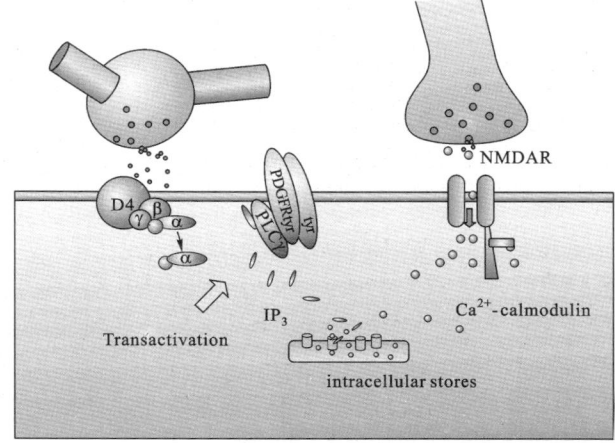

Fig.4.9 D4 receptor stimulation transactivates the PDGFR causing autophosphorylation at Y1021 of this receptor. Y1021 forms an SH2 binding site leading to PLCγ activation, the production of IP3 (inositol triphosphate), the release of intracellular Ca^{2+} and a Ca^{2+}-calmodulin-dependent inhibition of NMDA currents in CA1 hippocampal neurons.

GENERAL CITATIONS

Ali DW, Salter MW. 2001. NMDA receptor regulation by Src kinase signalling in excitatory synaptic transmission and plasticity. *Curr Opin Neurobiol*, 11: 336-342.

Kotecha SA, MacDonald JF. 2003. Signalling molecules and receptor transduction cascades that regulate NMDA receptor-mediated synaptic transmission. *Int Rev Neurobiol*, 54: 51-106.

Lisman J, Schulman H, Cline H. 2002. The molecular basis of CaMKII function in synaptic and behavioural memory. *Nat Rev Neurosci*, 3: 175-190.

Shah BH, Catt KJ. 2004. GPCR-mediated transactivation of RTKs in the CNS: mechanisms and consequences. *Trends Neurosci*, 27: 48-53.

Xia S, Miyashita T, Fu TF, Lin WY, Wu CL, Pyzocha L, et al. 2005. NMDA receptors mediate olfactory learning and memory in *Drosophila*. *Curr Biol*, 15: 603-615.

DISCOVERY CITATIONS

Bai D, Zhu G, Pennefather P, Jackson MF, MacDonald JF, Orser BA. 2001. Distinct functional and pharmacological properties of tonic and quantal inhibitory postsynaptic currents mediated by gamma-aminobutyric acid(A) receptors in hippocampal neurons. *Mol Pharmacol*, 59: 814-824.

Bayer KU, de Koninck P, Leonard AS, Hell JW, Schulman H. 2001. Interaction with the NMDA receptor locks CaMKII in an active conformation. *Nature*, 411: 801-805.

Hering H, Lin CC, Sheng M. 2003. Lipid rafts in the maintenance of synapses, dendritic spines, and surface AMPA receptor stability. *J Neurosci*, 23: 3262-3271.

Huang Y, Lu W, Ali DW, Pelkey KA, Pitcher GM, Lu YM, et al. 2001. CAKbeta/Pyk2 kinase is a signaling link for induction of long-term potentiation in CA1 hippocampus. *Neuron*, 29: 485-496.

Kotecha SA, Jackson MF, Al-Mahrouki A, Roder JC, Orser BA, MacDonald JF. 2003. Co-stimulation of mGluR5 and N-methyl-D-aspartate receptors is required for potentiation of excitatory synaptic transmission in hippocampal neurons. *J Biol Chem*, 278: 27742-27749.

Kotecha SA, Oak JN, Jackson MF, Perez Y, Orser BA, van Tol HH, et al. 2002. A D2 class dopamine receptor transactivates a receptor tyrosine kinase to inhibit NMDA receptor transmission. *Neuron*, 35: 1111-1122.

Kullmann DM. 2000. Spillover and synaptic cross talk mediated by glutamate and GABA in the mammalian brain. *Prog Brain Res*, 125: 339-351.

Lee FJ, Xue S, Pei L, Vukusic B, Chery N, Wang Y, et al. 2002. Dual regulation of NMDA receptor functions by direct protein-protein interactions with the dopamine D1 receptor. *Cell*, 111: 219-230.

Lei S, Czerwinska E, Czerwinski W, Walsh MP, MacDonald JF. 2001. Regulation of NMDA receptor activity by F-actin and myosin light chain kinase. *J Neurosci*, 21: 8464-8472.

Lu W, Man H, Ju W, Trimble WS, MacDonald JF, Wang YT. 2001. Activation of synaptic NMDA receptors induces membrane insertion of new AMPA receptors and LTP in cultured hippocampal neurons. *Neuron*, 29: 243-254.

Man HY, Lin JW, Ju WH, Ahmadian G, Liu L, Becker LE, et al. 2000. Regulation of AMPA receptor-mediated synaptic transmission by clathrin-dependent receptor internalization. *Neuron*, 25: 649-662.

Nong Y, Huang YQ, Ju W, Kalia LV, Ahmadian G, Wang YT, et al. 2003. Glycine binding primes NMDA receptor internalization. *Nature*, 422: 302-307.

Oak JN, Lavine N, van Tol HH. 2001. Dopamine D(4) and D(2L) Receptor stimulation of the mitogen-activated protein kinase pathway is dependent on trans-activation of the platelet-derived growth factor receptor. *Mol Pharmacol*, 60: 92-103.

Paoletti P, Ascher P. 1994. Mechanosensitivity of NMDA receptors in cultured mouse central neurons. *Neuron*, 13: 645-655.

Strutz-Seebohm N, Werner M, Madsen DM, Seebohm G, Zheng Y, Walker CS, et al. 2003. Functional analysis of *Caenorhabditis elegans* glutamate receptor subunits by domain transplantation. *J Biol Chem*, 278: 44691-44701.

Kainate Receptors

CHAPTER 5

Christophe Mulle

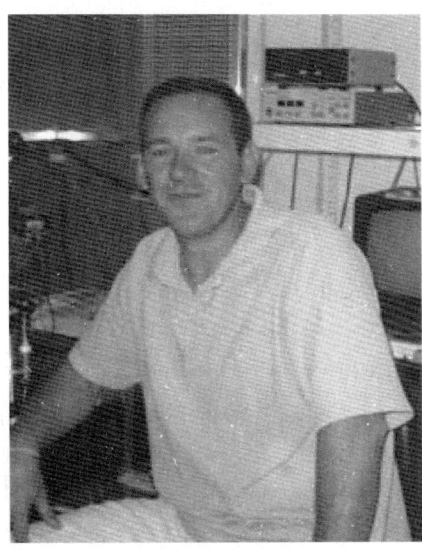

Dr. Mulle is a Professor and Director in the Department of "Physiologie Cellulaire de la Synapse", Université Victor Segalen Bordeaux 2, Bordeaux, France. He attended Université Laval, Québec, followed by the Institut Pasteur and The Salk Institute, San Diego.

MAJOR CONTRIBUTIONS

1. Mulle C, Sailer A, Perez-Otano I, Dickinson-Anson H, Castillo PE, Bureau I, Maron C, Gage FH, Mann JR, Bettler B, Heinemann SF. 1998. Altered synaptic physiology and reduced susceptibility to kainate-induced seizures in GluR6-deficient mice. *Nature*, 392: 601-605.

2. Bureau I, Dieudonne S, Coussen F, Mulle C. 2000. Kainate receptor-mediated synaptic currents in cerebellar Golgi cells are not shaped by diffusion of glutamate. *Proc Natl Acad Sci USA*, 97: 6838-6843.

3. Mulle C, Sailer A, Swanson GT, Brana C, O'Gorman S, Bettler B, Heinemann SF. 2000. Subunit composition of kainate receptors in hippocampal interneurons. *Neuron*, 28:475-484.

4. Jaskolski F, Coussen F, Nagarajan N, Normand E, Rosenmund C, Mulle C. 2004. Subunit composition and alternative splicing regulate membrane delivery of kainate receptors. *J Neurosci*, 24: 2506-2515.

5. Coussen F, Perrais D, Jaskolski F, Sachidhanandham S, Bockaert J, Marin P, Mulle C. 2006. Coassembly of two GluR6 kainate receptor splice variants within a functional protein complex. *Neuron*. (in press)

MAIN TOPICS

Kainate receptor subunits: functional properties of recombinant receptors

Postsynaptic kainate receptors : temporal integration of excitatory signals

Presynaptic kainate receptors : role in synaptic plasticity

A metabotropic function for kainate receptors

Subcellular localization and intracellular trafficking of kainate receptors

Kainate receptors during development

Kainate receptors in synaptic pathology

SUMMARY

Kainate receptors are ionotropic glutamate receptors composed of various combinations of five subunits GluR5, GluR6, GluR7, KA1 and KA2. Kainate receptors form cationic ion channels that can flux Ca^{2+} depending on mRNA editing of a glutamine in the channel pore region. Classical glutamate receptor ligands show poor selectivity for kainate receptors over AMPA receptors, although specific antagonists directed against GluR5 containing-receptors have recently been developped, and should prove very useful for the study of kainate receptor function in synaptic physiology and pathology. At variance with AMPA and NMDA receptors which mainly operate at post-synaptic site and are the key agents of fast glutamatergic synaptic transmission, kainate receptors play a variety of functions by acting at presynaptic, postsynaptic and extrasynaptic sites. At postsynaptic sites, kainate receptors are implicated in synaptic currents of small amplitude and slow decay kinetics that display prominent summation properties in response to repetitive stimualtions. Presynaptic kainate receptors regulate the release of GABA and glutamate at many different synapses. In doing so, they can facilitate presynaptic forms of short and long term synaptic plasticity. Finally, kainate receptors regulate neuronal excitability by inhibition of Ca^{2+}-dependent K^+ channels. While kainate receptors act by the opening of a cation channels, some of the functions of kainate receptors involve a metabotropic action through the coupling to a G-protein, independent of an ionotropic action. The molecular link between kainate receptors and G-protein coupling is not yet identified. The different functions of kainate receptors result from the activation of receptors located in a variety of neuronal subdomains. This raises the question of the polarized trafficking of kainate receptors to pre- and postsynaptic sites, and their stabilization in specific functional domains. Trafficking of kainate receptors to the plasma membrane greatly depends on kainate receptors subunits and splice variants. Splice variants mainly differ in their cytoplasmic C-ter domain, which binds scaffolding proteins of the post-synaptic density as well as adhesion proteins. Kainate receptors are expressed early during development and appear to play a role in the construction of synaptic networks. Finally, kainate receptors are likely involved in many neurological disorders, including neurodegenrative diseases such as epilepsy and stroke, and in inflammatory pain. Because of their role as regulators of the maturation and function of synaptic circuits, kainate receptors appear as very promising therapeutic targets.

KAINATE RECEPTOR SUBUNITS: FUNCTIONAL PROPERTIES OF RECOMBINANT RECEPTORS

Kainate receptors were identified as a novel family of glutamate receptors, following the cloning of five subunits by cDNA sequence homology with AMPA receptor subunits. These five subunits named GluR5, GluR6, GluR7, KA1 and KA2 are the product of five separate genes (grik1 to grik5). Each subunit is a transmembrane protein with a membrane topology similar to that of AMPA and NMDA receptor subunits. The N-terminal domain is extracellular and is followed by a series of 4 successive membrane domains (M1 to M4). M1, M3 and M4 are transmembrane domains, whereas M2 makes a short hair-pin like segment that dips into the lipid bilayer, and is crucial for the ion permeation activity of kainate receptors. The C-terminal domain is cytoplasmic, it shows a large variability between subunits and splice varants and interacts with a variety of cytoplasmic proteins important for receptor trafficking and transduction mechanisms. Glutamate, the most likely endogenous agonist of kainate receptors, binds within a pocket formed by two apposed segments in the N-terminal domain and in the extracellular loop between M3 and M4. Variations in the amino acid sequence of the glutamate binding domain account for differences in the pharmacological profile of kainate receptor subtypes. Crystal structures of the GluR5 and GluR6 kainate receptor ligand binding cores in complex with various agonists has now been solved. This has therapeutic potential in that it should help to design subtype-selective ligands and allosteric modulators.

Many of the properties of kainate receptors have been described in studies where recombinant subunits were expressed in heterologous cells in culture (such as HEK293 cells). GluR5, GluR6 and GluR7 are capable of forming functional cationic channels gated by glutamate, when expressed as homomers. In contrast, expression of KA1 and KA2 subunits does not yield homomeric channels but these subunits form high affinity binding sites for kainate in the range 5–15 nM. Co-expression studies followed by either electrophysiological or biochemical experiments have demonstrated the formation of many different combinations of heteromeric kainate receptors. GluR6/KA2 and GluR5/GluR6 kainate receptors probably compose at least part of the native kainate recetors. Co-assembly can change both the pharmacological and biophysical properties of kainate receptors. Recombinant kainate receptor channels are gated by glutamate, and by several natural or synthetic ligands, such as kainate or domoate. AMPA is not an agonist of GluR6 but can gate GluR5 or the heteromeric GluR6/KA2 kainate receptor. For understanding the pathophysioloigcal function of kainate receptors, it is important to stress that glutamate, the endogenous agonist, binds kainate receptors with an affinity in the 100 µM range, similar to that of AMPA receptors. It is yet not excluded that certain subtypes of native kainate receptors might bind the endogenous agonist with a very different affinity. The development of specific pharmacological tools should be instrumental to better define the function of kainate receptors in the physiology and pathology of brain functions. Specific agonists (ATPA) and antagonists for the GluR5 subunit (LY 382884, UBP 302) have been produced. It has however proven difficult to develop ligands for the other subunits, like the GluR6 subunit, even though it is probably a major player in synaptic functions attributed to kainate receptors. Crystal structure studies have in fact revealed that the agonist binding pocket of GluR6 is relatively small as compared to GluR5, and thus might not be able to accomodate ligands with a high affinity for the ligand binding site. AMPA and kainate receptors have been difficult to distinguish from each other with pharmacological agents, since many non-NMDA receptor antagonists such asCNQX, act on both types of receptors. To reveal kainate receptor function, the most widely used compound is GYKI 53655, a selective non competitive antagonist of AMPA receptors.

The GluR5 and GluR6 subunits, but not the other subunits, can undergo mRNA editing that changes an amino acid (from a glutamine to an arginine residue, thus dubbed the Q/R site) in the channel pore region, leading to changes in permeation properties. Editing of the Q/R site determines single channel conductance and calcium permeability, and transforms the rectification properties (I/V curve) of the channels from inward rectification to linear or slight outward rectification. Unlike the AMPA receptor subunit GluR2, which is fully edited in the brain, the extent of edition of GluR5 and GluR6, thus calcium permeability, can vary depending on neuronal populations or stages of neuronal development. Alternative splice variants of GluR5, GluR6 and GluR7 subunits also exist in the brain. These receptor proteins display distinct cytoplasmic C-terminal domains, they differ in their membrane trafficking properties and bind distinct subsets of interacting proteins (see below), but do not differ in their functional properties.

The composition of native kainate receptors is yet largely unknown. Kainate receptors are expressed widely throughout the nervous system, as indicated by in situ hybridization studies of mRNAs. The pattern of mRNA distribution supports the notion that native kainate receptors are heterogenous and that most combinations of the five kainate receptor subunits are possible in heteromeric receptors. The use of subunit-specific antibodies confirms that GluR6 can assemble with KA1 and KA2. In addition, electrophysiological comparisons of wild-type and knock-out mice for the GluR5, GluR6 and KA2 subunits indicate that GluR5/GluR6 and GluR6/KA2 assemblies exist in the brain. To date, much remains to be done to understand how the molecular composition of native kainate receptors relates to a specific fucntion or subcellular localization of kainate receptors.

POSTSYNAPTIC KAINATE RECEPTORS: TEMPORAL INTEGRATION OF EXCITATORY SIGNALS

Finding a physiological function for kainate receptors in the brain has long been hampered by the lack of pharmacological tools selective for these receptors. The use GYKI 53655 that antagonizes AMPA but not kainate receptors was of great help in this regard. Because kainate receptors are closely related to AMPA receptors, the key receptors in glutamatergic synaptic transmission, it was first assumed that these receptors could play a similar role. As shown in the next three paragraphs, the function of kainate receptors is more complex and varied. They do not play their major function by a fast depolarization of the postsynaptic membrane, but rather act as regulators of the activity of synaptic networks. At a post-synaptic level kainate receptors integrate synaptic activity and regulate neuronal excitability. At a presynaptic level, kainate receptors regulate the release of neurotransmitter, acting both as autoreceptors (release of glutamate) and heteroreceptors (release of GABA).

Functional kainate receptors can be activated exogenous agonists in most neuronal populations. It has taken much more time to find a physiological function for kainate receptors in synaptic transmission. The first evidence came from electrophysiological recordings in CA3 pyramidal cells of the hippocampus with stimulations elicited to release glutamate from mossy fibers. In these experiments, mossy fiber synaptic currents were almost completely abolished in presence of GYKI 53655. However, a small synaptic current with slow onset and decay kinetics was found to be mediated by kainate receptors. Additionally, these synaptic currents displayed prominent summation properties in response to repetitive stimulation, in a rate dependent manner, suggesting that KAR-EPSCs play a role in the temporal integration during repetitive synaptic stimulation. The reason for these unexpected properties is still unclear, but it was indicated that they were not due to an extrasynaptic localization of KARs. Mossy fibers contact CA3 pyramidal cells on proximal dendrites, within the stratum lucidum, whereas other glutamatergic afferents contact distal dendrites. Using puff application of kainate, the authors showed that functional kainate receptors were restricted to proximal dendrites, where mossy fibers make synaptic contacts with CA3 pyramidal cells.

Thus, at variance with AMPA receptors, postsynaptic kainate receptors are probably not present at all glutamatergic synapses in a given neuron. Another example of this selectivity is that of superficial dorsal horn neurons in the spinal cord, where kainate receptor-mediated EPSCs seem to be restricted to synapses formed by high-threshold nociceptive and thermoreceptive primary afferent fibers. In many cell types, it has not yet been possible to document synaptic currents mediated by kainate receptors, although selective agonists activate kainate receptor-mediated inward currents. This is the case in CA1 pyramidal neurons or in striatal medium spiny neurons. The existence of extrasynaptic kainate receptors, raises the question of the physiological conditions under which they can be activated by endogenous glutamate. Release of glutamate from nearby astrocytes was recently shown to be a nonsynaptic source of glutamate mediating activation of kainate receptors in hippocampal interneurons. Spillover of glutamate from neighbouring synapses during high frequency bursts of activity on presynaptic afferents is another potential source of glutamate to activate these receptors.

Nevertheless, the list of synapses where kainate receptors take part in excitatory synaptic current has built up over the last years: hippocampal and neocortical GABAergic interneurons and pyramidal cells, basolateral amygdala, spinal cord, cerebellar Purkinje cells and Golgi cells. At all these synapses, kainate receptor-mediated EPSCs display a relatively low amplitude as compared to the AMPA component, as well as slower onset kinetics. Related to their slower onset kinetics and smaller amplitude, it is possible that synaptic kainate receptors experience a lower occupancy by glutamate than AMPA receptors. This may result from a lower affinity for glutamate or from a location at some distance from glutamate release sites. However, the fact that glutamate transporter inhibition only results in limited changes on kainate receptor-mediated EPSCs indicate that kainate receptors contributing to these EPSCs might be present at perisynaptic sites rather than at a remote extrasynaptic location. The small amplitude of kainate receptor-mediated EPSCs suggest that these receptors are not essential for spike discharge following a single afferent stimulation. However, the slow time course of kainate receptor-mediated EPSCs, and possibly the non saturation of synaptic kainate receptors, allows prominent summation of EPSCs leading to temporal integration of synaptic inputs in conditions of repetitive afferent stimulations. An additional function for postsynaptic kainate receptors in the regulation of neuronal excitability by a non ionotropic action is now emerging. These findings will be discussed in paragraph 4.

PRESYNAPTIC KAINATE RECEPTORS: ROLE IN SYNAPTIC PLASTICITY

Activation of kainate receptors regulates transmitter release at many excitatory and inhibitory synapses. The use kainate and other kainate receptor agonists to activate presynaptic receptors has provided many examples for such a regulatory function. Many of these studies have initially focused on the hippocampus. The first evidence that presynaptic kainate receptors may modulate the release of glutamate came from pharmacological studies on synaptosomes. In hippocampal slices, bath application of kainate reduces the postsynaptic EPSC amplitude at synapses between Schaffer collaterals and CA1 pyramidal cells, decreases the presynaptic calcium signal and enhances paired pulse facilitation, indicating a presynaptic locus of regulation. Presynaptic kainate receptors also regulate the evoked release of GABA from inhibitory interneurons in the hippocampus. Evidence for a presynaptic regulatory function of presynaptic kainate receptors has then extended to several other brains regions including the cerebellum, the striatum, the nucleus accumbens, the amygdala and the spinal cord (reviewed in Chapter 7). Two important questions need to be resolved: (i) the physiological conditions under which these presynaptic kainate receptors are activated, and (ii) the mechanisms of action of presynaptic kainate receptor.

In comparison with the large number of studies in which kainate receptors were activated by exposure to exogenous agonists, there are few instances where glutamate released from endogenous sources was shown to act on presynaptic kainate receptors to modulate neurotransmitter release. The most studied example is the synapse between mossy fibers and CA3 pyramidal cells. At this synapse, nanomolar concentrations of kainate increase synaptic transmission whereas larger concentrations depress glutamate release. Under physiological conditions, glutamate released by mossy fibers act on kainate receptors (autoreceptors) to facilitate glutamate release. Kainate receptor stimulation leads to a frequency-dependent increase in the subsequent release of glutamate as indicated by the use of selective kainate receptor antagonists and mutant mice. A marked decrease in the extent of paired-pulse facilitation of mossy fiber EPSCs was observed for short time intervals (<40 ms) in GluR6$^{-/-}$ mice. By monitoring NMDA synaptic responses, the degree of high frequency facilitation (20-100 Hz) was decreased by the use of pharmacological agents that inhibit kainate receptors. The rapid action of synaptically released glutamate on subsequent EPSCs strongly suggests that kainate receptors are located close to synaptic release sites. The molecular composition of presynaptic kainate receptors at the mossy fiber synapse is still a matter of debate. Indeed, the GluR5 antagonist LY 283884, clearly depresses high frequency facilitation whereas no difference is observed between wild-type and GluR5$^{-/-}$ mice. Moreover, GluR5 mRNA is not detected in dentate granule cells that give rise to mossy fibers. Besides this fast acting regulation of glutamate release, presynaptic kainate receptors are also involved in other forms of presynaptic plasticity at this synapse. A characteristic feature of mossy fiber synaptic transmission is low frequency facilitation that develops with repetitive stimulation in the low frequency range (0.05 to 5 Hz), and that requires activation of CaMKII. Activation of kainate receptors does not induce but rather facilitates the extent of this form of short term synaptic plasticity, as indicated by the analysis of

GluR6$^{-/-}$ mice. Mossy fiber synapses also display a cAMP-dependent presynaptic form of long term synaptic potentiation that does not require activation of NMDA receptors, but depends on Ca^{2+} entry in the mossy fiber nerve terminal and subsequent activation of a Ca^{2+}-stimulated adenylyl cyclase AC8. Mossy fiber LTP is largely impaired in GluR6$^{-/-}$ mice but it can be rescued by increasing the excitability of mossy fibers or by strengthening the LTP induction protocol. The identity of presynaptic kainate receptors is there again a matter of debate, given the fact that LY 283884 and UBP 296, two GluR5 antagonists, antagonize mossy fiber LTP. Despite these uncertainties, it is well documented that activation of presynaptic kainate receptors plays a permissive role in short and long-term synaptic plasticity at the hippocampal mossy fiber synapse. Kainate receptors also contribute to different forms of long-term potentiation in the amygdala and in the auditory cortex, through GluR5 or GluR6 containing kainate receptors, but the mechanism have not yet been clearly examined.

What are the physiological conditions under which endogenous sources of glutamate can regulate GABAergic synaptic transmission through activation of kainate receptors? This was examined with much detail in paired recordings of hippocampal interneurons and CA1 pyramical cells. This work demonstrated that ambient glutamate released by basal activity, or stimulation of the stratum radiatum, facilitates GABAergic synapstic transmission by activating presynaptic kainate receptors. Astrocytes appear as another interesting potential source of glutamate that could contribute to the regulation of network activity. The facilitation of GABAergic synaptic transmission by endogenous glutamate contrasts with the inhibitory effects of exogenous application of kainate that was reported in most previous reports for this and other synapses. It is thus not clear if there are physiological conditions under which presynaptic kainate receptors can depress GABAergic synaptic transmission. One can speculate that this can happen under pathological conditions, such as stroke, which leads to a large glutamate overflow.

A METABOTROPIC FUNCTION FOR KAINATE RECEPTORS

In addition to ionotropic signaling involving kainate receptors, kainate and other agonists have been reported to show neuronal activities that are mediated by the coupling to G proteins. It was first reported that the mechanisms through which kainate receptors inhibit GABAergic synaptic transmission in the hippocampus was sensitive to pertussis toxin and to inhibitors of protein kinase C. These electrophysiological experiments were reinforced by biochemical experiments on hippocampal membranes demonstrating a coupling between kainate receptors and Gi/Go proteins. The possibility remains that these metabotropic type actions on GABAergic synaptic transmission involve, at least in part, an indirect mechanism, such as kainate-stimulated release of some endogenous compound which may then activate its own G-protein coupled receptor. Additional evidence for a metabotropic action of kainate receptors has recently been growing in experimental conditions where the independence of the effect observed on an ionic mechanism can be better controlled. For instance, in dorsal root ganglion neurons, exposure to kainate induces a G-protein dependent release of Ca^{2+} from internal stores, and inhibits K$^+$-induced Ca^{2+} increase. This effect is sensitive to pertussis toxin and to inhibitors of protein kinase C, and does not require ion permeation through the kainate receptor channel, although it depends on the presence of GluR5, which is an ion forming kainate receptor subunit. Finally, it has been shown that postsynaptic kainate receptors enhance CA1 pyramidal cell excitability by inhibiting the slow after hyperpolarization generated by a voltage-independent, Ca^{2+} dependent K$^+$ current (I$_{sAHP}$). This inhibition of I$_{sAHP}$ is prevented by inhibitors of G-protein dependent cascades, and is mimicked by a high frequency train of stimuli designed to activate Schaffer collaterals projecting onto CA1 pyramidal cells. Furthermore, a similar I$_{sAHP}$ mediated increase in CA3 pyramidal cell excitability was observed during bath application of KA. The modulation of I_{sAHP} by kainate exposure was lost in mice deficient for the GluR6 kainate receptor subunit. Thus evidence builds up that kainate receptors can operate in two distinct modes (i) by a well characterized ionotropic action and (ii) by an indirect regulation of ion channels through activation of G-proteins. The mechanisms underlying the metabotropic action of kainate receptors remain to be elucidated, as kainate receptors do not belong to the metabotropic glutamate receptor family, which comprises of 7TM receptors directly coupled to specific G-proteins. There is for yet no evidence that kainate receptors directly interact with G-proteins, and it is conceivable that the metabotropic action of kainate receptors necessitate a protein link (for instance a scaffolding protein) between the receptor to the G-protein.

SUBCELLULAR LOCALIZATION AND INTRACELLULAR TRAFFICKING OF KAINATE RECEPTORS

The control of cell-surface expression and delivery of glutamate receptors in defined functional domains has a key role in modifying the strength of excitatory synapses during synaptic plasticity and development. More generally, the function of glutamate receptors in neuronal networks is regulated by the identity and density of glutamate receptors in each functional domain.

The role of kainate receptors in synaptic transmission depends on their precise localization in pre-synaptic, postsynaptic and extrasynaptic domains. This has now been described in a large number of electrophysiological experiments. However, the paucity of specific kainate receptor antibodies suitable for immunogold labeling, has hampered studies designed at defining precisely the subcellular location of these receptors in various neuronal domains. A key question for cell biologists is that of the mechanisms of polarized trafficking of proteins either to axonal/ pre-synaptic compartments or dendritic/postsynaptic compartments. The simplest explanation would be

that kainate receptors with different subunit compositions would traffick to one or the other compartment. The analysis mutant mice deficient for GluR5, GluR6 and KA2 subunits have yet provided no clear indication of a link between subunit composition and polarized targeting of kainate receptors. At the mossy fiber synapse, it is nevertheless clear that pre- and post-synaptic kainate receptors have different pharmacological properties, thus likely different molecular composition.

The mechanisms that lead to differential insertion of kainate receptors in the plasma membrane have been characterized recently. These mechanisms depend on molecular determinants in the C-terminal domain of subunit splice variants, and on the heteromeric composition of kainate receptor. To decipher these mechanisms, experiments have used recombinant subunits fused to an epitope tag such as GFP which were transfected in cell lines or hippocampal neurons in culture. KA2 and GluR5c are not expressed at the plasma membrane as homomers. They have an RXR motif that mediates retention of several channels and receptors in the endoplasmic reticulum. This retention motif is masked through coassembly with other kainate receptor subunits. Disruption of these motifs results in exit from the ER and cell-surface expression. In contrast, GluR6a and GluR7a are highly expressed at the cell surface when assembled in homomeric channels. In addition, when assembled in heteromeric kainate receptors, GluR6a and GluR7a promote cell surface expression of subunits which are normally retained in the ER. This is ensured by a short forward trafficking signal in the C-terminal domain composed of a series of basic amino acid residues.

Kainate receptor and splice variants diverge at the cytoplasmic domain, opening the possibility that trafficking and subcellular localization of kainate receptors is regulated differentially by cytoplasmic proteins that interact with this region. For AMPA and NMDA receptors, these interactions are essential for the regulated trafficking and stabilization of receptors in postsynaptic compartments, especially during synaptic plasticity. Much less is known for kainate receptors, albeit a number of interacting proteins have now been characterized. As an example, proteins that contain a PDZ domain, such as PSD-95 interact with GluR6a and GluR5b, and might be important for targeting and stabilization of kainate receptors in the postsynaptic membrane. On the other hand, GluR6a also interacts *in vitro* and *in vivo* with cadherin-catenin adhesion complexes. Such an interaction might also be important in localizing kainate receptors at synapses during synapse formation, and perhaps more specifically, in perisynaptic domains.

KAINATE RECEPTORS DURING DEVELOPMENT

Several lines of evidence suggest a role for kainate receptors in neuronal development. Early reports detected kainate receptor subunit mRNAs in the brain at early developmental stages. In the rat by E14, high-affinity kainate sites are found throughout the grey matter, and are particularly abundant in the spinal cord and ventral forebrain structures. All genes undergo a surge of expression in the late embryonic/early postnatal period. In parallel, mRNA editing of GluR5 and GluR6 is developmentally regulated, suggesting that Ca^{2+} permeability may change during ontogeny. As an example, kainate receptors on DRG neurons from late embryonic and newborn rats are predominantly Ca^{2+} permeable but then become fully Ca^{2+} impermeable later during maturation. This switch in Ca^{2+} permeability matches the time course of RNA editing of the GluR5 subunit at the Q/R site. The GluR5 subunit is highly expressed around the period of birth in the somatosensory neocortex and in the thalamus. The time course of this GluR5 subunit expression is consistent with the period of greatest developmental plasticity in the somatosensory cortex. In the somatosensory cortex, developing thalamocortical synapses express postsynaptic kainate receptors as well as AMPA receptors, although the two types of receptors do not coexist at the same synapses. Moreover, during a critical period for experi-

ence-dependent plasticity, kainate receptor contribution to synaptic transmission decreases while AMPAR contribution increases, likely due to the loss of synaptic kainate receptors. Interestingly, at early postnatal stages, kainate synapses can be converted to AMPA synapses by a pairing stimulation designed to induce LTP. In addition, thalamocortical synaptic transmission is regulated by presynaptic kainate receptors at early developmental stages. Indeed, developing thalamocortical synapses exhibit short-term depression during high frequency trains (50-100 Hz), an effect blocked by the GluR5 antagonist LY 382884. GluR5 containing receptors present on thalamocortical axons are thus activated by synaptically released glutamate under conditions of brief intense activity. This regulation is absent after the first post-natal week, consistent with the large decrease in GluR5 mRNA expression in the adult thalamus. In the developing hippocampus, tonic activation of kainate receptors by endogenous glutamate strongly regulates both GABAergic and glutamatergic synaptic transmission. In doing so, kainate receptors control spontaneous network activity, which is a characteristic feature of immature neuronal networks thought to play an important role in the development of synaptic circuitry. Application of LY382884 results in a decrease in the frequency of network bursts, suggesting that endogenous activation of GluR5 subunit-containing kainate receptors is involved in burst initiation. The question remains as to the source glutamate and why this regulation disappears after the first post-natal week although kainate receptors are still expressed in the hippocampus. Finally, activation of kainate receptors regulates the motility of mossy fiber axonal filopodia in immature hippocampal slices. This regulation is likely to be physiological since synaptically released glutamate induced by electrical stimulation also causes bidirectional effects on filopodial motility at different developmental stages. From these data, the following two-step model for the role of kainate receptors in synaptogenesis has been proposed. At early stage-synaptic stimulation of kainate receptors enhances the motility of immature filopodia, thus facilitating filopodia to explore their environment and contact potential synaptic targets. At later stages, inhibition of the motility of filopodia which have contacted a target, facilitates the formation of mature synapses.

KAINATE RECEPTORS IN SYNAPTIC PATHOLOGY

Glutamate receptor activation is thought to be involved in neurologic disease due to their downstream effects on cell survival, genetic expression of axon guidance cues, synaptic connectivity/formation of networks, and neuronal excitability. Among glutamate receptors, kainate receptors are well known for their ability to cause excitotoxic cell death and to elicit seizures in animal models of temporal lobe epilepsy. Identification of therapeutic pharmacologic targets and development of kainate receptor antagonists remain central themes in epilepsy and stroke research.

Systemic or local administration of kainate to rodents has been widely used as a model of human temporal lobe epilepsy. Direct evidence for the involvement of kainate receptors in the generation of seizures comes from studies on kainate receptor knock-out mice. GluR6-deficient mice are less susceptible to seizures after kainate injection than wild-type mice. This is probably linked to the high expression level of kainate receptor in CA3 pyramidal cells that render this region particularly sensitive to the epileptogenic and neurotoxic effects of kainate. In keeping with these results, the lack of the GluR6 subunit prevents kainate-induced epileptiform bursts *in vitro*. In contrast the lack of GluR5, a subunit mainly expressed in GABAergic interneurons, renders hippocampal slices more sensitive to the epileptiform action of kainate. However these results apparently contradict pharmacological results obtained on epileptogenesis induced by the muscarinic agonist pilocarpine. Indeed, selective antagonists of GluR5 prevent epileptiform activity in the slice preparation and in the awake animal in the pilocarpine model. These apparently contradictory results likely reflect the fact that epilepsy results from a disbalance between excitation and inhibition that cause neocortical networks to switch from physioloigcal activity to epileptiform bursts. Further work will probably refine the conditions under which the usefulness of kainate receptor agonists and antagonists can be demonstrated.

Genetic studies are now starting to unravel possible links between kainate receptors and developmental disorders such as autism. The functional link between a polymorphism in GluR6 (and in some cases mutations in exonic regions) and these disease is not yet established. But, in view of growing evidence that kainate receptors play a crucial role in the development of synaptic circuitry, this subject is certainly worthwhile of future exploration. Two studies have also related a polymorphism in the GluR6 kainate receptor gene to the age of onset of Huntington's disease. Finally, kainate receptors have recently appeared as very promising targets in nociception. A full chapter will be devoted to the role of kainate receptors in nociception and inflammatory pain.

CONCLUSIONS AND FUTURE DIRECTIONS

Kainate receptors have thus emerged as glutamate receptors that can play a variety of functions in many different brain regions. In contrast to AMPA receptors, these receptors are clearly not absolutely required for fast excitatory synaptic transmission, but rather play a modulatory function in the regulation of synaptic networks. This regulation operates at presynaptic sites by the ability of kainate receptors to regulate in a bidirectional manner the release of neurotransmitters. This regulation also operates at a postsynaptic level, by integrating excitatory signals over time in response to repetitive stimulations, and by changing the level of neuronal excitability. Although many receptor subtypes likely exist in the brain, through various heteromeric combinations of subunits and splice variants, the link between these diverse subtypes and the specific functions of kainate receptors are not yet clear. These aspects clearly need further investigation, because it could help to identify targets for specific brain functions. Along these lines, much is expected from the development of specific pharmacological tools that might prove extremely useful in the treatment of several pathologies, including neurodegenerative disease and inflammatory pain.

GENERAL CITATIONS

Bortolotto ZA, Clarke VR, Delany CM, Parry MC, Smolders I, Vignes M, et al. 1999. Kainate receptors are involved in synaptic plasticity. *Nature*, 402: 297-301.

Collingridge GL, Isaac JT, Wang YT. 2004. Receptor trafficking and synaptic plasticity. *Nat Rev Neurosci*, 5: 952-962.

Huettner JE. 2003. Kainate receptors and synaptic transmission. *Prog Neurobiol*, 70: 387-407.

Jaskolski F, Coussen F, Mulle C. 2005. Subcellular localization and trafficking of kainate receptors. *Trends Pharmacol Sci*, 26: 20-26.

Lerma J. 2003. Roles and rules of kainate receptors in synaptic transmission. *Nat Rev Neurosci*, 4: 481-495.

DISCOVERY CITATIONS

Castillo PE, Malenka RC, Nicoll RA. 1997. Kainate receptors mediate a slow postsynaptic current in hippocampal CA3 neurons. *Nature*, 388: 182-186.

Contractor A, Swanson G, Heinemann SF. 2001. Kainate receptors are involved in short- and long-term plasticity at mossy fiber synapses in the hippocampus. *Neuron*, 29: 209-216.

Cossart R, Esclapez M, Hirsch JC, Bernard C, Ben-Ari Y. 1998. GluR5 kainate receptor activation in interneurons increases tonic inhibition of pyramidal cells. *Nat Neurosci*, 1: 470-478.

Frerking M, Ohliger-Frerking P. 2002. AMPA receptors and kainate receptors encode different features of afferent activity. *J Neurosci*, 22: 7434-7443.

Garcia EP, Mehta S, Blair LA, Wells DG, Shang J, Fukushima T, et al. 1998. SAP90 binds and clusters kainate receptors causing incomplete desensitization. *Neuron*, 21: 727-739.

Hirbec H, Francis JC, Lauri SE, Braithwaite SP, Coussen F, Mulle C, et al. 2003. Rapid and differential regulation of AMPA and kainate receptors at hippocampal mossy fibre synapses by PICK1 and GRIP. *Neuron*, 37: 625-638.

Jaskolski F, Coussen F, Nagarajan N, Normand E, Rosenmund C, Mulle C. 2004. Subunit composition and alternative splicing regulate membrane delivery of kainate receptors. *J Neurosci*, 24: 2506-2515.

Jiang L, Xu J, Nedergaard M, Kang J. 2001. A kainate receptor increases the efficacy of GABAergic synapses. *Neuron*, 30: 503-513.

Kamiya H, Ozawa S, Manabe T. 2002. Kainate receptor-dependent short-term plasticity of presynaptic Ca^{2+} influx at the hippocampal mossy fiber synapses. *J Neurosci*, 22: 9237-9243.

Kerchner GA, Wang GD, Qiu CS, Huettner JE, Zhuo M. 2001. Direct presynaptic regulation of GABA/glycine release by kainate receptors in the dorsal horn: an ionotropic mechanism. *Neuron*, 32: 477-488.

Kidd FL, Isaac JT. 1999. Developmental and activity-depe-ndent regulation of kainate receptors at thalamocortical synapses. *Nature*, 400: 569-573.

Li P, Wilding TJ, Kim SJ, Calejesan AA, Huettner JE, Zhuo M. 1999. Kainate-receptor-mediated sensory synaptic transmission in mammalian spinal cord. *Nature*, 397: 161-164.

Liu QS, Xu Q, Arcuino G, Kang J, Nedergaard M. 2004. Astrocyte-mediated activation of neuronal kainate receptors. *Proc Natl Acad Sci USA*, 101: 3172-3177.

Melyan Z, Wheal HV, Lancaster B. 2002. Metabotropic-mediated kainate receptor regulation of IsAHP and excitability in pyramidal cells. *Neuron*, 34: 107-114.

Melyan Z, Lancaster B, Wheal HV. 2004. Metabotropic regulation of intrinsic excitability by synaptic activation of kainate receptors. *J Neurosci*, 24: 4530-4534.

Mulle C, Sailer A, Perez-Otano I, Dickinson-Anson H, Castillo PE, Bureau I, et al. 1998. Altered synaptic physiology and reduced susceptibility to kainate-induced seizures in GluR6-deficient mice. *Nature*, 392: 601-605.

Rodriguez-Moreno A, Lerma J. 1998. Kainate receptor modulation of GABA release involves a metabotropic function. *Neuron*, 20: 1211-1218.

Rozas JL, Paternain AV, Lerma J. 2003. Noncanonical signaling by ionotropic kainate receptors. *Neuron*, 39: 543-553.

Schmitz D, Mellor J, Breustedt J, Nicoll RA. 2003. Presynaptic kainate receptors impart an associative property to hippocampal mossy fiber long-term potentiation. *Nat Neurosci*, 6: 1058-1063.

Tashiro A, Dunaevsky A, Blazeski R, Mason CA, Yuste R. 2003. Bidirectional regulation of hippocampal mossy fiber filopodial motility by kainate receptors: a two-step model of synaptogenesis. *Neuron*, 38: 773-784.

Yan S, Sanders JM, Xu J, Zhu Y, Contractor A, Swanson GT. 2004. A C-terminal determinant of GluR6 kainate receptor trafficking. *J Neurosci*, 24: 679-691.

Excitatory Amino Acid Neurotransmitter Regulation

CHAPTER 6

Rochelle Hines, Alaa El-Husseini

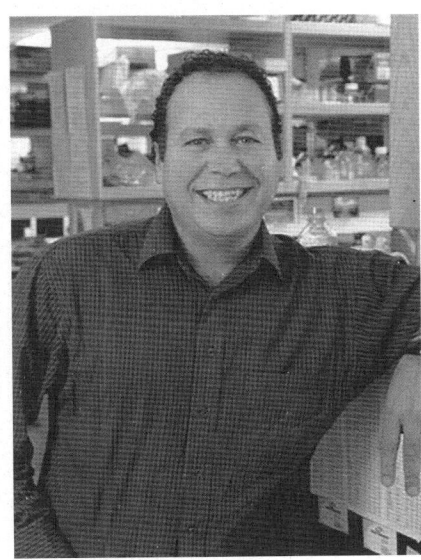

Dr. El-Husseini is an Assistant Professor and Invesitgator in the Brain Research Centre, University of British Columbia, Vancouver, Canada. He graduated from the University of Ain Shams and obtained a M.S. in Physiology at the University of Manitoba. After gaining a Ph.D. in Neuroscience at the University of British Columbia, he pursued postdoctoral training at the same institution, followed by postdoctoral training at the University of California.

Ms. Rochelle Hines is a graduate student in Dr. El-Husseini's laboratory.

MAJOR CONTRIBUTIONS

1. El-Husseini A, Schnell E, Chetkovich D M, Nicoll R, Bredt D S. 2000. PSD-95 drives maturation of excitatory synapses. *Science*, 290: 1364-1368.

2. El-Husseini A, Schnell E, Dakoji S, Sweeney N, Zhou Q, Prange O, Gauthier-Campbell C, Aguilera-Moreno A, Nicoll R, Bredt D S. 2002. Synaptic strength regulated by palmitate cycling on PSD-95. *Cell*, 108:849-863.

3. Prange O, Wong TP, Gerrow K, Wang YT, El-Husseini A. 2004. A balance between excitatory and inhibitory synapses is controlled by PSD-95 and neuroligin. *Proc Natl Acad Sci USA*, 101:13915-13920.

4. Huang K, Yanai A, Kang R, Arstikaitis P, Mullard A, Singaraja R, Haigh B, Gauthier-Campbell C, Hayden MR, El-Husseini A. 2004. Huntingtin interacting protein HIP14 is a palmitoyl transferase involved in palmitoylation and trafficking of multiple neuronal proteins. *Neuron*, 44:977-986.

5. Levinson JN, Cherry N, Huang K, Gerrow K, Kang R, Prange O, El-Husseini A. 2005. Neuroligins mediate excitatory and inhibitory synapse formation: involvement of PSD-95 and neurexin-1 beta in neuroligin-induced synaptic specificity. *J Biol Chem*, 280:17312-17319.

6. Lise MF, Wong TP, Trinh A, Hines RM, Liu L, Kang R, Hines DJ, Lu J, Goldenring JR, Wang YT, El-Husseini A. 2006. Involvement of myosin Vb in glutamate receptor trafficking. *J Biol Chem*, 281(6):3669-3678.

7. Gerrow K, Romorini S, Nabi SM, Colicos MA, Sala C, El-Husseini A. 2006. A preformed complex of postsynaptic proteins is involved in excitatory synapse development. *Neuron*, 49(4): 547-562.

8. Yanai A, Huang K, Kang R, Singaraja RR, Arstikaitis P, Gan L, Orban PC, Mullard A, Cowan CM, Raymond LA, Drisdel RC, Green WN, Ravikumar B, Rubinsztein DC, El-Husseini A, Hayden MR. 2006. Palmitoylation of huntingtin by HIP14 is essential for its trafficking and function. *Nat Neurosci*, 9(6): 824-831.

MAIN TOPICS

Developmental Regulation
   Profile of expression of receptor subunits
   Silent synapses
   Excitatory synapse formation and maturation
   Role of adhesion molecules in excitatory synapse
      formation
Regulation of Receptor Clustering
   Synaptic scaffolding proteins
   Transmembrane AMPA receptor regulatory proteins
   NARP, a secreted protein that regulates AMPA re-
      ceptor clustering
Regulation of Spine Dynamics and Morphology
   Shank and homer
   SPAR
Regulation of Receptor Sorting and Cycling
   Early sorting and assembly
   Molecular motors
Protein Modifications and Receptor Regulation
   Phosphorylation
   Palmitoylation
   Protein degradation

SUMMARY

Individual synapses vary enormously in their biochemical properties and functionality. The neurotransmitters released, the receptors activated, and the ensuing physiological responses are all variable, and susceptible to modification through a variety of mechanisms. The regulation of neurotransmitter receptors is a central mechanism by which the signaling properties of a synapse and a cell may be controlled. Excitatory neurotransmitter receptors are primarily localized to the postsynaptic dendritic compartment, anchored within the postsynaptic density (PSD). In their lifetime, receptors are subject to alternative splicing, differential sorting and compartmentalization. Moreover, these processes are influenced by activity driven protein trafficking, post-translational modifications and interaction with an overwhelmingly increasing number of proteins enriched at excitatory synapses. The diverse repertoire of regulatory mechanisms contributes to the amazing heterogeneity of synapse morphology and function in the central nervous system. Changes in receptor trafficking has been also implicated in shaping synaptic activity and plasticity, and defects in these processes may underlie several pathological states.

INTRODUCTION

Neurotransmission at excitatory synapses in the mammalian brain is primarily mediated by glutamate release from the presynaptic terminal, which is then bound by specific receptors in the postsynaptic terminal. Formation of excitatory synapses is thought to be mediated by adhesion molecules. Neurotransmitter receptors on the postsynaptic side are bound into a proteinaceous network of scaffolding proteins, adhesion molecules and signal transduction enzymes, collectively referred to as the post synaptic density (PSD). The presynaptic side is distinguished by machinery for glutamate production, compartmentalization into vesicles, and release. The spatial and temporal control that scaffolding proteins exert on signaling molecules in the PSD can have profound implications on synaptic transmission (Fig.6.1).

Several factors appear to control the number of specific receptor subunits present at the synapse. Recent studies showed that the expression of glutamate receptor subunits is tightly regulated in development with a switch in specific subunit expression. Remarkably, whereas NMDA-type glutamate receptor number at the synapse is relatively static, AMPA-type glutamate receptor cycling is very dynamic and is regulated by synaptic activity. Surface expression of glutamate receptors is controlled by a large family of interacting proteins that regulate receptor insertion, removal and degradation, thereby influencing synaptic strength. In this chapter, we summarize some of the new findings that unraveled the intricate control of excitatory neurotransmitter receptor dynamics regulating synaptic activity.

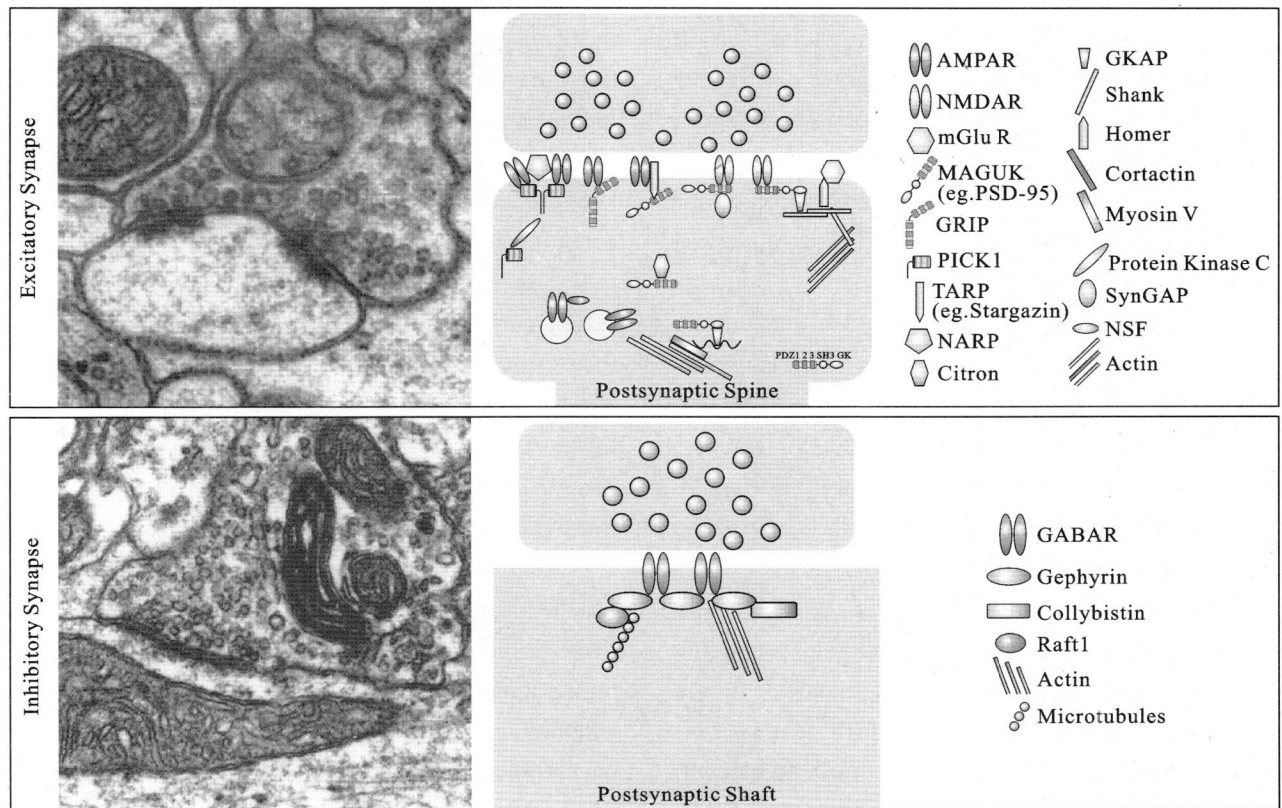

Fig.6.1 The postsynaptic density (PSD) of excitatory synapses is composed of neurotransmitter receptors that are bound into a meshwork of scaffolding proteins, adhesion molecules and signal transduction enzymes. Adhesion molecules are thought to initiate contact formation. Interaction with scaffolding proteins will lead to the recruitment of the numerous signaling proteins and neurotransmitter receptors that make up the PSD. Within the PSD, scaffolding proteins exert spatial and temporal control on receptors and signaling molecules influencing synaptic output. In contrast, few scaffolding proteins and effectors have been identified at inhibitory postsynaptic sites. The electron micrographs demonstrate the reduced PSD in an inhibitory synapse in comparison to the excitatory synapse which bears a thick, complex PSD.

DEVELOPMENTAL REGULATION

Profile of Expression of Receptor Subunits

Over the course of development, the subunit composition of neurotransmitter receptors changes dramatically, having profound influences on signal transmission. Some types of receptors are present in the embryonic brain, while others have dominant expression in the postnatal brain or in the adult brain.

The α-amino-3-hydroxy-5-methylisoxazolepropionic acid (AMPA) receptor family is a group of ionotropic glutamate receptors subunits including GluR1-GluR4. At embryonic day 15, the GluR1 subunit is detected in the whole brain. In general, during late embryonic and early postnatal development, levels of GluR1 increase progressively. GluR1 increases in the cerebral cortex but decreases in the striatum over the course of postnatal development. Early in postnatal development, GluR1 is transiently expressed in the cerebellum at specific time points. Through these early periods, both granule and Purkinje cells express GluR1; however from postnatal day 21 forward, GluR1 levels in these cell types are very low. GluR2/3 subunits are also present in embryonic development, whereas the GluR4 subunit only in late postnatal development and adulthood.

In addition, GluR2-4 subunits are subject to posttranscriptional mRNA editing. One edited site is an arginine residue which regulates calcium permeability of the GluR2 subunit. Additional editing involves substitution of glycine for arginine 764 in GluR2-4. This arginine to glycine conversion results in receptors with faster rates of recovery from desensitization. GluR mRNA subunits can also be spliced into two variants, referred to as flip and flop. Receptor complexes that contain flop variants show increased desensitization during glutamate application. Accordingly, the steady state currents of flop variants will be smaller than those of flip variants. In terms of development, the flip variant dominates before birth and continues to be expressed into adulthood. On the other hand, flop variants are in low abundance before postnatal day 8 and are up-regulated to about the same level as the flip forms in adulthood.

Functional AMPARs also exist in two basic forms: calcium-impermeable and calcium-permeable channels. The ion permeability is dictated by the presence of the GluR2 subunit, which renders heteromeric AMPAR complexes impermeable to calcium. AMPAR diversity is modulated by alternative RNA splicing and editing, and by targeting and trafficking of receptor subunits at dendritic spines. Because of GluR2's importance in dictating the ion flux at synaptic sites, its expression is tightly regulated. The GluR2 gene is under transcriptional control by the transcription factor neural restrictive silencer element (NRSE, also known as RE1), a gene silencing factor that prevents non-neuronal expression. Following transcription, GluR2 mRNAs are edited by double-stranded RNA-specific editase 1 (ADAR2). In addition GluR2 subunit expression can be dynamically regulated in response to activity beyond developmental time periods. The precise control of AMPAR composition is a critical factor in controlling synaptic plasticity.

N-methyl-D-aspartate (NMDA)-type receptor subunits include NR1, NR2A-D, NR3. The functional NR1 subunit is widely expressed in the brain throughout pre- and postnatal development. In contrast, the modulatory subunits NR2A-D display differential patterns throughout development. The NR2A subunit is widely expressed postnatally, while the NR2B subunit is broadly distributed throughout the embryonic brain, being limited to the forebrain at postnatal stages. The NR2C subunit appears postnatally, prominent in the cerebellum, whereas NR2D is mainly present in the diencephalon and brainstem during embryonic and neonatal periods. During the late prenatal and early postnatal periods, the NR3 subunit is abundant.

The metabotropic glutamate receptor (mGluR) family currently includes eight members, divided into three groups based on their sequence homology and enzyme specificity. mGluR1 and mGluR5 (group I) activate a G-protein coupled to phospholipase C. mGluR2, 3, and 8 receptor (group II) subunits favor activation by trans-1-aminocyclopentane-1,3-dicarboxylate, whereas 1,2-amino-4-phosphonobutyrate is the ideal agonist of mGluR4, 6, and 7 receptor subunits (group III). mGluRs demonstrate distinct regional and temporal regulation over the course of development. Group I subunits are minimally detected during embryonic development. The level of mGluR1 gradually increases during early postnatal periods. mGluR5 increases perinatally, peaking around postnatal day 14, and declines steadily into adulthood.

Differential patterns are also seen with group I mGluR splice variants. Three splice variants for mGluR1 have been identified, mGluR1α, mGluR1β and mGluR1c, which vary primarily in the length of their carboxyl-terminal tails. When compared to cells expressing mGluR1β or mGluR1c receptors, cells expressing mGluR1α show increased agonist potency and basal phospholipase C activity. Over the course of development, mGluR1α predominates, as mGluR1β and mGluR1c are not typically detected until adulthood. In contrast, mGluR5α declines with development, while the mGluR5β splice variant increase, dominating in adulthood.

In addition, group II and III mGluRs are differentially expressed during development. mGluR2 mRNA displays low levels at birth, increasing during postnatal development, whereas mGluR3 is high at birth and decreases during maturation to adult levels of expression. mRNA and protein expression for the mGluR4 subunit is low at birth and increases during postnatal development. Similarly, mGluR7a levels are highest during the first two postnatal weeks, and then decline in cortical regions. The tightly controlled temporal and spatial variation in patterns for excitatory receptor subunits and splice variants suggests that regulation of receptor composition influences synaptic function.

Silent Synapses

As evident from the first section, glutamatergic synaptic transmission undergoes significant changes during the course of development. It is thought that initially, glutamatergic transmission is primarily NMDAR-mediated, without any significant contribution of AMPARs. Due to the voltage-dependent magnesium block of NMDA channels, these early synapses are predominantly "silent" or inactive at resting membrane potentials. It has been indicated that the first glutamatergic synapses established in hippocampal pyramidal cells are "silent". The proportion of "silent" synapses decreases steadily between postnatal day 2 and postnatal day 5. Throughout development synapses acquire AMPARs with little change in NMDAR expression. The transformation of "silent" synapses into functional synapses is dependent upon the activation of NMDARs. Spontaneous activation of NMDA results in the rapid recruitment of AMPARs into silent synapses. NMDA activation also results in a significant increase in the frequency of AMPAR-mediated miniature excitatory postsynaptic currents. Thus awakening of "silent" synapses represents a mechanism by which activity can modulate synaptic signaling.

Excitatory Synapse Formation and Maturation

In addition to the tight control of glutamate receptor expression, several other mechanisms regulate the maturation of glutamatergic synapses (Fig.6.1). Most glutamate receptor subunits are localized to actin rich dendritic protrusions known as spines. There is considerable evidence that contact formation and structural remodeling of spines is regulated by several important classes of proteins including adhesion molecules involved in target recognition and initial contact

formation, and scaffolding proteins important for protein recruitment to excitatory synapses. These components are distinct from those involved in regulation of neurotransmitter receptor clustering at inhibitory synapses (Fig.6.1).

The formation and maturation of excitatory synapses is generally thought to be comprised of three successive steps where the necessary proteins are synthesized followed by their trafficking to initial sites of contact between the axonal growth cones and the dendrites of other cells. Maturation of these sites involves recruitment of neurotransmitter receptors and their interacting partners to form a functional synapse (Fig.6.2, see also the color plate). Current research suggests that the initial contact formation is regulated by adhesion molecules. Many adhesion systems are specifically enriched at excitatory synaptic contacts including: neural cell adhesion molecule (NCAM), SynCAM, the cadherin/catenin system, the cadherin like neuronal receptors, ephrin and the Ephrin receptor (EphR) tyrosine kinase system, and the β-neurexin/neuroligin system. Several of these proteins have been shown to regulate excitatory synapse formation.

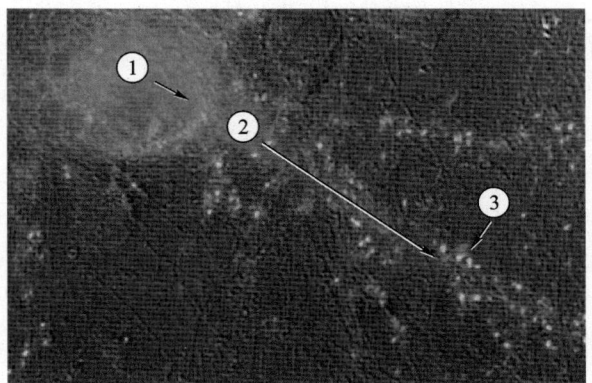

① Synthesis,   ② Trafficking   ③ Complex assembly,
Modification   Specification of
& Sorting   synaptic structure &
                                function

Fig.6.2 The construction of excitatory synapses is thought to involve three successive processes. Initially the necessary proteins are synthesized and sorted in the soma for delivery to axons and dendrites. This step is followed by trafficking to initial sites of contact between the axonal growth cones and dendrites. Finally, the maturation of these sites involves further recruitment of proteins, including neurotransmitter receptors and their interacting partners, resulting in a functional synapse.

Role of Adhesion Molecules in Excitatory Synapse Formation

A breakthrough in understanding the role of cell adhesion molecules in excitatory synapse formation stems from recent studies which demonstrated that heterologous expression of neuroligin-1 is sufficient to induce excitatory synapses. At cell-cell contact sites, neuroligins interact trans-synaptically with β-neurexins, and this interaction is thought to induce presynaptic differentiation and synapse formation. Further, this heterotypic interaction induces the differential recruitment of proteins to the pre- versus postsynaptic compartments.

The neuroligin family of adhesion molecules is comprised of four related genes in humans, known as neuroligin-1-4. Overexpression of neuroligin-1, -2, or -3 in cultured hippocampal neurons results in the formation of excitatory postsynaptic specializations. These specializations have been shown to contain glutamate neurotransmitter receptors. Importantly, these specializations were found to oppose presynaptic axon terminals equipped for the release of glutamate.

Although previously thought to specifically induce excitatory synapse formation, recent findings show that coupling of neuroligins to β-neurexins also regulates inhibitory synapse formation. These findings are supported by the recent discovery that endogenous neuroligin-1 is enriched at excitatory synapses whereas neuroligin-2 is mainly found at inhibitory synapses. Expression of β-neurexin on the surface of non-neuronal cells or via attachment to synthetic beads also induces the clustering of both excitatory and inhibitory postsynaptic receptors. In addition, overexpression of neuroligin-1, -2, or -3 in cultured hippocampal neurons results in the formation of inhibitory contacts. These results indicate that neuroligins are involved the formation of heterogeneous types of synapses.

Although neuroligins have become a hot topic of study, several other important adhesion molecules have been implicated in excitatory synapse formation.

Like neuroligins, SynCAM 1 is another cell adhesion molecule that has been shown to be sufficient to drive the formation of presynaptic terminals. SynCAM 1 is localized to both pre- and postsynaptic compartments and shares similarities with NCAM and the invertebrate molecules fasciclin II and apCAM. Expression of SynCAM 1 in non-neuronal cells induces the formation of presynaptic terminals when cocultured with neurons, similar to the effects seen with neuroligin. Further, the known protein interaction motifs in the cytosolic tails of SynCAM 1 and β-neurexins are highly conserved, suggesting further similarity between these cell adhesion systems. However, the downstream effectors for these systems are not clearly defined. Expression of the isolated cytoplasmic tail of SynCAM in neurons inhibited synapse assembly indicating that PDZ domain containing adaptor proteins may be involved synapse formation, perhaps analogous to the role of scaffolding proteins in neuroligin function. In contrast to neuroligins, SynCAM 1 over expression in hippocampal neurons has only been shown to specifically promote excitatory synaptic transmission, demonstrating that multiple cell adhesion systems may serve distinct functions.

An additional cell adhesion molecule, NCAM, is thought to be involved in early stages of synapse establishment, as well as subsequent maturation. 2–3 day old cultured neurons bear clusters of NCAM at the cell surface that are linked to trans-Golgi-derived organelles. Further, these organelles have been shown to rapidly translocate to pre- and postsynaptic sites after initial contact formation. This suggests that other molecules, such as neuroligins or SynCAM may be involved in contact initiation, followed by recruitment of NCAM and other proteins. NCAM also regulates excitatory synapse density and strength. Interestingly, synaptic activity modulates NCAM expression, with increases in the percentage of spines expressing NCAM following long term potentiation.

Members of the Eph receptor family of tyrosine kinases and ephrin ligands, have also been implicated in the development of mature excitatory synapses. Extensive analysis, using different combinations of double and triple knockouts of EphB1, EphB2, and EphB3, revealed that these receptors are involved in dendritic spine morphogenesis and synapse formation in the hippocampus. Altered spine formation in the EphBR mutants is also associated with reduced excitatory synapse density and reduced clustering of both NMDA and AMPA receptors. Although all of the aforementioned systems share the ability to regulate cell adhesion, each system appears to control specific steps of synapse formation and maturation. Further investigation of the functional, temporal and spatial attributes of these molecules with respect to synapse formation will reveal if they work in a cooperative and integrated manner. The growing body of research on cell adhesion molecules suggests that some molecules are required for the initial synaptogenic events, whereas others are then recruited to dictate what type of synapse is formed or whether the synapse should be stabilized, moving on to maturity. Further, cell adhesion molecules are coming to the forefront in the regulation of synaptic function beyond development, in adulthood, having implications for their potential roles in plasticity.

REGULATION OF RECEPTOR CLUSTERING

Synaptic Scaffolding Proteins

Another group of proteins thought to control excitatory synapse maturation are scaffolding proteins enriched at the PSD (Fig.6.3). Scaffolding proteins help to assemble large protein complexes at cellular junctions especially within the spine heads. Many of these proteins display dramatic structural plasticity, where protein interaction and subcellular distribution can be regulated in response to environmental and developmental cues. Scaffolding proteins generally contain multiple protein-protein interaction domains required for the assembly of large protein complexes. Scaffolding proteins can regulate the activity of ion channels by influencing their trafficking, endocytosis, subcellular localization, subunit composition and functional properties.

Membrane-associated guanylate kinases: the PSD-95 family of proteins

The membrane-associated guanylate kinase (MAGUK) family of proteins is of central importance to protein scaffolding in many cell types. MAGUKs are defined by the presence of a domain homologous to the yeast guanylate kinase (GK) domain, which is catalytically inactive. The GK domain is always preceded by a Src-homology-3 (SH3) domain. In addition, MAGUKs contain PDZ domains, which are named for the original proteins in which the motifs were identified (PSD-95, discs large, and zona occludens 1). PDZ domains bind the carboxyl-terminus of proteins or form dimers with other PDZ domain containing proteins. These domains are often arranged in tandem arrays or associated with other protein-protein interaction domains to form a protein scaffold. Protein multimerization may act to enhance clustering of binding proteins into large assemblies confined to specific sites, such as the PSD.

PSD-95 (postsynaptic density protein of 95 kDa) is the prototypical PDZ domain containing protein, and extensive research has been conducted on this family of proteins (Fig.6.3). The PSD-95 family is encoded by four genes — PSD-95 / synapse associated protein 90 (SAP90), postsynaptic density protein of 93 kDa (PSD-93) / chapsyn-110, synapse associated protein 102 (SAP102), and synapse associated protein 97 (SAP97), which are characterized by 3 PDZ domains, in addition to the SH3 and GK domain characteristic of MAGUKs.

Maturation of pre- and postsynaptic contacts through assembly of cell adhesion molecules and scaffolding proteins is critical for excitatory synapse formation. Importantly, PSD-95 plays a key role in regulating synapse fate with neuroligins. Studies in heterologous cells show that PSD-95 induces clustering of neuroligin-1 through PDZ-mediated interactions. Although PDZ-dependent interactions are required for clustering, these interactions are not essential for the synaptogenic activity of neuroligin. However, the number and morphology of synapses induced by neuroligin is regulated by PSD-95. This is due to the ability of PSD-95 to cluster, compartmentalizing it to specific contact sites. Consistent with this, overexpression studies show that PSD-95 accelerates clustering of several proteins including at early stages of development (Fig.6.4, see also the color plate).

These findings indicate that through recruitment of cell adhesion molecules and associated proteins, PSD-95 modulates the morphology of the PSD and presynaptic terminals and the number of excitatory synapses induced by cell adhesion molecules.

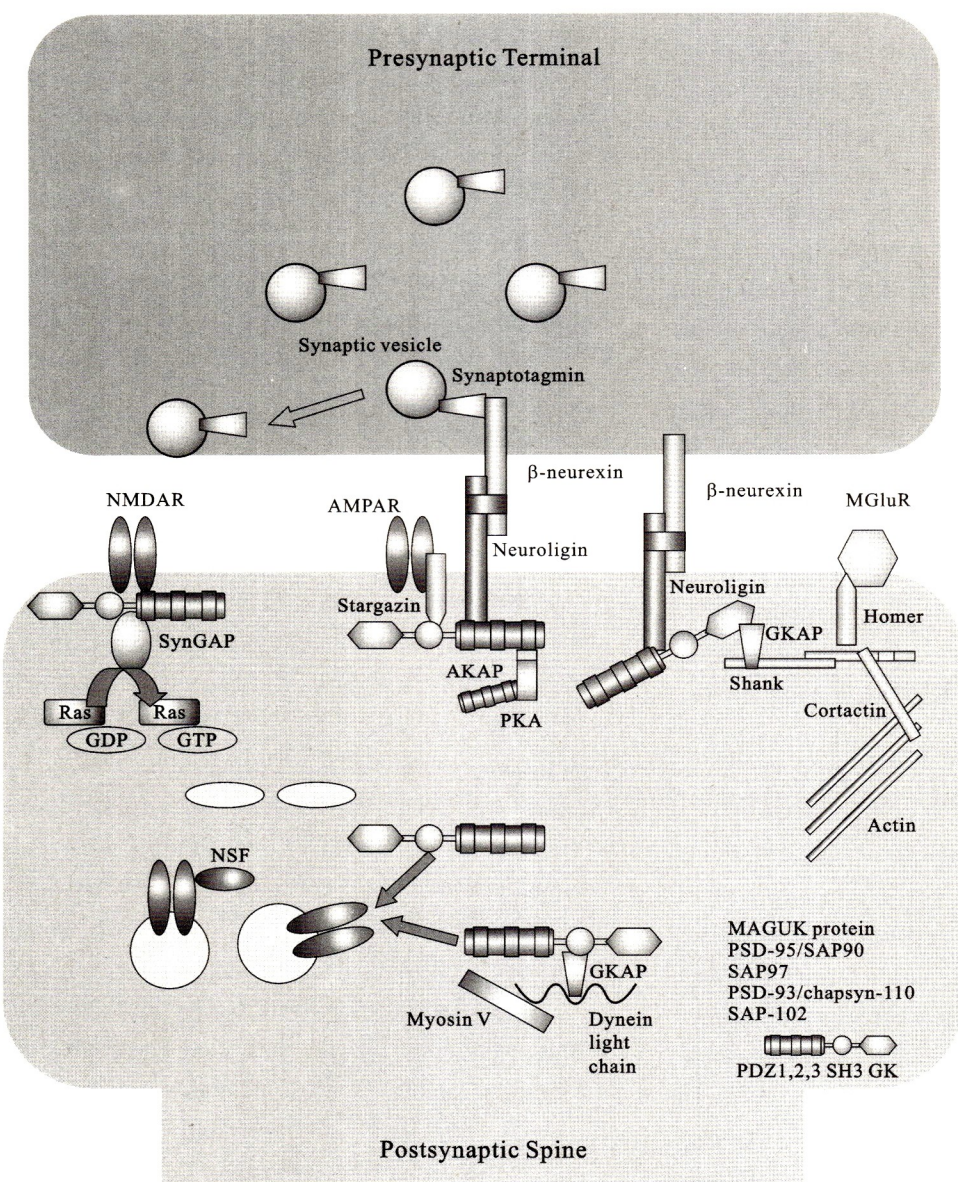

Fig.6.3 PSD-95 is a major player of the PSD, which performs multiple functions. Interaction of PSD-95 with NMDARs is thought to couple NMDARs to select signaling enzymes, which control neuronal function. PSD-95 also serves to cluster cell adhesion molecules such as neuroligins which regulate synapse formation and morphology. Association of PSD-95 with stargazin regulates AMPA receptor clustering at the synapse. PSD-95 may also participate in the dynamic regulation of AMPAR internalization dependent upon palmitate cycling of PSD-95. PSD-95 may regulate neurotransmitter receptor phosphorylation by recruitment of enzyme anchoring proteins such as AKAPs. Finally, coupling of PSD-95 to other scaffolding proteins such as GKAP may regulate the function of proteins involved in spine growth or maturation such as shank and Homer.

Although substantial evidence exists for an interaction between PSD-95 and NMDARs, it remains unclear how PSD-95 modulates NMDAR trafficking or function. Insertion of NMDARs at synaptic contact sites is not altered by mutations of the cytoplasmic tails of NMDAR subunits, by genetic disruption of PSD-95 or by interfering peptides that disperse synaptic clusters of PSD-95. These results demonstrate that the synaptic clustering of NMDARs by PSD-95 is not dependent upon PDZ-based interactions. Despite this, a recent study shows that expression of PSD-95 and NR1/NR2A subunits in heterologous cells increases the number of functional channels at the cell surface and the channel opening rate of NMDARs.

Although these results support a role for PSD-95 in NMDAR regulation in neurons, clear evidence for this role is still lacking.

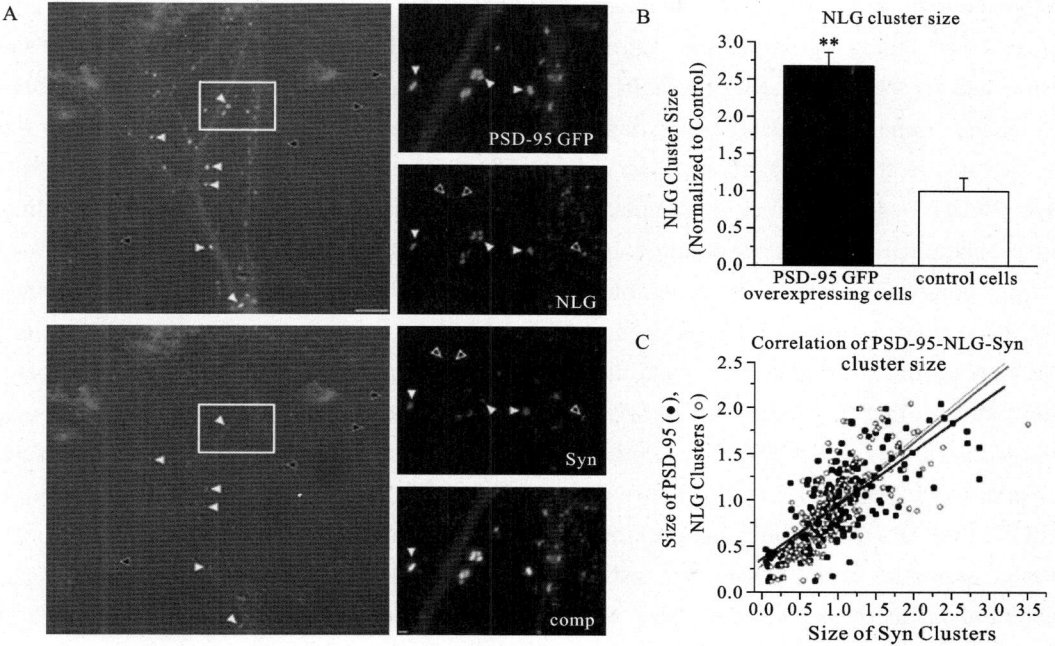

Fig.6.4 PSD-95 recruits neuroligins to the synapse and regulates presynaptic maturation. Hippocampal neurons were transfected with PSD-95 GFP and subsequently stained with antibodies specific to neuroligin subtypes 1 and 3. The synaptic marker synaptophysin was used to visualize presynaptic terminals. Left overview panel in A shows an overlay image of PSD-95 GFP (green), neuroligin (NLG; red), synaptophysin (Syn; blue) and a DIC image. Higher magnification micrographs of boxed regions are shown in panels to the right. A. Clusters of endogenous synaptic neuroligin were larger in neurons transfected with PSD-95 GFP (white arrowheads) than in untransfected control cells in the same field of view (black arrowheads). B. Bar graph summarizing the data of neuroligin cluster size. C. A linear correlation ($P < 0.0001$) between the size of PSD-95 GFP, NLG, and Syn clusters at single synapses.

In contrast to NMDARs, mounting evidence indicates that the clustering of AMPARs is regulated by PSD-95. This exogenous PSD-95 also increases the number of synaptic AMPARs. This effect seems paradoxical as PSD-95 does not directly bind AMPARs. Current research suggests that PSD-95 and AMPARs interact via stargazin, a member of the transmembrane AMPAR regulatory protein (TARP) family (to be discussed below).

Other protein scaffolds:GRIP, PICK-1

The PDZ-containing glutamate receptor interacting protein GRIP1/ABP binds to the carboxy-terminal PDZ motif of AMPAR subunits GluR2 and GluR3. It

is thought that GRIP1/ABP may serve to link AMPARs as cargoes to the microtubule transport system. Another protein associated with the GluR2 and GRIP1/ABP complex is liprin-α1. In turn, liprin-α1 interacts with a member of the kinesin superfamily KIF1, and GIT1, a GTPase-activating protein for the ADP-ribosylation factor family of small GTPases known to regulate protein trafficking and the actin cytoskeleton. Interfering with the GIT1-liprin-α1 interaction, by overexpression of a dominant-negative, reduces surface clustering of AMPARs *in vitro*.

Protein interacting with C kinase (PICK1) is another well characterized PDZ domain-containing scaffold protein. PICK1 interacts with the C-termini of AMPARs, and is found to be specifically colocalized with AMPARs at excitatory synapses. PICK1 induces clustering of AMPARs in heterologous expression systems. Viral expression of wild type PICK1 in hippocampal slices results in increased AMPAR-mediated excitatory postsynaptic current amplitude. Blockade of the PICK1 PDZ domain interactions produced opposite effects on synaptic strength and AMPAR rectification to those observed with wild type PICK1 overexpression. Immunocytochemical and biochemical analyses in cultured hippocampal neurons demonstrate that overexpression of wild type PICK1 causes a decrease in endogenous GluR2 surface expression, with no change in GluR1. These results indicate that regulation of AMPAR subunit composition involves PICK1 PDZ domain interactions. Specifically, PICK1 seems to reduce the GluR2 content of AMPARs at synaptic sites, resulting in the increased synaptic strength seen at resting membrane potentials with overexpression. This represents an interesting mechanism of regulating calcium permeability at synaptic sites, as the GluR2 subunit confers Ca^{2+} permeability to AMPARs.

Dynamic changes in Ca^{2+} are thought to occur through the exchange of synaptic GluR2-lacking and GluR2-containing receptors. It has been shown that two GluR2-interacting proteins, PICK1 and N-ethylmaleimide sensitive fusion protein (NSF), are specifically required for calcium-permeable AMPARs plasticity. Additionally, PICK1 has been shown to regulate the formation of extrasynaptic pools of GluR2-containing AMPARs that may be recycled into synapses during plasticity. Thus, PICK1 can regulate the calcium permeability of AMPARs at excitatory synapses by dynamically regulating the synaptic delivery of GluR2-containing receptors.

Transmembrane AMPA Receptor Regulatory Proteins

In addition to cytoplasmic interacting proteins, transmembrane AMPAR regulatory proteins (TARPs) have been recently characterized. TARPs are transmembrane proteins with four membrane-spanning domains

that interact with the transmembrane region of AMPARs. This family of proteins includes stargazin, γ-3, γ-4, and γ-8, all of which mediate the surface expression of AMPARs. Stargazin, the archetypal TARP, is critical for AMPAR targeting to synapses in cerebellar granule cells. Stargazin contains a carboxy-terminal PDZ binding region that interacts with PSD-95. Stargazin overexpression drastically increases the number of extra-synaptic AMPARs. Conversely, expression of a mutant stargazin lacking the PDZ-binding domain disrupts synaptic clustering of AMPARs in hippocampal cells, demonstrating the importance of this domain in synaptic targeting. In COS7 cells GluR1 is expressed poorly on the surface and is primarily retained in the endoplasmic reticulum. Coexpression with stargazin dramatically increases the surface fraction of GluR1. Upregulation of endoplasmic reticulum chaperone proteins both mimicked and occluded the effect of stargazin. These findings uncover a role for stargazin in AMPAR trafficking through the early compartments of the biosynthetic pathway in the endoplasmic reticulum. A recent study has shown that the AMPAR/TARP complex is not always stable at the synapse. Upon binding glutamate, AMPARs detach from TARPs to undergo internalization. Further, this regulated interaction with TARPs at the synapse may participate in activity-dependent turnover of AMPARs.

Beyond their role in AMPAR targeting, TARPs have also been implicated in modulation of channel function. Coexpression of GluR1 with stargazin markedly enhanced glutamate-induced currents in heterologous cell lines. This enhancement was also observed when stargazin was coexpressed with GluR2 homomeric channels, which typically produce only small or negligible currents. These results suggest that stargazin not only promotes AMPAR surface expression but also directly modulates AMPAR activity. Coexpression of stargazin with AMPAR subunits was also found to reduce receptor desensitization in response to glutamate. In addition, receptor deactivation rates were slowed, and the recovery from desensitization was accelerated. The correlation between desensitization and the stability of the AMPAR suggests that binding of stargazin may stabilize the receptor complex. Postsynaptic complexes of AMPARs and stargazin are more responsive to synaptically released glutamate when compared with receptors lacking interaction. The existence of functionally distinct synaptic AMPARs, based on their interaction with stargazin, may represent a mechanism for regulation of synaptic strength.

NARP, a Secreted Protein that Regulates AMPA Receptor Clustering

Another mode of regulation of excitatory synapse function involves neuronal activity-regulated pentraxin (NARP) protein, a secreted immediate-early gene (IEG) which is regulated by synaptic activity. NARP is part of a pentraxin complex that also includes neuronal pentraxin-1 (NP1). These proteins combine to form highly organized complexes, where the relative ratio of each protein in the complex is dependent upon the neuron's prior activity and developmental stage. These proteins interact via N-terminal coiled-coil domains, and contain C-terminal pentraxin domains which mediate association with AMPARs. In addition to its interaction with AMPARs, several other features of NARP are suggestive of a role in excitatory synaptogenesis. NARP is selectively enriched at excitatory synapses, and has been shown to form homomeric multimers and large cell surface clusters that co-localize with AMPAR subunits. Neurons overexpressing wild-type NARP show increased clustering of AMPARs. Transfection with dominant-negative NARP mutants results in selective binding of endogenous NARP and prevention of its synaptic accumulation, ultimately leading to decreased GluR1 subunit clustering. Despite their marked effect at excitatory synapses, neither dominant-negative or wild-type NARP overexpression influences the postsynaptic clustering of inhibitory synaptic proteins such as gephyrin.

REGULATION OF SPINE DYNAMICS AND MORPHOLOGY

The majority of glutamate receptor subunits are localized to actin rich dendritic protrusions known as spines. Spines are unique compartments because they lack microtubules, but contain varying amounts of smooth endoplasmic reticulum, ribosomes, and contain a large number of proteins that make up the PSD. The heterogeneity of spine morphology is apparent even on a single dendrite of a single neuron. Live imaging studies have revealed that spines are remarkably dynamic, being assembled or changing size and shape over timescales of seconds to minutes and of hours to days. Changes in spine size and morphology may be related to long-term changes in the function of a single synapse.   As the size of the spine head is proportional to the area of the PSD, to the number of postsynaptic receptors and to the number of docked vesicles, the growth of the spine head likely correlates with a strengthening of synaptic transmission. The strengthening or addition of synaptic contacts can impact overall cell signaling, increasing the propensity for action potential propagation via summation of multiple inputs.   The majority of the movement and morphological changes seen in spine heads are dependent upon actin remodeling. Because an important influence on spine morphology is activity, a link between receptor activation and the actin cytoskeleton will be important for regulation of these changes. Poised between the postsynaptic membrane embedded with receptors and the underlying cytoskeleton, the PSD is well positioned to provide this important link and influence spine morphology.

Shank and Homer

Several cytoskeleton associated proteins with multiple protein-protein interaction domains have been shown to regulate spine morphology. For instance, the Shank family of proteins is essentially constructed out of protein interaction motifs, including multiple ankyrin repeats, a Src-homology-3 (SH3) domain, a PDZ domain, a long proline-rich region and a sterile alpha motif (SAM) domain. These domains mediate multiple protein interactions in the PSD providing important links between NMDARs and mGluRs, inositol trisphosphate receptors (IP3Rs) in the smooth endoplasmic reticulum (sER) and the actin cytoskeleton via cortactin. Homer proteins are multimeric adaptors that crosslink group I mGluRs, IP3Rs and Shank at the synapse via EVH1 (enabled (Ena) / vasodilator-stimulated phosphoprotein (VASP) Homology 1) domains in Homer that interact with proline rich motifs. Overexpression of Shank results in enlargement and maturation of dendritic spines and enhancement of presynaptic function in cultured hippocampal neurons. Experiments employing a series of deletion constructs demonstrated that synaptic targeting and cooperation with Homer are necessary for Shank to exert its effects on spine morphology. In addition to morphological effects, the Shank / Homer complex influences the recruitment of related proteins to synaptic sites. For example, Shank and Homer mediate the recruitment of inositol triphosphate (IP(3)) and smooth endoplasmic reticulum into dendritic spines. Dominant-negative mutants of Shank cause reductions in spine density, which may result from alteration in spine stability or from inhibition of spine formation. Shank can thus influence spine morphology, mediated by the link between receptor activation and actin-based spine remodeling.

SPAR

Another PSD protein, spine-associated RapGAP (Rap-specific GTPase-activating protein) or SPAR, represents a more direct link between neurotransmitter receptors and cytoskeletal dynamics. As suggested by its name, SPAR is a GTPase-activating protein (GAP) and a member of the Rap family of small GTPases involved in regulation of the actin cytoskeleton and cell adhesion. SPAR consists of two distinct actin-interacting domains separated by a GAP domain and a PDZ domain, and followed by a guanylate kinase (GK) binding domain. In heterologous cells, SPAR reorganizes F-actin into large aggregates or dispersed clusters, and recruits PSD-95 to these structures. Interestingly, overexpression of SPAR in neurons enlarges dendritic spine heads and alters their morphology leading to thorny or multilobed shapes. SPAR-induced changes in spine-head width are dependent upon the GAP domain, the second actin-binding domain and the GK-binding domain. Expres-

sion of SPAR mutant constructs that act in a dominant-negative fashion, results in the conversion of mature spines into elongated, thin filopodia. Thus, both the actin-binding and RapGAP properties of SPAR influence spine morphology via the link between receptor mediated signaling and the actin cytoskeleton.

Currently, investigators have identified numerous molecules that regulate spine morphology (summarized in Table 6.1). Importantly, many of the identified spine morphogens have a link with the actin cytoskeleton, either directly, indirectly or via regulatory GTPases. An important avenue that warrants further investigation is whether the morphogens are also regulated in an activity dependent fashion that parallels spine formation, maturation and morphology.

REGULATION OF RECEPTOR SORTING AND CYCLING

Early Sorting and Assembly

As we have discovered, AMPARs are hetero-oligomeric complexes composed of different combinations of GluR1-4 subunits. Whereas GluR4-containing AMPARs are common in early postnatal development, GluR1–GluR2 or GluR2–GluR3 subunit combinations predominate in the mature hippocampus. The subunit combinations are dictated early in receptor trafficking, in the endoplasmic reticulum. The mechanism by which these combinations are determined is somewhat unclear, but is thought to depend on interactions between the luminal, amino-terminal domains of the receptor subunits. GluR1–GluR2 hetero-oligomers exit the endoplasmic reticulum rapidly, and are transported to the Golgi apparatus for glycosylation. On the other hand, GluR2–GluR3 hetero-oligomers are retained much longer in the endoplasmic reticulum. Interestingly, a portion of GluR2 subunits seems to dwell at the endoplasmic reticulum. This immature GluR2 pool is retained within the endoplasmic reticulum in an active manner, dependent upon the presence of an edited charged arginine residue lining the channel pore. Lack of glutamine editing to arginine in GluR1, GluR3, and GluR4 prevents their retention in this fashion.

Table 6.1   Molecules that regulate spine morphology.

Protein	Basic Cellular Function	Effect on Dendritic Spines
Contact Initiation and Spine Formation		
Neuroligins, β-neurexin	β-neurexin (pre) and neuroligin (post) mediate cell-to-cell contact at synaptic sites.	Clustering of β-neurexin leads to recruitment of synaptic vesicles; neuroligin promotes the recruitment of NMDARs and PSD-95.
SynCAM	Cell adhesion molecule localized to both sides of the synaptic cleft.	SynCAM induces the formation of presynaptic terminals.
Contact Stabilization, Maturation and Spine Morphogenesis		
PSD-95	Major component of PSD, scaffold that binds many proteins via multiple domains.	PSD-95 increases the number and size of spine heads, dependent upon PDZ domain interactions.
Shank	Multi-domain scaffold of PSD, binds to NMDAR, mGluR and provides link with actin.	Interaction with Homer via Shank's PDZ domain leads to increases in spine head size.
SPAR	Functions as a RapGAP inhibiting Rap activity; interacts with and reorganizes F-actin.	SPAR interacts with PSD-95 to reorganize F-actin and increase spine head size.
Ephrins, EphR	Ephrins are the ligand for the Eph receptor tyrosine kinase family.	EphrinB-EphB receptor regulates the morphogenesis and maturation of spines.
Ras	Small GTPase activated by receptor tyrosine kinases, leading to activation of the MAP kinase pathway.	Ras/MAP kinase activation is required for filopodia formation resulting from depolarizing stimuli.
Rac	Small GTPase that regulates the actin cytoskeleton through mediators (Pak kinase).	Blockade of Rac1 induces long, thin spines and inhibits spine head growth, and stability.
RhoA, Rho kinase/ROCK	Small GTPase that regulates the actin cytoskeleton throuth Rho kinase/ROCK.	Activation of Rho A can result in loss of spines. Inhibition of Rho kinase induces long spines.
Kalirin	Dual Rho Guanine nucleotide exchange factor (GEF), activates Rac and Rho's.	Catalytically inactive Kalirin (does not activate Rac1) blocks ephrin-induced spine development.
Neurabin I, Spinophilin (Neurabin II)	Actin binding proteins that promote F-actin crosslinking. Also contain PP1 binding domains, PDZ domains, and C-terminal coiled-coil domains.	Knockouts of Spinophilin show increases in spine density, expression of Neurabin I in cultured cells causes filopodial outgrowth, dependent upon actin binding domain.
Cadherin, β-catenin	Cadherin is a Ca^{2+}-dependent homophilic adhesion molecule that couples with the actin-cytoskeleton via β-catenin.	Blockade of cadherin results in elongation and bifurcation of spine head, and disruption of the distribution of postsynaptic proteins.
NCAM	Membrane protein implicated in adhesion between neurons, located both pre and postsynaptic.	Levels of postsynaptic NCAM expression regulate the number and strength of excitatory synaptic connections.

Export of AMPARs from the endoplasmic reticulum may further require interaction between the carboxy-terminal domain of the AMPAR subunits and other proteins. The GluR2 subunit contains a carboxy-terminal PDZ consensus motif that allows for interaction with several PDZ domain-containing proteins. GluR2's exit from the endoplasmic reticulum is thought to be regulated by carboxy-terminal interaction with protein interacting with C kinase-1 (PICK1). SAP97 interacts with a PDZ motif in the carboxy-terminal region of GluR1. It has been suggested that this interaction occurs early, before GluR1 exits

the endoplasmic reticulum. Indeed, interference with PDZ dependent interactions prevents normal synaptic targeting of GluR1.

In vivo, functional NMDARs contain both NR1 and NR2 subunits, which assemble to form a tetrameric complex. More specifically, a functional receptor is thought to be comprised of two homodimers of two NR1 subunits and two NR2 subunits. The homodimer formed by the NR2 subunits can contain either the same or different NR2 splice variants, and this is also true for NR1 splice variants. Due to the number of possible combinations, a single neuron can contain multiple NMDAR complexes. As with AM-PAR complexes, little is known about the mechanism dictating the assembly of NMDARs in the endoplasmic reticulum. It is still undetermined whether NMDA assembly is regulated, or whether it is dependent solely upon the availability of subunits. When expressed alone in heterologous cell lines, neither NR1 nor NR2 subunits form functional receptors. As opposed to being expressed at the cell surface, the ubiquitous NR1-1 splice variant was retained within the endoplasmic reticulum. Endoplasmic reticulum retention of NR1 is dependent upon two carboxy-terminal motifs: the RRR motif, which serves as a retention signal, and the PDZ-interacting domain, which serves as an exit signal.

Interactions between SAP102 and Sec8 have also been shown to be important for the delivery of NMDARs to the cell surface. SAP102 interacts with the PDZ-binding domain of Sec8. The Sec genes, originally characterized in yeast mutants lacking secretory activity, have also been shown to be important for eukaryotic secretion involving the exocyst complex. The exocyst, also known as the Sec6/8 complex, is implicated in exocytosis and consists of eight proteins (Sec3, Sec5, Sec6, Sec8, Sec10, Sec15, Exo70 and Exo84). Specifically, the exocyst is thought to direct intracellular membrane vesicles to their fusion targets on the plasma membrane. The association of NMDARs and SAP102 with the exocyst complex suggests that PDZ protein–receptor interactions occur early in the secretory pathway, playing an important role in receptor delivery to synapses. This interaction also demonstrates that PDZ-containing proteins modulate organization and targeting of macromolecular complexes before they reach the plasma membrane, further regulating receptor expression and function.

Regulation of the abundance of NMDARs and AMPARs at excitatory synapses is critical during changes in synaptic efficacy associated with learning and memory. In particular, AMPARs undergo continuous cycling into and out of the postsynaptic membrane. AMPARs inserted during LTP are thought to originate from an intracellular vesicular pool. Internalized AMPARs are sorted in early endosomes either to a specialized recycling endosome compartment for reinsertion to the plasma membrane or to late endosomes and lysosomes for degradation. Ras-like GTPases of the Rab family have been implicated as regulators of organelle transport and gluatamte receptor trafficking. Rabs are monomeric G-proteins that function as molecular switches to control many eukaryotic cell functions. Multiple Rab GTPases, such as Rab1, Rab4, Rab5, Rab7 and Rab11, have been identified to regulate ER to Golgi transport as well as the endocytosis and trafficking of receptors between early, late and recycling endosomes and lysosomes. Specifically, Rab GTPases have been shown to determine the subcellular distribution of transported cargos by regulating the movement of vesicles and organelles along cytoskeletal filaments.

Recent studies show that Rab 5, Rab 8, and Rab 11 are involved in regulation of AMPAR insertion and recycling. Increased recycling leads to increased AMPAR surface expression. Conversely, blocking endocytic recycling results in reduced surface expression of AMPARs, confining AMPARs to recycling compartments within the dendrites. Further, this endocytic recycling is required for the maintenance of AMPAR, but not NMDAR surface expression at excitatory synapses. This indicates that neurons maintain a reserve pool of AMPARs that are readily available for modifying synaptic strength. For example, LTP has been shown to promote not only AMPAR insertion but also the recycling of cargo from endocytic compartments.

Molecular Motors

Once receptor subunits have been sorted and assembled, they must be transported great lengths from the soma to the dendritic compartment. Most receptors are synthesized a great distance away from the synapse and require some method of transport to reach their final target. The microtubule cytoskeleton is responsible for the majority of long-range transport along the dendritic shaft. The microtubule transport network is constructed out of long hollow cylinders of α- and β-tubulins, upon which kinesins and dyneins move a variety of cargoes.

Kinesin superfamily proteins (KIFs) and dynein superfamily proteins are microtubule-dependent motors that slide along microtubules through ATP hydrolysis. The microtubules in axons are unipolar, with the "plus end" in the direction of the synapse. By contrast, the microtubules in dendrites have mixed polarity in the proximal region and unipolarity in the distal region, with the "plus end" toward the periphery. Kinesins are primarily responsible for plus-end-directed movement on microtubules, although a few family members power minus-end-directed transport; whereas dyneins, are primarily minus-end-directed microtubule motors.

Kinesins and dyneins drive the transport of a wide variety of organelles and vesicular cargoes including endoplasmic reticulum (ER), Golgi, endosomes, lysosomes, mitochondria and transport vesicles containing receptors and other proteins. Inhibition of microtubule motors, dynein or kinesin, reduces AMPAR-mediated responses, suggesting that microtubule transport is important for the dynamic regulation of AMPARs. It has also been shown that the AMPAR GluR2 subunit-interacting protein (GRIP1) can directly interact with kinesin heavy chains. This interaction is thought to specifically involve KIF1A, and may also involve liprin-α. In general, GRIP forms a link between AMPARs and kinesins that mediates microtubule-based transport to synaptic sites.

Kinesins have also been implicated in NMDAR transport to synaptic sites. KIF17 is a neuron specific kinesin, localized to dendrites and implicated in the transport of vesicles containing the NR2B subunit NMDARs from the cell body to postsynaptic sites. Selective transport is mediated by the KIF17 PDZ domain which interacts with a large protein complex including mLin-2 (CASK), mLin-7 (MALS/Velis), and the NR2B subunit.

Following transport down the dendrite along the microtubule cytoskeleton, receptors reach dendritic spines and must be specifically transported to the synaptic active zone in order to be functional. Transport within the spine occurs via non-microtubule based transport, as dendritic spines lack microtubular cytoskeletons. Spines are rich in highly motile actin filaments involved in structural remodeling and transport. Actin depolymerization results in the removal of AMPARs from synaptic sites. A protein originally identified in erythrocytes, red blood cell protein 4.1, has been suggested to be important for the transport of AMPARs within the spine. Members of the protein 4.1 family link the spectrin–actin cytoskeleton to the cell membrane through interaction with membrane-associated proteins. Interestingly, the neuronal isoform 4.1N interacts directly with the carboxy-terminal regions of GluR1 or GluR4. Further, the surface expression of these AMPAR subunits in heteorlogous cells is dependent upon interaction with protein 4.1.

In addition to transport within the spine, the actin cytoskeleton has recently been suggested to contribute to long range transport along the dendrite in parallel to the microtubule system. Transport along the actin cytoskeleton is mediated by the myosin family of motor proteins. With actin as a scaffold, myosins use the energy of ATP hydrolysis for movement of a variety of cargoes. Virtually all eukaryotic cells contain at least one of the several classes of myosins (I–XVII). The high degree of conservation suggests that myosins play an important role in cellular maintenance. The class V myosins have a role in organelle transport in yeast, melanocytes and neurons. Myosin Va and b are present in dendrites and spines, and have been shown to be associated with postsynaptic proteins. The tail domain of myosin Vb indirectly interacts with the M4 muscarinic acetylcholine receptors, suggesting a role for myosins in the recycling of these receptors. A recent work also revealed a role for myosin Vb in the transport of GluR1 subunit. Expression of a dominant negative form of myosin Vb resulted in perinuclear accumulation of GluR1, reducing its surface expression and clustering at the synapse (Fig.6.5, see also the color plate).

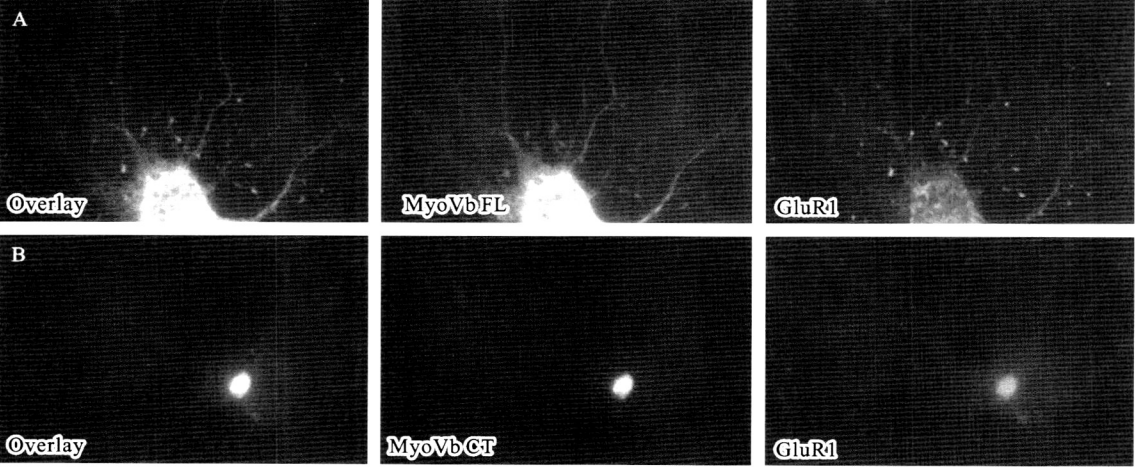

Fig.6.5 Involvement of myosin V motors in AMPAR trafficking. Effects of full length Myosin Vb (MyoVb FL) and a dominant negative form of Myosin Vb (C-terminal fragment; MyoVb CT) on trafficking of the AMPAR GluR1 subunit. Hippocampal neurons were transfected with either MyoVb FL or MyoVb CT and stained for GluR1. A. Left panel: overlay of MyoVb FL (green), and GluR1 (red). B. Left panel: overlay of MyoVb CT (green), and GluR1 (red). A. In neurons expressing MyoVb FL, GluR1 shows a normal distribution, and form clusters in the dendrites which are co-localized with the MyoVb FL. B. In neurons expressing the dominant negative form MyoVb CT, GluR1 is seen to accumulate in a perinuclear region containing MyoVb CT. A significant reduction in the number of GluR1 clusters was also observed. This suggests that MyoVb is required for proper trafficking of GluR1 from the soma to the synapse.

Two other types of myosins, myosin Va and myosin VI have been shown to be coupled to PDZ proteins. Myosin Va accumulates in dendritic spines and has been to associate with GKAP, a binding partner of PSD-95. This interaction would allow for the possible interaction and transport of several other proteins, including NMDA and AMPAR subunits. Myosin VI, on the other hand, binds SAP97, which in turn binds to the GluR1 subunit of AMPARs. Interestingly, expression of a dominant-negative myosin VI in vitro induces synapse loss. In addition, myosin VI deficient neurons demonstrate decreased numbers of synapses and alterations in dendritic spines *in vitro* and *in vivo*. Hippocampal neurons obtained from myosin VI deficient mice also show a defect in activity-induced endocytosis of AMPARs. These results are indicative of a possible role for actin-based transport in receptor recycling through interaction of PSD-95 family members and myosin motors.

Myosin II regulatory light chain co-localizes with NR1 in the dendritic spines of cultured hippocampal neurons and is found to complex with and modulate the function of multiple proteins including NR1, NR2A, B, and PSD-95 and modulate NMDAR function in vitro. Functional connectivity has also been shown between Rab proteins and motors of the actin cytoskeleton. This further implicates the actin cytoskeleton, mediated by Rabs and myosins in the transport of receptors within spines.

PROTEIN MODIFICATIONS AND RECEPTOR REGULATION

Phosphorylation

Kinases and Phosphatases in Receptor Regulation

Protein kinase activation, or phosphorylation, is a central mechanism of cellular regulation. This is especially true in the nervous system, where phosphorylation has been implicated in processes such as neurotransmitter synthesis and release, action potentials, ion channel conductance, and axonal transport. In addition to many other proteins, neurotransmitter receptors at the plasma membrane are highly regulated by phosphorylation. In fact, phosphorylation of ionotropic receptors is essential for structural and functional regulation of these important proteins.

Phosphorylation of AMPARs results in changes in receptor function and consequently, excitatory synaptic transmission. AMPAR mediated currents can be inhibited through the blockade of cAMP-dependent protein kinase (PKA). This result suggests that PKA may play a role in maintaining the basal level of AMPA-R function. Conversely, AMPAR mediated synaptic responses can be increased through expression of constitutively active calcium-calmodulin-dependent protein kinase II (CaMKII) or protein kinase C (PKC).

A large body of research has identified and characterized twelve distinct sites by which AMPARs are directly phosphorylated. The major phosphorylation sites of GluR1 are serine 831 and serine 845, located in the carboxy-terminal domain. Serine 845 is phosphorylated by cyclic-AMP dependent protein kinase (protein kinase A (PKA)), whereas serine 831 is phosphorylated by both PKC and CaMKII. Intracellular perfusion of PKA into heterologous cells expressing GluR1 resulted in potentiation of the peak amplitude of the whole-cell current, and regulated the open probability of the ion channel pore. Mutation of serine 845 to alanine abolishes this effect, demonstrating that this potentiation is dependent upon phosphorylation of serine 845 on GluR1 by PKA. Similarly, CaMKII has been shown to potentiate AMPA-R function in GluR1-transfected heterologous cells through regulation of the open-channel conductance. Analogously, mutation of serine 831 to alanine eliminates the potentiation induced by CaMKII and also reduces the basal response of GluR1 to glutamate application.

The GluR2 subunit also has two serine phosphorylation sites in its carboxy-terminal domain, serine 863 and serine 880. These phosphorylation sites are conserved in the carboxy-termini of GluR3 and GluR4c. PKC acts as the primary kinase for both serine 863 and serine 880. Interestingly, serine 880 is located in the carboxy-terminal region of GluR2 which has been shown to interact with PDZ protein scaffolds. Phosphorylation regulated interaction of GluR2 with PDZ-domain-containing proteins may act to modulate the synaptic targeting of AMPARs. In addition, the AMPAR-associated protein stargazin is phosphorylated and this phosphorylation promotes the synaptic trafficking of AMPARs. Activation of synaptic NMDARs can act to induce both stargazin phosphorylation and dephosphorylation through activation of kinases and phosphatases respectively. Stargazin phosphorylation is initiated by CaMKII and PKC, whereas stargazin dephosphorylation is achieved through activation of protein phosphatase 1 (PP1).

Tyrosine phosphorylation is the primary regulator of NMDAR activity. PSD-95, the NMDAR binding partner, associates with the Src family of non-receptor tyrosine kinases (SFKs). SFKs upregulate the function of NMDARs and are thought to act as a molecular hub on which various signalling pathways converge. SFKs link G-protein coupled receptors, receptor protein tyrosine kinase signaling, the Ras pathway and the cytokine and integrin receptor pathways to NMDARs, providing many potential avenues for modulation of receptor function. SFK activity is highly regulated through phosphorylation and dephosphorylation events that modulate SFK intramolecular interactions. For example, SFKs can be activated by protein tyrosine phosphatases (PTPs), or by extrinsic ligands that disrupt the intramolecular interactions.

The NR2B subunit of the NMDAR is the primary substrate for tyrosine-phosphorylation in the PSD. The NR2A receptor subunit is also subject to tyrosine-phosphorylation. These subunits are characterized by long intracellular carboxy-terminal tails with 25 tyrosine residues each; however it is unclear which tyrosine residues undergo phosphorylation, mediating the effects of SFKs on NMDAR function.

Organizing Kinases and Phosphatases: A-Kinase Anchoring Proteins (AKAPs)

In order to control postsynaptic signaling, scaffolding and anchoring proteins target protein kinases and phosphatases to distinct subcellular environments, where they can control the phosphorylation state of associated substrates. Recruitment of kinases and phosphatases provides temporal regulation of neurotransmission. A-kinase anchoring proteins (AKAPs) are archetypical scaffolding proteins that act to organize receptor signaling in the PSD. More specifically, AKAPs function to compartmentalize PKA as well as other important enzymes.

AKAPs dimerize with the N-terminus of PKA via an amphipathic helix of 14–18 residues. The compartmentalization of these dimmers is regulated by multiple targeting domains present on the AKAP protein. Many AKAP proteins are localized based on long-chain fatty acid modification such as myristolation, prenylation, and palmitoylation (to be discussed below) of specific protein domains. AKAP79/150 is anchored to the plasma membrane through sequences that bind phospholipids.

AKAP79/150 is enriched in the dendritic spines of neurons, specifically in the PSD fractions. AKAP79 forms a signaling complex, through interaction with the A subunit of the Ca^{2+}/calmodulin-dependent phosphatase PP2B and PKC, that regulates the phosphorylation and thus function of a variety of ion channels including both AMPA and NMDARs, L-type calcium channels, M-type potassium channels and aquaporin water channels. For example, anchored PKA promotes the phosphorylation of the GluR1 subunit, whereas anchored PP2B dephosphorylates this subunit at the same site. This complex allows for the integration of multiple second-messengers at postsynaptic membranes, leading to coordinated signaling.

Through interaction with PKA and PP2B, AKAPs regulate cAMP-dependent phosphorylation, which in turn controls the activity and surface expression of synaptic AMPARs. NMDAR activation causes the loss of PKA from the synapse and a reduction in AMPAR surface expression. Inhibition of PKA also results in reduced surface expression of AMPARs. Further, a disruption of the PKA–AKAP interaction results in a reduction in synaptic AMPARs in cultured neurons. The AKAP79/150 signaling complex indirectly binds the GluR1 subunit of the AMPAR via PSD-95 or SAP97. AKAP-anchored PP2B may also dephosphorylate the PSD-95-associated ubiquitin E3 ligase, MDM2, resulting in its activation. The outcome of this activation is ubiquitination of PSD-95, and dissociation of the AKAP complex from the AMPAR, leading to internalization. Thus anchored PKA and PP2B act in opposition, where phosphorylation maintains the surface expression and dephosphorylation signals the internalization of the AMPAR.

AKAPs have been shown to regulate AMPARs through a dopamine mediated mechanism. It has been shown that treatment with a dopamine receptor agonist enhances GluR1 phosphorylation, increasing its surface expression. Mutant AKAP79/150 or PSD-95, that fails to target synaptic sites, disrupts these effects of dopamine signaling on GluR1. Importantly, *in vivo* stimulation of dopamine release in the ventral tegmental area also results in increased GluR1 phosphorylation in the nucleus accumbens. When paired with the *in vitro* data, these results indicate that AMPAR dynamics may be regulated by the association of GluR1 with AKAP79/150 via PSD-95.

The interaction of NMDARs with multiple AKAPs is also suggestive of dynamic regulation of NMDAR signaling. In addition to mediating association with AMPAR's, PSD-95 connects AKAP79/150 to the NR2B subunit of the NMDARs. Additionally, the yotiao splice variant of AKAP350 binds to the cytoplasmic tail of the NR1 subunit of the NMDAR. Yotiao binding associates neuronal inositol triphosphate receptors (IP(3)R) with the NR1 subunit, providing a link between cAMP and calcium signaling. The modification of AKAP regulated protein complexes can thus result in dynamic alterations in the effects of glutamate signaling in the PSD.

Palmitoylation

Another mechanism mediating the trafficking of proteins to the plasma membrane is through the addition of long-chain fatty acids. Two well characterized lipid modifications include the co-translational addition of myristic acid to the amino-terminal glycine (myristoylaiton), and the post-translational attachment of prenyl groups to carboxy-terminal cysteine containing motifs (prenylation). In palmitoylation, palmitate is linked through thioester bonds to cysteine residues. This lipid modification increases hydrophobicity thus facilitating protein interaction with the membrane. Palmitoylation, in contrast to stable myristoylation and prenylation, is a reversible modification allowing for dynamic regulation of protein targeting.

PSD-95 is one prototypical palmitoylated protein. Palmitoylation of PSD-95 is essential for postsynaptic targeting. Alternative splicing of the amino-terminus of PSD-95 generates two isoforms, PSD-95α and PSD-95β. PSD-95α is palmitoylated, whereas PSD-95β which lacks amino-terminal cysteines is not palmitoylated and does not cluster ion channels. Other members of the PSD-95 family have different palmitoylation states that influence their functions. The PSD-95 family of membrane-associated guanylyl kinases (MAGUKs) includes PSD-93/Chapsyn-110, SAP-97/HDLG, and SAP-102, all of which contain similar protein-protein interaction domains. Although the amino-terminus of PSD-93 and SAP-102 both contain cysteines, only PSD-93 is palmitoylated and clusters ion channels. The amino-terminus of SAP-102 lacks surrounding hydrophobic amino acids that are required for palmitoylation. SAP-97 lacks amino-terminal cysteines, is not palmitoylated and does not act to cluster ion channels at postsynaptic sites. Attaching the amino-terminus of palmitoylated PSD-95 to SAP-97 instigates postsynaptic clustering of the chimera, further demonstrating the importance of this domain in the function of MAGUKs.

The ABP/GRIP (glutamate receptor interacting protein) family of scaffolding proteins is also palmitoylated. Similar to PSD-95, these scaffolding proteins contain multiple PDZ domains and act to organize signaling at excitatory synapses. ABP/GRIP proteins differ from PSD-95 family proteins in that they do not contain SH3 or guanylyl kinase domains. Further, ABP/GRIP proteins bind directly to AMPARs as opposed to NMDARs. Alternative splicing of the amino-terminus results in differential palmitoylation of specific isoforms of ABP/GRIP. As with PSD-95, only the palmitoylated isoform clusters at synapses, whereas the non-palmitoylated isoform creates intracellular clusters. The different palmitoylation states of ABP/GRIP may allow it to function as an anchor in AMPAR transport from intracellular sites to synaptic sites.

Many physiological stimuli alter protein palmitoylation levels, providing an important mechanism for regulating cell signaling at the synapse. On the presynaptic side, palmitate is added to several neurotransmitter vesicle proteins, thus regulating neurotransmitter release. On the postsynaptic side, synaptic scaffolding proteins that organize receptors are modified by palmitate, adapting the receptor clustering function of these proteins. Further, neurotransmitter receptors themselves are palmitoylated, adding another level of signal transduction regulation. As mentioned above, PSD-95 acts to cluster ion channels on the plasma membrane when overexpressed in heterologous cell lines. This clustering activity is dependent upon a pair of amino-terminal cysteine residues which are sites of palmitoylation. Mutation of the cysteine residues of PSD-95 prevents palmitoylation and ion channel clustering, causing accumulation in the perinuclear compartment. In neurons, palmitoylation is thought to initially target PSD-95 to transport vesicles. Blocking palmitoylation using 2-bromopalmitate disperses PSD-95/AMPAR clusters (Fig.6.6, see also the color plate). This result suggests that PSD-95 regularly alternates between palmitoylated and non-palmitoylated states, and that PSD-95 palmitoylation is necessary for AMPAR clustering. Prolonged synaptic activity accelerates depalmitoylation of PSD-95, resulting in enhanced AMPAR endocytosis. Further, these results demonstrate that PSD-95/ stargazin/AMPAR clusters are not stable structures, but instead maintain the capacity for reorganization and dynamic regulation.

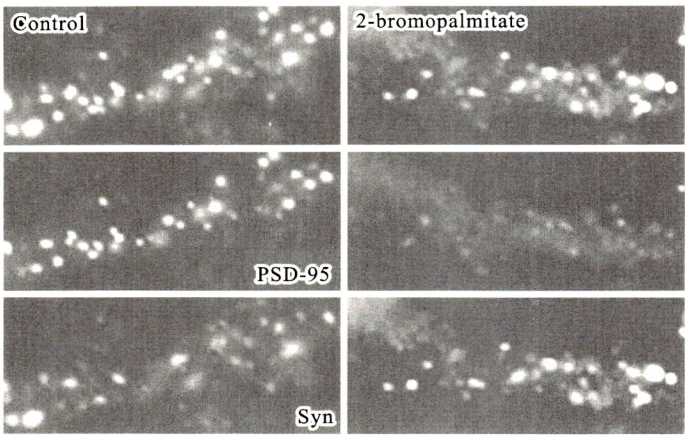

Fig.6.6 Modification of PSD-95 with the lipid palmitate is required for postsynaptic targeting. Effects of blocking protein palmitoylation on synaptic targeting of PSD-95. Hippocampal neurons were either treated with vehicle alone or with 100 μM 2-bromopalmitate, an agent that block protein palmitoylation, for 8 hours and then stained for PSD-95 (green) and synaptophysin (Syn) (red). Enlarged segments of dendrites are shown below. Normal distribution of PSD-95 clusters at synaptic sites. Treatment with 2-bromopalmitate, disperses synaptic clusters of PSD-95.

Protein Degradation

The rates of exocytosis and endocytosis determine the turn-over rate of membrane proteins including receptors. Endocytosis is mediated by cytoplasmic-coat proteins such as clathrin, which assemble into a pit-shaped invagination and slowly pinch the vesicle off from the surrounding membrane. Once removed from the membrane via endocytosis, receptors or other proteins can be sorted for reinsertion into the plasma membrane or for degradation. As with recycling and reinsertion, recent studies have demonstrated that the degradation process represents another organized mechanism to dynamically regulate excitatory neurotransmission.

The activity-dependent remodeling of the PSD is often associated with alterations in protein turnover. A recent study has demonstrated that increased protein turnover, resulting from synaptic activity corresponds with increases or decreases in ubiquitin conjugation of synaptic proteins. Further, long lasting activity-dependent changes were shown to require proteasome-mediated degradation. Ubiquitination involves the addition of ubiquitin to lysine groups in the target protein. First, ubiquitin forms a high-energy thioester bond with the ubiquitin-activating enzyme, termed E1. The activated ubiquitin is then transferred to a ubiquitin-conjugating enzyme (E2) and ligated to lysine residues in the substrate protein by a ubiquitin-ligase (E3). Proteins can be either mono-ubiquitinated or poly-ubiquitinated, and the extent of

unbiquitination determines the fate of the protein. Poly-ubiquitination targets proteins for proteasomal degradation. Degradation, in turn, alters downstream signaling to effectors such as CREB (cyclic AMP response element binding protein) and ERK-MAPK (extracellular signal regulated kinase—MAP kinase). On the other hand, the attachment of a single ubiquitin molecule to a substrate protein has been implicated in sorting of cargo proteins and internalization of cell surface receptors.

NMDAR targeting for either degradation or recycling is coordinated by distinct domains of NMDAR subunits. Membrane-proximal domains of NR1 and NR2 are important for protein internalization and transport to late endosomes for degradation. In contrast, distal C-terminal domains of NR2B mediate endocytosis and signal for protein recycling to the plasma membrane. These data suggest that NMDAR abundance at the synapse is regulated by the intracellular trafficking machinery mediated by specific domains present in individual subunits.

The scaffolding action of PSD-95 is another example of regulation via the ubiquitin-proteasome pathway. PSD-95 is ubiquitinated by the E3 ligase Mdm2 (murine double minute) in response to NMDAR activation. This ubiquitination results in the rapid removal of PSD-95 from synaptic sites through proteasome-dependent degradation. Blocking PSD-95 ubiquitination through mutation prevents NMDA-induced AMPAR internalization. Correspondingly, proteasome inhibitors also prevent NMDA-induced AMPAR endocytosis. From these results it has been suggested that ubiquitination of PSD-95 contributes to the regulation of AMPAR surface expression. Ubiquitination has been shown to be a general mechanism of targeting proteins for degradation, and can also serve to regulate intracellular trafficking. Further, activity can regulate the ubiquitin-proteasome system, providing control of protein turnover for the functional reorganization of synapses.

CONCLUSIONS

Recent findings revealed that the development of excitatory synapses involves specialized proteins that regulate synapse formation, receptor clustering and synaptic activity. Changes in synaptic activity are usually reflected in an overall change in the number of receptors available at the synapse. Moreover, long-lasting changes in synaptic activity are controlled by the number of synaptic AMPA receptors present at the synapse. Activity also modulates protein trafficking, clustering, recycling and degradation. The large number of proteins found clustered at excitatory synapses indicates that diverse mechanisms exist to fine tune synaptic function. Many of these molecules have been recently shown to directly influence synapse morphology and clustering of specific subunits of glutamate receptors. The recent identification of many receptor binding partners has begun to explain the mechanisms involved in glutamate receptor trafficking.

GENERAL CITATIONS

Bauman AL, Goehring AS, Scott JD. 2004. Orchestration of synaptic plasticity through AKAP signaling complexes. *Neuropharmacology*, 46:299-310.

Bredt DS, Nicoll RA. 2003. AMPA receptor trafficking at excitatory synapses. *Neuron*, 40:361-379.

Ehlers MD. 2002. Molecular morphogens for dendritic spines. *Trends Neurosci*, 25:64-67.

Ehlers MD. 2004. Deconstructing the axon: Wallerian degeneration and the ubiquitin-proteasome system. *Trends Neurosci*, 27:3-6.

El-Husseini Ael D, Bredt DS. 2002. Protein palmitoylation: a regulator of neuronal development and function. *Nat Rev Neurosci*, 3:791-802.

Hering H, Sheng M. 2001. Dendritic spines: structure, dynamics and regulation. *Nat Rev Neurosci*, 2:880-888.

Isaac JT. 2003. Postsynaptic silent synapses: evidence and mechanisms. *Neuropharmacology*, 45:450-460.

Kim E, Sheng M. 2004. PDZ domain proteins of synapses. *Nat Rev Neurosci*, 5:771-781.

Li Z, Sheng M. 2003. Some assembly required: the development of neuronal synapses. *Nat Rev Mol Cell Biol*, 4:833-841.

McGee AW, Bredt DS. 2003. Assembly and plasticity of the glutamatergic postsynaptic specialization. *Curr Opin Neurobiol*, 13:111-118.

Nakanishi S. 1992. Molecular diversity of glutamate receptors and implications for brain function. *Science*, 258:597-603.

Swope SL, Moss SJ, Raymond LA, Huganir RL. 1999. Regulation of ligand-gated ion channels by protein phosphorylation. *Adv Second Messenger Phosphoprotein Res*, 33:49-78.

Washbourne P, Dityatev A, Scheiffele P, Biederer T, Weiner JA, Christopherson KS, et al. 2004. Cell adhesion molecules in synapse formation. *J Neurosci*, 24:9244-9249.

Wenthold RJ, Prybylowski K, Standley S, Sans N, Petralia RS. 2003. Trafficking of NMDA receptors. *Annu Rev Pharmacol Toxicol*, 43:335-358.

Xiao B, Tu JC, Worley PF. 2000. Homer: a link between neural activity and glutamate receptor function. *Curr Opin Neurobiol*, 10:370-374.

DISCOVERY CITATIONS

Chih B, Engelman H, Scheiffele P. 2005. Control of excitatory and inhibitory synapse formation by neuroligins. *Science*, 307:1324-1328.

Ehlers MD. 2000. Reinsertion or degradation of AMPA receptors determined by activity-dependent endocytic sorting. *Neuron*, 28:511-525.

Ehlers MD. 2003. Activity level controls postsynaptic composition and signaling via the ubiquitin-proteasome system. *Nat Neurosci*, 6:231-242.

El-Husseini AE, Schnell E, Chetkovich DM, Nicoll RA, Bredt DS. 2000. PSD-95 involvement in maturation of excitatory synapses. *Science*, 290: 1364-1368.

El-Husseini AE, Craven SE, Chetkovich DM, Firestein BL, Schnell E, Aoki C, *et al.* 2000. Dual palmitoylation of PSD-95 mediates its vesiculotubular sorting, postsynaptic targeting, and ion channel clustering. *J Cell Biol*, 148:159-172.

El-Husseini Ael D, Schnell E, Dakoji S, Sweeney N, Zhou Q, Prange O, *et al.* 2002. Synaptic strength regulated by palmitate cycling on PSD-95. *Cell*, 108:849-863.

Gomez LL, Alam S, Smith KE, Horne E, Dell'Acqua ML. 2002. Regulation of A-kinase anchoring protein 79/150-cAMP-dependent protein kinase postsynaptic targeting by NMDA receptor activation of calcineurin and remodeling of dendritic actin. *J Neurosci*, 22:7027-7044.

Hawkins LM, Prybylowski K, Chang K, Moussan C, Stephenson FA, Wenthold RJ. 2004. Export from the endoplasmic reticulum of assembled N-methyl- d-aspartic acid receptors is controlled by a motif in the c terminus of the NR2 subunit. *J Biol Chem*, 279:28903-28910.

Hirbec H, Francis JC, Lauri SE, Braithwaite SP, Coussen F, Mulle C, *et al.* 2003. Rapid and differential regulation of AMPA and kainate receptors at hippocampal mossy fibre synapses by PICK1 and GRIP. *Neuron*, 37:625-638.

Huganir RL, Delcour AH, Greengard P, Hess GP. 1986. Phosphorylation of the nicotinic acetylcholine receptor regulates its rate of desensitization. *Nature*, 321:774-776.

Isaac JT, Nicoll RA, Malenka RC. 1995. Evidence for silent synapses: implications for the expression of LTP. *Neuron*, 15:427-434.

Lau LF, Huganir RL. 1995. Differential tyrosine phosphorylation of N-methyl-D-aspartate receptor subunits. *J Biol Chem*, 270:20036-20041.

Monyer H, Seeburg PH, Wisden W. 1991. Glutamate-operated channels: developmentally early and mature forms arise by alternative splicing. *Neuron*, 6:799-810.

O'Brien RJ, Xu D, Petralia RS, Steward O, Huganir RL, Worley P. 1999. Synaptic clustering of AMPA receptors by the extracellular immediate-early gene product Narp. *Neuron*, 23:309-323.

Osterweil E, Wells DG, Mooseker MS. 2005. A role for myosin VI in postsynaptic structure and glutamate receptor endocytosis. *J Cell Biol*, 168: 329-338.

Pak DT, Yang S, Rudolph-Correia S, Kim E, Sheng M. 2001. Regulation of dendritic spine morphology by SPAR, a PSD-95-associated RapGAP. *Neuron*, 31:289-303.

Prange O, Wong TP, Gerrow K, Wang YT, El-Husseini A. 2004. A balance between excitatory and inhibitory synapses is controlled by PSD-95 and neuroligin. *Proc Natl Acad Sci USA*, 101:13915- 13920.

Priel A, Kolleker A, Ayalon G, Gillor M, Osten P, Stern-Bach Y. 2005. Stargazin reduces desensitization and slows deactivation of the AMPA-type glutamate receptors. *J Neurosci*, 25:2682-2686.

Sala C, Piech V, Wilson NR, Passafaro M, Liu G, Sheng M. 2001. Regulation of dendritic spine morphology and synaptic function by Shank and Homer. *Neuron*, 31:115-130.

Sans N, Petralia RS, Wang YX, Blahos J 2nd, Hell JW, Wenthold RJ. 2000. A developmental change in NMDA receptor-associated proteins at hippocampal synapses. *J Neurosci*, 20:1260-1271.

Tomita S, Fukata M, Nicoll RA, Bredt DS. 2004. Dynamic interaction of stargazin-like TARPs with cycling AMPA receptors at synapses. *Science*, 303:1508-1511.

Xia H, Hornby ZD, Malenka RC. 2001. An ER retention signal explains differences in surface expression of NMDA and AMPA receptor subunits. *Neuropharmacology*, 41:714-723.

Spinal Glutamate Receptors

CHAPTER 7

Megumu Yoshimura

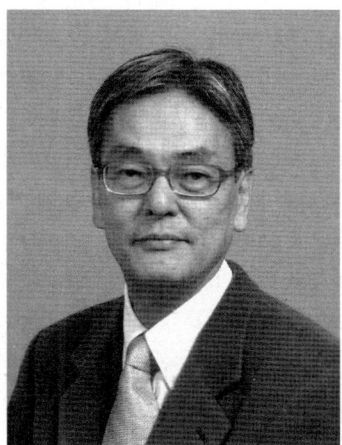

Dr. Yoshimura is a Professor and Chair in the Department of Integrative Physiology, Kyushu University, Fukuoka, Japan. He graduated from Kurume University, obtaining a M.D. in Medicine. He continued with his Ph.D. in Physiology at Kurume University.

MAJOR CONTRIBUTIONS

1. Furue H, Narikawa K, Kumamoto E, Yoshimura M. 1999. Responsiveness of rat substantia gelatinosa neurons to mechanical but not thermal stimuli revealed by *in vivo* patch-clamp recording. *J Physiol (London)*, 521:529-535.
2. Sonohata M, Furue H, Katafuchi T, Yasaka T, Doi A, Kumamoto E, Yoshimura M. 2004. Actions of noradrenaline on substantia gelatinosa neurones in the rat spinal cord revealed by *in vivo* patch recording. *J Physiol*, 555 (2): 515-526.
3. Yoshimura M, Furue H, Nakatsuk T, Matayoshi T, Katafuchi T. 2004. Functional reorganization of the spinal pain pathways in developmental and pathological conditions. In: Chadwick DJ and Goode J, eds. Novartis Foundation Symposium 261, *Pathological pain: From molecular to clinical aspects*. John Wiley & Sons, Ltd. 116-131.
4. Kato G, Furue H, Katafuchi T, Yasaka T, Iwamoto Y, Yoshimura M. 2004. Electrophysiological mapping of the nociceptive inputs to the substantia gelatinosa in rat horizontal spinal cord slices. *J Physiol (London)*, 560(1): 303-315.
5. Yoshimura M, Furue H, Nakatsuka H, Katafuchi T. 2004. Analysis of receptive fields revealed by *in vivo* patch-clamp recordings from dorsal horn neurons and in situ intracellular recordings from dorsal root ganglion neurons. In: Kumazawa T and Toide K, eds. The First International Pfizer Science and Research Symposium: Key Topic 2003: Central Mechanism of Neuropathic Pain. *Life Sciences*, 74: 2611-2618.

MAIN TOPICS

Fast excitatory synaptic transmission in the spinal dorsal horn

Slow excitatory synaptic current in dorsal horn neurons

In vivo patch-clamp analysis

Contribution of glutamate receptor subtypes to sensory transmission in the spinal dorsal horn

Presynaptic glutamate receptor

Metabotropic glutamate receptor

SUMMARY

The synapse of spinal dorsal horn neurons formed with primary afferents, interneurons or descending systems is the first step in the central nervous system (CNS) in which incoming sensory information is modified and integrated in differential manners according to the functional modality of the conversing inputs. Based on data obtained by immunohistochemical and electrophysiological examinations, all classes of primary afferents seem to release glutamate as a primary transmitter. Recently glutamate has also been shown to act at the terminals of primary afferents and GABAergic/glycinergic inhibitory interneurons, consequently modifying the strengthening of sensory transmissions. All types of ionotropic glutamate receptors, AMPA, Kainate and NMDA subtypes are expressed at the terminals; the AMPA receptor with GluR2 and GluR3 (GluR2/3) are expressed predominantly on myelinated fibers, while GluR2/4 are expressed predominantly on unmyelinated fibers. The termination of GluR2/3 positive afferents is in laminae II and IV, whereas GluR2/4 is found predominantly in laminae I and II. Spinal cord slice experiments have shown that the activation of presynaptic kainate receptors reduces the release of glutamate; data is consistent with that obtained from DRG-dorsal horn neurons co-culture preparations. In contrast, an activation of NMDA receptors is shown to produce hyperexcitability in sensory pathways by the release of substance P or glutamate from small diameter afferents. Similarly, a release of GABA and glycine is reported to be under the control of glutamate. In addition, metabotropic receptors are also expressed at primary afferents as well as spinal dorsal horn neurons. mGluR2/3-like immunoreactivities are found in L4 and L5 dorsal root ganglion neurons. The mGluR2/3 positive DRG neurons are small in diameter and also IB4 positive. These small afferents terminate preferentially in lamina IIi, which is consistent with the termination of IB4 positive afferents. mGluR4a—immunoreactive elements are seen in the dorsal horn, in particular in lamina II. The positive neurons found in dorsal root ganglion are small to medium in size. These presynaptic metabotropic receptors work synergistically or antagonistically with ionotropic receptors and control the release of glutamate from the primary afferents and interneurons, acting in concert to modify the nociceptive transmission in the spinal dorsal horn.

INTRODUCTION

The spinal pathway and functional role of primary afferents that convey nociceptive information to the CNS have been extensively examined by a combination of anatomical, immunohistochemical and physiological techniques which enable us to demonstrate a precise organization of the circuitry and ultra-structure of central terminals of a functionally characterized population of sensory fibers. To clarify how nociceptive information conveyed by the functionally diverse classes of primary afferents is modified, transmitters at afferent synapses with dorsal horn neurons are to be resolved. It is important in particular to determine whether functionally distinct classes of nociceptive as well as non-nociceptive afferents release distinct transmitters. Recent developments in whole cell recording techniques which have been adopted to spinal cord slice preparations have begun to disclose the characteristics of fast excitatory as well as inhibitory responses elicited in response to stimulation of primary afferents. Excitatory amino acids, in particular glutamate, have been proposed as a transmitter for the fast EPSP (excitatory postsynaptic potential, or EPSC in voltage clamp condition) at the afferent terminals based on both biochemical and physiological criteria.

Recently glutamate or related amino acids are also shown to have modulatory effects on the release of excitatory or inhibitory transmitters from both primary and interneuron terminals. These modulations are exerted through various glutamate receptor subtypes, including ionotropic and metabotropic receptors. Since glutamate is a prevalent transmitter, and since there is an excess of released glutamate which could diffuse to the vicinities of synapses, possibly affecting the strengthening of nociceptive transmission. Therefore, the identification of receptor subtypes involved in the modulations would be essential to develop a chemical producing analgesia.

This chapter reviews firstly the recent progress in the physiological, pharmacological and immunohistochemical properties of fast synaptic transmitter and their post-and pre-synaptic actions in dorsal horn neurons. Secondly, the slow synaptic responses that may contribute to the functional specificity of nociceptive

ceptive connections will be described. Lastly, recent progress in research on the post- and pre-synaptic ionotropic and metabotropic glutamate receptor subtypes will be discussed.

FAST EXCITATORY SYNAPTIC TRANSMISSION IN THE SPINAL DORSAL HORN

In spite of the fact that glutamate is a leading candidate as a transmitter for primary afferents, which has been demonstrated through several lines of evidence, the rigorous identification of glutamate as a transmitter could not be made with certainty until recently. High concentrations of glutamate and related enzymes are found in a subclass of DRG neurons. In early immunohistochemcal studies large DRG neurons are found to be labeled, whereas in other study few are labeled. On the other hand, a large number of labeled small neurons are also reported. This inconsistency might be due to at least in part, the difficulty in staining glutamate and its enzymes. Since the development

of slice patch recordings, a fast EPSC at the superficial dorsal horn, in particular the substantia gelatinosa (SG), has been shown to be mediated by the activation of the AMPA receptor subtype.

Primary afferent fibers terminated at the superficial dorsal horn are predominantly thinly myelinated Aδ and unmyelinated C fibers, only a few neurons are innervated by large Aδ afferents. In contrast, the deep dorsal horn is innervated by large Aβ and to some extent by Aβ afferents. The Aβ evoked EPSCs as well as Aδ and C afferent EPSCs are also blocked by the AMPA receptor antagonist, CNQX(Fig.7.1). The interaction of glutamate with non-NMDA receptors is likely to be responsible for the initial signaling of cutaneous sensory input in the dorsal horn. In addition, the Ia afferent excitation of motoneurons in the spinal ventral horn is also antagonized by a glutamate receptor antagonist. These observations support that the primary afferents, including muscle afferent, regardless of their sensory modalities release glutamate as a fast transmitter.

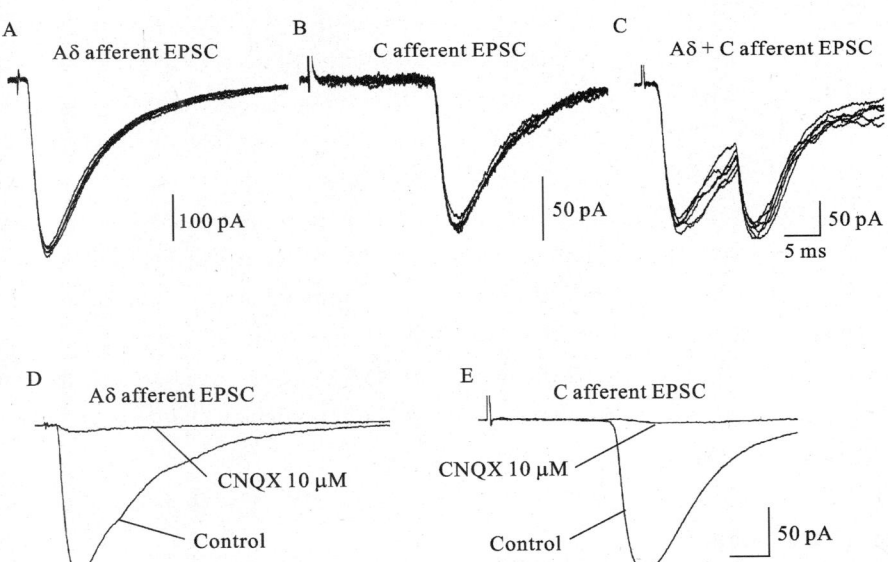

Fig.7.1 Aδ and C afferent-evoked synaptic responses in substantia gelatinosa neurons and its sensitivity to CNQX. Dorsal root stimulation evokes EPSCs mediated by Aδ (40 %), C (30 %) and Aδ + C (30 %) afferents. The Aδ and C afferent mediated EPSCs are blocked by CNQX (from Ataka et al., 2000; reproduced with permission).

In addition to the glutamate hypothesis, Holton and Holton (1954) provide evidence that adenosine triphosphate (ATP) is released from unmyelinated sensory fibers and suggest that ATP might be a transmitter of primary afferents in the spinal cord. Consistently with this notion, ATP is demonstrated electrophysiologically as a fast transmitter in a small proportion of primary afferent fibers. This notion is further supported by the fact that ATP is released by primary afferent stimulation into the spinal cord and the application of ATP produces a rapid excitation of dorsal horn neurons. However, the experiment performed by Bardoni is made using neonatal rats. ATP mediated fast EPSC has not been reported in matured rat spinal cords, suggesting a phenotypic change in releasable transmitters during maturation.

In addition to glutamate and ATP, aspartate is proposed to be a transmitter in the sensory pathway, in particular in spinal interneurons. Although the possibility of aspartate's role in transmission can't be excluded, recent electrophysiological data is still contradictory.

SLOW EXCITATORY SYNAPTIC CURRENT IN DORSAL HORN NEURONS

Under the current clamp condition, the contribution of NMDA receptors is tested in the synaptic responses at lamina II (substantia gelatinosa; SG) neurons by stimulation of Aδ and C afferents. A NMDA receptor antagonist, AP-5 has a small effect on the EPSPs, reducing the amplitude and decay phase slightly of the EPSPs.

However, the NMDA component becomes prominent even at a holding potential of –70 mV in the presence of GABA and glycine receptor antagonists, indicating that the duration of the dorsal root evoked EPSPs is limited or controlled by inhibitory currents. Consistently, the NMDA current shows a large amplitude comparable to the AMPA component when recorded at holding potentials of +40 mV and –70 mV, respectively, while in the presence of inhibitory receptor antagonists. Thus, the contribution of the NMDA component is as significant as those in other CNS synapses. However, the NMDA component is modified by inhibitory inputs lessening its significance in SG.

In addition to the slow EPSC mediated by the NMDA receptor, a much slower EPSC following the fast EPSCs is elicited in the majority of SG neurons. Repetitive focal stimulation applied to the SG or Aδ afferents elicit a slow EPSC that lasts for up to 5 s. The slow EPSC as well as a current evoked by the

application of aspartate reveal similar reversal potentials and show a marked outward rectification at holding potentials more negative than –30 mV, while the glutamate-induced current exhibites a relatively linear voltage relationship. In addition, the slow EPSCs are reversibly occluded during the aspartate-induced current but not by the glutamate-induced current. The slow EPSCs evoked by focal stimulation are slightly depressed but not abolished by CNQX with AP-5 (100 µM). Consistently, the aspartate- and glutamate-induced currents are also resistant to these antagonists. These observations suggest that a transmitter release, presumably from interneurons which are activated in part by Aδ afferents, mediates slow EPSCs and that an excitatory amino acid is presumably implicated in the generation of the slow EPSCs. These findings have been recorded with consistency although the receptor appears to differ from the known ligand-gated channels. C afferents are unlikely to contribute to the slow EPSC.

The glutamate-mediated slow synaptic current has been also reported in neonatal deep dorsal horn neurons. In this examination, Aδ and C but not Aδ afferent stimulation elicits a long lasting slow EPSC. Since the slow component is blocked by AP-5, deep dorsal horn neurons receive fast AMPA receptor mediated EPSCs and NMDA receptor mediated polysynaptic responses. The long time course is presumably due to a temporal summation of NMDA components(Fig.7.2). A slow EPSC mediated by temporal summation of NMDA receptor has not been reported in SG neurons, therefore, contribution of an NMDA receptor subtype is likely to be distinct between the superficial and deep dorsal horn.

IN VIVO PATCH-CLAMP ANALYSIS

The slice preparation is one useful method for analyzing synaptic transmission by the stimulation of a dorsal root. However, it is difficult to identify what kind of sensory modality is carried by afferent fibers in *in vitro* preparations. To address this problem, an *in vivo* patch-clamp recording method has been developed, which enable us to analyze synaptic current elicited by natural stimuli applied to the skin. In spite

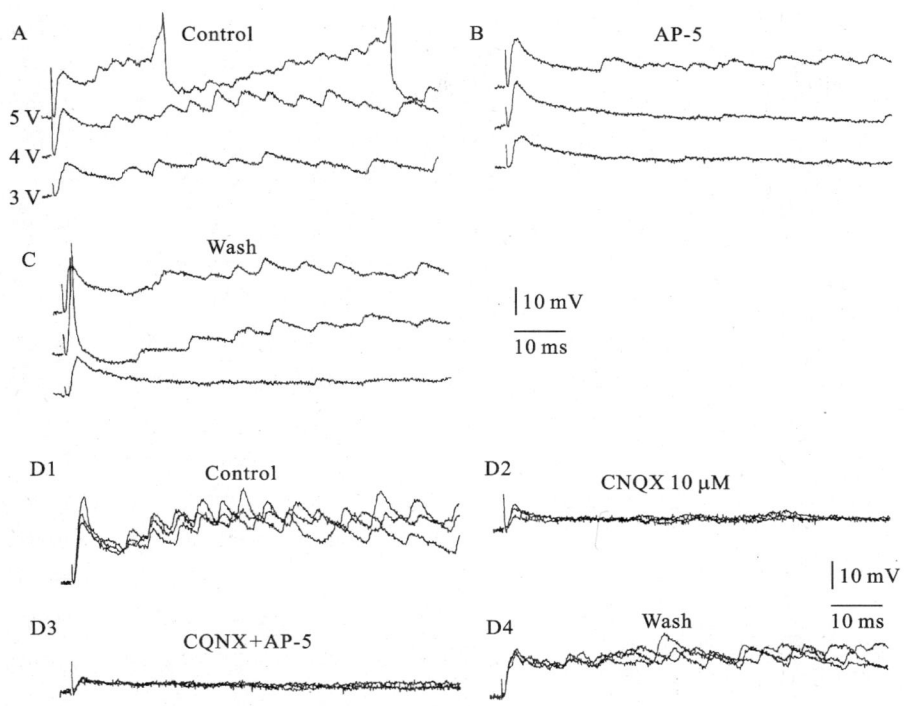

Fig.7.2 Dorsal root evoked mono- and polysynaptic responses in deep lamina neurons. Under the current clamp condition, increasing in stimulus intensity causes an increase in amplitude of monosynaptic EPSPs, which are followed by polysynaptic multi-peak EPSPs, probably due to a summation of EPSPs. NMDA receptor antagonist, AP-5 selectively depresses the polysynaptic but not the monosynaptic components (B). Both mono-and poly-synaptic components are depressed by CNQX (D2).

of these advantages, few laboratories are utilizing this method at present(see Chapter 33). This may be due at least in part, to difficulties in obtaining stable recordings from dorsal horn neurons, since recordings are hampered by movements of the spinal cord due to respiration and the pulsation of arteries. Synaptic responses evoked by mechanical noxious or non-noxious stimuli, thermal or chemical stimuli have been analyzed in the superficial and deep dorsal horn neurons. In SG neurons, mechanical noxious and non-noxious stimuli elicit a barrage of EPSCs which are completely blocked by the application of CNQX 20 μM, suggesting that both mechanical noxious and non-noxious sensations are transmitted by a release of glutamate. No slow synaptic current has been noticed in this experiment. The effect of CNQX can be direct but not through general circulation, since the block of EPSCs is very rapid as fast as that observed in slice preparation. Also the reversal of the effect is quite fast after the washout of CNQX.

Interestingly, no thermal response is observed in SG, in spite of the fact that the thermal sensation is conveyed by polymodal afferents, mainly C fibers, and those C afferent fibers terminate predominantly in SG as well as lamina I. Unresponsiveness of SG neu-

rons to thermal stimuli is not due to a bias that the recordings are made only from a subpopulation of SG neurons. Since recordings are made from wide varieties of neurons, including at least five distinct subtypes, which are consistent to those reported previously. In order to clarify where the thermal sensation is transmitted in the spinal cord, recordings are made from deeper laminae, lamina III-IV. About 20 % of deep dorsal horn neurons exhibit a barrage of EPSCs by thermal stimulation. The heat-evoked response is mediated by fast EPSCs but not by slow current. Although this response is also predicted to be mediated by peptide, such as substance P, the barrage of EPSCs are completely blocked by CNQX, after CNQX application, no residual response is detected, indicating that the heat sensation is solely mediated by glutamate through AMPA type receptors.

Noxious and non-noxious sensations also terminate in the deep laminae, all of those responses seem to be mediated by glutamate or related amino acids, since the responses are reversibly blocked by CNQX. However, the effect of CNQX takes a long time to affect the responses because of diffusion. Therefore, the assessment of the effect of CNQX should be made carefully.

CONTRIBUTION OF GLUTAMATE RECEPTOR SUBTYPES TO SENSORY TRANSMISSION IN THE SPINAL DORSAL HORN

It had been difficult to differentiate a synaptic response mediated by an activation of the kainite receptor; however, after the development of specific AMPA type receptor antagonist, kainite receptor mediated responses have been able to be investigated. For instance, the activation of kainite receptor mediated slow EPSCs in hippocampal neurons. In the spinal cord, Li (1999) has reported that high-intensity single-shock stimulation of primary afferent fibers, presumably C afferents produce a fast kainate-receptor-meidated EPSC in the superficial dorsal horn neurons. Activation of low-threshold afferent fibers only generates typical AMPA types EPSCs, indicating that kainite receptors are restricted to synapses formed with high-threshold nociceptive and thermoreceptive primary afferent fibers. In hippocampal neurons the kainite-receptor mediated EPSC has a much longer time course and required repetitive stimulation. These discrepancies could be due at least in part, to a kainite receptor subtype or the location of the receptor.

In neonatal spinal cords, a fast synaptic response mediated by a pure NMDA component has been reported. Similar synaptic organization in neonatal rat spinal cords has also been demonstrated, the synapses are silent under physiological condition, but it becomes functional in the presence of 5-HT. In the adult state, however, pure NMDA receptor mediated EPSCs are reduced significantly in number. Ca^{2+} permeable NMDA receptor activation would be essential to accelerate development of sensory circuitry or synaptic connectivity in the spinal dorsal horn.

PRESYNAPTIC GLUTAMATE RECEPTOR

Recent confocal and electron microscopy of double immunostaining studies reveal that primary afferent terminals express AMPA, kainite and NMDA receptors in lamina I-III. Not only excitatory synapses but also GABAergic and glycinergic terminals are en-

dowed with those receptors, suggesting a more complex modification of transmitter release by glutamate through various receptor subtypes in the sensory transmission. Kainate receptor subtype, GluR5 is present at high levels on small diameter primary afferent neurons that are considered to be nociceptive. Activation of presynaptic kainite receptors causes a decrease in glutamate release, while EPSCs evoked by dorsal horn neurons are not altered. Presynaptically expressed AMPA type receptors are classified further by staining using an antibody for the C termianus of glutamate receptor subunit 2 (GluR2) and GluR3 (GluR2/3) and with an antibody for GluR4. In dorsal roots, anti-GluR2/3 stain predominantly myelinated fibers, while anti-GluR4 or anti-GluR2/4 stains predominantly unmyelinated fibers. GluR2/3 positive neurons terminate in laminae III and IV, while positive GluR4 or positive GluR2/4 terminate in laminae I and II. GABAergic terminals are also immunostained with anti-GkuR2/4 and anti-GluR4 in laminae I and II, and deeper laminae are stained with anti-GluR2/3 (Fig.7.3).

A subtype of the AMPA receptor is known to be permeable to Ca^{2+}. In the spinal dorsal horn, activation of Ca^{2+} permeable AMPA receptors are expressed and play an important role in strengthening synaptic transmission. The functional significance of Ca^{2+} permeable AMPA receptors in pain processing is further tested by disrupting the genes encoding GluR1 or GluR2. AMPA receptors are critical determinants of nociceptive plasticity and inflammatory pain. A reduction in the number of Ca^{2+} permeable AMPA receptors and the density of AMPA channel currents in spinal neurons of GluR-A deficient mice is accompanied by a loss of nociceptive plasticity in *in vitro* and a reduction in acute inflammatory hyperalgesia in *in vivo*. Thus, this receptor is critically involved in activity-dependent changes in synaptic processing of nociceptive inputs.

METABOTROPIC GLUTAMATE RECEPTOR

Metabotropic glutamate receptors are G-protein-coupled receptors, which have been shown to be expressed in the spinal dorsal horn and play a role in

modulation of pain transmission(Fig.7.4). Activation of mGluR by local iontophoresis of a metabotropic

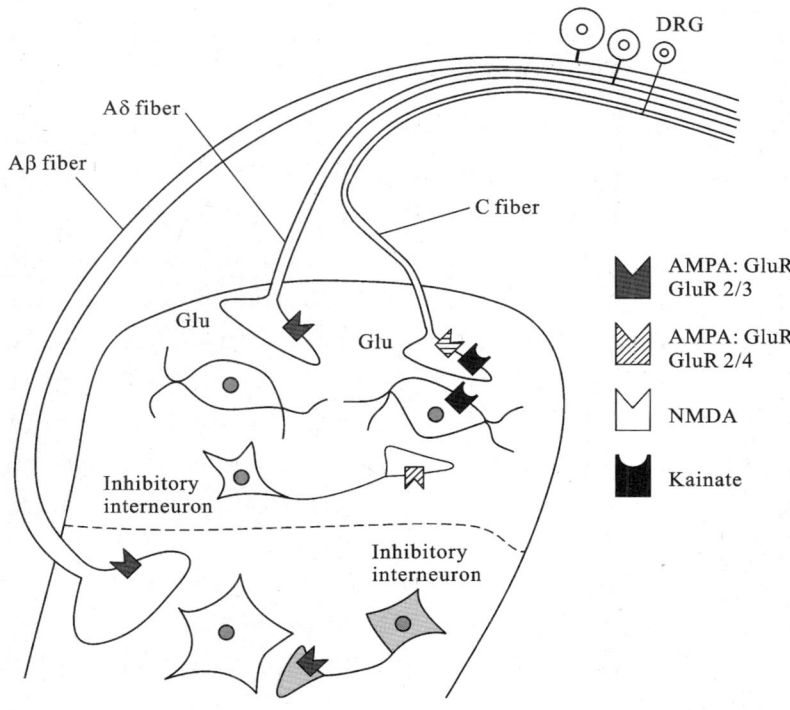

Fig.7.3 Schematic diagram of the expression of ionotropic glutamate receptor subtypes. Only distinguishing receptor subtypes are expressed in this schema, although AMPA, NMDA and kainate receptors are known to express at the postsynaptic membrane of the superficial and deep dorsal horn neurons, and the terminals of Aδ and C afferent fibers. GABAergic and glycinergic inhibitory interneurons are also endowed with those three types of the receptor.

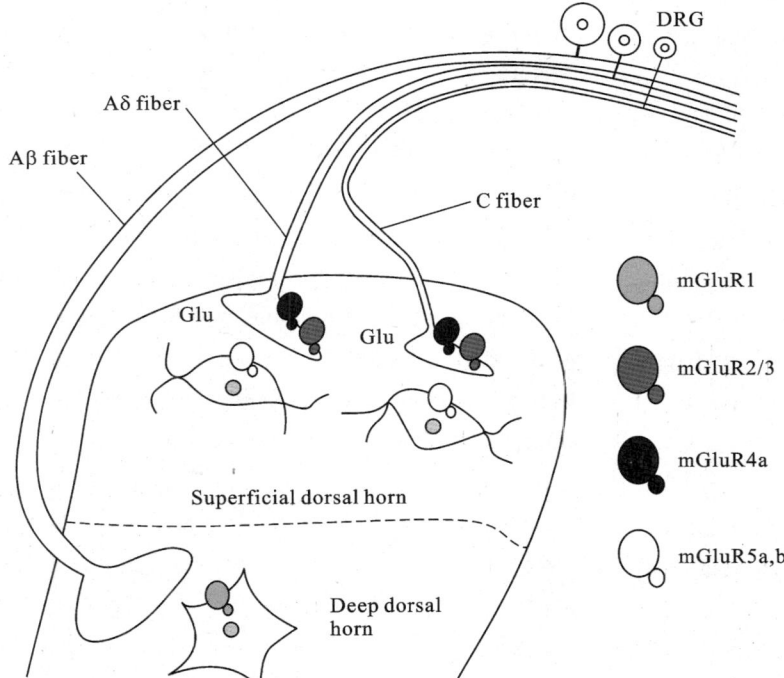

Fig.7.4 Schematic diagram of the expression of metabotropic glutamate receptor subtypes. Representative metabotropic receptors are drew in this schema.

glutamate receptor agonist, (1S, 3R)-1-amino-cyclopentane-1, 3-dicarboxylic acid (ACPD) enhances a response of dorsal horn neuron to ionotropic gluta-

mate receptor agonists (NMDA and kainite). With the application of ACPD there is also an increase in responses to non-noxious stimuli (brush, pressure) but not responses to noxious (pinch or squeeze) stimuli. These ACPD-mediated excitatory actions are blocked by a selective group 1 metabotropic receptor antagonist. These observations suggest a synergistic interaction between metabotropic and ionotropic receptors in the spinal dorsal horn. However, an underlying mechanism for the interaction is not resolved.

Localization of metabotropic receptor subtypes is investigated immunohistochemically. Antisera raised against mGluR5a, b intense immunoreactivity within the superficial dorsal horn is detected (lamina I and II). In contrast, anti-mGluR1a antibodies specifically immunolabeled both dendritic and somatic membranes of the deep dorsal horn neurons. mGluR1b immunoreactivity is prominent in lamina X. Thus, superficial dorsal horn neurons which receive predominantly noxious inputs from the periphery, preferentially express mGluR5a, b whereas deep dorsal horn neurons, in some of which are wide dynamic neurons, express predominantly the mGluR1 receptor subtype. By the introduction of a specific antiserum and with immunocytochemical techniques for light and electron microscopy, the presynaptic distribution of mGluR is also evident. Lamina II which receives small afferent fibers expresses a dense plexus of mGluR4a-immunorective elements. The immunostaining is composed of sparse immunoreactive fibers and punctate elements. No peirkaryal staining was seen. In addition, mGluR4a immunoreactivity is also detected in small to medium-sized neurons in dorsal root ganglia. These observations are consistent with the idea that the primary afferent, in particular, small Aδ and C nociceptive fibers expresses mGluR4a. A role of the receptor has, however, not been clarified. The localization of metabotropic glutamate receptors on primary afferent fibers is also demonstrated, particularly focusing on the mGluR2/3. mGluR2/3, positive dorsal root ganglion neurons are small in diameter. In the dorsal horn, mGluR2/3-like immunoreactivity is localized preferentially in lamina IIi and as well as with light staining in lamina III and IV. From the observation that some residual immunostaining occurs following rhizotomies, suggest that many but not all of these receptors are located on primary afferent fibers.

CONCLUSION AND FUTURE DIRECTIONS

In contrast to the efferent fibers which use acetylcholine, all classes of afferent fibers release glutamate as a principal transmitter. Glutamate acts not only postsynaptically but also presynaptically on dorsal horn neurons through various receptor subtypes, including ionotropic and metabotropic receptors. Leading to an idea that the processing and integration of nociceptive information in the spinal dorsal horn would be much more complicated than that previously thought. In addition to glutamate, small diameter afferent fibers, in particular nociceptive afferents, co-release peptides which contribute to a long lasting modification in excitability of dorsal horn neurons, although no such slow synaptic response mediated by a peptide has been observed in *in vivo* experiments so far. In the case of the AMPA receptor, the functional expression of the receptor is controlled by a second messenger system or by released ligand such as substance P receptor internalization. Therefore, various receptors, including peptide receptors expressed at the dorsal horn are further under control of such modification. Thus, in future directions, the identification of receptor subtypes and their properties as well as the search for their selective antagonists will be an essential step to better understanding the processing of nociceptive transmission and consequently the development of chemical analgesics. To address to these issues, using specific receptor knockout mice would be a useful method to understand the functional significance of receptors at the level of both behavioral and *in vivo* patch-clamp. Newly developed *in vivo* patch-clamp recording methods seem to be feasible as techniques to analyze the functional significance of eliminated receptors in combination with behavioral examinations. Recently, *in vivo* patch recording has been shown to be able to be done without anesthesia; in this method analysis of nociceptive transmission can be made without contamination of the effect of anesthetics.

GENERAL CITATIONS

Yoshimura M, Furue H, Nakatsuka T, Matayoshi T, Katafuchi T. 2004. Functional reorganization of the spinal pain pathways in developmental and pathological conditions. *Novartis Found Symp*, 261:116-124.

Yoshimura M, Furue H, Nakatsuka T, Katafuchi T. 2004. Analysis of receptive fields revealed by *in vivo* patch-clamp recordings from dorsal horn neurons and in situ intracellular recordings from dorsal root ganglion neurons. *Life Sci*, 74(21): 2611-2618.

DISCOVERY CITATIONS

Alvarez FJ, Villalba RM, Carr PA, Grandes P, Somohano PM. 2000. Differenntial distribution of metabotropic glutamate receptors 1a, 1b, and 5 in the rat spinal cord. *J Comp Neurol*, 422(3): 464-487.

Azkue JJ, Murga M, Fernandez-Capetillo O, Mateos JM, Elezgarai I, Benitez R, Osorio A, Diez J, Puente N, Bilbao A, Bidaurrazaga A, Kuhn R, Grandes P. 2001. Immunoreactivity of the group III metabotropic glutamate receptor subtype mGluR4a in the superficial laminae of the rat spinal dorsal horn. *J Comp Neurol*, 430 (4):448-457.

Baba H, Doubell TP, Moore KA, Woolf CJ. 2000. Silent NMDA receptor-mediated synapses are developmentally regulated in the dorsal horn of the rat spinal cord. *J Neurophysiol*, 83 (2): 955-962.

Bardoni R, Goldstein PA, Lee CJ, Gu JG, MacDermott AB. 1997. ATP P2X receptors mediate fast synaptic transmission in the dorsal horn of the rat spinal cord. *J Neurosci*, 17(14): 5297-5304.

Budai D, Larson AA. 1998. The involvement of metabotropic glutamate receptors in sensory transmission in dorsal horn of the rat spinal cord. *Neuroscience*, 83(2): 571-580.

Carlton SM, Hargett GL, Coggeshall RE. 2001. Localization of metabotropic glutamate receptors 2/3 on primary afferent axons in the rat. *Neuroscience*, 105(4): 957-969.

Castillo PE, Malenka RC, Nicoll RA. 1997. Kainate receptors mediate a slow postsynaptic current in hippocampal CA3

neurons. *Nature*, 388:182-186.

Coull JA, Boudreau D, Bachand K, Prescott SA, Nault F, Sik A, De Koninck P, De Koninck Y. 2003. Trans-synaptic shift in anion gradient in spinal lamina I neurons as a mechanism of neuropathic pain. *Nature*, 424: 938-942.

Dale N, Grillner S. 1986. Dual-component synaptic potentials in the lamprey mediated by excitatory amino acid receptors. *J Neurosci*, 6 (9):2653-2661.

Fitzgerald M. 1989. The course and termination of primary afferent fibers. In: Wall PD, Melzack R, eds. *Textbook of Pain*. New York: Churchill Kivingstone. 46-62.

Furue H, Narikawa K, Kumamoto E, Yoshimura M. 1999. Responsiveness of rat substantia gelatinosa neurones to mechanical but not thermal stimulation revealed by *in vivo* patch-clamp recording. *J Physiol*, 521(2): 529-535.

Fyffe REW. 1984. Afferent fibers. In: Davidoff RA, ed. *Handbook of the Spinal Cord*. New York: Dekker. 79-136.

Graham BA, Brichta AM, Callister RJ. 2004. *In vivo* responses of mouse superficial dorsal horn neurones to both current injection and peripheral cutaneous stimulation. *J Physiol (Lond)*, 561(3): 749-763.

Grudt TJ, Perl ER. 2002. Correlations between neuronal morphology and electrophysiological features in the rodent superficial dorsal horn. *J Physiol (Lond)*, 540 (1):189-207.

Gu JG, Albuquerque C, Lee CJ, MacDermott ABBY. 1996. Synaptic strengthening through activation of Ca^{2+} permeable AMPA receptors. *Nature*, 381; 793-796.

Hartmann B, Ahmadi S, Heppenstall PA, Lewin GR, Schott C, Borchardt T, Seeburg PH, Zeilhofer HU, Sprengel R, Kuner R. 2004. The AMPA receptor subunits GluR-A and GluR-B reciprocally modulate spinal synaptic plasticity and inflammatory pain. *Neuron*, 44 (4): 637-650.

Holton AF, Holton P. 1954. The capillary dilator substances in dry powders of spinal roots: a possible role of adenosine triphosphate in chemical transmission from nerve endings. *J Physiol*, 126: 125-141.

Jahr CE, Jessell TM. 1983. ATP excites a subpopulation of rat dorsal horn neurons. *Nature*, 304: 730-733.

Jahr CE, Jessell TM. 1985. Synaptic transmission between dorsal root ganglion and dorsal neurons in culture: antagonism of epsp's and glutamate excitation by kynurenate. *J Neurosci*, 5: 2281-2289.

Jahr CE, Yoshioka K. 1986. Ia afferent excitation of motoneu-rons in the in vitro new-born rat spinal cord is selective antagonized by kynurenate. *J Physiol (Lond)*, 370:515-530.

Jessell TM, Dodd J. 1986. Neurotransmitters and differenti-ation antigens in subsets of sensory neurons projecting to the spinal dorsal horn. In: Martin JB, Barcheas JD. eds, *Neuropeptides in Neurologic and Psychiatric Disease.* New York: Raven Press. 111-131.

Keast JR, Stephensen TM. 2000. Glutamate and aspartate im-munoreactivity in dorsal root ganglion cells supplying vis-ceral and somatic targets and evidence for peripheral ax-onal transport. *J Comp Neurol*, 424(4):577-587.

Kerchner GA, Wilding TJ, Huettner JE, Zhuo M. 2002. Kai-nate receptor subunits underlying presynaptic regulation of transmitter release in the dorsal horn. *J Neurosci*, 22 (18): 8010-8017.

Kerchner GA, Wilding TJ, Li P, Zhuo M, Huettner JE. 2001. Presynaptic kainite receptors regulate spinal sensory transmission. *J Neurosci*, 21 (1): 59-66.

Li P, Kershner GA, Sala C, Wei F, Huettner JE, Sheng M, Zhuo M. 1999. AMPA receptor-PDX interactions in facilitation of spinal sensory synapses. *Nat Neurosci*, 11: 972-977.

Li P, Wilding TJ, Kim SJ, Calejesan AA, Huettner JE, Zhuo M. 1999. Kainate-receptor-mediated sensory synaptic trans-mission in mammalian spinal cord. *Nature*, 397: 161-164.

Li P, Zhuo M. 1998. Silent glutamatergic synapses and noci-ception in mammalian spinal cord. *Nature*, 393: 695-698.

Light AR, Willcockson HH. 1999. Spinal laminae I-II neurons in rat recorded *in vivo* in hole cell, tight seal configuration: properties and opioid responses. *J Neurophysiol*, 82: 3316-3326.

Liu H, Mantyh PW, Basbaum AI. 1997. NMDA-receptor regu-lation of substance P release from primary afferent noci-ceptors. *Nature*, 386:721-724.

Liu XG, Morton CR, Azkue JJ, Zimmermann M, Sandkuhler J. 1998. Long-term depression of C- fibre-evoked spinal field potentials by stimulation of primary afferent A delta-fibres in the adult rat. *Eur J Neurosci*, 10(10):3069-3075.

Lu CR, Hwang SJ, Phend KD, Rustioni A, Valtschanoff JG. 2002. Primary afferent terminals in spinal cord express presynaptic AMPA receptors. *J Neurosci*, 22 (21): 9522-9529.

Lu CR, Willcockson HH, Phend KD, Lucifora S, Darstein M, Valtschanoff JG, Rustioni A. 2005. Ionotropic glutamate receptors are expressed in GABAergic terminals in the rat superficial dorsal horn. *J Comp Neurol*, 486 (2):169-178.

Ma KK, Howe R. 1991. Glutamate-immunoreactivity in the trigeminal and dorsal root ganglia, and intraspinal neurons and fibres in the dorsal horn of the rat. *Histochem J*, 23(4): 171-179.

Maxwell DJ, Rethelyi M. 1987. Ultrastructure and synaptic connections of cutaneous afferent fibers in the spinal cord. *Trends Neurosci*, 10: 117-123.

Miller BA, Woolf CJ. 1996. Glutamate-mediated slow synaptic currents in neonatal rat deep dorsal horn neurons *in vitro. J Neurophysiol*, 76(3): 1465- 1476.

Narikawa K, Furue H, Kumamoto E, Yoshimura M. 2000. *In vivo* patch-clamp analysis of EPSCs evoked in rat substan-tia gelatinosa neurons by cutaneous mechanical stimulation. *J Neurophysiol*, 84: 2171-2174.

Sonohata M, Furue H, Katafuchi T, Yasaka T, Doi A, Kumamoto E, Yoshimura M. 2000. Actions of noradrenalin on substantia gelatinosa neurones in the rat spinal cord re-vealed by *in vivo* patch recording. *J Physiol (Lond)*, 555(2):515-526.

Vignes M, Collingridge GL. 1997. The synaptic activation of kainate receptors. *Nature*, 388:179-182.

Wanaka A, Shiotani Y, Kiyama H, Matsuyama T, Kamada T, Shiosaka S, Tohyama M. 1987. Glutamate-like immunor-eactive structures in primary sensory neurons in the rat de-tected by a specific antiserum against glutamate. *Exp Brain Res*, 65(3):691-694.

Willis Jr. WC, Coggeshall RE. 2004. *Sensory Mechanisms of the Spinal Cord.* 3rd ed. 155-184.

Yajiri Y, Yoshimura M, Okamoto M, Takahashi H, Higashi H. 1997. A novel slow excitatory postsynaptic current in sub-stantia gelatinosa neurons of the rat spinal cord in vitro. *Neuroscience*, 76: 673-688.

Yoshimura M, Jessell TM. 1989. Primary afferent-evoked synaptic responses and slow potential generation in rat substantia gelatinosa neurons in vitro. *J Neurophysiol*, 62: 96-108.

Yoshimura M, Jessell TM. 1990. Amino acid-mediated EPSCs at primary afferent synapses with substantia gelatinosa neurones in the rat spinal cord. *J hysiol*, 430: 315-335.

Yoshimura M, Nishi S. 1993. Excitatory amino acid receptors involved in primary afferent-evoked polysynaptic EPSPs of substantia gelatinosa neurons in the adult rat spinal cord slice. *Neurosci Lett*, 143:131-134.

Yoshimura M, Nishi S. 1995. Primary afferent-evoked glycine- and GABA-mediated IPSPs in substantia gelatinosa neurones in the rat spinal cord *in vitro*. *J Physiol*, 482(1): 29-38.

Yoshioka K, Jessell TM. 1984. ATP release from the dorsal horn of rat spinal cord. *Soc Neurosci Abst*, 10:993.

Youn DH, Randic M. 2004. Modulation of excitatory synaptic transmission in the spinal substantia gelatinosa of mice deficient in the kainate receptor GluR5 and/or GluR6 subunit. *J Physiol (Lond)*, 555(Pt 3):683-698.

Glutamate Kainate Receptor in Pain Transmission and Modulation

CHAPTER 8

Min Zhuo

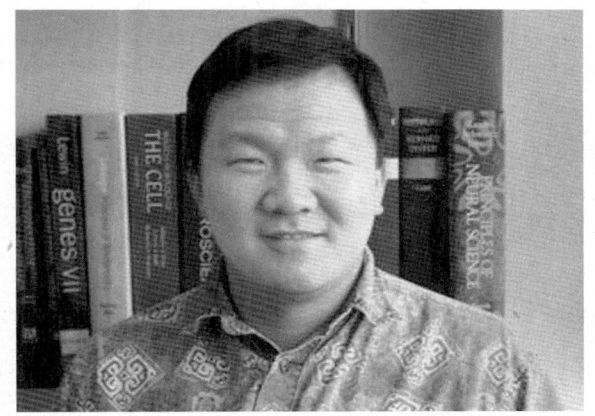

cingulate cortex. *J Neurophysiology*, 94:1805-1813.

Dr. Zhuo is a Professor of Physiology and Neuroscience, in the University of Toronto. He is also the Michael Smith Chair in Neuroscience and Mental Health, and the Canada Research Chair in Pain and Cognition. He obtained a Ph.D. in Pharmacology, from the University of Iowa and conducted postdoctoral work at Columbia and Stanford Universities.

MAJOR CONTRIBUTIONS

1. Li P, Zhuo M. 1998. Silent glutamatergic synapses and nociception in mammalian spinal cord. *Nature* 393:695-698.

2. Li P, Wilding TJ, Kim SJ, Calejesan AA, Huettner JE, Zhuo M. 1999. Kainate receptor-mediated sensory synaptic transmission in mammalian spinal cord. *Nature*, 397:161-164.

3. Kerchner G A, Wang G D, Qiu C-S, Huettner J E, Zhuo M. 2001. Direct presynaptic regulation of GABA/Glycine release by kainate receptors in the dorsal horn: an ionotropic mechanism. *Neuron*, 32:477-488 (Comment in: *Neuron*. 2001, 32(3): 376-378.)

4. Ko S, Zhao M-G, Toyoda H, Qiu C S, Zhuo M. 2005. Altered behavioral responses to noxious stimuli and fear in GluR5- or GluR6 deficient mice. *J Neuroscience*, 25:977-984.

5. Wu L J, Zhao M, Toyada H, Ko S, Zhuo M. 2005. Kainate receptor-mediated synaptic transmission in the adult anterior

MAIN TOPICS

Peripheral KA receptors in sensory transmission

Postsynaptic KA receptors mediate sensory nociceptive synaptic transmission

Presynaptic KA receptors regulate excitatory sensory transmission

Presynaptic regulation of spinal inhibitory transmission: a balance of excitatory vs. inhibitory influences

KA receptor desensitization dictates the time course of KA-triggered transmitter release

KA triggers release of both GABA and glycine

KA action occurs by an ionic mechanism

Synaptic glutamate triggers a KA and GABAB receptor-mediated suppression of spinal inhibitory transmission

A cellular mechanism for presynaptic KA receptor-mediated regulation of transmitter release

KA receptors and The Gate theory

SUMMARY

Glutamate is the major excitatory transmitter in the spinal cord dorsal horn. At postsynaptic sites, subtypes of glutamate receptors are important for mediating sensory synaptic responses. While AMPA and NMDA receptors are likely expressed in all sensory synapses, kainate(KA) receptors are expressed mainly in synapses receiving high-threshold sensory inputs.

In addition to its postsynaptic role, presynaptic KA receptors are important for regulation of both excitatory and inhibitory transmission within the dorsal horn. In the spinal cord dorsal horn, excitatory sensory fibers often terminate adjacent to sites of GABA and glycine release. Glutamate released from sensory fibers caused a KA and GABA_B receptor-dependent suppression of inhibitory transmission in spinal slices, providing evidence for a new role of KA receptors in regulating sensory transmission. Genetic studies using selective KA subtype receptor knockout mice found that KA receptors are important for persistent inflammatory pain as well as emotional responses to pain.

INTRODUCTION

Glutamate is the major excitatory transmitter at primary afferent synapses, where it conveys sensory information to the central nervous system via postsynaptic AMPA (α-amino-3-hydroxy-5-methyl-isoxozole propionic acid), NMDA (N-methyl-D-aspartate), and KA receptors on spinal cord dorsal horn neurons. In addition to postsynaptic receptors, many neurons express on their presynaptic terminals ionotropic receptors that are thought to regulate transmitter release, including receptors for transmitters as well as autoreceptors for the transmitter(s) released by the terminal itself. Much recent effort has focused on KA receptors as possible presynaptic regulators of transmission. In the hippocampus, for example, presynaptic KA receptor activation appears to reduce release of both glutamate and GABA (γ-aminobutyric acid). At primary afferent synapses in the spinal cord, in addition to the postsynaptic KA receptors that contribute to EPSCs evoked by high-threshold dorsal root fiber stimulation, there are KA receptors expressed presynaptically by dorsal root ganglion (DRG) neurons.

It is well-known that KA can depolarize a subset of dorsal root fibers. In addition, the electrophysiological properties of KA receptors were first described in acutely dissociated DRG neurons. Defining a physiological role for these receptors has gained

progress, in part due to the development of selective agonists and antagonists as well as generation of gene knockout mice. In this chapter, I will focus on the possible roles of KA receptors in the spinal cord dorsal horn by focusing on three major areas: (i) peripheral roles of KA receptors; (ii) postsynaptic KA receptor mediated sensory synaptic responses; (iii) presynaptic modulatory roles of KA receptors; (iv) presynaptic KA receptors as a balance mechanism for excitatory and inhibitory transmission.

PERIPHERAL KA RECEPTORS IN SENSORY TRANSMISSION

Considering the high density of KA receptors in small-size DRG cells, it is predictable KA receptors also exists in peripheral sensory terminals. KA receptors, along with other ionotropic glutamate receptors, have been localized on subpopulations of unmyelinated and myelinated sensory axons in normal skin. Activation of these receptors results in nociceptive behaviors and contributes to inflammatory pain.

There is also evidence that peripheral KA receptors undergo upregulation after inflammatory injury. At 48 h following complete Freund's adjuvant (CFA)-induced inflammation, the proportions of unmyelinated axons labeled for KA receptors were 48% as compared with 27% in the non-inflamed paw, suggesting that peripheral KA receptors may contribute to peripheral sensitization.

POSTSYNAPTIC KA RECEPTORS MEDIATE SENSORY NOCICEPTIVE SYNAPTIC TRANSMISSION

For many years, it is believed that excitatory synaptic transmission is mainly carried out by AMPA receptors in central sensory neurons. In the spinal cord dorsal horn, many studies using non-selective antagonists conclude that the roles of AMPA receptors, although KA receptor mediated, if any, are also blocked by this antagonist. The development of selective receptor antagonists and gene knockout mice permit reexamination of KA receptors in spinal synaptic transmission.

Using a selective AMPA receptor antagonist antagonist GYKI 53655, it has then been demonstrated that postsynaptic KA receptor can contribute to synaptic transmission. In the spinal cord dorsal horn neurons, KA receptor-mediated synaptic currents were detected by stimulation of high-threshold sensory fibers, providing the first evidence for KA receptor mediated synaptic transmission in the central nervous system. To detect if KA receptor may also expressed in spinal local inetrneurons, recordings from retrograde labeled neurons has been performed, and KA receptor- mediated currents can be detected from spinothalamic projecting cells. The contribution of postsynaptic KA receptors to nociceptive or pain transmission is further supported by two additional pieces of evidence: (i) KA receptor mediated sensory synaptic responses are sensitive to inhibition of opioid mu receptors, application of selective opioid receptor agonist DAMGO inhibited KA receptor mediated responses; (ii) in behavioral experiments, blockade of both AMPA and KA receptors by CNQX produced greater inhibition of behavioral nociceptive responses than inhibiting AMPA receptors alone.

Thus, postsynaptic glutamate receptors in spinal sensory synapses are not homogenous. In synapses receiving low-threshold sensory inputs, AMPA receptors are the major postsynaptic receptors. In synapses receiving high-threshold sensory inputs, both AMPA and KA receptors are involved, although the percentage contribution of KA receptors is smaller than that of AMPA receptors (Fig.8.1).

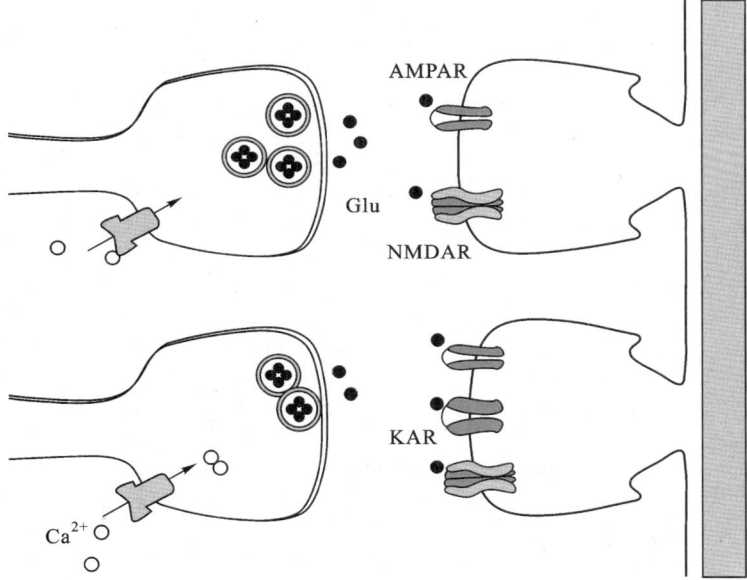

Fig.8.1   KA receptors are selectively expressed in spinal sensory synapses that receive high-threshold sensory inputs. While AMPA and NMDA receptors are expressed in all sensory synapses.

PRESYNAPTIC KA RECEPTORS REGULATE EXCITATORY SENSORY TRANSMISSION

The roles of KA receptors in spinal sensory synaptic transmission are not just limited to sensory synaptic transmission. Evidence from electrophysiological experiments in cultured neurons as well as spinal cord slices consistently suggest that activation of KA receptors at the central terminals of primary afferent sensory neurons inhibit the release of glutamate. For example, Kerchner, Huetner and Zhuo have examined the synapses formed by DRG neurons onto dorsal horn neurons (DRG → spinal synapses) in co-culture (Fig.8.2). Excitatory neurotransmission was monitored by recording NMDA receptor-mediated EPSCs in dorsal horn neurons, and DRG → spinal synapses were activated with a bipolar stimulating electrode in a theta glass pipette, placed against the cell body of a nearby, synaptically-coupled DRG neuron. Under the microscope, DRG cells chosen for stimulation were typically of the smaller size (<20 μm diameter). Fixed-latency, NMDA receptor-mediated EPSCs could be evoked in these conditions. KA (10 μM) reversibly suppressed evoked EPSC amplitude at DRG → spinal synapses. The KA receptor is likely containing GluR5 subunits, since ATPA, a selective GluR5 KA receptor agonist, did inhibit DRG → spinal transmission. To direct confirm the involvement of GluR5 KA receptors, ATPA's effect were also repeated in culture neurons from GluR5 knockout mice. ATPA produced inhibitory effects were completely inhibited.

Sensory transmission in a dish
DRG-dorsal horn neuron co-cultures

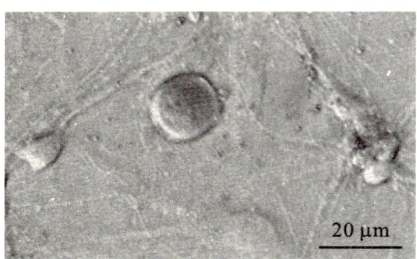

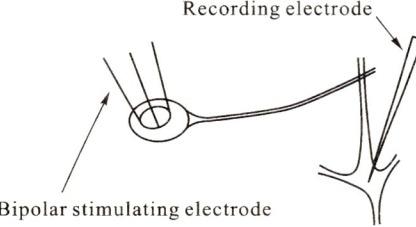

Fig.8.2 A diagram for DRG-dorsal horn neuron co-cultures. A photograph of co-cultured DRG and dorsal horn neurons and a diagram showing placement of recording and stimulating electrodes illustrate the experimental system.

In sum, presynaptic KA receptors on small diameter DRG cells can regulate glutamate release at primary afferent synapses. Thus KA receptors, in addition to mediating postsynaptic responses at those synapses, may also modulate somatosensory input into the spinal cord by acting on primary afferent fibers themselves. In addition, because the DRG → spinal synapse is a critical target for clinical treatment of pain, we suggest that selective activation of DRG KA receptors with appropriate agonists may represent a novel strategy for pain control.

PRESYNAPTIC REGULATION OF SPINAL INHIBITORY TRANSMISSION: A BALANCE OF EXCITATORY VS. INHIBITORY INFLUENCES

Inhibitory transmission in the spinal cord dorsal horn plays an important role in sensory transmission and modulation. In culture neurons recordings, KA receptor mediated currents can be recorded from many spinal local neurons. One important function for KA receptors in these neurons is to regulate releases inhibitory transmitters such as GABA and glycine in the spinal cord. To test for the presence of presynaptic KA receptors at spinal dorsal horn inhibitory synapses, we examined the effect of KA receptor activation on spontaneous miniature inhibitory postsynaptic currents (mIPSCs). Recordings were obtained from dorsal horn neurons in dissociated culture to allow for more rapid and complete exchange of the extracellular medium than is possible during acute slice recordings. Speed of exchange is an important consideration, because KA receptors exhibit prominent desensitization. Recordings were made in the presence of 500 nM tetrodotoxin (TTX), which blocked all voltage-gated Na^+ current, as well as SYM2206 (100 μM) and AP-5 (25 μM) to block AMPA and NMDA receptors, respectively. Neurons were voltage-clamped at 0 mV and perfused intracellularly with a low-Cl^- pipette solution. In these conditions, mIPSCs appeared as outward currents at a background frequency of 3.8 ± 0.4 s^{-1}. Upon application of KA (10 μM), this frequency increased to 850 ± 100 % of the control value during the first four seconds of the exposure, suggesting that KA acted at a presynaptic locus. In addition, co-application of KA with the non-selective AMPA/KA receptor antagonist CNQX (100 μM) resulted in no significant change in mIPSC frequency compared to control.

KA was consistent in its ability to trigger GABA/glycine release. We tested whether this effect could be mimicked by the endogenous agonist glutamate. We found that 30 μM glutamate was sufficient to enhance mIPSC frequency to a similar extent as 10 μM KA, when applied in the presence of TTX, SYM2206, AP-5, and metabotropic glutamate receptor (mGluR) antagonists, including the mGluR$_{1a}$-selective antagonist LY367385 (50 μM), the mGluR$_5$-selective antagonist MPEP (2 μM), and the group II/III mGluR antagonist CPPG (500 μM). Because we did not observe a subpopulation of cells in which KA or glutamate did not affect mIPSC frequency, and because dorsal horn neuronal cultures contain excitatory as well as inhibitory neurons, we conclude that these agonists stimulated inhibitory terminals that impinged on both types of postsynaptic cells.   Unlike KA receptors in the DRG cells, KA receptors in dorsal horn neurons were largely insensitive to the GluR5 subunit-preferring KA receptor-selective agonist ATPA (2 μM).

KA Receptor Desensitization Dictates the Time Course of Ka-triggered Transmitter Release

KA typically triggered a burst of mIPSCs that subsided during a 10 s exposure. This decline in mIPSC frequency over time might result from KA receptor desensitization, metabotropic inhibition of release through activation of presynaptic GABA$_B$ autoreceptors, or depletion of the readily-releasable pool of synaptic vesicles. In cultures exposed to the lectin conconavalin A (con A), which selectively removes desensitization of KA receptors, mIPSC frequency remained high throughout a 20 s KA application, suggesting that KA receptor desensitization played a large role in the waning of the KA-triggered mIPSC burst in control conditions.

By contrast, GABA$_B$ receptors did not contribute to the decay of KA-triggered mIPSC bursts. mIPSC frequency varied similarly over time whether KA was applied in control conditions or in the continual presence of the GABA$_B$ receptor antagonist CGP55845 (10 μM). Even in cultures treated with con A, CGP55845 had no effect on the time course of KA-triggered mIPSC bursts, a result mimicked when

elevated extracellular [KCl] was used instead of KA as the trigger for vesicle release. Further arguing against a role for GABA$_B$ receptors, KA and KCl each enhanced mIPSC frequency to a similar degree in the presence or absence of the GABA$_B$ receptor agonist baclofen (5–10 μM). Whereas it remains possible that GABA released consequent to KA receptor stimulation may activate GABA$_B$ receptors, such activation clearly did not underlie the waning of mIPSC frequency during KA exposure.

KA Triggers Release of Both Gaba and Glycine

Glycine and GABA are probably co-packaged in and co-released from spinal interneurons. Bicuculline and strychnine each blocked a portion of IPSCs evoked by extracellular stimulation (eIPSCs), and a combination of the two antagonists blocked eIPSCs completely, suggesting that both GABA and glycine were released from individual cultured dorsal horn neurons and contributed to postsynaptic currents. We predicted that GABAergic and glycinergic mIPSCs would be regulated similarly by presynaptic KA receptor activation. Indeed, in the presence of strychnine (500 nM), KA enhanced mIPSC frequency in all nine neurons tested. Similarly, in the presence of bicuculline (5 μM), KA increased mIPSC frequency in six of eight experiments; in two, no change in frequency was noted. Of side interest, whereas bicuculline and strychnine each depressed mIPSC frequency when applied alone, neither antagonist produced any significant effect on mIPSC amplitude, suggesting that individual mIPSCs were typically mediated by GABA or glycine, but not both. Such a phenomenon has been attributed to differential clustering of the two receptor types at postsynaptic sites, not to differential release of GABA and glycine.

KA Action Occurs by an Ionic Mechanism

We sought to determine how presynaptic KA receptor activation is linked to GABA/glycine release. Among various possible models, three include these. First,

Na^+ entry through KA receptors may depolarize nerve terminals, causing voltage-gated Ca^{2+} channel activation, Ca^{2+} entry, and vesicle fusion. Second, if axon terminals contain Ca^{2+}-permeable KA receptors, Ca^{2+} entry and transmitter release could be achieved in the absence of membrane depolarization or Ca^{2+} channel activity, as has been proposed at hippocampal interneuron–interneuron synapses. Third, KA receptors may be linked metabotropically to the transmitter release machinery. To distinguish between these models, we first examined the ability of KA to enhance mIPSC frequency when extracellular Na^+ was replaced entirely by N-methyl-D-glutamine. Although background mIPSC frequency and amplitude were similar in this condition compared to control, KA no longer enhanced mIPSC frequency. This observation suggests that Na^+ entry through activated KA receptors was essential, and that even if those receptors were Ca^{2+}-permeable, KA receptor-mediated Ca^{2+} entry was not sufficient to trigger transmitter release. Confirming that depolarization could indeed trigger GABA/glycine release and that removal of extracellular Na^+ per se did not interfere with this process, elevating extracellular [KCl] to 20 mM in Na^+-free medium induced a large, sustained enhancement of mIPSC frequency. Although we do not formally exclude a more complex coupling between KA receptors and transmitter release, our findings indicate a requirement for an ionic component in KA action, most likely reflecting the ability of Na^+ entry to occur directly through ionotropic KA receptors.

We next tested the Ca^{2+}-dependence of KA-induced GABA/glycine release. The standard extracellular solution contained 2 mM Ca^{2+} and 2 mM Mg^{2+}. Lowering this Ca^{2+} to Mg^{2+} ratio from 2:2 to 1.5:2.5 resulted in a significant reduction in the ability of 10μM KA to evoke mIPSC bursts while leaving background mIPSC frequency unaffected. These data suggest that KA-triggered GABA/glycine release, but not spontaneous quantal release, was sensitive to changes in extracellular [Ca^{2+}]. To identify a role for voltage-gated Ca^{2+} channels in mediating the effects

of KA, we first applied 50 μM $CdCl_2$, a concentration sufficient to block voltage-gated Ca^{2+} currents in cultured dorsal horn neurons with little to no effect on the magnitude of KA-induced currents; in this condition, KA was unable to trigger an increase in mIPSC frequency. Whereas the L-type Ca^{2+} channel antagonist nimodipine had no effect on KA-induced GABA/glycine release, the selective N-type antagonist ω-conotoxin GVIA and the P/Q-type antagonist ω-conotoxin MVIIC (which also weakly blocks N-type channels) each partially blocked the phenomenon. These data are consistent with the prevalence of N- and P/Q-type voltage-gated Ca^{2+} channels, but not L-type channels, on presynaptic axon terminals in the spinal cord. Because a combination of ω-conotoxin GVIA and ω-conotoxin MVIIC did not completely prevent KA action, it remains possible that other Ca^{2+} channel subtypes, such as R-type channels, may play some role.

Taken together, these data support a model in which GABA/glycine release is triggered by Na^+ entry through activated KA receptors and opening of presynaptic voltage-gated Ca^{2+} channels. Although we note that the magnitude of somatic depolarization induced by 10 μM KA was small—too small, indeed, to cause detectable activation of voltage-gated Ca^{2+} channels in the current-clamped portion of the membrane—the magnitude of depolarization in axon terminals could be larger. At terminals, input resistance is greater than at the cell body, and KA receptors may be more densely expressed; such factors may underlie the ability of KA to cause sufficient terminal depolarization to activate presynaptic voltage-gated Ca^{2+} channels.

Synaptic Glutamate Triggers a KA and GABA_B Receptor-mediated Suppression of Spinal Inhibitory Transmission

We next examined whether these effects of KA receptor activation could be reproduced in a more intact preparation using synaptic glutamate, instead of exogenously-applied agonists, as the trigger. Intracellular recordings were achieved from superficial dorsal horn

A

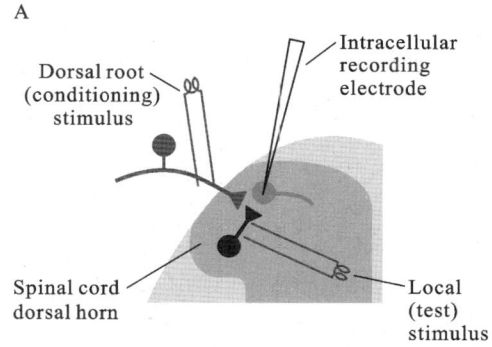

B   Stimulation protocol

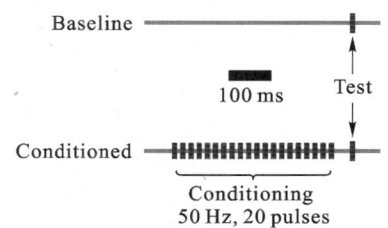

C

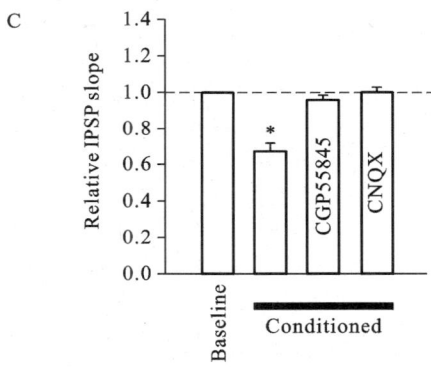

Fig.8.3 Synaptic glutamate from sensory fibers suppresses inhibitory transmission in the dorsal horn through KA and GABA$_B$ receptor activation. A. A diagram illustrates the placement of recording and stimulating electrodes in a transverse spinal cord slice. Intracellular recordings were performed from dorsal horn neurons, and stimulating electrodes were placed in the dorsal root, to activate sensory fibers, and in the dorsal horn, to activate inhibitory interneurons. B. The stimulation protocols are illustrated for baseline and conditioned responses. C. Pooled data illustrate the effects of conditioning on the slope of the rising phase of IPSPs evoked by test stimulation in control conditions or in the presence of CGP55845 (10 μM) or CNQX (20 μM). *, significant difference from baseline.

neurons in spinal cord slices from adult rats, and two stimulating electrodes were introduced, one locally in the dorsal horn and one in the attached dorsal root.

the presence of SYM2206 and AP-5, local stimulation produced a hyperpolarizing inhibitory postsynaptic potential (IPSP) that was sensitive to picrotoxin (20 μM) and strychnine (1 μM), indicating that this stimulation activated local GABA- and glycinergic interneurons (Fig.8.3). By contrast, stimulation of excitatory sensory fibers in the dorsal root produced no response when the stimulus intensity was below the threshold needed to activate fibers eliciting EPSCs mediated by postsynaptic KA receptors.

Because primary afferent sensory fibers release glutamate in the vicinity of GABA- and glycine-containing boutons in the superficial dorsal horn, we hypothesized that dorsal root stimulation may activate presynaptic KA receptors on spinal interneurons and thereby modulate inhibitory transmission. Indeed, when a conditioning stimulus train (50 Hz, 20 pulses) was delivered to the dorsal root, both the amplitude and the slope of the rising phase of an IPSP generated 50 ms later by local stimulation were reduced relative to the baseline, unconditioned response. The conditioning train itself triggered no EPSP or IPSP. In the presence of CNQX (20 μM) instead of SYM2206, conditioning did not affect IPSPs, suggesting that KA receptor activation was necessary. Furthermore, conditioning produced no effect in the presence of CGP55845 (10 μM). Thus, in agreement with the effects of KA detailed above in cultured neurons, inhibitory transmission in spinal slices was downregulated by synaptic glutamate through a mechanism involving KA receptors and GABA$_B$ receptors.

A Cellular Mechanism for Presynaptic KA Receptor-mediated Regulation of Transmitter Release

In the model illustrated in Fig.8.4, we show the detailed examination of a mechanism linking presynaptic KA receptor activation to changes in transmitter release probability. This mechanism most likely involved an ionotropic action of KA receptors, which by permitting Na$^+$ entry, led to terminal depolarization, voltage-gated Ca^{2+} channel activation, and Ca^{2+}-dependent vesicle fusion. In this way, presynaptic KA receptor activation enhanced GABA/glycine release from dorsal horn neurons to an extent that could activate a negative-feedback pathway, mediated by GABA$_B$ autoreceptors, inhibiting subsequent evoked

release. Such a pathway appears to exist physiologically, as synaptically-released glutamate was able to suppress spinal inhibitory transmission in a KA and GABA$_B$ receptor-dependent fashion.

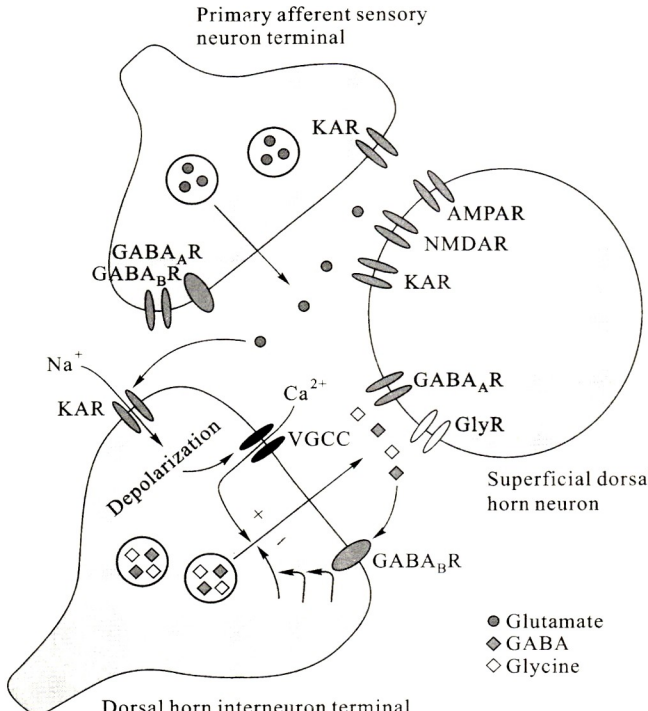

Primary afferent sensory neuron terminal

Superficial dorsal horn neuron

Dorsal horn interneuron terminal

● Glutamate
◆ GABA
◇ Glycine

Fig.8.4   Presynaptic KA receptors regulate spinal inhibitory transmission. A model of a synaptic glomerulus depicts the proposed function of presynaptic KA receptors at dorsal horn inhibitory synapses. These receptors, which can be activated by glutamate released from primary afferent sensory fibers, mediate Na$^+$ entry and terminal depolarization, triggering opening of voltage-gated Ca^{2+} channels (VGCC) and Ca^{2+}-dependent vesicle fusion. GABA released in this manner may activate presynaptic GABA$_B$ autoreceptors, reducing action potential-dependent transmitter release. Previous work has shown that sensory neuron terminals contain GABA$_A$ and GABA$_B$ receptors (Malcangio and Bowery, 1996), indicating that sensory neurons and dorsal horn interneurons engage in reciprocal heterosynaptic regulation of transmitter release. Other studies have documented additional roles for KA receptors in spinal sensory transmission. Along with AMPA and NMDA receptors, KA receptors mediate a component of the postsynaptic response of dorsal horn neurons to high-threshold sensory fiber stimulation. In addition, sensory fibers themselves express presynaptic KA receptors that regulate glutamate release.

KA RECEPTORS AND THE GATE THEORY

Regulation of inhibitory transmission in the dorsal horn is essential for proper processing of pain and other sensory information; for instance, agonists of GABA$_A$ and GABA$_B$ receptors are antinociceptihve, and spinal administration of antagonists induces chronic pain. In their gate control theory of pain, Melzack and Wall (1965) proposed that pain transmission in the dorsal horn is enhanced by the activity of nociceptive sensory fibers, but suppressed by the activity of nonnociceptive fibers that may act in concert with local inhibitory neurons; the balance between enhancement and suppression determines the setting of a "gate" that permits or restricts the relay of nociceptive information from the spinal cord to higher

brain centers. We suggest that the ability of glutamate released from sensory fibers to regulate GABA/glycine release via presynaptic KA receptors could represent one component of gate control. Finally, our data broaden the known roles of KA receptors in spinal sensory pathways. We previously showed that KA receptors mediate a component of the postsynaptic response of dorsal horn neurons to high-threshold primary afferent sensory fiber stimulation. Antagonists that block these postsynaptic KA receptors and the presynaptic KA receptors on dorsal horn interneurons would be expected to have analgesic properties. We have also reported that sensory fibers themselves express presynaptic KA receptors, that activation of those receptors with exogenous agonists suppressed sensory transmission. Because the KA receptors on peripheral sensory neurons could be pharmacologically separated from those expressed on spinal neurons, manipulation of spinal KA receptors with selective agonists and antagonists could represent a viable therapeutic strategy for the treatment of pain.

GENETIC AND PHARMACOLOGICAL INHIBITION OF KA RECEPTORS AND PAIN

Due to the lack of selective KA receptor antagonists in commercial companies, the studies of KA receptors in behavioral pain are highly limited. Very often drugs used are non-selectively affected both AMPA and KA receptors. It is hard to make conclusion of the roles of KA receptors in pain based on the data of mixed receptor antagonists. Considering the general roles of AMPA and KA receptors in pain related central transmission and modulation, it is expected that antagonists reduce pain in animal models and humans. However, it is also clear that inhibition of both AMPA and KA receptors are likely to lead to many central side effects in patients.

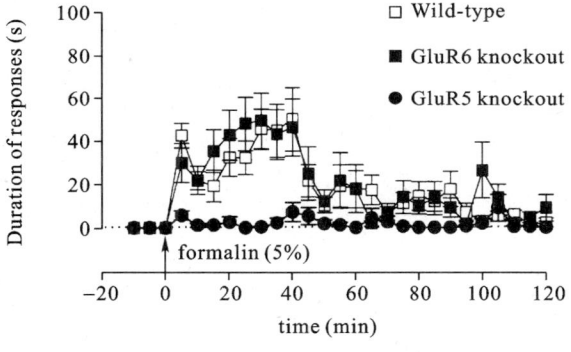

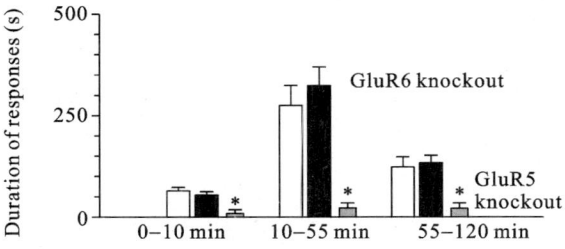

Fig.8.5   Reduced response to formalin in GluR5, but not GluR6, knockout mice A. Behavioral responses to formalin injection, plotted in 5-min intervals, in wild type mice as compared to GluR5 and GluR6 knockout mice. B. Data from (A) grouped into three phases.

Use of genetically manipulated mice provides a better mechaninistic study of KA receptors roles in

pain. Genetic deletion of GluR5 and Glu6 lead to selective changes in behavioral responses to noxious stimuli. While behavioral responses to capsaicin or inflammatory pain were significantly reduced in mice lacking GluR5 but not GluR6 subunits, mice lacking GluR6 but not GluR5 showed a significant reduction in fear memory(Fig.8.5). Learning-related synaptic potentiation was significantly reduced in the lateral amygdala of GluR6 but not GluR5 knockout mice. These findings provide evidence that distinct KAR subtypes contribute to chemical/inflammatory pain and fear memory. Selectively targeting different KAR subtypes may provide a useful strategy for treating persistent pain and fear-related mental disorders.

CONCLUSIONS AND FUTURE DIRECTIONS

Cumulative evidence has been reported for the involvement of glutamate KA receptors in physiological functions of the CNS such as physiological pain, fear, anxiety, learning and memory. Understanding the molecular, cellular and neuronal circuits changes of glutamate KA receptors in various regions of the brain not only provide basic information for brain functions, but provide potential new drug targets for treating different mental diseases. Future studies to investigate the exact signaling pathways for the regulation and plasticity of KA receptors are needed. The use of modern genetic approaches combined with traditional pharmacological, physiological and behavioral studies will facilitate the investigation of KA receptors.

GENERAL CITATIONS

Bleakman D, Lodge D. 1998. Neuropharmacology of AMPA and KA receptors. *Neuropharmacology*, 37: 1187-1204.

Bleakman D. 1999. KA receptor pharmacology and physiology. *Cell Mol Life Sci*, 56: 558-566.

Frerking M, Nicoll R A. 2000. Synaptic KA receptors. *Curr Opin Neurobiol*, 10: 342-351.

Lerma J. 2003. Roles and rules of KA receptors in synaptic transmission. *Nat Rev Neurosci*, 4: 481-495.

Zhuo M. 2004. Central plasticity in pathological pain. *Novartis Found Symp*, 261: 132-145. (discussion 145-154)

Huettner J E, Kerchner G A, Zhuo M. 2002. Glutamate and the presynaptic control of spinal sensory transmission. *Neuroscientist*, 8: 89-92.

DISCOVERY CITATIONS

Youn D H, *et al*. 2005. Altered long-term synaptic plasticity and KA-induced Ca$^{(2+)}$ transients in the substantia gelatinosa neurons in GLU(K6)-deficient mice. *Brain Res Mol Brain Res*, 142:9-18.

Kerchner G A, Wilding T J, Huettner J E, Zhuo M. 2002. KA receptor subunits underlying presynaptic regulation of transmitter release in the dorsal horn. *J Neurosci*, 22: 8010-8017.

Kerchner G A, Wilding T J, Li P, Zhuo M, Huettner J E. 2001. Presynaptic KA receptors regulate spinal sensory transmission. *J Neurosci*, 21: 59-66.

Kerchner G A, Wang G D, Qiu C S, Huettner J E, Zhuo M. 2001. Direct presynaptic regulation of GABA/glycine release by KA receptors in the dorsal horn: an ionotropic mechanism. *Neuron*, 32: 477-488.

Wu L J, Zhao M G, Toyoda H, Ko S, Zhuo M. 2005. KA receptor-mediated synaptic transmission in the adult anterior cingulate cortex. *J Neurophysiol*, 94: 1805-1813.

Dominguez E, *et al*. 2005. Two prodrugs of potent and selective GluR5 KA receptor antagonists actives in three animal models of pain. *J Med Chem*, 48: 4200-4203.

Lu C R, *et al*. 2005. Ionotropic glutamate receptors are expressed in GABAergic terminals in the rat superficial dorsal horn. *J Comp Neurol*, 486: 169-178.

Ko S, Zhao M G, Toyoda H, Qiu C S, Zhuo M. 2005. Altered behavioral responses to noxious stimuli and fear in glutamate receptor 5 (GluR5)- or GluR6-deficient mice. *J Neurosci*, 25: 977-984.

MacDermott A B. 2001. Glutamate and GABA: a painful combination. *Neuron*, 32: 376-378.

Sailer A, *et al*. 1999. Generation and analysis of GluR5(Q636R) KA receptor mutant mice. *J Neurosci*, 19: 8757-8764.

Li P, *et al*. 1999. KA-receptor-mediated sensory synaptic transmission in mammalian spinal cord. *Nature*, 397: 161-164.

Agrawal S G, Evans R H. 1986. The primary afferent depolarizing action of KA in the rat. *Br J Pharmacol*, 87: 345-355.

Ault B, Hildebrand L M. 1993. Activation of nociceptive reflexes by peripheral KA receptors. *J Pharmacol Exp Ther*, 265: 927-932.

Huettner J E. 1990. Glutamate receptor channels in rat DRG neurons: activation by KA and quisqualate and blockade of desensitization by Con A. *Neuron*, 5: 255-266.

Sato K, Kiyama H, Park H T, Tohyama M. 1993. AMPA, KA and NMDA receptors are expressed in the rat DRG neurones. *Neuroreport*, 4: 1263-1265.

Part III Neuropeptides, ATP, Retrograde Messengers and Opioids

Neuropeptides

CHAPTER 9

Xu Zhang, Lan Bao

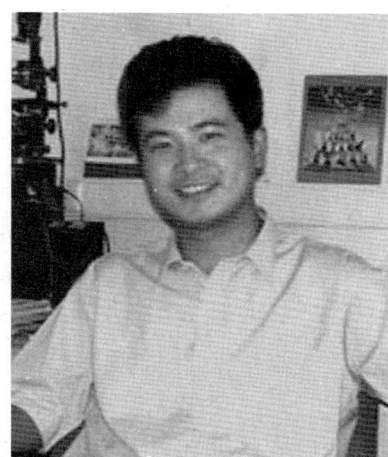

Dr. Xu Zhang, is a Principal Investigator and Professor in the Laboratory of Sensory System, Institute of Neuroscience, Chinese Academy of Sciences, China. He obtained a MD degree from 4th Military Medical University, China, and then got a Ph.D. in the Department of Neuroscience, Karolinska Institute, Sweden.

MAJOR CONTRIBUTIONS

1. Guan JS, Xu ZZ, Gao H, He SQ, Ma GQ, Sun T, Wang LH, Zhang ZN, Lena I, Kitchen I, Elde R, Zimmer A, He C, Pei G, Bao L, Zhang X. 2005. Interaction with vesicle luminal protachykinin regulates surface expression of δ-opioid receptors and opioid analgesia. *Cell*, 122: 619-631.
2. Yang L, Zhang FX, Huang F, Lu YJ, Li GD, Bao L, Xiao HS, Zhang X. 2004. Peripheral axotomy induces trans-synaptic modification of channels, receptors and signaling pathways in rat dorsal spinal cord. *Eur J Neurosci*, 19: 871-883.
3. Xiao HS, Huang QH, Zhang FX, Bao L, Lu YJ, Guo C, Yang L, Huang WJ, Fu G, Xu SH, Cheng XP, Yan Q, Zhu ZD, Zhang X, Chen Z, Han ZG, Zhang X. 2002. Identification of gene expression profile of dorsal root ganglion in the rat peripheral axotomy model of neuropathic pain. *Proc Natl Acad Sci USA*, 99: 8360-8365.

4. Tong YG, Wang HF, Ju G, Grant G, Hökfelt T, Zhang X. 1999. Increased uptake and transport of cholera toxin B-subunit in dorsal root ganglion neurons after peripheral axotomy: possible implications on sensory sprouting. *J Comp Neurol*, 404: 143-158.
5. Zhang X, Bao L, Arvidsson U, Elde R, Hökfelt T. 1998. Localization and regulation of the delta-opioid receptor in dorsal root ganglia and spinal cord of the rat and monkey: Evidence for association with the membrane of large dense-core vesicles. *Neuroscience*, 82: 1225-1242.

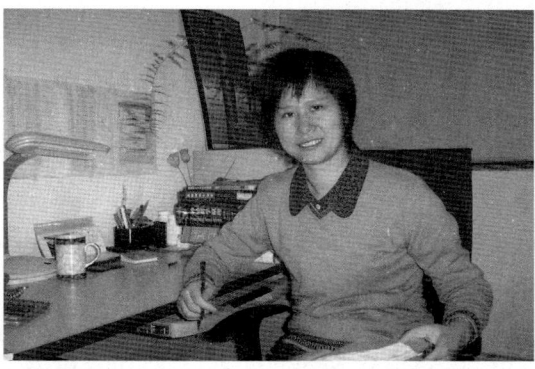

Dr. Lan Bao, is a Principal Investigator and Professor in the Laboratory of Molecular Cell Biology, Institute of Biochemistry and Cell Biology, Chinese Academy of Sciences, China. She obtained a MD degree from 4th Military Medical University (FFMU), China, and continued on to a Ph.D., Department of Aerospace Physiology, FFMU.

MAJOR CONTRIBUTIONS

1. Guan JS, Xu ZZ, Gao H, He SQ, Ma GQ, Sun T, Wang LH, Zhang ZN, Lena I, Kitchen I, Elde R, Zimmer A, He C, Pei G, Bao L, Zhang X. 2005. Interaction with vesicle luminal protachykinin regulates surface expression of δ-opioid receptors and opioid analgesia. *Cell*, 122: 619-631.
2. Bao L, Jin SX, Zhang C, Wang LH, Xu ZZ, Zhang FX,

Wang LC, Ning FS, Cai HJ, Guan JS, Xiao HS, Xu ZDQ, He C, Hokfelt T, Zhou Z, Zhang X. 2003. Activation of delta-opioid receptors induces receptor insertion and neuropeptide secretion. *Neuron*, 37: 121-133.

3. Bao L, Wang HF, Cai HJ, Tong YG, Jin SX, Lu YJ, Grant G, Hökfelt T, Zhang X. 2002. Peripheral axotomy induces only very limited sprouting of coarse myelinated afferents into inner lamina II of rat spinal cord. *Eur J Neurosci*, 16: 175-185.

4. Bao L, Kopp J, Zhang X, Xu ZQD, Zhang LF, Wong H, Walsh J and Hökfelt T. 1997. Localization of neuropeptide Y Y1 receptors in cerebral blood vessels. *Proc Natl Acad Sci USA*, 94: 12661-12666.

MAIN TOPICS

Substance P and its receptor

Opioid-peptides and their receptors

Cholecystokinin and its receptors

Neuropeptide Y and its receptors

Other neuropeptides and G-protein-coupled receptors

SUMMARY

Neuropeptides are expressed in the dorsal root ganglion neurons and dorsal spinal cord neurons. Peripheral nociceptive stimuli cause the release of neuropeptides to modulate the sensory transmission. Neuropeptide substance P is known to be involved in the modulation of nociception and inflammatory pain. Opioid-peptides and their receptors play important roles in pain inhibition. The cholecystokinin and its receptors represent an endogenous peptide system to counteract the opioid system. Furthermore, a large number of neuropeptide receptors are recently identified in dorsal root ganglion neurons and their functions need to be analyzed.

INTRODUCTION

Neuropeptides have long been of interested in studies on the modulation of pain transmission. Small neurons in the dorsal root ganglion (DRG) express neuropeptides, such as substance P, calcitonin gene-related peptide and somatostatin. In the superficial dorsal horn of the spinal cord, enkephalin, dynorphin, neuropeptide Y, cholecystokinin, neurotensin and other types neuropeptides are expressed in the interneurons. The expression of neuropeptides in DRG neurons is regulated by factors that are expressed in the peripheral tissues, such as nerve growth factor.

Neuropeptides are synthesized in the cell bodies of primary sensory neurons. Synthesized neuropeptides are packed into the large dense-core vesicles (LDCVs) in the regulated secretory pathway at the trans-Golgi network. These neuropeptide-containing LDCVs are transported to the peripheral terminals in the skin and the central terminals in the superficial dorsal horn of the spinal cord. They are stored in these secretory vesicles, and are released upon peripheral nociceptive stimulations or activation of certain types of neurotransmitter/neuromodulator receptors. The stimulus-triggered increase in the intracellular Ca^{2+} is required for the exocytosis of neuropeptide-containing LDCVs. In contrast to the exocytosis-site of synaptic vesicles at the presynaptic membrane of nerve terminals, the exocytosis of neuropeptides occurs on the plasma membrane outside the presynaptic membrane. In addition, neuropeptides can be released from the cell bodies of the sensory neurons.

Neuropeptide receptors are members of the superfamily of G-protein-coupled receptors with seven transmembrane domains. A number of neuropeptide receptors are expressed in DRG neurons and interneurons in the spinal dorsal horn. Neuropeptide receptors are synthesized in the cell bodies of primary sensory neurons. Most neuropeptide receptors are sorted into the constitutive pathway in the trans-Golgi network and are inserted into the plasma membrane spontaneously. However, recent studies show that certain types of receptor can be sorted into the regulated secretory pathway and associate with the membrane of LDCVs, allowing stimulus-induced membrane insertion of the receptors. Moreover, the receptors can be preferably localized at cell bodies or terminals, suggesting that there are intrinsic mechanisms to regulate the localization of neuropeptide receptors in primary sensory neurons. The regulatory mechanisms and their functional significances in pain transmission remain to be understood.

Following the stimulation of the receptor-specific

neuropeptide, in most cases, activated receptors are internalized via the endosomes. The internalized receptors are further processed in either the recycling pathway for the re-sensitization or the degradation pathway for the desensitization. Understanding of molecular and cellular mechanisms for the receptor re-sensitization or desensitization is one of the major research interests in both pain study and neurobiological studies.

In this chapter we will focus on substance P, opioid peptides, cholecystokinin, neuropeptide Y and their receptors that are normally expressed in DRG neurons and/or dorsal spinal cord neurons. Their potential functions in the modulation of nociceptive transmission will be discussed.

SUBSTANCE P AND ITS RECEPTOR

Substance P is the best-known neuropeptide involving in modulation of pain transmission. Von Euler and Gaddum discovered this peptide in 1931. Leeman's laboratory identified its sequence in 1970. Together with substance K, substance P belongs to tachykinin peptides coded by the preprotachykinin-A gene. This peptide was identified in small DRG neurons with immunohistochemistry. Double-immunolabeling shows that substance P is co-localized with calcitonin gene-related peptide in these neurons. These peptides are often packed into the same LDCVs at the trans-Golgi network in the cell bodies and are transported to the peripheral terminals of C fibers in peripheral tissues and to the central terminals in laminae I–II of the spinal cord (Fig.9.1). These peptide-containing LDCVs are stored in the terminals and peptides can be released upon neural firing and specific chemical stimulations.

Peripheral tissue injury and inflammation cause the release of substance P in the peripheral tissues. Electrophysiological experiments indicate that substance P seems not to directly sensitize cutaneous nociceptors; it contributes to the peripheral hyperalgesia indirectly via its pro-inflammatory effects, including vasodilatation and histamine release from mast cells. Nociceptive stimuli cause release of substance P from the terminals of C-fibers in laminae I–II of the spinal cord. Substance P released from the central terminals acts on dorsal spinal cord neurons expressing substance P/neurokinin 1 receptor. Mantyh and his colleagues show that substance P causes internalization of neurokinin 1 receptor. Specific antagonists can block this excitatory effect of substance P on dorsal-horn neurons.

It has been generally accepted that substance P plays roles in the nociception and inflammatory pain. Studies in genetically mutated mice show that mice that lack either substance P or neurokinin 1 receptors do not respond to moderate or severe pain. However, the precise role of tachykinins in the nociceptive response of the spinal cord remains controversial, because substance P receptor antagonists cannot reduce human pain, and the nociceptive defect in substance P gene knockout mice appears to be mainly involved in supraspinal mechanisms and peripheral pro-inflammatory effects. Therefore, the physiological function of substance P in the dorsal spinal cord remains to be further elucidated.

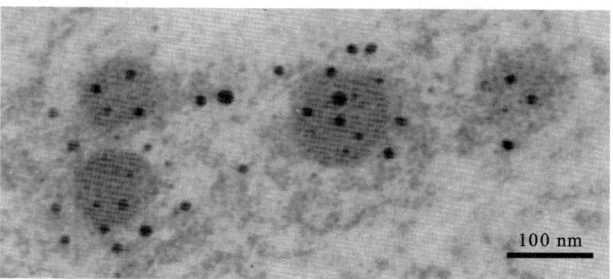

Fig.9.1   Triple-immunogold labeling shows the colocalization of substance P (15 nm gold particles), calcitonin gene-related peptide (10 nm) and galanin (5 nm) in the large dense-core vesicles in the terminal of C fiber in lamina II of the spinal cord of the rat.

OPIOID-PEPTIDES AND THEIR RECEPTORS

The most established clinical treatment that acts through neuropeptide receptors is the administration of morphine to patients with pain. The discovery of several endogenous peptide ligands for opioid receptors in the mid 1970s established the link between pain and opioid-peptides. Enkephalins, dynorphins, and other opioid-peptides are found in interneurons in the dorsal horn of the spinal cord, where they modulate incoming nociceptive impulses. Opioid-peptides are also found in several brain regions on the ascending or descending pathways that are responsible for the nociception/pain transmission or modulation, such as the periaqueductal grey matter. Importantly, a recent study reveals a regulatory mechanism of opioid analgesia. Downstream regulatory element antagonistic modulator (DREAM) is a calcium-sensing protein and inhibitor of prodynorphin transcription under basal conditions. Deletion of this gene results in reduced pain behaviour, being presumably due to the high concentrations of dynorphin A in the spinal cord of these mutated mice. This result suggests that manipulation of endogenous opioid peptides is a viable way to achieve analgesia.

One of the most important discoveries in pain study has been the identification of the opioid receptors in the pain pathways. Three major types of opioid receptors, μ-, δ-, κ-opioid receptors, have been cloned. Morphine primarily acts at μ-opioid receptors, enkephalin at δ-opioid receptors and dynorphin at κ-opioid receptors. These opioid receptors are expressed in neurons in DRG and the dorsal spinal cord. Therefore, they are both pre-synaptic and post-synaptic receptors in the dorsal spinal cord. In most cases, these opioid receptors directly mediate inhibitory effects on pain transmission. Substance P-containing small neurons express both μ-and δ-opioid receptors. In small DRG neurons δ-opioid receptors are localized in the cytoplasm and are often associated with LDCVs (Fig.9.2, see also the color plate), in contrast to the cell surface localization of μ-opioid receptors. δ-opioid receptors are inserted into the plasma membrane following agonist and nociceptive stimulations. It is interesting that agonists of μ-opioid receptor, [D-Ala^2, N-Me-Phe^4, Gly-ol^5]-enkephalin (DAMGO), endomorphin, methadone and fentanyl, but not morphine, induce internalization of surface μ-opioid receptors. The internalized μ-opioid receptors are recycled to the cell surface and resensitized. In contrast, δ-opioid receptor agonists induce δ-opioid receptor internalization and the

internalized receptors are mainly degraded in lysosomal compartments. The mechanisms underlying the differential trafficking of opioid receptors are unclear.

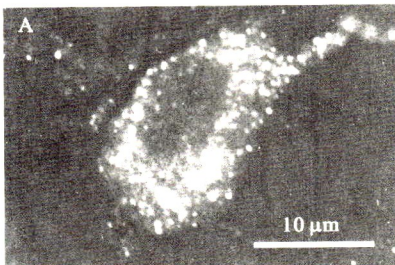

dorsal root gangalion

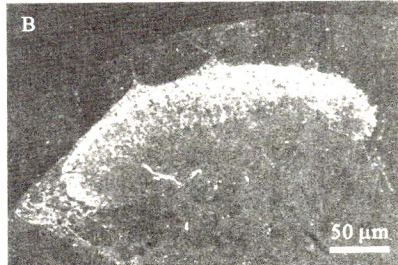

dorsal horn of spinal cord

Fig.9.2 A. Double-immunofluorescence labeling shows co-localization of δ-opioid receptor (in green) and calcitonin gene-related peptide (in red) in LDCVs in the cell body of a small neuron in the mouse dorsal root ganglion. B. The colocalization is seen in the terminals of C fibers in laminae I–II of the mouse spinal cord.

Recent studies show the interaction among different types of opioid receptor. For instance, μ-opioid receptor interacts with δ-opioid receptor, and this receptor interaction may be involved in the development of morphine tolerance. Therefore, when opioid receptors are genetically deleted, complex effects on pain behavior are seen. The mice lacking δ-opioid receptor or enkephalin do not develop morphine tolerance. Despite these findings, the hope for novel peptide ligands to replace morphine has not been fulfilled. Blockage of δ-opioid receptor while activating μ-opioid receptors is one of the potential strategies for increasing the efficiency of morphine analgesia while reducing the risk of development of morphine tolerance. Thus, understanding of the molecular and cellular mechanisms of opioid receptor trafficking remains at the center of pain research, and will help to develop new opioid therapies in pain treatments.

CHOLECYSTOKININ AND ITS RECEPTORS

In the spinal cord and the brain, the opioid systems can be counteracted by other endogenous peptide systems. The representative system is composed of cholecystokinin and its receptors. Only very low levels of cholecystokinin have been detected in DRG neurons under normal circumstance. In the superficial dorsal horn of the spinal cord, cholecystokinin is expressed in interneurons and often co-localized with μ-opioid receptor. In situ hybridization shows that its receptors, cholecystokinin A and B receptor, are present in DRG neurons. Cholecystokinin is shown to be pronociceptive, and antagonists of cholecystokinin B receptor are shown to be antinociceptive. In agreement, the mice deficient in cholecystokinin B receptor show reduction in mechanical sensitivity and hyperalgesia to thermal nociceptive stimuli. Cholecystokinin is probably an opioid antagonist. It has been shown that cholecystokinin system interacts with opioid system. Deletion of cholecystokinin B receptor in the mice results in an upregulation of the endogenous opioid system. Thus, cholecystokinin system is the interesting target of new drugs for pain treatment.

NEUROPEPTIDE Y AND ITS RECEPTORS

Neuropeptide Y is wildly expressed in the central nervous system and in the sympathetic neurons that innervate the blood vessels. This neuropeptide is normally not expressed in DRG neurons. However, its receptor, Y1 receptor, is expressed in small DRG neurons and interneurons in the inner lamina II of the spinal cord. These receptors are localized in the plasma membrane of the cell bodies of small DRG neurons containing calcitonin gene-related peptide (Fig.9.3, see also the color plate). In the dorsal spinal cord, Y1 receptors are expressed in GABAergic interneurons, and localized in the plasma membrane of the cell bodies and the dendrites. Another subtype of neuropeptide Y receptor, Y2 receptor, is identified in

medium-sized or large DRG neurons containing calcitonin gene-related peptide in rat and to localize in different subpopulation of DRG neurons with Y1 receptor. Intrathecal administration of neuropeptide Y induces spinal analgesia. A substantial decrease in pain threshold is seen in the mice lacking Y1 receptor.

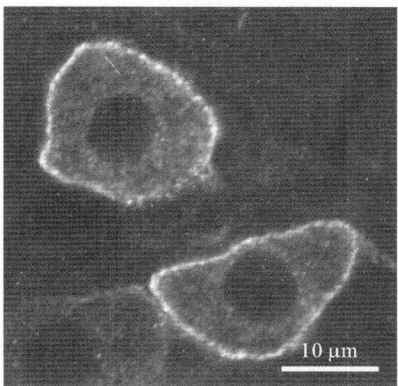

Fig.9.3   Immunofluorescence labeling shows that neuropeptide Y Y1 receptor is localized on the cell surface of the cell body of small neurons in the mouse dorsal root ganglion.

OTHER NEUROPEPTIDES AND G-PROTEIN-COUPLED RECEPTORS

A large G-protein-coupled receptor subfamily comprising 50 members that are related to MAS1, Mas-related genes (*mrgs*), is identified in DRG neurons. The results from in situ hybridization show that mrgAs and mrgD are specifically expressed in distinct subpopulations of small DRG neurons. At least mrgA1 and A4 can be activated by the RFamide neuropeptides NPFF and NPAF, respectively. Intrathecal administration of NPFF enhances the morphine analgesia.

Another recently identified subfamily of G-protein-coupled receptor in small DRG neurons is the sensory neuron-specific G-protein-coupled receptors (SNSRs). Proenkephalin A peptide fragment and bovine adrenal medulla peptide 22 (BAM22) activate these receptors, suggesting that SNSRs are involved in the modulation of nociception.

GENERAL CITATIONS

Abdelhamid E E, Sultana M, Portoghese P S, Takemori A E.
   1991. Selective blockage of delta opioid receptors prevents

the development of morphine tolerance and dependence in mice. *J Pharmacol Exp Ther*, 258: 299-303.

Bauerfeind R, Huttner W B. 1993. Biogenesis of constitutive secretory vesicles, secretory granules and synaptic vesicles. *Curr Opin Cell Biol*, 5: 628-635.

Bean A J, Zhang X, Hokfelt T. 1994. Peptide secretion: what do we know? *Faseb J*, 8: 630-638.

Hökfelt T. 1991. Neuropeptides in perspective: the last ten years. *Neuron*, 7: 867-879.

Hökfelt T, Bartfai T, Bloom F. 2003. Neuropeptides: opportunities for drug discovery. *Lancet Neurol*, 2: 463-472.

Hökfelt T, Zhang X, Wiesenfeld-Hallin Z. 1994. Messenger plasticity in primary sensory neurons following axotomy and its functional implications. *Trends Neurosci*, 17: 22-30.

Rupniak N M, Kramer M S. 1999. Discovery of the antidepressant and anti-emetic efficacy of substance P receptor (NK1) antagonists. *Trends Pharmacol Sci*, 20: 485-490.

Todd A J, Spike R C. 1993. The localization of classical transmitters and neuropeptides within neurons in laminae I-III of the mammalian spinal dorsal horn. *Prog Neurobiol*, 41: 609-645.

Waldhoer M, Bartlett S E, Whistler J L. 2004. Opioid receptors. *Annu Rev Biochem*, 73:953-990.

Woolf C J, Salter M W. 2000. Neuronal plasticity: increasing the gain in pain. *Science*, 288: 1765-1769.

DISCOVERY CITATIONS

Bao L, Jin S X, Zhang C, Wang L H, Xu Z Z, Zhang F X, Wang L C, Ning F S, Cai H J, Guan J S, *et al*. 2003. Activation of delta opioid receptors induces receptor insertion and neuropeptide secretion. *Neuron*, 37: 121-133.

Cao Y Q, Mantyh P W, Carlson E J, Gillespie A M, Epstein C J, Basbaum A I. 1998. Primary afferent tachykinins are required to experience moderate to intense pain. *Nature*, 392: 390-394.

Chang M M, Leeman S E. 1970. Isolation of a sialogogic peptide from bovine hypothalamic tissue and its characterization as substance P. *J Biol Chem*, 245: 4784-4790.

Cheng H Y, Pitcher G M, Laviolette S R, Whishaw I Q, Tong K I, Kockeritz L K, Wada T, Joza N A, Crackower M, Goncalves J, *et al*. 2002. DREAM is a critical transcriptional repressor for pain modulation. *Cell*, 108, 31-43.

De Felipe C, Herrero J F, O'Brien J A, Palmer J A, Doyle C A, Smith A J, Laird J M, Belmonte C, Cervero F, Hunt S P. 1998. Altered nociception, analgesia and aggression in mice lacking the receptor for substance P. *Nature*, 392: 394-397.

Dong X, Han S, Zylka M J, Simon M I, Anderson D J. 2001. A diverse family of GPCRs expressed in specific subsets of nociceptive sensory neurons. *Cell*, 106: 619-632.

Fields H L, Emson P C, Leigh B K, Gilbert R F, Iversen L L. 1980. Multiple opiate receptor sites on primary afferent fibres. *Nature*, 284: 351-353.

Hökfelt T, Kellerth J O, Nilsson G, Pernow B. 1975. Substance P: localization in the central nervous system and in some primary sensory neurons. *Science*, 190: 889-890.

Jung L J, Scheller R H. 1991. Peptide processing and targeting in the neuronal secretory pathway. *Science*, 251: 1330-1335.

Kerekes N, Landry M, Rydh-Rinder M, Hokfelt T. 1997. The effect of NGF, BDNF and bFGF on expression of galanin in cultured rat dorsal root ganglia. *Brain Res*, 754: 131-141.

Kessler J A, Black I B. 1980. Nerve growth factor stimulates the development of substance P in sensory ganglia. *Proc Natl Acad Sci USA*, 77: 649-652.

Kurrikoff K, Koks S, Matsui T, Bourin M, Arend A, Aunapuu M, Vasar E. 2004. Deletion of the CCK2 receptor gene reduces mechanical sensitivity and abolishes the development of hyperalgesia in mononeuropathic mice. *Eur J Neurosci*, 20: 1577-1586.

Lamotte C, Pert C B, Snyder S H. 1976. Opiate receptor binding in primate spinal cord: distribution and changes after dorsal root section. *Brain Res*, 112: 407-412.

Lembo P M, Grazzini E, Groblewski T, O'Donnell D, Roy M O, Zhang J, Hoffert C, Cao J, Schmidt R, Pelletier M, *et al*. 2002. Proenkephalin A gene products activate a new family of sensory neuron—specific GPCRs. *Nat Neurosci*, 5: 201-209.

Levine J D, Fields H L, Basbaum A I. 1993. Peptides and the primary afferent nociceptor. *J Neurosci*, 13: 2273-2286.

Lindsay R M, Harmar A J. 1989. Nerve growth factor regulates expression of neuropeptide genes in adult sensory neurons. *Nature*, 337: 362-364.

Liu H, Brown J L, Jasmin L, Maggio J E, Vigna S R, Mantyh P

W, Basbaum A I. 1994. Synaptic relationship between substance P and the substance P receptor: light and electron microscopic characterization of the mismatch between neuropeptides and their receptors. *Proc Natl Acad Sci USA*, 91: 1009-1013.

Naim M, Spike R C, Watt C, Shehab S A, Todd A J. 1997. Cells in laminae III and IV of the rat spinal cord that possess the neurokinin-1 receptor and have dorsally directed dendrites receive a major synaptic input from tachykinin-containing primary afferents. *J Neurosci*, 17: 5536-5548.

Naveilhan P, Hassani H, Lucas G, Blakeman K H, Hao J X, Xu X J, Wiesenfeld-Hallin Z, Thoren P, Ernfors P. 2001. Reduced antinociception and plasma extravasation in mice lacking a neuropeptide Y receptor. *Nature*, 409: 513-517.

Nawa H, Hirose T, Takashima H, Inayama S, Nakanishi S. 1983. Nucleotide sequences of cloned cDNAs for two types of bovine brain substance P precursor. *Nature*, 306: 32-36.

Nitsche J F, Schuller A G, King M A, Zengh M, Pasternak G W, Pintar J E. 2002. Genetic dissociation of opiate tolerance and physical dependence in delta-opioid receptor-1 and preproenkephalin knock-out mice. *J Neurosci*, 22: 10906-10913.

Otten U, Goedert M, Mayer N, Lembeck F. 1980. Requirement of nerve growth factor for development of substance P-containing sensory neurones. *Nature*, 287: 158-159.

Panula P, Kalso E, Nieminen M, Kontinen V K, Brandt A, Pertovaara A. 1999. Neuropeptide FF and modulation of pain. *Brain Res*, 848: 191-196.

Polgar E, Shehab S A, Watt C, Todd A J. 1999. GABAergic neurons that contain neuropeptide Y selectively target cells with the neurokinin 1 receptor in laminae III and IV of the rat spinal cord. *J Neurosci*, 19: 2637-2646.

Pommier B, Beslot F, Simon A, Pophillat M, Matsui T, Dauge V, Roques B P, Noble F. 2002. Deletion of CCK2 receptor in mice results in an upregulation of the endogenous opioid system. *J Neurosci*, 22: 2005-2011.

Tsao P I, von Zastrow M. 2000. Type-specific sorting of G protein-coupled receptors after endocytosis. *J Biol Chem*, 275: 11130-11140.

von Euler U S, Gaddum J H. 1931. An unidentified depressor substance in certain tissue extracts. *J Physiol*, 72: 74-87.

Zhang X, Bao L, Arvidsson U, Elde R, Hökfelt T. 1998. Localization and regulation of the delta-opioid receptor in dorsal root ganglia and spinal cord of the rat and monkey: evidence for association with the membrane of large dense-core vesicles. *Neuroscience*, 82: 1225-1242.

Zhang X, Bao L, Xu Z Q, Kopp J, Arvidsson U, Elde R, Hökfelt T. 1994. Localization of neuropeptide Y Y1 receptors in the rat nervous system with special reference to somatic receptors on small dorsal root ganglion neurons. *Proc Natl Acad Sci USA*, 91: 11738-11742.

Zhang X, Dagerlind A, Elde R P, Castel M-N, Broberger C, Wiesenfeld-Halin Z, Hökfelt T. 1993a. Marked increase in cholecystokinin B receptor messenger RNA levels in rat dorsal root ganglia after peripheral axotomy. *Neuroscience*, 57: 227-233.

Zhang X, Nicholas A P, Hökfelt T. 1993b. Ultrastructural studies on peptides in the dorsal horn of the spinal cord. I. Co-existence of galanin with other peptides in primary afferents in normal rats. *Neuroscience*, 57: 365-384.

Zhang X, Shi T, Holmberg K, Landry M, Huang W, Xiao H, Ju G, Hökfelt T. 1997. Expression and regulation of the neuropeptide Y Y2 receptor in sensory and autonomic ganglia. *Proc Natl Acad Sci USA*, 94: 729-734.

Zhu Y, King M A, Schuller A G, Nitsche J F, Reidl M, Elde R P, Unterwald E, Pasternak G W, Pintar J E. 1999. Retention of supraspinal delta-like analgesia and loss of morphine tolerance in delta opioid receptor knockout mice. *Neuron*, 24: 243-252.

Zimmer A, Zimmer A M, Baffi J, Usdin T, Reynolds K, Konig M, Palkovits M, Mezey E. 1998. Hypoalgesia in mice with a targeted deletion of the tachykinin 1 gene. *Proc Natl Acad Sci USA*, 95: 2630-2635.

ATP and Its Receptors in Pain

CHAPTER 10

Terumasa Nakatsuka, Jianguo G. Gu

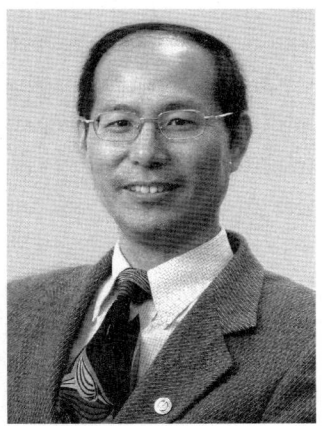

Dr. Gu is an Associate Professor at the Department of Oral & Maxillofacial Surgery & Diagnostic Sciences, College of Dentistry and McKnight Brain Institute, University of Florida, Gainesville, FL, USA. He graduated from Shanghai Medical University, Shanghai, China and obtained a PhD, Department of Pharmacology, University of Manitoba, Canada.

MAJOR CONTRIBUTIONS

1. Gu JG, MacDermott AB. 1997. Activation of ATP P2X receptors elicits glutamate release from sensory neuron synapses. *Nature*, 389: 749-753.
2. Nakatsuka T, Gu JG. 2001. ATP P2X receptor-mediated enhancement of glutamate release and evoked EPSCs in dorsal horn neurons of the rat spinal cord. *J Neurosci*, 21: 6522-6531.
3. Nakatsuka T, Furue H, Yoshimura M, Gu JG. 2002. Activation of central terminal vanilloid receptor-1 receptors and alpha beta-methylene-ATP-sensitive P2X receptors reveals a converged synaptic activity onto the deep dorsal horn neurons of the spinal cord. *J Neurosci*, 22: 1228-1237.
4. Nakatsuka T, Tsuzuki K, Ling JX, Sonobe H, Gu JG. 2003. Distinct roles of P2X receptors in modulating glutamate release at different primary sensory synapses in rat spinal cord. *J Neurophysiol*, 89: 3243-3252.

5. Chen M, Gu JG. 2005. A P2X receptor-mediated nociceptive afferent pathway to lamina I of the spinal cord. *Mol Pain*, 1: 4.

MAIN TOPICS

ATP-induced painful sensations

P2X receptors on sensory ganglion neurons

P2X receptors on the central terminals of primary afferents

P2X receptors on spinal cord dorsal horn neurons

P2X receptors in inflammatory pain

P2X receptors in neuropathic pain

Sensory functions of P2Y receptors

SUMMARY

In the somatosensory system, ATP released from tissues serves as a sensory mediator to elicit impulses at peripheral terminals of primary afferent fibers and to modulate sensory synaptic transmission at central sites in the spinal cord dorsal horn. The sensory effects of ATP are mainly mediated by P2X and P2Y receptors, two purinergic receptor subfamilies that are expressed on primary afferent fibers. Both receptor subtypes have been indicated to be involved in nociceptive signaling, transmission and regulation. Thus, these receptors may represent a promising target for therapeutic management of pain.

INTRODUCTION

ATP is a nucleotide that plays essential roles in cells. Intracellular ATP serves as a primary energy source for most activities of living cells. ATP can also be released to extracellular space to function as an intercellular chemical messenger. Actions of extracellular ATP are mediated by ATP receptors expressed on plasma membranes of cells. ATP receptors belong to purinergic receptor family, a multifunctional receptor family classified into P1 receptor (for adenosine) and P2 receptor (for ATP and other nucleotides). On pharmacological and molecular biological bases, P2 receptors can be further classified into two subfamilies, P2X receptor family and P2Y receptor family.

P2X receptor family consists of at least seven P2X subunits ($P2X_1$–$P2X_7$). Each P2X subunit has two transmembrane domains with a cysteine rich extracellular loop, which contains the ATP binding site (Fig.10.1A). Each functional P2X receptor is composed of three or more P2X subunits, forming a pore structure that is permeable to cations including Ca^{2+}. Therefore, P2X receptor family is a ligand-gated ion channel family. Assembled from the 7 P2X subunits, at least 11 subtypes of functional P2X receptors can be formed in heterologous expression system. These 11 P2X receptors are homomeric $P2X_1$ to $P2X_7$ receptors, heteromeric $P2X_{1/5}$, $P2X_{2/3}$, $P2X_{2/6}$, and $P2X_{4/6}$. More functional P2X receptors may be assembled from P2X subunits. While ATP activates all functional P2X receptors, α, β-methylene ATP, a metabolically stable ATP analog preferentially activates $P2X_1$, $P2X_3$, $P2X_{1/5}$, $P2X_{2/3}$, $P2X_{4/6}$ receptors. Several other ATP analogs, including 2-methylthio-ATP (2MeSATP), adenosine-5'-O-(3-thiotriphosphate (ATPγS), and 2', 3'-O-(benzoyl-4-benzoyl)-ATP (BzATP), are also agonists for P2X receptors. Kinetically, homomeric $P2X_1$ and $P2X_3$ receptors desensitize rapidly after activation but other P2X receptors have weak or little desensitization. Suramin and pyridoxal-phosphate-6-azophenyl-2', 4'-disulphonic acid tetrasodium (PPADS) are broad spectrum antagonists for all P2X receptors except $P2X_7$ receptor.

Trinitrophenyl-adenosine triphosphate (TNP-ATP), on the other hand, was shown to be highly selective to block $P2X_1$, $P2X_3$, and $P2X_{2/3}$ receptors. Cyclic pryridoxine-4, 5-mono-phsophate-6-azo-phenyl-2', 5'-disulfonate (MRS2220) bolocks $P2X_1$ receptors but has no effect on $P2X_2$ or $P2X_4$ receptors. Recently, A-317491 has been identified as a potent antagonist for $P2X_3$ and $P2X_{2/3}$ receptors. Di-inosine pentaphosphate (Ip5I) is much more potent to block $P2X_1$ and $P2X_3$ receptors than to block $P2X_{2/3}$ receptors and is useful to distinguish between $P2X_3$ and $P2X_{2/3}$ receptors. Brilliant Blue G is a selective blocker of $P2X_7$ receptors. Brilliant Blue G blocks $P2X_7$ receptors in nanomolar range, although $P2X_2$ and $P2X_4$ receptors are blocked in the micromolar range and other subtypes are unaffected. Oxidized ATP irreversibly blocks $P2X_1$, $P2X_2$, and $P2X_7$ receptors.

P2Y receptors are G protein-coupled receptors. These receptor proteins contain typical features of G-protein-coupled receptors including seven predicted hydrophobic transmembrane domains (Fig.10.1B). At least 8 subtypes of P2Y receptors, including $P2Y_1$, $P2Y_2$, $P2Y_4$, $P2Y_6$, $P2Y_{11}$, $P2Y_{12}$, $P2Y_{13}$, and $P2Y_{14}$, have been identified so far in mammals. Based on intracellular signaling pathways coupled with P2Y receptor activation, they can be categorized into two major classes. The first class includes $P2Y_1$, $P2Y_2$, $P2Y_4$, $P2Y_6$, and $P2Y_{11}$; they predominantly couple to Gq protein and lead to the activation of phospholipase C. The second class includes $P2Y_{12}$, $P2Y_{13}$, and $P2Y_{14}$; they couple to Gi protein and cause the inhibition of adenylyl cyclase and regulation of ion channels. In addition to ATP, the principal physiological agonists of P2Y receptors also include ADP, UTP, UDP, and 2-methyltio-ADP (2-MeSADP). Suramin acts as an antagonist at most P2Y-receptors with the exception of $P2Y_4$ receptors. PPADS has been shown to block $P2Y_1$, $P2Y_4$ and $P2Y_6$ receptors. Reactive blue 2 is an antagonist of $P2Y_1$, $P2Y_4$, $P2Y_6$, and $P2Y_{11}$ receptors. The nucleotide analogue 2'-deoxy-N^6-methyladenosine-3',5'-bisphosphate (MRS 2179) seems to be a potent and selective antagonist at $P2Y_1$ receptor.

Sensory functions of ATP have long been proposed before the identifications of its receptors. Holton and Holton (1953) first showed over half century ago that sensory neurons could release ATP and suggested that ATP might function as a chemical messenger to transfer sensory information. This idea was not greatly appreciated until three decade later after the demonstration of ATP-induced membrane depolarizing currents in both sensory ganglion neurons and spinal cord dorsal horn neurons. Since the first identification and cloning of cDNAs encoding P2X receptors in 1994, a great body of evidence has been accumulated to indicate that ATP and P2X receptors are involved in a variety of pain mechanisms. P2Y receptors are also widely expressed in somatosensory system including primary afferent fibers and dorsal horn neurons. The potential nociceptive functions of P2Y receptors have just been explored recently. This chapter will introduce nociceptive functions of ATP and its receptors to pain researchers who are not specified in purinergic system.

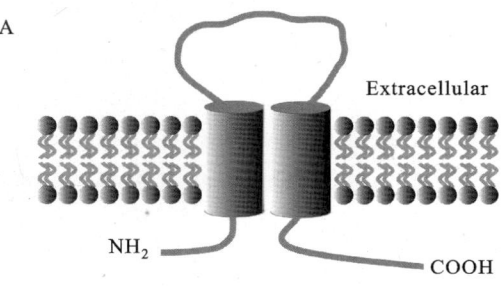

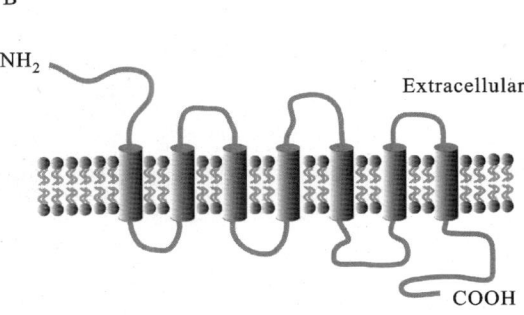

Fig.10.1 Structures of P2 receptors. A. P2X subunits have two transmembrane domains with a cysteine rich extracellular loop which contains the ATP binding site. B. P2Y receptors are G-protein-coupled receptors including seven predicted hydrophobic transmembrane domains.

ATP-INDUCED PAINFUL SENSATIONS

Algogenic or pain-producing actions of ATP were observed on the human blister base preparation sev-

eral decades ago. When ATP was injected intradermally into the backs of human volunteers, it evoked weal and flare responses in a dose dependent manner. Injections of ATP into the forearms of human volunteers produced a persistent painful sensation, unlike histamine which only produced transient pain or itch on some occasions (Fig.10.2). ATP-induced painful sensations in humans were not relieved by indomethacin, doxantrazole and cimetidine. More recently, pain-producing effects of ATP were studied in details in human volunteers. When ATP was delivered to the forearm skin of volunteers, it produced a modest burning pain sensation, which began within 20 seconds and was maintained for several minutes. Persistent delivery of ATP led to desensitization within 12 min but the recovery was almost 1 hour later. ATP also caused an increase in blood flow, as assessed using a laser Doppler flow meter. Pain induced by ATP was suggested to be dependent on capsaicin-sensitive sensory neurons since the pain was reduced in the skin treated repeatedly with topical capsaicin. It was shown that painful sensations were much enhanced when ATP was injected into the skin after solar radiation. These findings indicate that ATP produces burning pain by activating nociceptors of capsaicin-sensitive afferent fibers. Thus, ATP is an activator of nociceptors and endogenous ATP may be a mediator of pain in somatosensory and trigeminal sensory systems. Similar to human studies, nociceptive behaviors were observed in animals following a subplantar injection of ATP or α, β-methylene ATP. Desensitization of capsaicin-sensitive peripheral nerves with a subplantar injection of capsaicin abolished the nociceptive behaviors in animals subsequently injected with α, β-methylene ATP. While exogenous ATP has been shown to provoke painful sensations in both humans and animals, no direct evidence has been obtained to show that endogenously released ATP produces painful sensations in humans or animals. Normally, endogenous ATP levels at extracellular space are kept very low due to the high activity of ecto-nucletidase, which can rapidly metabolize ATP. However, intracellular ATP levels are near 10 mM. Therefore, a large amount of ATP can be released during tissue damage, which may stimulate nociceptive neurons expressing ATP receptors. This possibility was tested by a study using a co-culture of skin cells and primary afferent neurons. It was found that skin cell damage caused action potential firing in adjacent primary afferent neurons. The action was eliminated by enzymatic degradation of ATP, desensitization or blockade of P2X receptors. This finding suggests that ATP from the cytosol of damaged cells can provide a rapid signal to initiate nociceptive response through P2X receptor activation.

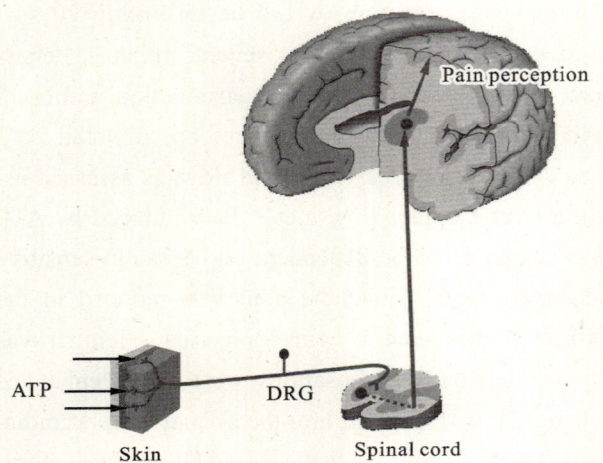

Fig.10.2 ATP and pain. ATP released from damaged cells stimulates P2X receptors on peripheral terminals of primary afferents and initiates pain.

P2X RECEPTORS ON SENSORY GANGLION NEURONS

The cell bodies of primary afferent fibers or sensory ganglion neurons have been used as a model for studying nociceptors. In neurons isolated from dorsal root ganglions of rats and cats, ATP was shown to evoke inward currents. The inward currents showed rapid activation, but decay phase displayed very distinct kinetics in different cells, from fast and complete desensitization to little desensitization. Based on desensitization rates and patterns, ATP-evoked currents were classified into three basic phenotypes, fast, slow, and mixed current types. Molecular cloning of P2X receptors, particularly $P2X_3$ receptors, has led to a better understating of molecular substrates for

ATP-activated inward currents and their potential sensory functions. In fact, $P2X_3$ receptor has been the main focus in studying nociceptive functions of P2X receptor family. $P2X_3$ receptor was identified and cloned from dorsal root ganglion (DRG) neurons. The channel transcript was present in a subset of sensory ganglion neurons, but it was not observed in other tissues, including sympathetic neurons, enteric neurons, and central nervous system.

$P2X_3$-immunoreactivity was shown predominantly on IB4-poisitive and TRPV1-ir positive neurons, suggesting a nociceptive function of P2X3 receptors. One of the key findings suggesting nociceptive functions of $P2X_3$ receptors was $P2X_3$ receptor-mediated excitation of tooth-pulp nociceptive neurons. ATP-evoked currents on tooth-pulp nociceptive neurons were shown to be similar to those of heterologously expressed channels containing $P2X_3$ subunits. Furthermore, $P2X_3$-ir was found on both cell bodies and afferent fiber endings of tooth-pulp nociceptors. On the other hand, non-nociceptive neurons of muscle stretching afferent fibers were lack of $P2X_3$-ir although they also responded to ATP. Thus, the study demonstrated that nociceptive and non-nociceptive sensory ganglion neurons express distinct P2X receptors. Nociceptive functions of $P2X_3$ receptors were further supported by pain behavioral assessment performed on $P2X_3$-knockout mice.

In heterologous expression system, ATP and α, β-methylene ATP evoked rapidly desensitizing currents in $P2X_3$ receptor expressing cells and they evoked slowly desensitizing currents in cells co-expressed $P2X_3$ and $P2X_2$ subunits. The slow P2X currents were mediated by heteromeric $P2X_{2/3}$ receptors. In somotosensory system, *in situ* hybridization revealed that small-sized DRG neurons predominantly possessed mRNAs for $P2X_3$, medium-sized neurons expressed mRNAs for both $P2X_2$ and $P2X_3$ subunits, and large-sized DRG neurons did not express detectable $P2X_3$ mRNAs. Thus, $P2X_3$ receptor subunits on small-sized sensory neurons may be assembled as homomeric $P2X_3$ receptors, which may account for fast current phenotype observed in many small-sized DRG neurons. On the other hand, P2X$_3$ receptor subunits may be assembled together with P2X$_2$ subunits to form P2X$_{2/3}$ receptors in medium-sized DRG neurons, which may account for slow current phenotype observed in these neurons. The co-expression of homomeric P2X$_3$ and heteromeric P2X$_{2/3}$ in the same neurons was thought to account for the mixed currents shown in some medium-sized DRG neurons.

While nociceptive functions of homomeric P2X$_3$ receptors were well supported by their expression patterns, it remains unclear about the sensory functions of heteromeric P2X$_{2/3}$ receptors. P2X$_{2/3}$ receptors appeared to be mainly expressed on capsaicin-insensitive DRG neurons. This suggests that these receptors may not be involved in physiological pain conditions. However, the potential role of P2X$_{2/3}$ in pathological pain states has been suggested in animal models. It was found that α, β-methylene ATP injection into rat plantar surface produced mechanical allodynia along with nocifensive behavior and thermal hyperalgesia. Interestingly, the mechanical allodynia evoked by α, β-methylene ATP remained in neonatal capsaicin-treated rats. Because neonatal capsaicin treatment selectively removed the subpopulation of nociceptive neurons that express TRPV1 and homomeric P2X$_3$ receptors, the allodynia induced by α, β-methylene ATP was suggested to be mediated by P2X$_{2/3}$ receptors rather than homomeric P2X$_3$ receptors.

The expression of P2X receptors other than P2X$_3$ and P2X$_{2/3}$ subtypes has been explored on DRG neurons. Immunoreactivities for P2X$_1$ to P2X$_6$ receptors have all been found on sensory ganglion neurons. The combination of patch-clamp recordings with immunostaining for P2X$_1$ and P2X$_3$ receptor subunits on acutely dissociated DRG neurons showed that ATP could evoke rapidly desensitizing currents not only in DRG neurons with P2X$_3$-immunoreactivity, but also in the neurons with P2X$_1$-immunoreactivity alone. Kinetics of ATP-activated current was also shown significantly different between P2X$_1$-ir DRG neurons and P2X$_3$-ir DRG neurons. These results suggested that P2X$_1$ receptors also contributed to fast currents evoked by ATP. For α, β-methylene ATP-evoked slow currents, a recent study has indicated that in addition to P2X$_{2/3}$ receptors, other P2X receptors may contribute to these slow currents. This conclusion was based on the effects of TNP-ATP, a potent antagonist of P2X$_1$, P2X$_3$, and P2X$_{2/3}$ receptors, on α, β-methylene ATP-induced currents in acutely dissociated DRG neurons. It was found that in a subpopulation of DRG neurons, α, β-methylene ATP-evoked slow currents could not be blocked by TNP-ATP, but could be inhibited by PPADS. Based on pharmacological and electrophysiological profiles, the TNP-ATP-resistant slow currents were suggested to be mediated by P2X$_{4/6}$ and/or P2X$_{1/5}$ receptors. The sensory functions of these P2X receptors remain to be studied.

P2X RECEPTORS ON THE CENTRAL TERMINALS OF PRIMARY AFFERENTS

Functional subgroups of primary afferent fibers terminated in different lamina regions of the dorsal horn. The central terminals of primary afferent fibers are presynaptic sites of the first sensory synapses within the spinal cord dorsal horn. Many receptors on these terminals play a role in modulating sensory synaptic transmission. P2X receptor-immunoreactivity associated with central terminals of primary afferents has been examined using antibodies against P2X$_1$, P2X$_2$, and P2X$_3$ subunits. The immunoreactivity of P2X$_3$ receptors was observed in the inner portion of substantia gelatinosa and was reduced subsequent to dorsal rhizotomy, as well as subsequent to neonatal capsaicin treatment. P2X$_1$ and P2X$_2$ immunoreactivities in afferent central terminals were also found in superficial laminae. The immunostaining for P2X$_3$ receptor subunit was colocalized with that for TRPV1 receptor or lectin IB4 in the inner portion of substantia gelatinosa. When saporin-conjugated IB4 was injected into rat sciatic nerve to chemically remove IB4-positive neurons, the immunostaining for P2X$_3$ receptor were almost completely disappeared in the spinal cord. To demonstrate the role of presynaptic P2X receptors at sensory synapses, effects of ATP and its analogs on glutamatergic synaptic transmission were examined using a DRG-dorsal horn co-culture system. It was shown that activation of P2X receptors localized at presynaptic terminals on DRG neurons resulted in increased frequency of spontaneous glutamate release as well as directly elicited action potentials at the terminals to cause glutamate release. Patch-clamp experiments performed on spinal cord slice preparations further showed that distinct subtypes of P2X receptors were located at presynaptic terminals that innervate several different laminas, including lamina I, substantia gelatinosa (lamina II), and lamina V neurons. Moreover, the activation of these P2X receptors enhanced glutamate release in different fashions (Fig.10.3). In substantia gelatinosa neurons, the modulation of glutamate release by presynaptic P2X receptors was mainly transient. In contrast, P2X receptor-mediated modulation of glutamate release was long-lasting in lamina I and lamina V neurons. Pharmacologically, both transient and long-lasting types of modulation were blocked by PPADS. Transient modulation was not observed in the presence of TNP-ATP, suggesting that homomeric P2X$_3$ receptors may be involved in presynaptic modulation in substantia gelatinosa neurons. In lamina V neurons, P2X receptor-mediated long-lasting modulation of glutamate release remained in the presence of TNP-ATP. In addition, the removal of P2X$_3$ recep-

tor-expressing afferent terminals by the targeting toxin saporin-conjugated IB4 or by surgical removal of superficial dorsal horn did not affect presynaptic P2X receptor-mediated long-lasting modulation of glutamate release in lamina V neurons. The pharmacological profiles appeared to be consistent with the involvement of P2X$_{4/6}$ or P2X$_{1/5}$ receptors. Differences among P2X repressing afferent fibers in superficial lamina (lamina I & II) and lamina V also include capsaicin-sensitivity. In superficial laminas, P2X expressing afferent central terminals were derived from capsaicin-sensitive primary afferents, while P2X-expressing central terminals in lamina V were from capsaicin-insensitive Aδ primary afferents. Although P2X$_3$-expressing central terminals only directly make synapses in lamina II, inputs from these afferent terminals could recruit both excitatory and inhibitory synaptic activities and polysynaptically conveyed the activity to lamina V neurons. These polysynaptic inputs, together with monosynaptic inputs that were carried by P2X-expressing/ capsaicin-insensitive afferent fibers, were shown to converge on lamina V neurons (Fig.10.3). This convergence could produce temporal summation in the same lamina V neurons. It has been suggested that this convergence may lead to the development of hyperactivity in deep dorsal horn neurons following tissue inflammation and nerve injury.

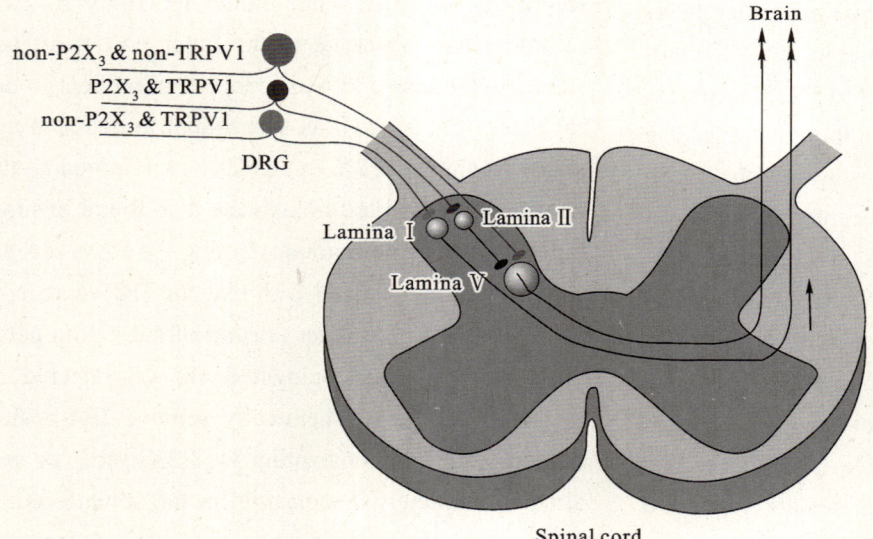

Fig.10.3 P2X receptors in central terminals of primary afferents. The schematic diagram illustrates three P2X-puringeric sensory pathways to lamina I, II, and V of the spinal cord dorsal horn. The pathway to lamina II is the afferent fibers expressing both P2X$_3$ and TRPV1 receptors. The P2X receptor subtypes of two other pathways had pharmacological properties distinct from P2X$_3$ containing receptors.

P2X RECEPTORS ON SPINAL CORD DORSAL HORN NEURONS

The first observation of ATP actions on sensory neurons was made on both primary afferent neurons and dorsal horn neurons. It was shown that in a subpopulation of cultured dorsal horn neurons, ATP produced a rapid and marked depolarization accompanied with action potentials. All P2X mRNAs except $P2X_3$ were widely distributed in the spinal cord dorsal horn. $P2X_2$, $P2X_4$, and $P2X_6$ were strongly expressed in superficial laminae, while all P2X mRNAs except $P2X_3$ sparsely distributed in deep dorsal horn. In acutely dissociated dorsal horn neurons from superficial lamina, ATP evoked slowly desensitizing inward currents but α, β-methylene ATP was not effective. It was found that the ATP-evoked currents on dorsal horn neurons were sensitive to the block by suramin and PPADS. ATP was able to evoke Ca^{2+} transients in the presence of La^{3+} to block voltage gated Ca^{2+} channels suggested that postsynaptic P2X receptors on dorsal horn neurons are highly Ca^{2+}-permeable. In a small population of dorsal horn neurons of superficial lamina, it was found that EPSCs could not be completely blocked by glutamate receptor antagonists but can be blocked by addition of P2X receptor antagonists suramin and PPADS. This result suggested that P2X receptors were localized at postsynaptic sites of a small population of dorsal horn neurons to mediate sensory synaptic transmission. The subtypes of P2X receptors on dorsal horn neurons remain unclear due to the lack of selective P2X receptor antagonists for different P2X receptor subtypes. In the spinal cord slice preparations, application of ATP evoked inward currents. However, it was not clear whether the ATP-evoked inward current in this study was mediated by P2X receptors on dorsal horn neurons or secondary response in the slice preparations. In fact, most investigators have failed to elicit P2X currents in brain and spinal cord slice preparations. The reason for unable to demonstrate functional P2X receptors in tissue slice preparations remains unclear. One possibility is that P2X receptors are mainly expressed on presynaptic terminals and the levels of P2X receptors on cell bodies are very low. The expression of P2X receptors on presynaptic terminals of dorsal horn inhibitory neurons have been demonstrated using cultured neurons from neonatal rats. It was shown that ATP increased the frequency of miniature inhibitory postsynaptic currents (mIPSCs) mediated by $GABA_A$ receptors in subpopulation of the dorsal horn neurons. These presynaptic effects were inhibited by suramin, PPADS, and reactive blue and were not reproduced by UTP or ADP-β-S, suggesting the involvement of P2X receptors rather than of P2Y receptors. ATP reversibly increased the amplitude of electrically evoked GABAergic IPSCs and changed paired-pulse ratio without affecting IPSC kinetics. The effects of ATP might be mediated by P2X receptors having a pharmacological profile dominated by the $P2X_2$ subtype. These findings suggest that presynaptic P2X receptors underlie an inhibitory action of ATP on a subset of GABAergic interneurons involved in the spinal processing of nociceptive information. Furthermore, using synaptic bouton preparations, it was demonstrated that activation of P2X receptors facilitated glycine release from the nerve terminals of glycinergic interneurons projecting onto substantia gelatinsa neurons. The increase of spontaneous glycine release by ATP required extracellular Ca^{2+} but not the operation of the voltage-gated Ca^{2+} channels. The effects of ATP were completely abolished by suramin and PPADS and the actions of ATP were not affected by NEM, which blocks the function of G proteins. The glycinergic miniature IPSC frequency was increased by 2MeSATP, but not by α, β-methylene ATP, and that both suramin and PPADS blocked the facilitatory effect of ATP, suggest that the purinorecptors involved are likely to be $P2X_2$ receptors. While functional P2X receptors have been confirmed to be present on the spinal cord dorsal horn, perhaps mainly on presynaptic terminals of inhibitory neurons, their roles in nociception remain to be studied.

P2X RECEPTORS IN INFLAMMATORY PAIN

Co-administration of ATP or α, β-methylene ATP with formalin, carrageenan, or complete Freund's adjuvant (CFA) into the rat hindpaw strongly enhanced nociceptive behaviors in rodents. Both ATP and α, β-methylene ATP specifically activated the peripheral terminals of Aδ and C-fiber nociceptors in *in vitro* skin-nerve preparation. In addition, P2X receptor agonists produced elevated ongoing activities in C-mechanoheat nociceptors under carrageenan inflammation. These results provide evidence in support of P2X receptor-mediated augmentation of inflammatory pain sensations. The ablation of $P2X_3$ gene resulted in the loss of rapidly desensitizing ATP-activated currents in DRG neurons. In these $P2X_3$ knock-out mice, formalin-induced pain behavior was reduced although the deletion of $P2X_3$ gene caused the enhancement of thermal hyperalgesia in chronic inflammation. The intrathecal treatment with P2X receptor antagonists, PPADS or TNP-ATP suppressed both of formalin- and capsaicin-induced nociceptive behaviors in mice. Similarly, the intrathecal administration of $P2X_3$ receptor antisense oligonucleotide significantly decreased nociceptive behaviors observed after CFA, formalin or α, β-methylene ATP into the rat hindpaw. These results have demonstrated that activation of $P2X_3$ receptors contributes to the expression of chronic inflammatory states and that relief of chronic pain may be achieved by selective blockade of $P2X_3$ receptor activation. Recently, a selective antagonist for $P2X_3$ and $P2X_{2/3}$ receptors, A-317491, has been developed. Consist with previous observations using $P2X_3$ antisense, intraplantar and intrathecal injections of A-317491 produced dose-related antinociception in chronic thermal hyperalgesia under CFA inflammation. A-317491 was also very effective in reducing the number of nocifensive events triggered by formalin injection into rat hindpaw.

Mechanisms by which P2X receptors are involved in inflammatory pain have been explored. It was shown that peripheral inflammation enhanced the expression of $P2X_2$ and $P2X_3$ receptors in DRG neurons, caused large increase in ATP-activated rapidly- and slowly-desensitizing currents, and altered the voltage dependence of P2X receptors (Fig.10.4B). The increase in ATP responses gave rise to large depolarizations that exceeded the threshold of action potentials in inflamed DRG neurons. Thus, up-regulation of P2X receptors may sensitize ATP signaling via P2X receptors and thereby may contribute to inflammatory pain state. Although it remains unclear how inflammation resulted in P2X receptor up-regulation, one mechanism could be up-regulation of P2X receptors by growth factors. Nerve growth factors are known to be increased during inflammation. Intrathecal administration of GDNF or NGF was found to increase the number of $P2X_3$-positive neurons in both cervical and lumbar DRG rats. GDNF treatment also increased $P2X_3$ immunoreactivity in inner substantia gelatinosa in the spinal cord while $P2X_3$ expression in control animals was restricted to a narrow band of primary afferent terminals within inner substantia gelatinosa of the spinal cord. More interestingly, NGF treatment induced novel pattern of $P2X_3$ expression, with intense immunoreactivity in axons projecting to lamina I and to the ventro-medial afferent bundle beneath the central canal. The change in $P2X_3$ expression patterns may be important in $P2X_3$ involvement of inflammatory pain. In addition to up-regulation by growth factors, modulation of P2X receptors by inflammatory mediators may be another important mechanism for sensitizing nociceptive signaling pathways via ATP and P2X receptors. A number of inflammatory mediators were found to directly modulate P2X receptor-mediated currents. For example, currents mediated by homomeric $P2X_3$ and heteromeric $P2X_{2/3}$ receptors were significantly potentiated by substance P and bradykinin. The effects were mimicked by phorbol ester and blocked by inhibitors of protein kinases. These results suggest that inflammatory mediators may sensitize nociceptors through phosphorylation of $P2X_3$ and $P2X_{2/3}$ receptors.

In addition to $P2X_3$ receptors, $P2X_7$ receptor has

drawn a great attention in inflammatory pain. $P2X_7$ receptor is expressed predominantly in immune cells. In mice lacking $P2X_7$ receptors, inflammatory hypersensitivity is completely absent to both mechanical and thermal stimuli, while normal nociceptive processing is preserved. The knockout mice were unimpaired in their ability to produce mRNA for pro- IL-1β, and cytometric analysis of cytokines from knockout mice following CFA inflammation insult suggested a selective effect of the gene deletion on release of IL-1β and IL-10, with systemic reductions in adjuvant-induced increases in IL-6 and MCP-1. Thus, $P2X_7$ receptor may play a common upstream transductional role via its regulation of mature IL-1β production in the development of inflammatory pain state.

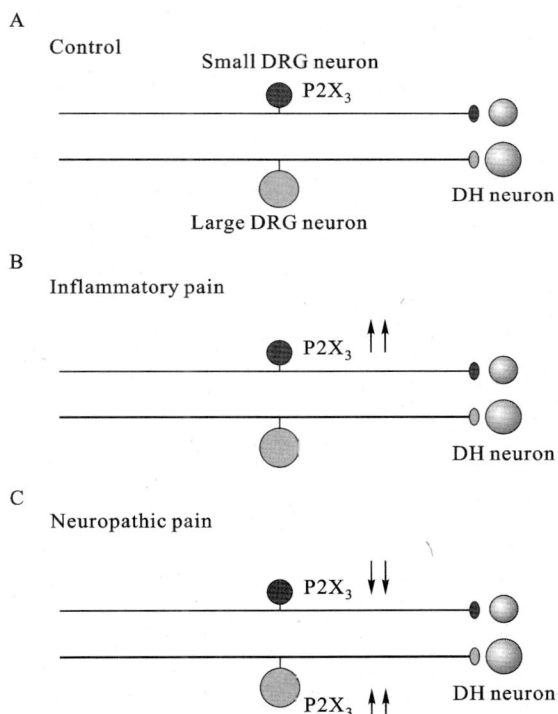

Fig.10.4 $P2X_3$ receptors in chronic pain. A. In normal conditions, $P2X_3$ receptors are expressed predominantly on small sized DRG neurons. B. $P2X_3$ receptors on small-sized DRG neurons are up-regulated following peripheral inflammation. C. Both down-regulation and up-regulation of $P2X_3$ receptor in DRG neurons have been observed after peripheral nerve injury. In small-sized DRG neurons, the number of cells expressing $P2X_3$ was significantly reduced, while $P2X_3$ immunoreactivity and $P2X_3$-like responses were detected in a subset of large sized DRG neurons after peripheral nerve injury.

P2X RECEPTORS IN NEUROPATHIC PAIN

Several lines of evidence implicated that P2X receptors may be involved in neuropathic pain. It has been shown that $P2X_3$ receptor expression was alternated in DRG neurons after peripheral nerve injury. The population of $P2X_3$ mRNA-expressing neurons in DRGs largely increased 3 days after transection of the tibial and common peroneal nerves. On the other hand, in dying DRG neurons following nerve injury, the number of $P2X_3$ mRNA-expressing neurons was significantly reduced. This result suggested that axotomized DRG neurons decreased $P2X_3$ expression, but $P2X_3$ mRNA expression increased in adjacent intact DRG neurons after peripheral nerve injury. P2X3 receptor expression and function were examined in DRG neurons obtained from spinal nerve ligation model rats exhibiting neuropathic pain. In small-sized neurons, there was a significant reduction in the number of cells that were sensitive to α, β-methylene ATP. $P2X_3$ immunoreactivity and $P2X_3$-like responses were detected in a subset of larger-sized DRG neurons and the number and amplitude of these responses were unchanged after spinal nerve ligation. While there appears to be a decrease in $P2X_3$ receptors following spinal nerve ligation, certain subsets of small and large DRG neurons maintain $P2X_3$ receptor expression and function (Fig.10.4C). DRGs with attached dorsal roots were removed and ectopic discharges were recorded from teased dorsal root fascicles. It was found that some axotomized afferent neurons developed ongoing discharges (ectopic discharges) following spinal nerve ligation. Chronically axotomized DRG neurons displaying ectopic discharges enhanced their activity after application of ATP or α, β-methylene ATP. This ATP-induced enhancement of ectopic discharges was significantly blocked by P2X receptor antagonists. This result suggests that purinergic sensitivity is developed in DRG neurons following chronic axotomy of peripheral nerve.

P2X$_3$ receptor has been used as a therapeutic target to treat neuropathic pain in experimental animals. The intrathecal treatment with P2X$_3$ receptor antisense oligonucleotide reduced mechanical allodynia after spinal nerve ligation. Intrathecal delivery of A-317491 also attenuated mechanical allodynia in both the chronic constriction injury and spinal nerve ligation models of neuropathy. These data suggest that activation of P2X$_3$ receptors strongly contribute to the expression of neuropathic pain state and P2X$_3$ receptor provides a therapeutic target for neuropathic pain.

P2X$_7$ receptor was up-regulated in human DRGs and injured nerves obtained from chronic neuropathic pain patients, suggesting the potential involvement of P2X$_7$ receptors in neuropathic pain. Consistent with this idea, the ablation of P2X$_7$ gene reduced neuropathic pain following partial nerve ligation in mice. Thus, P2X$_7$ receptor may provide a therapeutic target

for treatment of neuropathic pain conditions. P2X$_4$ receptors have also been suggested to be involved in neuropathic pain. It has been demonstrated that the expression of P2X$_4$ receptor strikingly increased in the spinal cord after peripheral nerve injury, and these P2X$_4$ receptor expression was induced in hyperactive microglia. The role of P2X$_4$ receptor-expressing microglia in neuropathic pain states was demonstrated by intraspinal administration of microglia in which P2X$_4$ receptors had been induced and stimulated, which produced tactile allodynia in naive rats. On the other hand, the intraspinal administration of P2X$_4$ receptor antisense, which decreased the induction of microglia P2X$_4$ receptors, significantly suppressed tactile allodynia after peripheral nerve injury. Thus, activation of P2X$_4$ receptors in hyperactive microglia may be necessary for tactile allodynia after peripheral nerve injury (Fig.10.5).

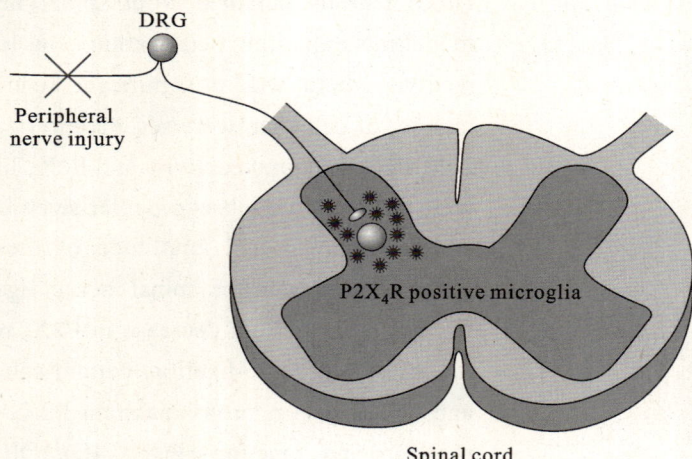

Fig.10.5 P2X$_4$ receptors in spinal hyperactive in neuropathic pain. Peripheral nerve injury causes microglial cells to congregate, and to produce P2X$_4$ receptors. The resulting neuropathic pain is suppressed by inhibiting P2X$_4$ receptors, and is mimicked by infusing microglia that bear activated P2X$_4$ receptors into the intact spinal cord.

SENSORY FUNCTIONS OF P2Y RECEPTORS

P2Y receptors have been shown to have nociceptive, non-nociceptive, and anti-nocicptive functions. mRNAs for several P2Y receptors including P2Y$_1$, P2Y$_2$, P2Y$_4$ and P2Y$_6$ were found to be expressed in dorsal root ganglions, nodose ganglions, and trigeminal ganglions. P2Y$_1$ receptors were localized on over 80% of these sensory ganglion neurons, preferentially on the small-sized neurons. P2Y$_4$ receptors were preferentially expressed on medium- and large-sized neurons. There are good overlap between P2Y$_1$ receptor expression and P2X$_3$ expression, about 80% of P2X$_3$ receptor-positive neurons stained for P2Y$_1$ receptor in DRG, TG and NG while only 30% stained for the P2Y$_4$ receptor. Subpopulations of P2Y$_1$-immunoreactive neurons were co-expressed with NF200, CGRP and IB4. Most P2Y$_4$ receptor-positive neurons were co-expressed with NF200 and only a few P2Y$_4$ receptor-positive neurons were co-expressed with CGRP or with IB4.

P2Y has been implicated to play a role in mechanical sensory signaling. It has been shown that the frequency of touch-induced action potentials from frog sensory nerve fibers was increased by P2 receptor agonists applied at peripheral nerve endings. Contribution of P2Y receptors in mechanical sensory transduction was further supported by the finding that a significant proportion of low threshold slowly and rapidly adapting $A\delta$ fibers could be activated by P2Y receptor agonist UTP. The activation of peripheral $P2Y_1$ receptors appeared to participate in the generation of sensory action potentials by light touch.

Potential nociceptive functions of P2Y receptors have been explored. Using skin-nerve preparations from adult mice, it was shown that P2Y receptor signaling could lead to action potential firing in primary afferent fibers. UTP activated sustained action potential firing in about half of C fibers in a concentration-dependent manner. The effect was mediated by $P2Y_2$ and/or $P2Y_4$ receptors, but not by $P2Y_6$ receptors because the $P2Y_6$ agonist UDP was unable to activate C fibers. In comparison to C fibers, few thinly myelinated $A\delta$ fibers were activated by UTP. The majority of the UTP-sensitive C and $A\delta$ fibers responded to capsaicin with a barrage of action potentials, whereas the UTP-insensitive fibers were largely unresponsive to capsaicin. Furthermore, the majority of the UTP-sensitive C fibers and all of the UTP-sensitive $A\delta$ fibers also responded to P2X receptor agonist α, β-methylene ATP, indicating that P2Y and P2X receptors are widely co-expressed. These results suggest that P2Y receptor subtypes may be involved in nociceptive signaling on capsaicin-sensitive and P2X-expressing cutaneous sensory nerve endings.

Sensitization of nociceptors by P2Y receptors may be a mechanism by which P2Y receptors are involved in nociception. Recent studies demonstrated that ATP through activation of P2Y could enhance TRPV1 receptor-mediated responses and the effect involved PKC. For example, exposing embryonic sensory neurons in culture to ATP did not increase the release of immunoreactive substance P or CGRP from sensory neurons, but pre-exposing sensory neurons to ATP prior to the administration of capsaicin resulted in a significant augmentation of release evoked by capsaicin. This sensitizing action of ATP was mimicked by P2Y receptor agonists 2-2-chloroadenosine triphosphate and UTP. Pretreatment of sensory neurons with a selective PKC inhibitor attenuated the augmentation of capsaicin-induced peptide release by ATP. This suggests that PKC is involved in modulating TRPV1 receptors following P2Y receptor activation. Consistent with these results, in cells expressing TRPV1 receptors and $P2Y_1$ receptors, ATP increased the capsaicin-evoked currents through $P2Y_1$ receptor activation and PKC-dependent pathway. P2Y mediated modulation of TRPV1 receptor functions may sensitize thermal responses. Indeed, in the presence of ATP, the temperature threshold for TRPV1 receptor activation was reduced from 42 degrees to 35 degrees, such that non-noxious thermal stimuli were capable of activating TRPV1 receptors. This may be a novel mechanism by which ATP initiates nociceptive signals when a large amount of ATP is released from damaged cells during tissue injury. Consistent with this idea, it was found that ATP-induced thermal hyperalgesia was abolished in mice lacking TRPV1 receptors. However, this study showed that $P2Y_2$ receptors, rather than $P2Y_1$ receptors, were involved in the potentiation of TRPV1 receptor activity. The involvement of $P2Y_2$ was supported by the in situ hybridization experiments showing the co-expression of TRPV1 mRNA with $P2Y_2$ mRNA in rat lumbar DRGs. These data indicate the importance of metabotropic $P2Y_2$ receptors in nociception through TRPV1 receptors.

Different from these excitatory actions of P2Y receptors on primary afferent neurons, the inhibitory effects of P2Y receptors were observed in spinal cord dorsal horn. For example, in the presence of ATP, slow depolarization of substantia gelatinosa neurons following repetitive stimulation of C-fibers was suppressed. Inhibition of the amplitude of slow depolarization by ATP showed a concentration-dependent manner. The inhibitory effect of ATP was mimicked by P2Y selective agonist UTP, but not by P2X receptor selective agonist α, β-methylene ATP. These results suggest that at spinal cord level, ATP may inhibit C-fiber nociceptive transmission to the spinal cord dorsal horn via P2Y receptor activation. This idea was supported by the effects of intrathecal administration of P2Y receptor agonists on nociception in both normal rats and rat model of neuropathic pain. In normal rats, it was shown that intrathecal administration of UTP and UDP, but not UMP or uridine, significantly elevated the mechanical nociceptive thresholds during paw pressure test. Similarly, UTP and UDP significantly prolonged the thermal nociceptive latency in the tail-flick test of normal rats. In rats of neuropathic pain model following sciatic nerve ligation, allodynia in these animals were alleviated by UTP and UDP. These results suggest that activation of UTP-sensitive $P2Y_2$ and/or $P2Y_4$ receptors and the UDP-sensitive $P2Y_6$ receptor produces inhibitory effects on nociceptive transmission. One of underlying mechanisms of P2Y receptor-mediated antinociception may be through inhibition of voltage-gated Ca^{2+} at presynatpic terminals of primary afferent fibers. It was shown that UTP, ADP, and ATP depressed N-type Ca^{2+} current in small-sized DRG neurons and this effect could be largely abolished by $P2Y_1$ receptor antagonists. $P2Y_1$ receptor-mediated inhibition of N-type Ca^{2+} current was shown to involve in the α, β subunit of $G_{q/11}$ proteins. These results raised a possibility that through inhibition of voltage-gated Ca^{2+} channels on the central terminals of nocicpetive afferent fibers, activation of P2Y receptors may lead to decreases in glutamate release form afferent fibers and thereby reduce nociceptive inputs to the spinal cord dorsal horn.

CONCLUSION

Evidence has now been accumulated to indicate sensory functions of P2X and P2Y receptors. P2X subtypes including $P2X_3$, $P2X_{2+3}$, $P2X_4$ and $P2X_7$ are shown to be involved in pathological pain conditions including both inflammatory pain and neuropathic pain. Nociceptive functions of P2X receptors other than the above mentioned subtypes remain to be ex-

plored. P2Y receptors may have nociceptive functions through the coupling of intracellular signaling pathways, leading to sensitization of nociceptors. Thus, both P2X and P2Y receptors may serve as therapeutic targets for pain treatment.

GENERAL CITATIONS

Gu JG. 2003. P2X receptor-mediated modulation of sensory transmission to the spinal cord dorsal horn. *Neuroscientist*, 9: 370-378.

Kennedy C. 2005. P2X receptors: targets for novel analgesics? *Neuroscientist*, 11: 345-356.

Khakh BS, Burnstock G, Kennedy C, King BF, North RA, Seguela P, Voigt M, Humphrey PP. 2001. International union of pharmacology. XXIV. Current status of the nomenclature and properties of P2X receptors and their subunits. *Pharmacol Rev*, 53: 107-118.

Koles L, Furst S, Illes P. 2005. P2X and P2Y receptors as possible targets of therapeutic manipulations in CNS illnesses. *Drug News Perspect*, 18: 85-101.

North RA. 2002. Molecular physiology of P2X receptors. *Physiol Rev*, 82: 1013-1067.

Ralevic V, Burnstock G. 1998. Receptors for purines and pyrimidines. *Pharmacol Rev*, 50: 413-492.

Tsuda M, Inoue K, Salter MW. 2005. Neuropathic pain and spinal microglia: a big problem from molecules in "small" glia. *Trends Neurosci*, 28: 101-107.

Vial C, Roberts JA, Evans RJ. 2004. Molecular properties of ATP-gated P2X receptor ion channels. *Trends Pharmacol Sci*, 25: 487-493.

von Kugelgen I, Wetter A. 2000. Molecular pharmacology of P2Y-receptors. *Naunyn Schmiedebergs Arch Pharmacol*, 362: 310-323.

DISCOVERY CITATIONS

Bardoni R, Goldstein PA, Lee CJ, Gu JG, MacDermott AB. 1997. ATP P2X receptors mediate fast synaptic transmission in the dorsal horn of the rat spinal cord. *J Neurosci*, 17: 5297-5304.

Bland-Ward PA, Humphrey PP. 1997. Acute nociception mediated by hindpaw P2X receptor activation in the rat. *Br J Pharmacol*, 122: 365-371.

Bleehen T, Keele CA. 1977. Observations on the algogenic actions of adenosine compounds on the human blister base preparation. *Pain*, 3: 367-377.

Chen CC, Akopian AN, Sivilotti L, Colquhoun D, Burnstock G, Wood JN. 1995. A P2X purinoceptor expressed by a subset of sensory neurons. *Nature*, 377: 428-431.

Chen M, Gu JG. 2005. A P2X receptor-mediated nociceptive afferent pathway to lamina I of the spinal cord. *Mol Pain*, 1: 4.

Chessell IP, Hatcher JP, Bountra C, Michel AD, Hughes JP, Green P, Egerton J, Murfin M, Tsuda M, Shigemoto-Mogami Y, Koizumi S, Mizokoshi A, Kohsaka S, Salter MW, Inoue K. 2003. P2X$_4$ receptors induced in spinal microglia gate tactile allodynia after nerve injury. *Nature*, 424: 778-783.

Cockayne DA, Hamilton SG, Zhu QM, Dunn PM, Zhong Y, Novakovic S, Malmberg AB, Cain G, Berson A, Kassotakis L, Hedley L, Lachnit WG, Burnstock G, McMahon SB, Ford AP. 2000. Urinary bladder hyporeflexia and reduced pain-related behaviour in P2X$_3$-deficient mice. *Nature*, 407: 1011-1015.

Collo G, North RA, Kawashima E, Merlo-Pich E, Neidhart S, Surprenant A, Buell G. 1996. Cloning OF P2X5 and P2X6 receptors and the distribution and properties of an extended family of ATP-gated ion channels. *J Neurosci*, 16: 2495-2507.

Cook SP, Vulchanova L, Hargreaves KM, Elde R, McCleskey EW. 1997. Distinct ATP receptors on pain-sensing and stretch-sensing neurons. *Nature*, 387: 505-508.

Coutts AA, Jorizzo JL, Eady RA, Greaves MW, Burnstock G. 1981. Adenosine triphosphate- evoked vascular changes in human skin: mechanism of action. *Eur J Pharmacol*, 76: 391-401.

Gerevich Z, Borvendeg SJ, Schroder W, Franke H, Wirkner K, Norenberg W, Furst S, Gillen C, Illes P. 2004. Inhibition of N-type voltage-activated calcium channels in rat dorsal root ganglion neurons by P2Y receptors is a possible mechanism of ADP-induced analgesia. *J Neurosci*, 24: 797-807.

Gu JG, MacDermott AB. 1997. Activation of ATP P2X receptors elicits glutamate release from sensory neuron synapses. *Nature*, 389: 749-753.

Hamilton SG, McMahon SB, Lewin GR. 2001. Selective activation of nociceptors by P2X receptor agonists in normal and inflamed rat skin. *J Physiol*, 534: 437-445.

Holton FA, Holton P. 1953. The possibility that ATP is a transmitter at sensory nerve endings. *J Physiol,* 119: 50-51.

Hugel S, Schlichter R. 2000. Presynaptic P2X receptors facilitate inhibitory GABAergic transmission between cultured rat spinal cord dorsal horn neurons. *J Neurosci*, 20: 2121-2130.

Jahr CE, Jessell TM. 1983. ATP excites a subpopulation of rat dorsal horn neurones. *Nature*, 304: 730-733.

Krishtal OA, Marchenko SM, Pidoplichko VI. 1983. Receptor for ATP in the membrane of mammalian sensory neurones. *Neurosci Lett*, 35: 41-45.

Lewis C, Neidhart S, Holy C, North RA, Buell G, Surprenant A. 1995. Coexpression of P2X2 and P2X3 receptor subunits can account for ATP-gated currents in sensory neurons. *Nature*, 377: 432-435.

McGaraughty S, Wismer CT, Zhu CZ, Mikusa J, Honore P, Chu KL, Lee CH, Faltynek CR, Jarvis MF. 2003. Effects of A-317491, a novel and selective P2X$_3$/P2X$_{2/3}$ receptor antagonist, on neuropathic, inflammatory and chemogenic nociception following intrathecal and intraplantar administration. *Br J Pharmacol*, 140: 1381-1388.

Moriyama T, Iida T, Kobayashi K, Higashi T, Fukuoka T, Tsumura H, Leon C, Suzuki N, Inoue K, Gachet C, Noguchi K, Tominaga M. 2003. Possible involvement of P2Y$_2$ metabotropic receptors in ATP-induced transient receptor potential vanilloid receptor 1-mediated thermal hypersensitivity. *J Neurosci*, 23: 6058-6062.

Nakamura F, Strittmatter SM. 1996. P2Y1 purinergic receptors in sensory neurons: contribution to touch- induced impulse generation. *Proc Natl Acad Sci USA*, 93: 10465-10470.

Nakatsuka T, Furue H, Yoshimura M, Gu JG. 2002. Activation of central terminal vanilloid receptor-1 receptors and alpha beta-methylene-ATP-sensitive P2X receptors reveals a converged synaptic activity onto the deep dorsal horn neurons of the spinal cord. *J Neurosci*, 22: 1228-1237.

Okada M, Nakagawa T, Minami M, Satoh M. 2002. Analgesic effects of intrathecal administration of P2Y nucleotide receptor agonists UTP and UDP in normal and neuropathic pain model rats. *J Pharmacol Exp Ther*, 303: 66-73.

Paukert M, Osteroth R, Geisler HS, Brandle U, Glowatzki E, Ruppersberg JP, Grunder S. 2001. Inflammatory mediators potentiate ATP-gated channels through the P2X(3) subunit. *J Biol Chem*, 276: 21077-21082.

Richardson J, Peck WL, Grahames CB, Casula MA, Yiangou Y, Birch R, Anand P, Buell GN. 2005. Disruption of the P2X$_7$ purinoceptor gene abolishes chronic inflammatory and neuropathic pain. *Pain*, 114: 386-396.

Souslova V, Cesare P, Ding Y, Akopian AN, Stanfa L, Suzuki R, Carpenter K, Dickenson A, Boyce S, Hill R, Nebenuis-Oosthuizen D, Smith AJ, Kidd EJ, Wood JN. 2000. Warm-coding deficits and aberrant inflammatory pain in mice lacking P2X$_3$ receptors. *Nature*, 407: 1015-1017.

Tominaga M, Wada M, Masu M. 2001. Potentiation of capsaicin receptor activity by metabotropic ATP receptors as a possible mechanism for ATP-evoked pain and hyperalgesia. *Proc Natl Acad Sci USA*, 98: 6951-6956.

Tsuzuki K, Kondo E, Fukuoka T, Yi D, Tsujino H, Sakagami M, Noguchi K. 2001. Differential regulation of P2X$_3$ mRNA expression by peripheral nerve injury in intact and injured neurons in the rat sensory ganglia. *Pain*, 91: 351-360.

Vulchanova L, Riedl MS, Shuster SJ, Stone LS, Hargreaves KM, Buell G, Surprenant A, North RA, Elde R. 1998. P2X$_3$ is expressed by DRG neurons that terminate in inner lamina II. *Eur J Neurosci*, 10: 3470-3478.

Xu GY, Huang LY. 2002. Peripheral inflammation sensitizes P2X receptor-mediated responses in rat dorsal root ganglion neurons. *J Neurosci*, 22: 93-102.

Yoshida K, Nakagawa T, Kaneko S, Akaike A, Satoh M. 2002. Adenosine 5'-triphosphate inhibits slow depolarization induced by repetitive dorsal root stimulation via P2Y purinoceptors in substantia gelatinosa neurons of the adult rat spinal cord slices with the dorsal root attached. *Neurosci Lett*, 320: 121-124.

Opioid Receptors

CHAPTER 11

Zhizhong Z. Pan

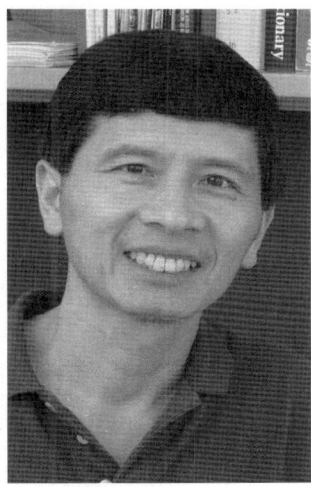

Dr. Pan is an Associate Professor, in the Departments of Anesthesiology and Pain Medicine, and Biochemistry and Molecular Biology, University of Texas, Houston, USA. He graduated from Jiangxi University and continued with graduate studies at the Chinese Academy of Sciences, obtaining a M.S. in Physiology. After gaining a Ph.D. in Neuroscience at Oregon Health Sciences University, he continued postdoctoral training at the University of California at San Francisco.

MAJOR CONTRIBUTIONS

1. Pan ZZ, Tershner SA, Fields HL. 1997. Cellular mechanism for anti-analgesic action of agonists of the kappa-opioid receptor. *Nature*, 389(6649): 382-385.
2. Pan ZZ, Hirakawa N, Fields HL. 2000. A cellular mechanism for the bidirectional pain-modulating actions of orphanin FQ/nociceptin. *Neuron*, 26(2): 515-522.
3. Pan ZZ. 2003. κ-Opioid receptor-mediated enhancement of the hyperpolarization-activated current (Ih) through mobilization of intracellular calcium in rat nzucleus raphe magnus. *J Physiol (Lond)*, 548(3): 765-775.
4. Bie B, Peng Y, Zhang, Y, Pan ZZ. 2005. Cyclic AMP-med-

iated mechanisms for pain sensitization during opioid withdrawal. *J Neurosci* 25(15): 3824-3832.
5. Ma JY, Zhang Y, Kalyuzhny AE, Pan ZZ. 2006. Emergence of functional κ-opioid receptors induced by chronic morphine. *Mol. Pharmacol.* 69: 1137-1145.

MAIN TOPICS

Molecular structure

Endogenous peptides and opioid compounds

Signal transduction pathways

Internalization

Cellular actions

Behavioral functions and interactions

Receptor trafficking

SUMMARY

Opioid receptors have drawn enormous research interests because they mediate opioid actions that are highly relevant to clinical treatment of pain and drug addiction. Opioid receptors are among those early receptor systems discovered in the CNS. Cloning of the members of the opioid receptor family, mainly mu, delta and kappa receptors, reveals that they belong to the super family of G protein-coupled receptors with seven transmembrane domains. While the divergent sequence on the amino terminus of different types of opioid receptors contributes to selective ligand binding, sequence differences in the carboxyl tail account for their differential interactions with intracellular kinases, effectors and trafficking-regulating proteins. Most endogenous opioid peptides are not selective at each receptor, but sufficiently selective opioid compounds have been developed for studies on the function of each opioid receptor type. All opioid receptors couple, mostly through $G_{i/o}$ proteins, to potassium channels and calcium channels, and to multiple second messenger pathways that mediate short-term and long-term changes in cell functions. All opioid receptors produce similar or identical cellular actions that usually inhibit cellular and synaptic activities, including membrane hyperpolarization, inhibition of calcium conductance and reduction of neurotransmitter release. The major system actions of opioid receptors are analgesia and reward, which are the focus of majority basic and clinical studies of opioids. These system actions are primarily mediated by the mu receptor, whereas the functions of kappa and delta receptors are much less clear. The fact that different types of opioid receptors share similar cellular actions but have distinct system actions can be largely attributed to their differential synaptic and cellular locations in a specific neuronal circuit. Importance of functional interactions between opioid receptor types and particularly, agonist-induced opioid receptor trafficking, is increasingly recognized, and the underlying mechanisms are rigorously investigated in current opioid research.

INTRODUCTION

Opium derived from poppies has been used for centuries to treat pain and mood-related problems. The main ingredient of opium is morphine, which is still being widely used clinically today to control moderate to severe pain. Morphine and derivatives generally referred to as opioids had been used for many years with no knowledge of how they worked in humans. Our understanding of opioid actions in human bodies historically began with the discovery of endogenous opioid receptors in early 1970's. In the next three decades, our knowledge of opioid receptors and their actions has mushroomed and is still exponentially growing at present. Perhaps because opioid actions are closely related to clinical practice and to problems of drug abuse in the modern society, tremendous ef-

forts have been made to understand cellular and molecular mechanisms underlying opioid receptor-mediated actions on many functions of the CNS. Cloning of several different types of opioid receptors represents a remarkable leap in our understanding of molecular and neurobiological mechanisms for opioid receptor functions. Today, opioid receptors and their endogenous peptides constitute a neurotransmitter system that is one of the best-studied and known neurotransmission systems in the CNS. Opioid receptors and peptides have broad distribution throughout the CNS, suggesting that the opioid neurotransmission system is involved in the regulation and modulation of many CNS functions. As we know today, opioid receptors mediate two major behavioral actions: pain inhibition and reward. Opioid receptors also have a variety of other actions, many of which comprise unwanted side effects associated with the use of large doses of exogenous opioids. These actions include immune modulation, neuroendocrine regulation, cognitive functions, gastrointestinal inhibition, respiratory depression, sedation, and nausea. Research into each of these opioid actions has provided enormous information with respect to the role of opioid receptors in a certain regulating or modulating function, particularly in the areas of pain modulation and reward function of the brain. As all actions of exogenous and endogenous opioids are mediated through opioid receptors, a fundamental issue to understanding of the mechanisms for opioid actions is to demonstrate the function of an opioid receptor in a given cell, including its molecular structure, the intracellular second messenger systems it couples to convey extracellular stimulation to intracellular responding mechanisms, the action of the effectors it couples to on cell function, and its regulation in membrane density by various acute and chronic stimulating environment. This Chapter will cover these important functions of opioid receptors by outlining critical steps in our understanding of these functions of opioid receptors, emphasizing recent findings and progress in the field. Regarding opioid actions, this Chapter, understandably, will focus on the role of opioid receptors in modulation of pain in pain-related central neurons.

MOLECULAR STRUCTURE

The existence of endogenous opioid receptors was first suggested by the work of Goldstein *et al.* who, using redioligand binding, demonstrated stereospecific recognition of opioid compounds in their actions. In 1973, three laboratories independently identified specific opioid binding sites (opioid receptors) in the brain by demonstrating high affinity and stereoselective binding of opioid compounds to brain tissues. Based on the findings that different classes of opioid compounds produce distinct behavioral effects, Martin and his colleagues defined three different types of opioid receptors associated with three types of opioid agonists used: μ for morphine-like, κ for ketocyclozocine-like drugs and σ for the drug SKF-10,147. A year later, another opioid receptor termed δ receptor was identified by Lord *et al.* in mouse vas deferens. The σ receptor was later found to mediate naloxone-irreversible effects and is no longer considered as a part of the opioid receptor family. Subsequent studies have confirmed the other three types of opioid receptors, namely, μ, δ, and κ. Representing a major step in opioid research, the δ-opioid receptor (DOR) was first cloned by Evans' and Kieffer's groups in 1992, followed a year later by the cloning of μ- (MOR) and κ-opioid receptors (KOR) by several laboratories. In 1994, several groups reported identification of yet another opioid receptor, ORL-1. Currently, although there is a discrepancy regarding the total number of opioid receptor subtypes, MOR, DOR and KOR are generally accepted as the three major opioid receptors that mediate primary actions of opioids in the CNS.

The cloning of opioid receptors reveals the molecular nature of opioid receptors and their structural relationship to other membrane receptors. Opioid receptor family belongs to the super family of G protein-coupled receptors that typically have seven hydrophobic transmembrane domains (Fig.11.1, see also the color plate). Extensive studies have demonstrated the molecular biology of opioid receptors. The three opioid receptors share extensive homologies in their sequences, having a roughly 60% identical amino acid

sequence. Highly conserved are the sequences of membrane-spanning domains 2, 3 and 7, while the sequences of transmembrane domains 1, 4, 5 and 6 are less homologous. Sequence homology is significantly high in the intracellular loops of all three opioid receptors, supporting the notion that they all interact with similar Gi/Go proteins. The most unique region of the sequence is at the amino and carboxyl termini with differences in both amino acid sequences and sizes. The unique extracellular amino end of the sequence probably contributes to specific ligand binding of a certain opioid receptor type. The divergent carboxyl terminus in the sequence of opioid receptors may contribute to differential properties in receptor phosphorylation and internalization. It may imply differential interactions of different opioid receptors with intracellular signal transduction pathways. All three opioid receptors have extracellular glycosylation sites and intracellular phosphorylation sites. Current molecular biology studies of opioid receptors use point mutation techniques to understand the molecular functions of specific residues or segments in the sequence. From these studies, considerable insights have emerged regarding amino acid residues responsible for affinity and selectivity in ligand binding, G protein coupling and phosphorylation by protein kinases. These areas are beyond the scope of this Chapter. Readers are referred to references in General Readings for details.

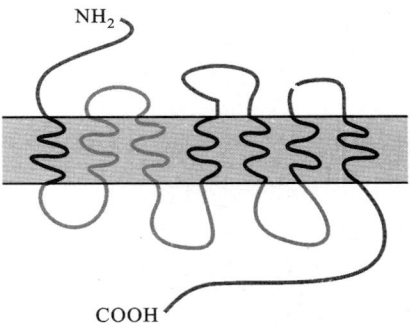

Fig.11.1 Molecular structure of opioid receptors. Lines indicate the degree of sequence homology among MOR, KOR and DOR. Red, unique; green, high homology; blue, low homology.

Another important feature of opioid receptors, similar to other G protein-coupled receptors, is functional interaction between each other on cell membrane. Fully functional KOR and DOR can form a heterodimer that has distinct ligand binding and functional properties. Heterodimerization of MOR and DOR exists in native cells and occupancy by a DOR antagonist increases the signaling activity and analgesic function of MOR.

ENDOGENOUS PEPTIDES AND OPIOID COMPOUNDS

Historically, endogenous opioid peptides were identified after the discovery of opioid receptors. In 1975, Hugh *et al.* first reported the identification of endogenous opioid peptides termed enkephalins in the brain. The observation that the opioid antagonist naloxone reversed the analgesia induced by electrical stimulation of certain brain sites suggested that endogenous opioid peptides were released during the analgesia. Subsequent studies led to the discovery of other two members in the family of endogenous opioid peptides, β-endorphins and dynorphins. All these peptides produce potent analgesic effect *in vivo*. Soon after, the genes that encode for the three members of the opioid peptide family were cloned, establishing the molecular sources of the opioid peptides. The three precursors are proopiomelanocortin for β-endorphins, proenkephalin for enkephalins and prodynorphin for dynorphins. Each precursor encodes multiple copies of different opioid peptides, producing a different mix of endogenous opioid peptides. Binding studies demonstrate that none of these endogenous opioid peptides are selective at a certain type of opioid receptors, with β-endorphins preferring MOR, enkephalins preferring DOR/MOR and dynorphins preferring KOR (Table 11.1). In contrast, endogenous peptides for ORL_1 are selective over the other three receptors. More recently, two new and closely related endogenous opioid peptides, termed endomorphin-1 and endomorphin-2, have been discovered in the brain. The endomorphins display considerably high affinity and selectivity for MOR over DOR and KOR, and produce potent analgesia *in vivo*.

Our understanding of the biological functions of opioid receptors is profoundly facilitated by the development and synthesis of exogenous opioid compounds that are much more selective than those endogenous peptides. Those compounds allow detailed studies on the binding characteristics of each opioid receptor type and their tissue distributions in the brain and peripherals. Specifically, typical and highly selective agonists include DAMGO for MOR, DPDPE and deltorphin for DOR, and U69,593 for KOP (Table 11.1). Significant progress in functional studies of opioid receptors has been achieved by the availability of highly selective antagonists. Such important antagonists include CTAP for MOR, naltrindole and naltriben for DOR and nor-BNI for KOP. These selective opioid compounds have contributed enormously to illustration of opioid receptor functions in previous *in vitro* and *in vivo* studies. They represent one of the best pharmacological tools available for studies of neurotransmitter systems in the CNS, and are still widely used in current research into opioid receptor functions in various physiological and pathological conditions.

Table 11.1 Commonly used opioid peptides and compounds.			
Receptors	Endogenous peptides	Exogenous compounds	
		Agonists	Antagonists
MOR	β-endorphins	DAMGO	CTAP
	Enkephalins		CTOP
	Endomorphin-1		β-Funaltrexamine
	Endomorphin-2		
KOR	Dynorphins	U69,593	nor-BNI
		U50,488	
DOR	Enkephalins	DPDPE	Naltrindole
		Deltorphin	Naltriben
			BNTX
ORL_1	Nociceptin	$[Arg^{14},Lys^{15}]$-	UFP-101
	Nocistatin (antagonist)	Nociceptin	

SIGNAL TRANSDUCTION PATHWAYS

As a member of the G protein-coupled receptor family, opioid receptors produce their effects through coupled G proteins in most known opioid actions. It has been well established that all three types of opioid receptors couple to pertussis toxin-sensitive Gi/Go proteins and produce downstream effects mostly via Giβ/γ subunits of the G proteins. There is also substantial evidence showing opioid receptors coupling to stimulatory Gs proteins, particularly after chronic exposure of opioid receptors to opioid agonists. However, biochemical evidence for such Gs coupling remains to be demonstrated.

The most prominent and best-characterized signal transduction pathway coupled via G proteins to opioid receptors is the cAMP-protein kinase A (PKA) pathway. All opioid receptors activated by acute application of opioid agonists consistently inhibit, mostly via Giβ/γ, the activity of adenylyl cyclase (AC) that catalyzes the production of intracellular cAMP. While acute opioids inhibit AC activity, persistent stimulation of MOR with chronic opioids induces a compensatory increase or up-regulation in AC activity to pre-opioid levels, and upon removal of opioid agonists, the AC activity further increases to even higher levels. This molecular adaptation to chronic opioids in AC activity and resultant intracellular level of cAMP has been demonstrated later in many brain regions, and has been widely regarded as a molecular model for adaptations that account for the cellular mechanisms of opioid tolerance and withdrawal (see chapter 30). Recent studies focus on the function of different AC isoforms in actions of acute and chronic opioids in specific brain areas. There are a total of nine AC isoforms identified, whose brain distributions and synaptic locations are highly specific, indicating complex and multiple pre- and post-synaptic actions of the enzyme isoforms. In cell lines *in vitro*, acute activation of MOR inhibits the activity of ACI, ACV, ACVI and ACVIII isoforms. These AC isoforms are likely substrates for upregulation by chronic opioids. For example, chronic morphine increases expression of ACI and ACIII mRNA and proteins in locus coeruleus. ACIII immunoreactivity is increased by chronic morphine in dorsal raphe nucleus. In a recent study of neurons in the nucleus raphe magnus (NRM), a critical brainstem area for opioid analgesia, we have shown that chronic morphine upregulates the mRNA level of ACVI and ACVIII and increases the immunoreactivity of ACV/VI. The detailed mechanisms underlying the chronic opioid-induced AC supersensitization have yet to be elucidated.

Another G protein-regulated signal transduction pathway functionally coupled to MOR is the phospholipase A_2 (PLA_2) pathway. All three opioid receptors expressed in cell lines functionally couple to the PLA_2 pathway to release arachidonate in a pertussis toxin-dependent manner. In neurons of the periaqueductal gray (PAG), activation of MOR inhibits presynaptic GABA release in GABAergic terminals through the PLA_2-arachidonic acid pathway. We have recently demonstrated that the PLA_2 pathway is also involved in MOR-mediated inhibition of glutamate release from presynaptic terminals in central amygdala neurons. Thus, the PLA_2 pathway mediates opioid inhibition of presynaptic release of both glutamate and GABA in central neurons.

Other signal transduction pathways coupled to or activated by opioid receptors are the phospholipase C (PLC) pathway as well as various protein kinase pathways, including protein kinase C (PKC) , calcium/calmodulin-dependent protein kinase II (CaMKII), mitogen-activated protein kinases and G protein-coupled receptor kinases (GRKs). Acute and chronic stimulation of opioid receptors may activate these protein kinases, which then phosphorylate opioid receptors at multiple phosphorylation sites on the carboxyl terminus and third intracellular loop. Phosphorylation and dephosphorylation of opioid receptors play a crucial role in receptor binding affinity, efficiency of coupling to G proteins, receptor internalization and downstream effects.

Fig.11.2 illustrates the main signal transduction pathways and ion channels coupled to opioid receptors.

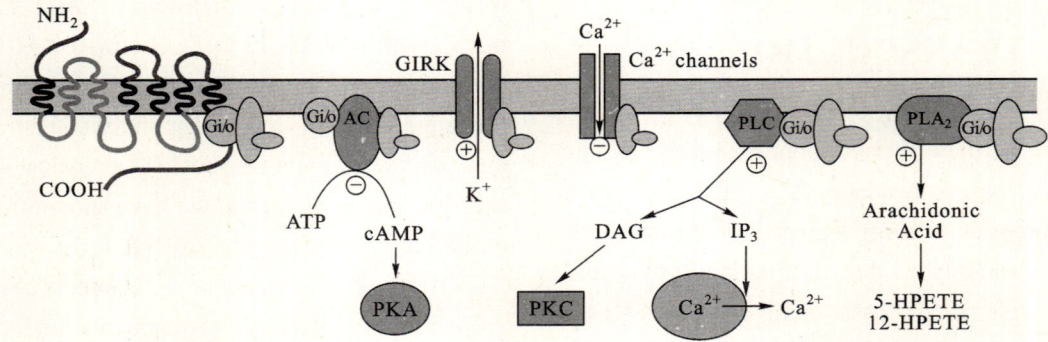

Fig. 11.2   Ion channels and signal transduction pathways coupled to opioid receptors through Gi/o proteins. Circled plus sign indicates activation and circled minus sign indicates inhibition. AC, adenylyl cyclase; DAG, diacylglycerol; GIRK, inwardly rectifying potassium channel; IP$_3$, inositol 1,4,5-triphosphate; PKA, protein kinase A; PKC, protein kinase C; PLA$_2$, phospholipase A$_2$; PLC, phospholipase C.

INTERNALIZATION

Receptor internalization generally employs a process of classic endocytosis in which receptors move from plasma membrane to intracellular compartments. Opioid receptors, like other G protein-coupled receptors, undergo rapid internalization within minutes after agonist binding. It is a key process to regulate receptor density on surface membrane and thereby agonist effects in response to agonist activation. Our knowledge on receptor internalization has dramatically improved in recent years through extensive studies. Current understanding of opioid receptor internalization is largely based on the findings in β-adrenoceptors. Thus, once agonist-bound, an opioid receptor is phosphorylated by a GRK, which uncouples the receptor from G proteins and promotes the receptor binding with arrestin. This binding associates the arrestin-bound receptor with clathrin-coated pits, where the receptor is internalized to endosomes through endocytosis (Fig. 11.3). Therefore, it appears that agonist binding triggers the event of receptor internalization, and GRK phosphorylation and arrestin binding play a critical role in the process. A decrease in receptor internalization would increase the number of available receptors on surface membrane and enhance agonist response, and vice versa. For example, in mice lacking β-arrestin, which would reduce receptor internalization, morphine analgesia mediated primarily through MOR is significantly potentiated and prolonged.

A particular interesting feature of opioid receptor internalization is its agonist dependence. Different MOR agonists with similar potency in G protein activation and AC inhibition remarkably differ in induction of MOR internalization. Among commonly used MOR agonists, DAMGO, methadone and etorphin potently stimulate MOR internalization, whereas morphine does not induce apparent MOR internalization. These observations indicate that binding of opioid receptors with different agonists causes differential conformational changes that can affect the receptor interaction with intracellular regulating proteins, resulting in various efficacy for receptor internalization. They also suggest that receptor internalization is independent on receptor efficacy for other coupled effectors. Among the three opioid receptors, MOR and DOR consistently internalize upon agonist activation. For KOR expressed in cell lines, human KOR readily internalizes whereas rat or mouse KOR does not internalize in comparable conditions. Studies with point and truncation mutations suggest that opioid receptor internalization is largely dependent on the carboxyl terminus of the receptor sequence. This is implied by the divergent sequence in the carboxyl tail. Interestingly, in a chimera of MOR combined with a DOR carboxyl tail, morphine causes internalization.

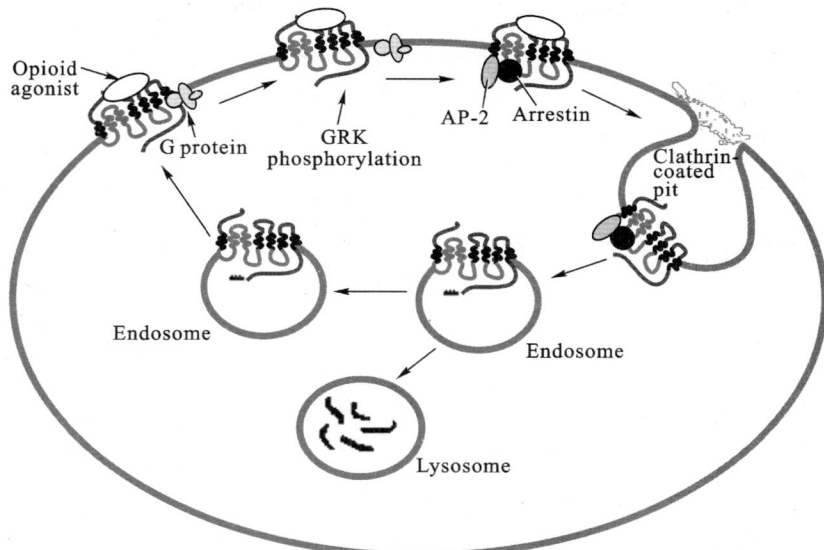

Fig.11.3 Pathways of opioid receptor internalization and trafficking. Binding of an opioid agonist to an opioid receptor induces receptor phosphorylation by the G protein-coupled receptor kinase (GRK), which leads to receptor dissociation from the G protein and increased receptor binding affinity for arrestin. The receptor bond to arrestin and to other regulatory proteins such as AP-2 is moved to clathrin-coated pit where classic endocytosis occurs. The internalized receptor in endosomes is subject to a sorting process and is trafficked either to lysosomes for degradation or to a recycling pathway for membrane insertion and resensitization.

CELLULAR ACTIONS

All opioid receptors produce similar to identical cellular actions in central neurons. These actions are generally inhibitory to neuronal activity or excitability. Both presynaptic and postsynaptic actions have been extensively studied in the CNS. Cellular actions produced by acute opioid agonists include inhibition of AC and production of cAMP, activation of cell-hyperpolarizing potassium (K^+) channels, inhibition of calcium channels, inhibition of neurotransmitter release, release of intracellular calcium (Ca^{2+}) and activation of various protein kinases.

As discussed above, opioid inhibition of AC activity and cAMP production has been extensively described in cell lines and in neurons of brain areas associated with opioid analgesia and opioid addiction. As the basal level of AC activity and intracellular cAMP is rather low, most studies examined opioid actions on conditions of stimulated AC activity and elevated cAMP level by either AC activators or chronic opioid-induced AC sensitization. Exogenous cAMP analogs generally have two direct actions on central neuron functions. First, they increase neurotransmitter release in central neurons from both glutamatergic and GABAergic terminals. Second, they enhance the membrane-depolarizing current, hyperpolarization-activated current (I_h) mediated by the cation channel termed HCN channels. The molecular mechanism for cAMP augmentation of HCN channel conductance has been demonstrated in a previous study, which showed that cAMP binding to the cyclic nucleotide-binding domain of the HCN channel removes its inhibition on a core transmembrane domain. I_h is an important membrane current in control of resting membrane potential, cell excitability and firing patterns. In contrast to the effects of exogenous cAMP analogs, physiological effects of intracellular cAMP that is increased by chronic opioids *in vivo* have only recently been reported. Chronic morphine increases presynaptic GABA release through an up-regulated cAMP pathway. In a recent study, we have shown that chronic morphine increases presynaptic glutamate release and augments the I_h in the same neuron, both through an up-regulated cAMP cascade.

Opioid activation of the inwardly rectifying K^+ conductance is a major inhibitory action of opioids on central neurons. Williams *et al.* first reported that enkephalin inhibits cell firing by opening K^+ channels. Later studies established that both MOR and DOR couple through G proteins to K^+ channels. Coupling of KOR to K^+ channels was not demonstrated until 1993, when KOR activation was shown to increase K^+ conductance in spinal neurons. Thus, activation of all opioid receptors on postsynaptic membrane opens the same inwardly rectifying K^+ channels and inhibits neuronal activity. This opioid action is widely distributed in neurons throughout the brain, including those involved in pain modulation, such as neurons in the brainstem as demonstrated by our previous studies.

Another main action of all opioid receptors is inhibition of Ca^{2+} channels. This opioid action has been described in many different types of neurons. With regard to pain modulation, MOR activation inhibits Ca^{2+} channels only in small-sized nociceptive neurons in trigeminal ganglia. This opioid action could represent one of the main mechanisms for opioid inhibition of pain at spinal levels.

The third major action of all opioid receptors is inhibition of neurotransmitter release. This is a presynaptic effect through opioid receptors on axon terminals. Nicoll *et al.* first described opioid inhibition of GABA synaptic release in hippocampal neurons and introduced the notion of disinhibition as a general mechanism for opioid actions in the CNS. Subsequently, a large number of studies have demonstrated that all three types of opioid receptors inhibit presynaptic release of neurotransmitters, including GABA, glutamate and acetylcholine, in a variety of central neurons and peripheral preparations. Opioid inhibition of GABA synaptic transmission becomes the most widespread presynaptic opioid effect in the CNS. It is generally agreed that this effect and opioid hyperpolarization of GABAergic neurons account for most excitatory actions of opioids in the CNS through the mechanism of disinhibition. For example, we have illustrated that MOR agonists produce antinociception in the brainstem by disinhibiting or activating pain-inhibiting output neurons through inhibition of both presumably GABAergic interneurons and GABA

synaptic transmission. Regarding the presynaptic mechanism for the opioid action, while both activation of K^+ conductance and inhibition of Ca^{2+} conductance are implicated, a more recent study shows that MOR activation inhibits GABA release by activating the PLA_2 signaling pathway and opening 4-AP-sensitive K^+ channels through arachidonic acid metabolites in PAG neurons. Recently, we also show that MOR activation inhibits glutamate release via the PLA_2 pathway and 4-AP-sensitive K^+ channels in central amygdala neurons. Thus, activation of the PLA_2 pathway and the 4-AP-sensitive K^+ channels could be the common mechanism for opioid inhibition of both glutamate and GABA release in central neurons.

Evidence for opioid release of intracellular Ca^{2+} is mostly from studies on transfected cell lines. Substantial data suggest opioid receptor-mediated mobilization of intracellular Ca^{2+} from Ca^{2+} stores in a Ca^{2+} influx-dependent or independent manner. The generally recognized mechanism suggests that opioid receptors are coupled to the PLC pathway through pertussis toxin-sensitive G proteins. Upon activation, opioid receptors stimulate the PLC, which promotes the production of diacylglycerol (DAG) and inositol 1,4,5-triphosphate (IP_3). The later triggers Ca^{2+} release from intracellular stores. Despite the evidence, the physiological effect of opioid-mediated Ca^{2+} increase in the intracellular space has been unclear. Our recent study demonstrates that KOR activation in brainstem neurons enhances the maximum conductance of the I_h by mobilizing Ca^{2+} from intracellular stores in an extracellular Ca^{2+}-dependent manner.

Several lines of evidence from studies of transfected cells indicate opioid receptor-mediated activation of PKC. A likely mechanism involves the PLC pathway and PKC activation by DAG. Although the evidence from transfected cell systems for opioid activation of PKC is ample, little data are available regarding an opioid effect directly due to PKC activation in native neurons. One example for this opioid action is the finding that MOR agonists enhance NMDA currents through PKC activation. Several studies also show that chronic morphine activates PKC in the CNS and it may contribute to the mechanisms of opioid tolerance. Detailed mechanisms for chronic opioid-mediated PKC activation remain to be demonstrated.

As cellular actions of acute opioids become clear, most current opioid studies are focusing on chronic opioid-induced cellular adaptations in these acute opioid actions in order to understand the neurobiological mechanisms underlying clinical and social problems associated with chronic use of opioid drugs, such as analgesic tolerance, physical dependence and drug addiction.

BEHAVIORAL FUNCTIONS AND INTERACTIONS

At the system level, opioids have two major actions: analgesia and reward. This section will focus on opioid receptor-mediated pain modulation.

The mechanisms of opioid analgesia have been extensively studied. Opioid receptors are expressed abundantly in all brain areas and the spinal cord that are involved in pain transmission and modulation. It is known for long time that MOR agonists such as morphine are strong analgesics and are still widely used as the primary choice for the treatment of moderate to severe pain, such as cancer pain. In mice lacking MOR, morphine-mediated analgesia, physical dependence and reward are lost, demonstrating that MOR is primarily responsible for mediating major behavioral actions of opioids. Depending on the synaptic location of MOR in different brain sites and spinal cord, cellular mechanisms for MOR-mediated behavioral analgesia may vary, but should be mediated by the cellular actions described above. In the NRM, we have characterized the mechanisms for MOR agonist-mediated analgesia in the brainstem NRM. Two MOR actions are involved. The first is inhibition of presynaptic GABA release in one type of NRM neurons (termed primary cells) that lacks postsynaptic MOR. The second action is membrane hyperpolarization of the other type of neurons (termed secondary cells) expressing postsynaptic MOR. Thus, based on previous behavioral work, we have proposed that MOR activation produces analgesia by (i) disin-

hibiting or activating primary cells and presumably their descending pain-inhibiting pathways, and (ii) inhibiting secondary cells and their putative descending pain-facilitating projections (Fig.11.4). Similar disinhibition mechanism has been proposed for the activation of output neurons in the PAG during opioid analgesia. The mechanism for opioid analgesia in the spinal cord is less clear due to poorly defined local neuronal circuitry, but it appears that both presynaptic inhibition of primary afferents and postsynaptic hyperpolarization of pain-transmitting neurons are involved.

The function of KOR is much less understood at present. Many *in vivo* studies show that KOR agonists applied systemically or intrathecally have some analgesic effect, which is much weaker than MOR agonists. KOR agonist U50,488-induced analgesia is abolished in mice lacking KOR, indicating the KOR role in KOR agonist-induced analgesia. Whether MOR is involved in KOR agonist-induced analgesia remains unclear. Brainstem application of KOR agonists has little effect on baseline pain threshold. However, there is a large amount of literature demonstrating that KOR activation can oppose MOR-mediated effects in many system actions of opioids, including analgesia, reward and learning/memory. As described above, MOR and KOR share the same cellular actions. Then, why does KOR activation produce such distinct or even opposite system effects? Using the NRM as a model of MOR-mediated analgesia, we have demonstrated the cellular mechanism for the functional antagonism of MOR and KOR. We found that while MOR is exclusively localized on secondary cells in the NRM, KOR is present only in primary cells and its activation hyperpolarizes these cells by opening K^+ channels. Because MOR-mediated activation (disinhibition) of primary cells is required for MOR agonist-induced analgesia, KOR-mediated inhibition of primary cells opposes the MOR effect on these cells and antagonizes MOR-mediated analgesia (Fig.11.4). Thus, it appears that despite the same cellular actions, different types of opioid receptors produce distinct system effects due to their differential cellular and synaptic locations.

The function of DOR is more perplexing. Abundant DOR immunoreactivity has been illustrated in brainstem areas crucial for opioid analgesia, such as the PAG and the NRM, and in the spinal cord, but no DOR-mediated cellular effect has been reported in neurons of the brainstem areas in normal conditions. Only in spinal cord neurons have both a cellular effect (inhibition of glutamate synaptic transmission) and behavioral analgesia been observed under control conditions. Behaviorally, DOR agonists produce little to weak analgesic effect. This can be largely attributed to the lack of DOR actions normally in the brain areas and only contribution from spinal DOR. In DOR knockout mice, while DOR agonist-mediated spinal analgesia is abolished, its supraspinal analgesia retains and is insensitive to DOR antagonists. This retained supraspinal analgesia is reversed by MOR antagonist, arguing that the DOR agonist-induced supraspinal analgesia in DOR knockout mice is mediated by MOR. These findings question the receptor selectivity of commonly used DOR agonists when applied *in vivo* and emphasize the importance of functional interactions between opioid receptor types in an *in vivo* system.

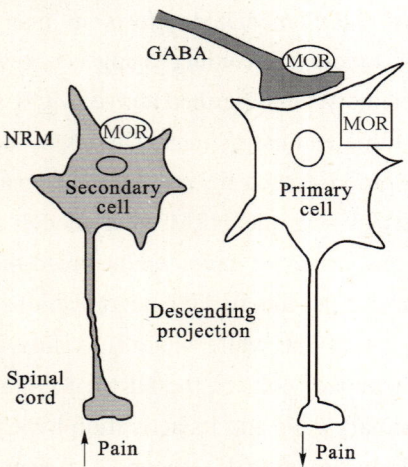

Fig.11.4 Schematic illustration of the mechanisms for MOR-mediated analgesia and for functional antagonism between MOR and KOR in the NRM. Activation of primary cells inhibits spinal pain transmission, whereas activation of secondary cells facilitates spinal pain. MOR agonists produce analgesia by (i) reducing presynaptic GABA release in primary cells and thereby disinhibiting (activating) these cells and their descending pain-inhibiting pathway, and (ii) hyperpolarizing secondary cells and removing their descending pain-facilitating actions. KOR agonists oppose MOR-mediated analgesia by hyperpolarizing primary cells that are activated by MOR agonists.

RECEPTOR TRAFFICKING

Presently, it is increasingly recognized that opioid receptors, like other G protein-coupled receptors, are dynamically and rapidly regulated by the mechanisms of receptor trafficking. Generally, receptor trafficking refers to a series of processes and pathways that mediate the translocation of receptors from surface plasma membrane to intracellular compartments and then back to surface membrane. Two forms of receptor trafficking are recognized: vertical trafficking and horizontal trafficking. Vertical trafficking deals with receptors moving between surface membrane and intracellular compartments, while horizontal trafficking concerns receptor movement between intrasynaptic structures and extrasynaptic locations on surface membrane. Receptor trafficking controls receptor functions by actively regulating the membrane density of receptors available for activation and intracellular pool of receptors available for membrane insertion.

A number of recent studies have reported opioid receptor trafficking induced by interactions between opioid receptor types. In cultured cortical neurons and native spinal neurons, 48 hours exposure to morphine significantly increases both the surface density of DOR on postsynaptic membrane and spinal analgesia induced by intrathecally applied DOR agonist. Swim stress induces DOR trafficking from cytoplasmic compartments to plasma membrane on presynaptic terminals in the PAG. Chronic morphine induces DOR-mediated inhibition of GABA release in PAG neurons. In vagas neurons of dorsal motor nucleus, activation of the cAMP-PKA pathway traffics MOR to surface membrane of GABAergic terminals and inhibits GABA release. Our recent study also shows that chronic morphine induces the emergence of functional DOR on surface membrane of putative GABAergic terminals in the NRM and that DOR agonists, ineffective in opioid naïve rats, inhibit presynaptic GABA release, produce analgesia and reduce morphine tolerance.

The mechanisms that regulate opioid receptor

trafficking are hot topics intensively investigated in current opioid research. Receptor internalization, the first step in receptor trafficking, is currently the best characterized trafficking process. In contrast, little is known regarding the mechanisms regulating the trafficking process of internalized receptors. These regulating processes are key to determining the trafficking of internalized receptors to either lysosomes for degradation or to a recycling pathway for membrane insertion and resensitization. While several proteins have been found important in the process, our understanding of intracellular pathways and regulating mechanisms for receptor trafficking is still at the infant stage. In vagas neurons, the MOR trafficking in GABAergic terminals can be induced by cAMP-PKA activation. The DOR trafficking in GABAergic terminals of PAG neurons is dependent on β-arrestin.

CONCLUSION AND FUTURE DIRECTIONS

Since the discovery and cloning of opioid receptors, decades of research has remarkably advanced our knowledge on the opioid rector system in terms of its molecular structure, endogenous ligands, signal transduction pathways, cellular actions, behavioral functions and regulating mechanisms. Today, it is one of the best-characterized receptor systems in the CNS. Current research is mostly focusing on the regulating mechanisms for opioid receptor functions and agonist-induced plastic changes in relation to clinically relevant diseases and problems caused by chronic use of opioids, such as analgesic tolerance, physical dependence and drug addiction.

Future studies at molecular level will identify more proteins and regulating mechanisms for opioid receptor trafficking and intracellular pathway sorting. The molecular mechanisms underlying differential regulation of opioid receptor trafficking by different opioid agonists binding to the receptors also will be intensively pursued. Studies at cellular level will further investigate functional adaptations and interactions between different types of opioid receptors with

regard to neuronal functions in specific brain areas and the spinal cord. Behavioral studies will remain a critical step to validate molecular and cellular findings and hypotheses in an intact system *in vivo*. These multi-disciplinary studies will further improve our understanding of opioid receptor functions in acute and chronic opioid conditions, and ultimately will lead to significantly improved opioid therapies for various types of pain and considerably more efficacious new analgesics with much less side effects.

GENERAL CITATIONS

Akil H, Owens C, Gutstein H, Taylor L, Curran E, Watson S. 1998. Endogenous opioids: overview and current issues. *Drug Alcohol Depend*, 51:127-140.

Fields H. 2004. State-dependent opioid control of pain. *Nat Rev Neurosci*, 5:565-575.

Henderson G, McKnight AT. 1997. The orphan opioid receptor and its endogenous ligand — nociceptin/orphanin FQ. *Trends Pharmacol Sci*, 18:293-300.

Kieffer BL. 2000. Opioid receptors: from genes to mice. *J Pain*, 1:45-50.

Law PY, Wong YH, Loh HH. 2000. Molecular mechanisms and regulation of opioid receptor signaling. *Annu Rev Pharmacol Toxicol*, 40:389-430.

Liu-Chen LY. 2004. Agonist-induced regulation and trafficking of kappa opioid receptors. *Life Sci*, 75:511-536.

Pan ZZ. 1998. mu-Opposing actions of the kappa- opioid receptor. *Trends Pharmacol Sci*, 19:94-98.

Williams JT, Christie MJ, Manzoni O. 2001. Cellular and synaptic adaptations mediating opioid dependence. *Physiol Rev*, 81:299-343.

DISCOVERY CITATIONS

Akil H, Mayer DJ, Liebeskind JC. 1976. Antagonism of stimulation-produced analgesia by naloxone, a narcotic antagonist. *Science*, 191:961-962.

Arvidsson U, Dado RJ, Riedl M, Lee JH, Law PY, Loh HH, *et al.* 1995. delta-Opioid receptor immunoreactivity: distribution in brainstem and spinal cord, and relationship to biogenic amines and enkephalin. *J Neurosci*, 15:1215-1235.

Avidor-Reiss T, Nevo I, Saya D, Bayewitch M, Vogel Z. 1997.

Opiate-induced adenylyl cyclase superactivation is iso-zyme-specific. *J Biol Chem*, 272: 5040-5047.

Bie B, Peng Y, Zhang Y, Pan ZZ. 2005. cAMP-mediated mechanisms for pain sensitization during opioid with-drawal. *J Neurosci*, 25:3824-3832.

Bohn LM, Lefkowitz RJ, Gainetdinov RR, Peppel K, Caron MG, Lin FT. 1999. Enhanced morphine analgesia in mice lacking beta-arrestin 2. *Science*, 286:2495-2498.

Bonci A, Williams JT. 1997. Increased probability of GABA release during withdrawal from morphine. *J Neurosci*, 17:796-803.

Brandt M, Gullis RJ, Fischer K, Buchen C, Hamprecht B, Moroder L, *et al*. 1976. Enkephalin regulates the levels of cyclic nucleotides in neuroblastoma × glioma hybrid cells. *Nature*, 262:311-313.

Browning KN, Kalyuzhny AE, Travagli RA. 2004. Mu-opioid receptor trafficking on inhibitory synapses in the rat brain-stem. *J Neurosci*, 24:7344-7352.

Cahill CM, Morinville A, Lee MC, Vincent JP, Collier B, Beaudet A. 2001. Prolonged morphine treatment targets delta opioid receptors to neuronal plasma membranes and enhances delta-mediated antinociception. *J Neurosci*, 21:7598-7607.

Chen L, Huang LY. 1991. Sustained potentiation of NMDA receptor-mediated glutamate responses through activation of protein kinase C by a mu opioid. *Neuron*, 7:319-326.

Commons KG. 2003. Translocation of presynaptic delta opioid receptors in the ventrolateral periaqueductal gray after swim stress. *J Comp Neurol*, 464:197-207.

Fukuda K, Kato S, Morikawa H, Shoda T, Mori K. 1996. Functional coupling of the delta-, mu-, and kappa-opioid receptors to mitogen-activated protein kinase and arachi-donate release in Chinese hamster ovary cells. *J Neuro-chem*, 67:1309-1316.

Glaum SR, Miller RJ, Hammond DL. 1994. Inhibitory actions of delta 1-, delta 2-, and mu-opioid receptor agonists on excitatory transmission in lamina II neurons of adult rat spinal cord. *J Neurosci*, 14:4965-4971.

Goldstein A, Lowney LI, Pal BK. 1971. Stereospecific and non-specific interactions of the morphine congener levorphanol in subcellular fractions of mouse brain. *Proc Natl Acad Sci USA*, 68:1742-1747.

Goldstein A, Tachibana S, Lowney LI, Hunkapiller M, Hood

L. 1979. Dynorphin-(1-13), an extraordinarily potent opi-oid peptide. *Proc Natl Acad Sci USA*, 76:6666-6670.

Gomes I, Gupta A, Filipovska J, Szeto HH, Pintar JE, Devi LA. 2004. A role for heterodimerization of mu and delta opiate receptors in enhancing morphine analgesia. *Proc Natl Acad Sci USA*, 101:5135-5139.

Greengard P, Jen J, Nairn AC. Stevens CF. 1991. Enhancement of the glutamate response by cAMP- dependent protein ki-nase in hippocampal neurons. *Science*, 253:1135-1138.

Grudt TJ, Williams JT. 1993. kappa-Opioid receptors also in-crease potassium conductance. *Proc Natl Acad Sci USA*, 90:11429-11432.

Hack SP, Bagley EE, Chieng BC, Christie MJ. 2005. Induction of delta-opioid receptor function in the midbrain after chronic morphine treatment. *J Neurosci*, 25:3192-3198.

Hughes J, Smith TW, Kosterlitz HW, Fothergill LA, Morgan BA, Morris HR. 1975. Identification of two related penta-peptides from the brain with potent opiate agonist activity. *Nature*, 258:577-580.

Ingram SL, Williams JT. 1994. Opioid inhibition of I_h via ade-nylyl cyclase. *Neuron*, 13:179-186.

Jolas T, Nestler EJ, Aghajanian GK. 2000. Chronic morphine increases GABA tone on serotonergic neurons of the dorsal raphe nucleus: association with an up-regulation of the cy-clic AMP pathway. *Neuroscience*, 95:433-443.

Jordan BA, Devi LA. 1999. G-protein-coupled receptor het-erodimerization modulates receptor function. *Nature*, 399:697-700.

Keith DE, Murray SR, Zaki PA, Chu PC, Lissin DV, Kang L, *et al*. 1996. Morphine activates opioid receptors without causing their rapid internalization. *J Biol Chem*, 271:19021-19024.

Liu JG, Anand KJ. 2001. Protein kinases modulate the cellular adaptations associated with opioid tolerance and depend-ence. *Brain Res Brain Res Rev*, 38:1-19.

Loh HH, Tseng LF, Wei E, Li CH. 1976. beta-endorphin is a potent analgesic agent. *Proc Natl Acad Sci USA*, 73:2895-2898.

Lord JA, Waterfield AA, Hughes J, Kosterlitz HW. 1977. En-dogenous opioid peptides: multiple agonists and receptors. *Nature*, 267:495-499.

Martin WR, Eades CG, Thompson JA, Huppler RE, Gilbert PE. 1976. The effects of morphine-and nalorphine-like drugs in the nondependent and morphine-dependent chronic spinal dog. *J Pharmacol Exp Ther*, 197:517-532.

Matthes HW, Maldonado R, Simonin F, Valverde O, Slowe S, Kitchen I, *et al*. 1996. Loss of morphine-induced analgesia, reward effect and withdrawal symptoms in mice lacking the mu-opioid- receptor gene. *Nature*, 383:819-823.

Nestler EJ, Aghajanian GK, 1997, Molecular and cellular basis of addiction. *Science*, 278:58-63.

Nicoll RA, Alger BE, Jahr CE. 1980. Enkephalin blocks inhibitory pathways in the vertebrate CNS. *Nature*, 287:22-25.

North RA, Williams JT, Surprenant A, Christie MJ. 1987, Mu and delta receptors belong to a family of receptors that are coupled to potassium channels. *Proc Natl Acad Sci USA*, 84:5487-5491.

Pan ZZ. 2003. Kappa-opioid receptor-mediated enhancement of the hyperpolarization-activated current (*I*(h)) through mobilization of intracellular calcium in rat nucleus raphe magnus. *J Physiol*, 548:765-775.

Pan ZZ, Williams JT, Osborne PB. 1990. Opioid actions on single nucleus raphe magnus neurons from rat and guinea-pig in vitro. *J Physiol*, 427:519-532.

Pan ZZ, Tershner SA, Fields HL. 1997. Cellular mechanism for anti-analgesic action of agonists of the kappa-opioid receptor. *Nature*, 389:382-385.

Pert CB, Snyder SH. 1973. Opiate receptor: demonstration in nervous tissue. *Science*, 179:1011-1014.

Sharma SK, Klee WA, Nirenberg M. 1975. Dual regulation of adenylate cyclase accounts for narcotic dependence and tolerance. *Proc Natl Acad Sci USA*, 72:3092-3096.

Simon EJ, Hiller JM, Edelman I. 1973. Stereospecific binding of the potent narcotic analgesic (3H) Etorphine to rat-brain homogenate. *Proc Natl Acad Sci USA*, 70:1947-1949.

Sternini C, Spann M, Anton B, Keith DE Jr, Bunnett NW, von

Zastrow M, *et al*. 1996. Agonist-selective endocytosis of mu opioid receptor by neurons in vivo. *Proc Natl Acad Sci USA*, 93:9241-9246.

Taddese A, Nah SY, McCleskey EW. 1995. Selective opioid inhibition of small nociceptive neurons. *Science*, 270:1366-1369.

Terenius L. 1973. Stereospecific interaction between narcotic analgesics and a synaptic plasm a membrane fraction of rat cerebral cortex. *Acta Pharmacol Toxicol (Copenh)*, 32:317-320.

Vaughan CW, Ingram SL, Connor MA, Christie MJ. 1997. How opioids inhibit GABA-mediated neurotransmission. *Nature*, 390:611-614.

Wainger BJ, DeGennaro M, Santoro B, Siegelbaum SA, Tibbs GR. 2001. Molecular mechanism of cAMP modulation of HCN pacemaker channels. *Nature*, 411:805-810.

Whistler JL, Chuang HH, Chu P, Jan LY, von Zastrow M. 1999. Functional dissociation of mu opioid receptor signaling and endocytosis: implications for the biology of opiate tolerance and addiction. *Neuron*, 23:737-746.

Williams JT, Egan TM, North RA. 1982. Enkephalin opens potassium channels on mammalian central neurones. *Nature*, 299:74-77.

Zadina JE, Hackler L, Ge LJ, Kastin AJ. 1997. A potent and selective endogenous agonist for the mu-opiate receptor. *Nature*, 386:499-502.

Zhu W, Pan ZZ. 2005. Mu-opioid-mediated inhibition of glutamate synaptic transmission in rat central amygdala neurons. *Neuroscience*, 133:97-103.

Zhu Y, King MA, Schuller AG, Nitsche JF, Reidl M, Elde RP, *et al*. 1999. Retention of supraspinal delta-like analgesia and loss of morphine tolerance in delta opioid receptor knockout mice. *Neuron*, 24:243-252.

Retrograde Messengers

CHAPTER 12

Min Zhuo[*]

MAJOR CONTRIBUTIONS

1. Zhuo M, Small SA, Kandel ER, Hawkins RD. 1993. Nitric oxide and carbon monoxide produce activity-dependent long- term synaptic enhancement in hippocampus. *Science*, 260: 1946-1950.
2. Zhuo M, Meller ST, Gebhart GF. 1993. Endogenous nitric oxide is required for tonic cholinergic inhibition of spinal mechanical transmission. *Pain*, 54:71-78.
3. Zhuo M, Hu Y, Schultz C, Kandel ER, Hawkins RD. 1994. Role of guanylyl cyclase and cGMP-dependent protein kinase in long-term potentiation in hippocampus. *Nature*, 368: 635-639.
4. Zhuo M. 1997. A diffusible neuronal messenger in the brain: nitric oxide. In: *Fudan Lectures in Neurobiology*, 13:41-50. (Review)
5. Zhuo, M, Laitinen, JT, Li, X-C, Kandel, ER, Hawkins, RD. 1998. Tests of the roles of nitric oxide and carbon monoxide in long-term potentiation in the hippocampus. *Learning & Memory*, 5:467-480.

MAIN TOPICS

Feedback control as a key mechanism for brain functions

NO, an important diffusible messenger

Retrograde messengers: a family of diffusible molecules in the brain

NO

CO

Other retrograde messengers

Molecular targets and downstream signaling pathways

Soluble guanylate cyclase (sGC)

cGMP-dependent protein kinase (PKG)

cGMP-related phosphodiesterases

Presynaptic vesicle-related proteins

cGMP-gated ion channels

Activity-dependent and biphasic modulation

LTP

L-LTP

LTD

Brain functions

Memory and fear

Persistent pain

Other functions

SUMMARY

In the neuronal circuit, feedback control is an important mechanism to maintain the stability of the circuit. Among many different signaling molecules, diffusible, gaseous messengers such as nitric oxide (NO) and carbon monoxide (CO) serve as key retrograde messengers in central excitatory synapses. Due to its rapid synthesis and non-vesicle dependent release, these gaseous messengers play different roles in synaptic transmission, in particular the plasticity. In this chapter, we will use NO and CO as two major examples of retrograde messenger families to explore their roles in central plasticity. We will discuss the synthesis of NO and CO, molecular target and downstream signaling proteins for NO and CO. Finally, we will also review the physiological functions of NO and CO in learning & memory, sensory transmission and pain, and cortical functions.

---

* The introduction of Dr. Zhuo, please refer to Chapter 8.

INTRODUCTION

Feedback control or "retrograde" signaling is common in the circuit to control the amount of information to pass by. In the brain, just like the computer, feedback controls are commonly used. At the systemic level, feedback inhibitory controls through projecting fibers control sensory inputs entering into the spinal cord, such as descending modulatory systems (see Chapter 27). At local circuit levels, neurotransmitters or neuro-modulator including neuropeptides can be released and then acti on presynaptic terminals, to achieve "retrograde" controls. These types of control can be positive or negative. In the case of positive control, retrograde messengers can enhance neurotransmitter release. For negative feedback control, retrograde messengers reduce transmitter release, thus reducing synaptic transmission. In this chapter, we will discuss the new classes of retrograde messengers that act locally between presynaptic terminals and postsynaptic spines. Unlike classic transmitters, retrograde messengers are not vesicle released nor do they require specialized release machinery. Among several retrograde messengers, we will focus on gaseous retrograde messengers such as nitro oxide (NO) and carbon monoxide (CO).

FEEDBACK CONTROL AS A KEY MECHANISM FOR BRAIN FUNCTIONS

Before we discuss retrograde messengers, it is important for us to examine a few examples of feedback control mechanisms at the systemic and synaptic levels (see Fig. 12.1). At the systemic level, for example, sensory transmission from the periphery to the brain can undergo feedback modulation at different levels of sensory central relays. In the spinal cord dorsal horn, spinal dorsal horn neurons receive sensory inputs from the periphery through activation of primary sensory afferent fibers. Dorsal horn neurons relay this information to supraspinal nuclei through ascending projection pathways. In the mean time, sensory dorsal

horn neurons also receive innervations of projecting fibers from supraspinal structures. These descending projection fibers form synaptic connections presynaptically and postsynaptically on dorsal horn sensory synapses. These descending modulation is biphasic. For inhibitory modulation, activation of descending pathways reduces dorsal horn responses to peripheral sensory stimulation; for facilitatory modulation, activation of descending modulates increase responses of dorsal horn neurons to peripheral stimuli. Such bipha-

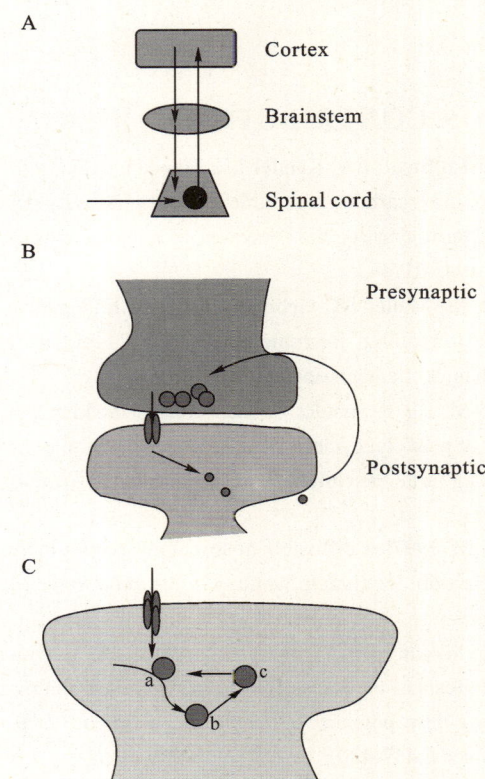

Fig.12.1 Feedback control as key mechanisms for neuronal synapses, circuits and inside cells. A. A diagram showing the descending modulatory systems of sensory transmission in the spinal cord. Descending projecting fibers the cortex, midbrain and brainstem exert biphasic modulation on spinal sensory transmission. By activating descending facilitatory or inhibitory systems, animals are able to enhance their detection of peripheral stimuli or reduce pain. B. Retrograde modulation of presynaptic release of transmitter by diffusible small molecules. C. Feedback control among intracellular messengers and proteins within a cell. The production of **b** molecule by activation of **a** proteins (e.g., cyclases) triggers the activity of a downstream protein **c**; the increased activity of **c** then modulates the activity of **a**.

sic modulation is physiologically important, descending inhibition is likely to contribute to reduced pain, while facilitatory modulation enhances the ability to detect potentially important or dangerous stimuli.

Feedback modulation at the synaptic level is the focus of this chapter, such as the role of NO and CO in synaptic LTP and LTD. LTP and LTD are two major forms of central plasticity that are thought to mimic synaptic changes during learning and memory. Alternation in presynaptic transmitter releases and/or postsynaptic glutamate receptor mediated responses are believed to contribute to synaptic potentiation or depression.

In addition to neuron-neuron communication, feedback controls are also widely found inside cells, including neurons (Fig.12.1C). Thus, it is commonly believed that the feedback control is essential for physiological functions, and disruption of such fine feedback controls will lead to pathological conditions.

NO, AN IMPORTANT DIFFUSIBLE MESSENGER

NO as a novel intracellular and intercellular messenger has drawn much attention from scientists. The study of NO has been greatly brought forward by a finding by Bredt and Snyder at John Hopkins University that NO synthase (NOS) activity is calcium-CaM dependent. Unlikely traditional neurotransmitters and modulators, NO has its own unique properties: (i) its release through a non-vesicle mechanism; (ii) it is membrane permeable; (iii) it has a very-short half life. These properties give NO a wide range of physiological functions in both animals and humans. It can serve as an important signal and release rapidly, and yet inactivate quickly. It also reaches target proteins in all directions without the requirement of receptors. Many studies consistently find that NO is involved in the central nervous system, immunological system, cardiovascular system, sensory system, digestive system, as well as in sexual behavior. Furthermore, NO also serves as a bad role in pathological diseases, such as hypertension, stroke, septic shock and other degenerative diseases of the brain. Understanding physio-

logical mechanisms of NO not only provide mechanisms of various systems, but also providean important basis for clinical treatment of disease.

RETROGRADE MESSENGERS: A FAMILY OF DIFFUSIBLE MOLECULES IN THE BRAIN

NO

Arginine is the precursor for NO production in the body (see Fig. 12.2A). NO is formed by neurons in the brain. NOS have different isoforms in mammalian system: including neuronal NOS (nNOS), endothelial NOS (eNOS), macrophage NOS, hepatic NOS, and cytochrome P-450 reductase. Although each isoform may be named after their primary location, their distributions can overlap. For example, eNOS is found in the brain as well.

Activation of NOS is calcium-calmodulin (CaM) dependent (Fig. 12.3A). NMDA or glutamate induces production of NO in different regions of the brain. For example, both in hippocampus and spinal cord, NMDA application induce NO release. In the cerebellum, glutamate induces fast release of NO which is thought to be important for cerebellar LTD. NOS also is regulated by other neurotransmitters such as acetylcholine and bradykinin. In the hippocampus, NO generated in carbachol treated slices modulate the rate of occurrence of muscarinic rhythmic slow activity. Nerve growth factor may also regulate NO activity, which subsequently affects gene-regulation of cells. NOS is widely distributed in the central nervous system, from the spinal cord to the neocortex. In the superficial layer of neocortex, NO coexist with other transmitters such as NPY and somaostatin. In hippocampus, NO is found in CA3 and CA1 pyramidal cells and granules cells in dentate gyrus. Interestingly, different subtypes of NOS are located in various regions. In CA1 pyramidal neurons, endothelial NOS is rich while nNOS is less. NOS terminals in dorsal horn of the spinal cord, in particular laminae II. The wide distribution of NOS indicates that NO may play various roles in physiological functions of the brain.

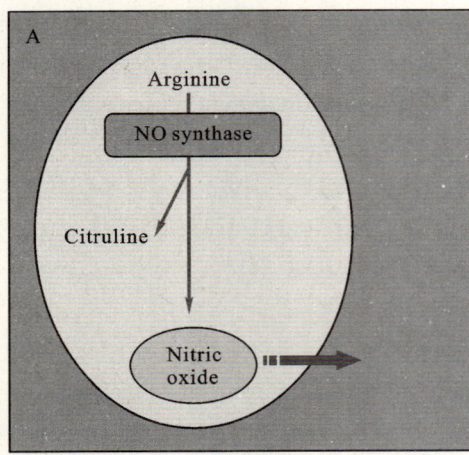

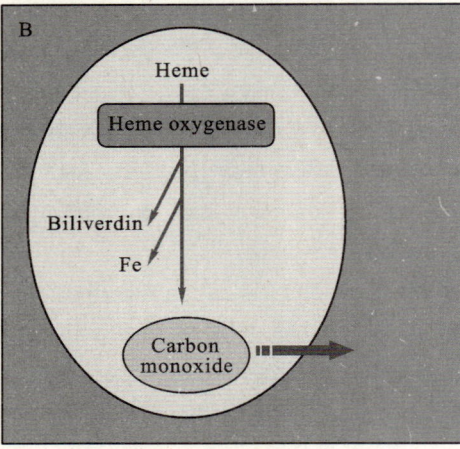

Fig.12.2 The production of NO and CO. Arginine is the precursor for NO production in the body. NO is formed by neurons in the brain. NOS has different isoforms in mammalian system: including neuronal NOS, endothelial NOS, macrophage NOS, hepatic NOS, and cytochrome P-450 reductase.

CO

CO is generated by heme oxygenase (HO) (Fig. 12.2B). HO cleaves the porphyrin ring of heme to form biliverdin, which then is reduced by biliverdin reductase to bilirubin. Ferrous ion is released and a one-carbon fragment produces as CO. HOs exist in two different forms: HO-1 and HO-2. HO-1 is induced by different cellular stimuli such as stress.

Although it is thought that HO-2 is not inducible, HO-2 can be activated by calcium-dependent manner in neurons (Fig. 12.3B). HO-2 is phosphorylated by casein kinase-2 (CK2), and this phosphorylation leads to activation of HO-2. Because protein kinase C activates CH2 in neurons, it is thus conceivable that neuronal activity that lead to the membrane depolariza-

tion and trigger calcium influx will activate HO-2 in neurons. Furthermore, it is recently found that calmodulin binds with nanomolar affinity to HO-2 in a calcium-dependent manner, causing activation of HO-2 activity in neurons. These rather classic signaling pathways provide mechanism for production of CO upon neuronal activity, indicating the important role of CO in many physiological functions of the brain.

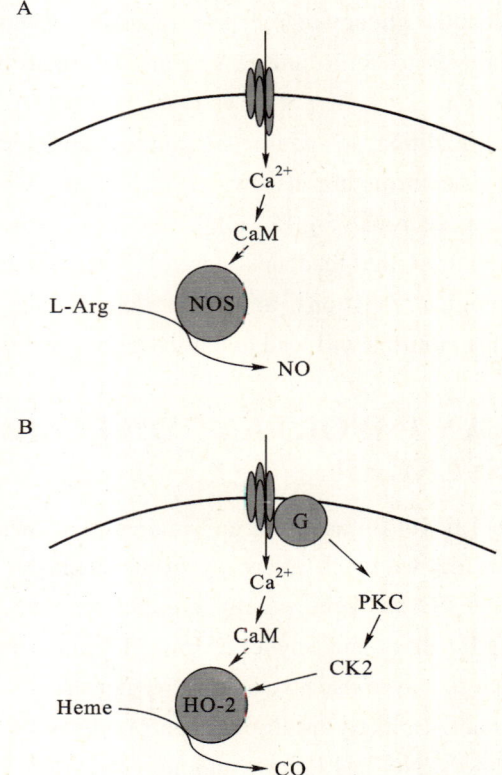

Fig.12.3 Activation and production of NO and CO. A. NOS is activated by calcium-calmodulin-dependent manner. Due to its sensitivity to calcium-calmodulin, NOS can be activated subsequent to many signaling pathways, such as activation of NMDA receptors, L-type voltage calcium channels, and activation of cholinergic muscarinic receptors. B. HO-2 is activated by calcium-dependent manner in neurons as NOS. HO-2 can be phosphorylated by casein kinase-2 (CK2), and this phosphorylation leads to activation of HO-2.

Other Retrograde Messengers

In addition to NO and CO, other molecules or peptides have been suggested as retrograde messengers in the central nervous system. They include: arachidonic acid, PAF, cannabinoids and BDNF.

MOLECULAR TARGETS AND DOWNSTREAM SIGNALING PATHWAYS

Soluble Guanylate Cyclase (sGC)

One of major target proteins for NO and CO in neurons are soluble GCs (Fig.12.4). Activation of sGCs by NO and CO lead to the production of cGMP, an important second messenger in neurons. This pathway is thought to be important for the LTP which is sensitive to inhibition of NOS. Inhibition of sGCs produced dose-dependent inhibition of LTP. cGMP produces a long-lasting depression in the cerebellum by an activity-dependent mechanism. 8-Br-cGMP, a membrane-permeable cGMP anaglous, produced a long- lasting depression of AMPA mediated responses when paired with the activity. Bath application of cGMP analogues or postsynaptic application of cGMP into the Purkinje cells induces a long-lasting depression of parallel-fiber mediated EPSP, indicating that activation of soluble GC of Purkinje cells is important for LTD. Furthermore, this cGMP-induced depression occludes normal LTD, suggesting that they share the same mechanisms. Since cGMP analogues only produce depression when paired with parallel fiber stimulation, the cGMP-induced depression is activity dependent, neither cGMP analogues nor weak stimulation alone produce significant LTD. Application of cGMP analog such as 8-Br-cGMP paired with weak synaptic activity induced LTP. A series of cGMP analog developed by Roger Tsien in University of San Diego provide helpful approaches for investigating roles of cGMP. For these analogues, they will be degraded by cGMP-phosphodiesterases within the neurons, so the drug mimics physiological increases of the cGMP after stimulation.

sGC is also phosphorylated (and activated) by PKC and by cAMP-dependent protein kinase. Because PKC is activated in LTP, it is thus possible that sGC phosphorylation by PKC may contribute to its activation during hippocampal LTP, in addition to activation by retrograde messenger NO and CO.

Tetanus application induced a transient rise in cGMP, reaching a maximum at 10 s and decreasing below basal levels 5 min after the tetanus, remaining below basal levels after 60 min. sGC activity increased 5 min after tetanus and returned to basal levels at 60 min. The decrease in cGMP was due to sustained tetanus-induced increase in cGMP-degrading phosphodiesterase activity, which remained activated 60 min after tetanus.

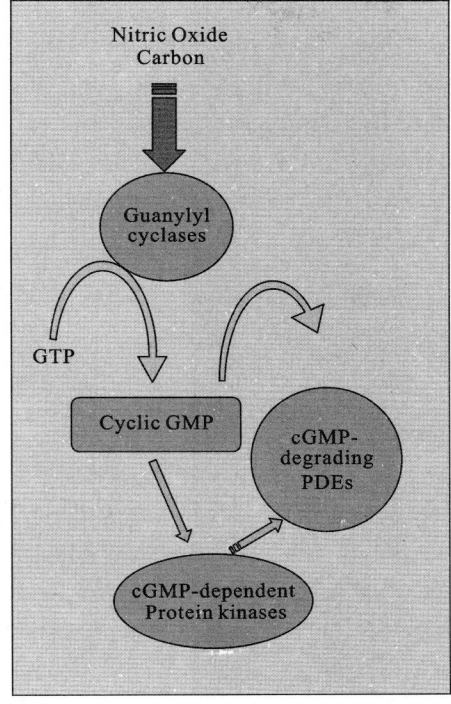

Fig.12.4 cGMP signaling pathways as the major downstream signaling pathways for NO and CO. One major target protein for NO and CO in neurons are soluble GCs. Activation of sGCs by NO and CO lead to the production of cGMP, an important second messengers in neurons. Among them, cGMP-dependent proteins kinases are thought to be important for cGMP-dependent synaptic potentiation.

cGMP-dependent Protein Kinase (PKG)

One key downstream protein for cGMP is cGMP-dependent protein kinase (PKG) (Fig. 12.5). In the cerebellum, it is believed that cGMP produces its effects by stimulating PKG. PKG is found 20 to 40 folds higher in the cerebellum than in the other region of the brain. PKG is cytoplasmic, and found is rich in the Purkinje cells. Consistently, a substrate for PKG has also been found which similar a distribution in the central nervous system. Pharmacological studies using a selective PKG inhibitor found that activation of PKG is important for the induction of cerebellar LTD. Pretreatment with a PKG inhibitor KT5823 antagonizes the desensitization of AMPA responses by 8-Br-cGMP. KT5823 blocks tACPD-induced suppression of AMPA mediated responses. The effect of KT5823 is selective for the induction, since KT5823 applied after the induction of LTD does not prevent LTD, indicating the expression of LTD does not require constitutive activation of PKG. In the hippocampus, Zhuo and Kandel found that inhibitor of PKG prevent the induction of LTP. Application of selective activator of PKG induced LTP. Genetic deletion of PKGI significantly reduced LTP in the hippocampus, supporting the roles of PKG in hippocampal LTP.

cGMP-related Phosphodiesterases

In addition to PKGs, cGMP-dependent phosphodiesterases (PDEs) are another improtant downstream signaling protein. Transcripts for subunits of several types of cGMP specific phosphodiesterase are found in the mammalian brain. What makes more important for the possible function of cGMP-dependent PDEs is that the activity of cGMP-PDEs can also contribute to the activity of sGSs. Thus, this interaction forms a feedback loop for activation of sGC in neurons. According to this hypothesis, the neuronal activity such as tetanic stimulation lead to activation of NO and/or CO, and to increased content of cGMP, which then activate PKG, which, in turn, will activate cGMP-degrading PDEs. Activation of cGMP-degrading PDEs then reduces or lowers the level of cGMP in the cells.

PRESYNAPTIC VESICLE-RELATED PROTEINS

In addition to cGMP-dependent signaling pathways, NO can affect presynaptic complexed release machinery to enhance transmitter release (Fig. 12.5). NO increases formation of the VAMP/SNAP-25/syntaxin 1a core complex and inhibits the binding of n-src 1 to syntaxin 1a. Both effects are likely to lead to en-

hancement of vesicle docking/fusion, and release of neurotransmitters. This signaling pathway is likely to be cGMP-independent. However, NO and/or CO may regulate phosphorylation of VASP through sGC and PKG pathways, and then contribute to aggregation of synaptophysin in presynaptic terminals.

cGMP-GATED ION CHANNELS

Not all targets of cGMP require the involvement of PKG. Cyclic nucleotide-gated (CNG) channels are calcium-permeable, nonspecific cation channels that can be activated directly by cGMP/and cAMP (Fig. 12.5). Two isoforms of these CNG channels are found in the hippocampal neurons, and genetic deletion of OCNC1 lead to reduced LTP.

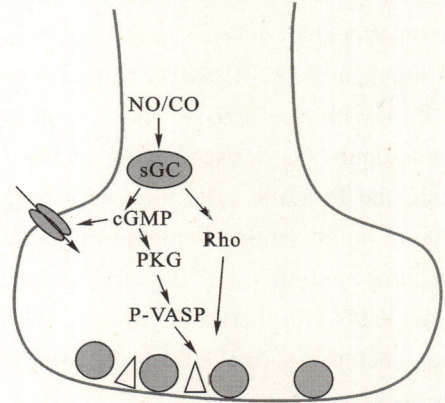

Fig.12.5 Presynaptic mechanism for NO and CO producing effects.

ACTIVITY-DEPENDENT AND BIPHASIC MODULATION

LTP

The first lines of evidence supporting the involvement of NOS in the LTP induction are pharmacological experiments using selective inhibitors blocking the metabolism of NO. For example, NOS inhibitors, hemoglobin that scavenges NO, etc. Because field recordings of EPSPs are seemly easy to be performed and thus commonly used in these studies. However, it is very difficult to standardize the individual slices used for the LTP studies. Nevertheless, the effects of NOS inhibition have been reported by many investigators. One carveat for these traditional electrophysiological experiments is the limited knowledge of the amount of inhibition of NOS activity. Few parallel biochemical experiments above been performed to evaluate the amount of NOS activity inhibited in these experimental conditions. The second line of evidence supporting NOS activity in LTP is the use of genetically mutanted mice. Single deletion of NOS leads to no change or reduction of LTP, while double knockout of NOS produces greater inhibition of LTP. Unlike pharmacological approaches, in these experiments, the overall NOS activity is abolished due to gene deletion. Finally, the evidence for NO as a retrograde messengers come from experiments using direct application of NO to the brain slices. Paired NO application with weak synaptic activity caused LTP. This effect is insensitive to the blockade of NMDA receptors, indicating that NO effects are downstream from NMDA receptors as suggested.

Considering the lack of complete inhibition of LTP by inhibition of NOS, it is thus proposed that some other messengers may also contribute to LTP. CO comes as another retrograde messenger candidate. Inhibition of the CO synthesis enzyme activity blocked the induction of LTP. Genetic deletion of HO-2, however, did not affect LTP under one condition, suggesting that the role of HO-2 in LTP may be compensate by other signaling proteins. Unfortunately, no double knockout or triple knockout studies have been pursued aggressively. It remains unknown if new gene deletion may lead to complete inhibition of LTP. Application of CO with synaptic activity leads to prolonged synaptic potentiation.

L-LTP

Although LTP is suggested as long-lasting potentiation, most of studies of LTP are limited to 45–60 min after the induction, due to the limitation of recording techniques. L-LTP is thought to more closely relate to long-term memory, although very strong induction protocol is needed. Furthermore, the recordings are highly technically difficult, and it is difficult to perform well control experiments as regulate LTP, such

as two-pathway experiments. In the case of L-LTP, inhibition of NO produces no significant reduction of synaptic potentiation, while inhibition of CO production produces greater inhibition.

LTD

Long-term depression, has been found in the hippocampus. It has been suggested that these types of synaptic depression may serve to prevent saturation of synaptic transmission caused by LTP. Recent studies raise the possibility that some retrograde messengers may also be involved in synaptic depression: (i) electrophysiological studies find that LTD accompanied decrease of transmitters release from presynaptic terminals; (ii) the induction of depression requires postsyanptic NMDA and/or mGluRs. The possible existence of diffusible messengers is raised by a report by Bolshakov and Siegelbaum (1994). In that report, they found that while the induction of LTD in the CA1 region of the hippocampus is postsynaptic, the expression of LTD is presynaptic. Therefore, as in the case of LTP in the CA1 region of the hippocampus, postsynaptic activation must release some diffusible messengers that then act on the presynaptic terminals. The first candidate is NO. NO has been suggested as a messenger in LTD by some investigators. NO synthase inhibitor L-MMNA pretreatment prevent the induction of hippocampal LTD. However, this was not observed by another group which employed a longer pretreatment of L-MMNA. Application of NO during low-frequency stimulation of presynaptic fibers (0.25 Hz) produces a long-lasting depression of synaptic transmission. This depression is NMDA-receptor independent and is not affected by GABA receptor blocker. Unlike NO, CO has not been reported to contribute to LTD.

BRAIN FUNCTIONS

Memory and Fear

One key function of possible hippocampal LTP is spatial memory. Inhibition of systemic NOS activity affected the formation of spatial memory in Morris water maze test. However, due to the nonselective distribution of NOS inhibitors, it is difficult to conclude that the defects are due to inhibition of hippocampal LTP, or other general side-effects of these inhibitors. A better study was performed using locally administered NOS inhibitors into the hippocampus. Application of N-omega-nitro-L-arginine into the dorsal hippocampus affected the manner in which the rats were searching the submerged platform during training, but did not affect the efficiency to find the spatial location of the escape platform. Hippocampal NO-synthase inhibition did not affect the learning of a new platform position in the same water tank (i.e. reversal learning). Moreover, no treatment effects were observed in the probe trials (i.e. after acquisition and after reversal learning), indicating that the rats treated with N-omega-nitro-L-arginine had learned the spatial location of the platform. These findings were obtained under conditions where the NO synthesis in the dorsal hippocampus was completely inhibited. On the basis of the present data it was concluded that hippocampal NO is not critically involved in place learning in rats.

Similarly, in Pavlovian conditioned fear tests, inhibition of NOS by different NOS inhibitors failed to block the acquisition or extinction of Pavlovian fear conditioning. However, NOS inhibitors did reduce locomotor activity and cause a corresponding increase in the expression of contextual freezing. It is concluded that NOS activity is not required for either the acquisition or expression of contextual fear conditioning.

One possible difficulty for these studies is that no parallel biochemical studies have been performed to assure the inhibition of NOS activity within the hippocampus. Indeed, many nonselective NO synthase inhibitors have produced contradictory results in learning experiments. However, these drugs also produced blood pressure changes, as NO is an endothelial-derived relaxing factor. A novel NO synthase inhibitor, 7-nitro indazole (7-NI), as a dose (30 mg/kg i.p.) shown previously to inhibit neuronal NO synthase by 85% without affecting blood pressure, pro-

duced amnesic effects both in a water maze and in an 8-arm radial maze.

Persistent Pain

NO has been reported to be important in nociceptive transmission, both peripherally and centrally. In the spinal cord, NO is produced as a result of activation of NMDA receptors. NO diffuses to presynaptic terminals, stimulates soluble guanylyl cyclase and increases the content of cGMP. Finally, cGMP causes the enhancement of transmitter release from presynaptic terminals by an activity-dependent mechanism. A NO sensitive enhancement of glutamate release by NMDA application has been reported in the spinal cord. Interestingly, both analgesic and algesic effects of NO have been reported in the spinal cord. It is unclear whether biphasic effects of NO in the spinal cord depend on the activity of presynaptic fibers frequency. The activity-dependent mechanism may explain input specificity for windup and LTP in the spinal cord.

Other Functions

NO and CO have been implicated in many different functions, although many of their effects may not be through retrograde signaling pathways.

CONCLUSIONS AND FUTURE DIRECTIONS

Studies of retrograde messengers provide important information about the neuronal process at the net work level. Activity-dependent synaptic depression and potentiation by these retrograde messengers allow inter-cellular communications within a range of neurons. Although the study of retrograde messengers in synaptic LTP proved to be difficult, just as to demonstrate how LTP in the CA1 may enhance spatial learning and memory. However, if we recognize the complexity of the central nervous systems, it is not too difficult to understand why a simple model of LTP can not explain learning and memory. For the roles of retrograde messengers in the brain functions, we are almost facing the similar situation. Studies using reduced preparations such as neuronal cultures and brain slices will never mimic physiological conditions *in vivo*. Thus, demonstration of negative or positive effects of retrograde messengers in reduced preparation should be used to exclude or directly argue the effects of retrograde messengers *in vivo*. Thus, much work will need to be done with retrograde messengers in terms of their physiological functions, and implications of their functions in pathological conditions.

GENERAL CITATIONS

Alger BE. 2002. Retrograde signaling in the regulation of synaptic transmission: focus on endocannabinoids. *Prog Neurobiol*, 68:247-286.

Baranano DE, Snyder SH. 2001. Neural roles for heme oxygenase: contrasts to nitric oxide synthase. *Proc Natl Acad Sci USA*, 98:10996-11002.

Boehning D, Snyder SH. 2003. Novel neural modulators. *Annu Rev Neurosci*, 26:105-131.

Bredt DS, Snyder SH. 1994. Nitric oxide: a physiologic messenger molecule. *Annu Rev Biochem*, 63: 175-195.

Hawkins RD, Zhuo M, Arancio O. 1994. Nitric oxide and carbon monoxide as possible retrograde messengers in hippocampal long-term potentiation. *J Neurobiol*, 25:652-665.

Schuman EM, Madison DV. 1994. Nitric oxide and synaptic function. *Annu Rev Neurosci*, 17:153-183.

Tao HW, Poo M. 2001. Retrograde signaling at central synapses. *Proc Natl Acad Sci USA*, 98:11009-11015.

DISCOVERY CITATIONS

Arancio O, Kandel ER, Hawkins RD. 1995. Activity-dependent long-term enhancement of transmitter release by presynaptic 3',5'-cyclic GMP in cultured hippocampal neurons. *Nature*, 376:74-80.

Blackshaw S, Eliasson MJ, Sawa A, Watkins CC, Krug D, Gupta A, *et al.* 2003. Species, strain and developmental variations in hippocampal neuronal and endothelial nitric oxide synthase clarify discrepancies in nitric oxide-dependent synaptic plasticity. *Neuroscience*, 119:979-990.

Boehning D, Sedaghat L, Sedlak TW, Snyder SH. 2004. Heme oxygenase-2 is activated by calcium-calmodulin. *J Biol Chem*, 279:30927-30930.

Boehning D, Moon C, Sharma S, Hurt KJ, Hester LD, Ronnett GV, *et al.* 2003. Carbon monoxide neurotransmission activated by CK2 phosphorylation of heme oxygenase-2. *Neuron*, 40:129-137.

Bredt DS, Hwang PM, Snyder SH. 1990. Localization of nitric oxide synthase indicating a neural role for nitric oxide. *Nature*, 347:768-770.

Bredt DS, Glatt CE, Hwang PM, Fotuhi M, Dawson TM, Snyder SH. 1991. Nitric oxide synthase protein and mRNA are discretely localized in neuronal populations of the mammalian CNS together with NADPH diaphorase. *Neuron*, 7:615-624.

Chien WL, Liang KC, Teng CM, Kuo SC, Lee FY, Fu WM. 2003. Enhancement of long-term potentiation by a potent nitric oxide-guanylyl cyclase activator, 3-(5-hydroxymethyl-2-furyl)-1-benzyl-indazole. *Mol Pharmacol*, 63:1322-1328.

Cummings JA, Nicola SM, Malenka RC. 1994. Induction in the rat hippocampus of long-term potentiation (LTP) and long-term depression (LTD) in the presence of a nitric oxide synthase inhibitor. *Neurosci Lett*, 176:110-114.

Dinerman JL, Dawson TM, Schell MJ, Snowman A, Snyder SH. 1994. Endothelial nitric oxide synthase localized to hippocampal pyramidal cells: implications for synaptic plasticity. *Proc Natl Acad Sci USA*, 91:4214-4218.

Frisch C, Dere E, Silva MA, Godecke A, Schrader J, Huston JP. 2000. Superior water maze performance and increase in fear-related behavior in the endothelial nitric oxide synthase-deficient mouse together with monoamine changes in cerebellum and ventral striatum. *J Neurosci*, 20:6694-6700.

Gelperin A. 1994. Nitric oxide mediates network oscillations of olfactory interneurons in a terrestrial mollusc. *Nature*, 369:61-63.

Ingi T, Chiang G, Ronnett GV. 1996. The regulation of heme turnover and carbon monoxide biosynthesis in cultured primary rat olfactory receptor neurons. *J Neurosci*, 16:5621-5628.

Ingi T, Cheng J, Ronnett GV. 1996. Carbon monoxide: an endogenous modulator of the nitric oxide-cyclic GMP signaling system. *Neuron*, 16:835-842.

Keefer EW, Gramowski A, Gross GW. 2001. NMDA receptor-dependent periodic oscillations in cultured spinal cord networks. *J Neurophysiol*, 86: 3030-3042.

Kleppisch T, Wolfsgruber W, Feil S, Allmann R, Wotjak CT, Goebbels S, *et al*. 2003. Hippocampal cGMP-dependent protein kinase I supports an age- and protein synthesis-dependent component of long-term potentiation but is not essential for spatial reference and contextual memory. *J Neurosci*, 23:6005-6012.

Klyachko VA, Ahern GP, Jackson MB. 2001. cGMP- mediated facilitation in nerve terminals by enhancement of the spike afterhyperpolarization. *Neuron*, 31:1015-1025.

Knowles RG, Palacios M, Palmer RM, Moncada S. 1989. Formation of nitric oxide from L-arginine in the central nervous system: a transduction mechanism for stimulation of the soluble guanylate cyclase. *Proc Natl Acad Sci USA*, 86:5159-5162.

Meffert MK, Premack BA, Schulman H. 1994. Nitric oxide stimulates $Ca^{(2+)}$-independent synaptic vesicle release. *Neuron*, 12:1235-1244.

Meffert MK, Calakos NC, Scheller RH, Schulman H. 1996. Nitric oxide modulates synaptic vesicle docking fusion reactions. *Neuron*, 16:1229-1236.

Michel T, Li GK, Busconi L. 1993. Phosphorylation and subcellular translocation of endothelial nitric oxide synthase. *Proc Natl Acad Sci USA*, 90: 6252- 6256.

Nathanson JA, Scavone C, Scanlon C, McKee M. 1995. The cellular Na^+ pump as a site of action for carbon monoxide and glutamate: a mechanism for long-term modulation of cellular activity. *Neuron*, 14:781-794.

Pape HC, Mager R. 1992. Nitric oxide controls oscillatory activity in thalamocortical neurons. *Neuron*, 9:441-448.

Poss KD, Thomas MJ, Ebralidze AK, O'Dell TJ, Tonegawa S. 1995. Hippocampal long-term potentiation is normal in heme oxygenase-2 mutant mice. *Neuron*, 15:867-873.

Savchenko A, Barnes S, Kramer RH. 1997. Cyclic-nucleotide-gated channels mediate synaptic feedback by nitric oxide. *Nature*, 390:694-698.

Smith SL, Otis TS. 2003. Persistent changes in spontaneous firing of Purkinje neurons triggered by the nitric oxide signaling cascade. *J Neurosci*, 23: 367-372.

Wang HG, Lu FM, Jin I, Udo H, Kandel ER, de Vente J, *et al*. 2005. Presynaptic and postsynaptic roles of NO, cGK, and RhoA in long-lasting potentiation and aggregation of synaptic proteins. *Neuron*, 45:389-403.

Williams SE, Wootton P, Mason HS, Bould J, Iles DE, Riccardi D, *et al*. 2004. Hemoxygenase-2 is an oxygen sensor for a calcium-sensitive potassium channel. *Science*, 306: 2093-2097.

Yuen PS, Doolittle LK, Garbers DL. 1994. Dominant negative mutants of nitric oxide-sensitive guanylyl cyclase. *J Biol Chem*, 269:791-793.

Part IV Inhibitory Transmission and Plasticity

Inhibitory Transmission

CHAPTER 13

Tian-Le Xu

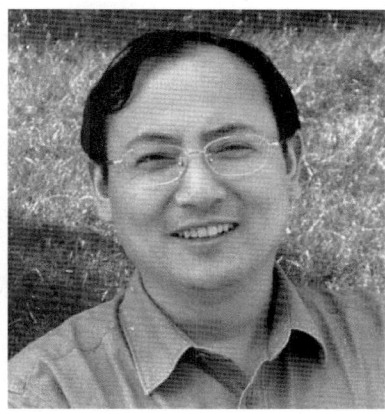

Dr. Xu is an Investigator and Chief in the Laboratory of Synaptic Physiology, Institute of Neuroscience, Chinese Academy of Sciences, Shanghai, China. He graduated from The Fourth Military Medical University and obtained a M.S. in Histology and embryology. He received a Ph.D. in Anatomy and Neurobiology from The Fourth Military Medical University.

MAJOR CONTRIBUTIONS

1. Lu H, Xu TL. 2002. The general anesthetic pentobarbital slows desensitization and deactivation of the glycine receptor in the spinal dorsal horn neurons. *J Biol Chem*, 277:41369-41378.

2. Li Y, Wu LJ, Legendre P, Xu TL. 2003. Asymmetric cross-inhibition between GABA$_A$ and glycine receptors in rat spinal dorsal horn neurons. *J Biol Chem*, 278:38637-38645.

3. Li YF, Wu LJ, Li Y, Xu TL. 2003. Mechanisms of H$^+$ modulation of glycinergic response in the rat sacral dorsal commissural neurons. *J Physiol (London)*, 552:73-87.

4. Wu LJ, Duan B, Mei YD, Gao J, Chen JG, Zhuo M, Xu L, Wu M, Xu TL. 2004. Characterization of acid-sensing ion channels in dorsal horn neurons of rat spinal cord. *J Biol Chem*, 279:43716-43724.

5. Gao J, Duan B, Wang DG, Deng XH, Zhang GY, Xu L, Xu TL. 2005. Coupling between NMDA receptor and acid-sensing ion channel contributes to ischemic neuronal death. *Neuron*, 48:635-646.

MAIN TOPICS

Inhibitory transmitters and transporters
Inhibitory receptors and their regulation
Co-release and cross-talk of GABA and glycine
The postsynaptic chloride homeostasis
Plasticity of the inhibitory transmission
Functions of the inhibitory transmission

SUMMARY

The operation of neuronal networks crucially depends on functions of the inhibitory transmission. This is accomplished largely by disinhibition of excitatory principal neurons whose activities are under dual tonic control of local-circuit interneurons and inhibitory projection neurons coming from neural command centers. According to this view, disinhibition is permissive, and excitatory input to principal neurons serves mainly a modulatory role. Thus, the inhibitory neurons control both the activity of principal neurons and their firing frequency by feedforward and feedback inhibition. Inhibitory inputs also control the timing of principal cell discharge and are thought to play a pivotal role in the generation of network oscillations. Finally, the yin-yang relationship between the excitatory and inhibitory transmissions is played out on the tightrope of a delicate balance, and imbalances between them lead to serious disorders.

INTRODUCTION

Synaptic transmission refers to the propagation of signals from one nerve cell to another. This occurs at a specialized cellular structure known as the synapse. Although electrical synapses exist in the nervous system, the most common type of synapse is the chemical synapse. The chemical synapse can be either excitatory or inhibitory in nature. Although most studies of synaptic transmission focus on excitatory synapses, inhibitory transmission by γ-aminobutyric acid (GABA) and glycine has become one of the most fascinating areas in neuroscience in recent years. In general, inhibitory transmission plays a fundamental role in controlling neuronal excitability and information processing, neuronal plasticity, and network synchronization in the central nervous system (CNS). The regulation of inhibitory transmission at molecular, cellular and systematic levels has yielded much information for investigation of disease states and for pharmacological and therapeutic intervention in inhibitory systems. In this Chapter, I will introduce the inhibitory transmission at several rapidly growing aspects.

INHIBITORY TRANSMITTERS AND TRANSPORTERS

GABA and glycine are the most important inhibitory neurotransmitters in the CNS. As a neurotransmitter, GABA is ubiquitous in the brain while glycine is mainly distributed in the brainstem and spinal cord. GABA was reported to be present in the vertebrate brain in 1950 and it was identified as a neurotransmitter in the early 1970s. GABA is present at high concentrations throughout the CNS. It has been estimated that 30%–40% of all CNS neurons utilize GABA as their primary neurotransmitter. This amino acid is synthesized from glutamate in a reaction catalyzed by glutamic acid decarboxylase (GAD) (Fig. 13.1A). Like most neurotransmitters, GABA is stored in synaptic vesicles and is released in a Ca^{2+}-dependent manner upon depolarization of the presynaptic membrane. Following release into the synaptic cleft,

GABA binds to and activates receptors on the postsynaptic membrane. GABA is cleared up by reuptake into presynaptic terminals and/or surrounding glial cells via highly specific transmembrane GABA transporters (GATs) (Fig.13.1A). This is the major mechanism for terminating the synaptic actions of GABA. Such transport requires extracellular Na^+ and Cl^- ions; two Na^+ and one Cl^- ion are transported for each GABA molecule. Four distinct genes encoding GATs, named GAT-1, GAT-2, GAT-3, and BGT-1 have been identified using molecular cloning. GATs contribute to

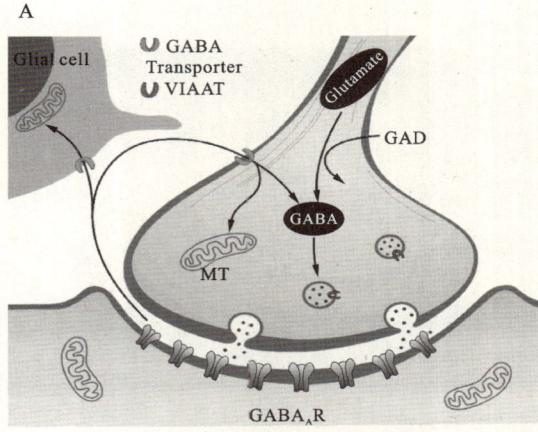

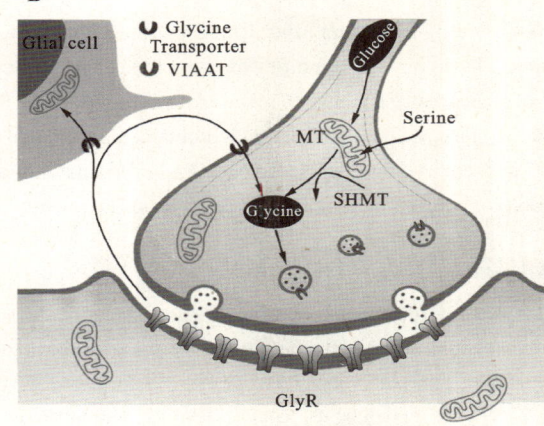

Fig.13.1 Synthesis, release, and reuptake of the inhibitory neurotransmitter GABA and glycine. A. GABA is synthesized from glutamate by GAD. B. Most of the glycine in the mammalian CNS is synthesized from glucose through serine in the mitochondria. High-affinity transporters terminate the actions of these transmitters. GABA$_A$R, GABA$_A$ receptor; GAD, the enzyme glutamic acid decarboxylase; GlyR, glycine receptor; MT, mitochondria; SHMT, the enzyme serine transhydroxymethylase; VIAAT, the vesicular inhibitory amino acid transporter.

modulate phasic (synaptic) and tonic (non-synaptic) GABA-mediated inhibition and GABA spillover. Consequently, altered GATs activity and/or expression are likely involved in the pathophysiology of at least two major human diseases: epilepsy and ischemia.

Glycine has been known to be an inhibitory neurotransmitter for about 40 years. Unlike GABA's ubiquitous distribution in the CNS, glycine is the major inhibitory neurotransmitter in the brainstem and spinal cord, where glycine is involved in the processing of motor and sensory information. Most of the glycine in the mammalian CNS is synthesized *de novo* from glucose through serine in the mitochondria, and this reaction is catalyzed by the enzyme serine transhydroxymethylase (SHMT), a pyridoxal phosphate-dependent enzyme (Fig.13.1B). Pyridoxal phosphate is a derivative of vitamin B_6. Just like GABA, glycine is released from nerve endings in a Ca^{2+}-dependent fashion. Glycine is then removed from the synaptic cleft by reuptake via Na^+/Cl^--dependent, high-affinity glycine transporters (GlyTs) (Fig.13.1B). Two GlyTs have been cloned so far: GlyT1 and GlyT2. GlyT1 is widely expressed in glial cells and is thought to control extracellular glycine concentration and regulate excitatory synapses via the glycine binding site on the NMDA receptors. GlyT2 is largely localized to the presynaptic terminals of glycinergic neurons in the brain stem and spinal cord, and is thought to provide the principal glycine uptake mechanism at glycinergic synapses. The unique expression patterns of GlyT1 and GlyT2 suggest they perform distinct functions. Indeed, studies on GlyT1 and GlyT2 knockout mice revealed different effects on glycinergic synaptic transmission. Moreover, the chronic effects of GlyT1 inhibitor sarcosine and GlyT2 inhibitor ALX-1393 on miniature inhibitory postsynaptic currents (mIPSCs) were studied in cultured spinal neurons. We found that sarcosine increased the frequency of overall mIPSCs without affecting the ratio of glycinergic, mixed and GABAergic mIPSCs, whereas ALX-1393 changed the ratio by increasing the proportions of GABAergic and mixed mIPSCs without affecting

overall mIPSC frequency. We propose that inhibition of GlyT1 by sarcosine increased overall mIPSC frequency via the activation of presynaptic glycine receptors (GlyRs), while inhibition of GlyT2 by ALX-1393 changed the ratio of glycinergic, mixed and GABAergic mIPSCs by shifting the balance of inhibitory transmitters in vesicles towards GABA.

In addition to the inhibitory action, glycine produces excitatory effects, by serving as an essential co-agonist of glutamate at the NMDA subtype glutamate receptors. The origin of glycine bound to NMDA receptors has not been fully elucidated, but either transmitter overspilling from adjacent glycinergic synapses or non-vesicular glycine release from adjacent glial cells has been suggested to play a role in glycine site saturation of NMDA receptors.

INHIBITORY RECEPTORS AND THEIR REGULATION

As mentioned above, GABA is the most abundant inhibitory neurotransmitter in the CNS. GABA activates three major classes of receptors, termed $GABA_A$, $GABA_B$ and $GABA_C$ receptors, and of which the $GABA_A$ and $GABA_C$ are ionotropic, while the $GABA_B$ are metabotropic receptors.

The $GABA_A$ and $GABA_C$ receptors are both ligand-gated Cl^- ion channels which are composed of five subunits, and each subunit has four transmembrane (TM) domains (Fig.13.2A). Activation of $GABA_A$ and $GABA_C$ receptors causes influx of Cl^- ion and hyperpolarization of the post-synaptic membrane and thus, inhibition of neuronal excitability. So far, a total of 6α, 4β, 3γ, one δ, one ε, one π subunits of $GABA_A$ receptors ($GABA_A$Rs) and 3ρ subunits of $GABA_C$ receptors have been cloned and sequenced from the mammalian nervous system. Recently, evidence was presented for the existence of an additional θ subunit. Furthermore, additional structural complexity exists due to alternative splicing of subunits. Despite this multitude of subunits, certain combinations are preferred. The subunit compositions and ratios of $GABA_A$Rs are shown in Fig.13.2B. It seems

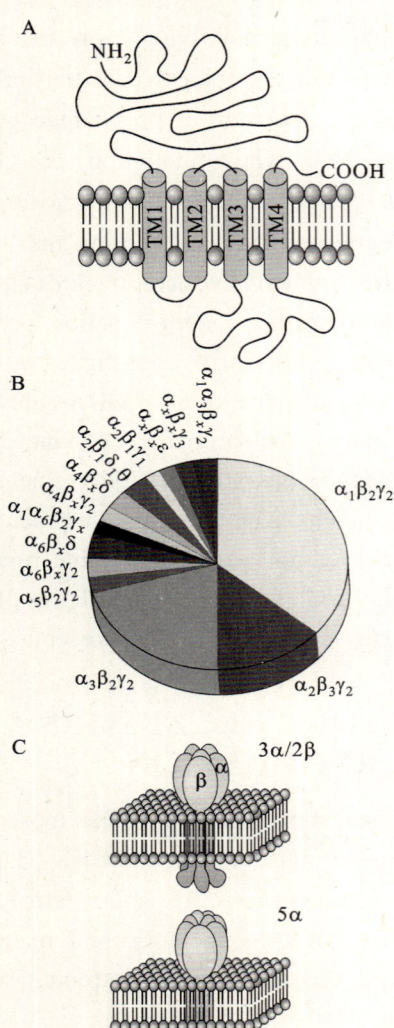

Fig.13.2 Structure and subunit compositions of GABA$_A$Rs and GlyRs. A. GABA$_A$R and GlyR subunit has the similar membrane topology with four transmembrane domains. B. A pie chart representing the approximate abundance of GABA$_A$Rs in the rat brain. Subscript *x* indicates the type of α, β or γ subunit that is currently not clear. C. Arrangement of α and β GlyR subunits in the heteromeric (top) and homomeric receptors (bottom). The stoichiometry is 3α:2β and 5α, respectively (Figures A and C were modified from Legendre, 2001).

that most functional GABA$_A$Rs in the CNS contain at least α- and β-subunits, plus a γ- or δ- subunit. In contrast to the large diversity of GABA$_A$Rs, GABA$_C$ receptors are mainly homo-oligomeric, made up of either ρ1 or ρ2 subunits. The ρ subunits do not assemble with α and β subunits to form a receptor. Thus, the composition of GABA$_C$ receptors is different to GABA$_A$Rs. Accordingly, GABA$_A$ and GABA$_C$ receptors are biochemically and pharmacologically dif-

ferent. GABA is an order of magnitude less potent at GABA$_A$ than GABA$_C$ receptors. GABA$_A$Rs are selectively blocked by the alkaloid bicuculline and are modulated by benzodiazepines, steroids, barbiturates, and divalent ion Zn^{2+}. More importantly, the stability and activity of GABA$_A$Rs at synapses are dynamically regulated through interacting with a range of diverse proteins, including cytoskeletal elements, microtubule-binding proteins, protein kinases, kinase-anchoring proteins and other signaling molecules. Identification of the signaling pathways that regulate the GABA$_A$Rs exo-and endocytosis will determine the relevance of this process for synaptic inhibition. GABA$_A$Rs are also phosphorylated by several protein kinases, including PKC, PKA, Ca^{2+}/calmodulin dependent protein kinase II (CaMKII) and tyrosine kinases. The importance of this modulation for synaptic inhibition will be best assessed in animals where the phosphorylation of individual receptor subunits is ablated by mutation.

GABA$_C$ receptors are not blocked by bicuculline, and benzodiazepines, steroids or barbiturates do not modulate them either. Instead, GABA$_C$ receptors are activated by Z-4-aminobut-2-enoic acid (*cis*-aminocrotonic acid, CACA) and CAMP (*cis*-2-(aminomethyl)cyclopropanecarboxylic acid) and they are selectively blocked by TPMPA ((1, 2, 5, 6-tetrahydropyridin-4-yl) methylphosphinic acid). GABA$_C$ receptors are found in many CNS locations, including the retina, cerebellum, hippocampus, optic tectum, and spinal cord. However, because very little is known about the functions of these receptors, and because no specific chemical modulators for the GABA$_C$ receptors are available, it is not discussed further in this Chapter.

GABA$_B$ receptors are seven transmembrane receptors that activate the second messenger systems phospholipase C and adenylate cyclase and regulate K^+ and Ca^{2+} ion channels via G proteins. These receptors are selectively activated by (R)-(−)-baclofen and the phosphinic acid analogue of GABA, CGP27492 ((3-aminopropyl) phosphinic acid). The phosphonic and sulphonic acid analogues of (R)-(−)-baclofen, phaclofen and saclofen antagonize these receptors selectively. To date, three subunits have been cloned and are termed as $GABA_BR_{1a}$, $GABA_BR_{1b}$ and $GABA_BR_2$. $GABA_B$ receptors are hetero-oligomeric receptors, made up of a $GABA_BR_{1a}$ or $GABA_BR_{1b}$ subunit and a $GABA_BR_2$ subunit.

$GABA_B$ receptors are expressed on both presynaptic and postsynaptic membrane. Compared with $GABA_ARs$, postsynaptic $GABA_B$ receptors produce a slower but longer-lasting form of inhibition, an effect largely ascribed to the opening of inwardly rectifying K^+ channels. In addition, inhibitory postsynaptic potentials (IPSPs) mediated by $GABA_B$ receptors require much stronger stimulation or stimuli of longer duration and higher frequency. These findings have led to the conclusion that the synaptic location of these receptor subtypes may differ. $GABA_ARs$ are believed to localize properly at the synapse, respond directly to the GABA release of a single quantum of neurotransmitter. In contrast, $GABA_B$ receptors may be extrasynaptic, sensing the overspilled GABA after high-intensity or prolonged, high frequency stimuli. On the presynaptic side, $GABA_B$ receptors function as autoreceptors or heteroreceptors located on GABAergic or glutamatergic terminals to regulate GABA and glutamate release, respectively.

GlyRs are also ligand-gated Cl^- ion channels and contain five subunits. Each subunit has four α-helical transmembrane domains (TM1-TM4). To date, four α-subunits (α1 to α4) and one β-subunit have been identified, and of which α- and β-subunit can form heteromeric and homomeric functional receptors with the stoichiometry of 3α:2β and 5α, respectively (Fig. 13.2C). Moreover, GlyR subunit composition experiences developmental changes. By around postnatal day 20 in rat, for example, GlyR subunit composition was completely switched from α2-homomers to α1β-heteromers. GlyR β-subunit distributes widely throughout the embryonic and adult CNS and is responsible for anchoring GlyRs to the subsynaptic cytoskeleton via cytoplasmic protein gephyrin. The broad expression profile is somewhat puzzling given that β-subunit does not form functional receptor in the absence of α-subunit.

Similar to the $GABA_ARs$, a number of exogenous and endogenous substances are found to have modulatory effects on GlyRs. These include the well-known GlyR antagonist strychnine, divalent Zn^{2+}, and intracellular protein kinases such as PKA, PKC and CaMKII. Accumulating evidence indicates that such protein kinase-dependent regulation of the GlyR has important functional consequences. For example, we have shown that CaMKII mediates the coupling between Ca^{2+} entry via AMPA and NMDA receptors to the functional enhancement of GlyRs. Moreover, our *in vitro* studies demonstrate that two endogenous antinociceptive neurotransmitters, 5-HT and noradrenalin, enhance the GlyR response through alterations of the intracellular PKC and PKA activities, respectively. More recently, prostaglandins E_2 (PGE_2), an important mediator of pain and inflammation, was found to reduce inhibitory glycinergic synaptic transmission at low nanomolar concentrations, whereas $GABA_A$, AMPA and NMDA receptor-mediated transmission remained unaffected. Inhibition of GlyRs occurred via a postsynaptic mechanism involving the activation of EP_2 receptors, cholera-toxin-sensitive G-proteins and PKA. Via this mechanism, PGE_2 may facilitate the transmission of nociceptive input through the spinal dorsal horn to higher brain areas where pain becomes conscious. Furthermore, the selective effect of PGE_2 on glycinergic transmission was mediated by a specific GlyR subtype, GlyR α3 (Fig.13.3). In addition, the amplitude of glycineinduced Cl^- currents (I_{Gly}) was enhanced after intracellular application of G-protein βγ dimer or after activation of a G protein-coupled receptor. However, the $GABA_AR$-mediated currents recorded in the same cells were unaffected by G-protein activation. These differential regulation profiles between GlyRs and $GABA_ARs$ suggest that both receptors have distinct functional roles.

Volatile anaesthetics and alcohol clearly affect GlyRs by allosteric mechanisms, but the kinetics of the interactions is still poorly understood, and there may be multiple allosteric binding sites. We reported the first evidence that pentobarbital slows the desensi-

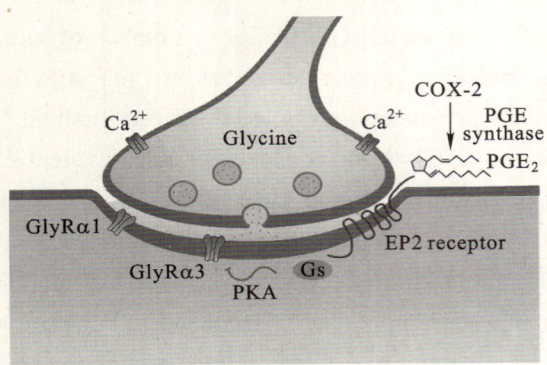

Fig.13.3 Modulation of PGE$_2$ on GlyRs. PGE$_2$ acts on post-synaptic EP2 receptors and activates intracellular PKA via G-protein Gs, resulting in PKA-dependent phosphorylation and inhibition of the GlyR α3 subunit (Motified from Zeilhofer, 2005).

tization and deactivation of the GlyRs in the rat spinal dorsal horn neurons (Fig.13.4A), and hypothesized that GlyRs and glycinergic neurotransmission may

play an important role in the modulation of general anesthesia in the mammalian spinal cord. In addition, we have investigated the effects of changes in extracellular pH on glycinergic miniature inhibitory postsynaptic currents (mIPSCs) as well as I_{Gly} in mechanically dissociated spinal dorsal horn neurons with native synaptic boutons preserved. Our results support a "conformational coupling" model for H$^+$ modulation of the GlyRs (Fig.13.4B) and suggest that H$^+$ may act as a novel modulator for inhibitory neurotransmission in the mammalian spinal cord. Local decrease in pH under such pathophysiological conditions as inflammation and ischemia could elicit pain, although the precise mechanism is not clear. Thus it would be very interesting to know whether the H$^+$ inhibition of glycinergic transmission may contribute to the pain that occurs in inflammatory and/or ischemic conditions.

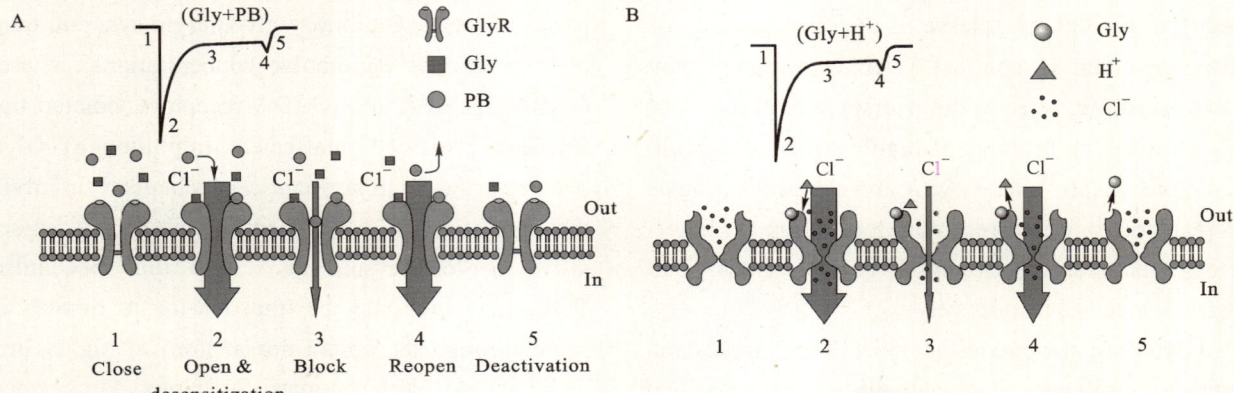

Fig.13.4 Schematic diagram illustrating the possible mechanisms by which the general anesthetic pentobarbital (PB) and H$^+$ modulate the GlyRs. A. 1, the GlyR channel closes before binding the ligand; 2, the binding of glycine (Gly) and PB leading to the channel opening allows a large amount of Cl$^-$ to flux intracelluarly. Subsequently, GlyR desensitizes, resulting in the decrease of Cl$^-$ flux. 3, a PB molecule blocks the opening channel, which accelerates the macroscopic desensitization of I_{Gly}. 4, the PB molecule is removed, and the channel reopens which increases the Cl$^-$ flux. 5, the agonist, Gly, and the modulator, PB, are removed, resulting in the closure of GlyR channel and the deactivation of I_{Gly}. B. H$^+$ competitively binds to the GlyRs (2), inducing a global conformational change of the GlyRs, and closing the pore domain (3). After washout, the remaining glycine activates the channel again and induces a rebound current because the unbinding rate of H$^+$ is faster than that of Gly (4) (Figure A was modified from Lu and Xu, 2002; Figure B was modified from Li *et al.*, 2003).

CO-RELEASE AND CROSS-TALK OF GABA AND GLYCINE

GABA and glycine are two distinct inhibitory neurotransmitters and they act at separate receptors. At the level of spinal cord and brain stem, the content of GABA and glycine of presynaptic terminals is developmentally changeable. For example, there is a de-

velopmental shift from GABAergic to glycinergic synapses in the spinal cord and auditory brain stem neurons accompanying with the postnatal maturation of the CNS. Interestingly, a reverse synapse transition from glycinergic to GABAergic was observed in the spinal dorsal neurons after periphery nerve injury.

Using dissociated rat spinal dorsal horn neurons with attached presynaptic terminal boutons, we have characterized the co-release of GABA and glycine. Our study supports the idea that GABA- and glycine-mediated cotransmissions might be a general principle of inhibition, especially in the mammalian spinal cord. Due to the difference between the decay time course of GABAergic and glycinergic mIPSCs, the co-release of GABA and glycine would finely tune their inhibitory effect *in vivo*. The findings raise many outstanding questions. How do the effects of the two transmitters summate? What are the pre- and postsynaptic mechanisms that determine the relative proportion and the variability of GABA *vs* glycine component of synaptic transmission? What is the physiological significance of co-transmission? So answers to these questions will be important.

A complex interaction between GlyRs and GABA$_A$Rs was reported. Cross-inhibition between GlyRs and GABA$_A$Rs was found in dissociated CA1 pyramidal neurons, whilst cross-sensitization was observed with carp third-order neurons. Recently, we have explored the mechanisms of the functional cross-talk between GlyRs and GABA$_A$Rs by analyzing cross-inhibition between I_{Gly} and GABA-induced Cl$^-$ currents (I_{GABA}) in spinal cord neurons, using whole-cell patch-clamp recording. Our results showed that cross-inhibition is asymmetric between GABA$_A$Rs and GlyRs and that glycine-induced inhibition of GABA$_A$ responses depends largely on phosphatase 2B activity and subsequent protein dephosphorylation processes. This process may be important for regulating inhibitory synaptic strength when neurons receive both GABAergic and glycinergic transmitters. Indeed, the GABAergic component of inhibitory neurotransmission at mixed synapses may be upregulated in individuals suffering from heritable disorders of glycinergic neurotransmission. Thus the cross-inhibition between GABA$_A$Rs and GlyRs could break excessive inhibition, reflecting the activity balance and plasticity of the neurons when receiving fast inhibitory co-transmissions. Interestingly, activity-dependent physical and functional interaction between phosphatase 2B and GABA$_A$Rs is necessary and sufficient for inducing LTD at hippocampal CA1 inhibitory synapses. Although co-release of GABA and glycine has not yet been detected in the hippocampus, a functional cross-inhibition has been shown for hippocampal GABA$_A$Rs and GlyRs. Whether or not the phosphatase 2B-dependent cross-inhibition between GABA$_A$Rs and GlyRs could regulate the synaptic transmission and plasticity remains to be established.

Recently, a functional cross-inhibition has also been shown for cortical GABA$_A$Rs and GlyRs. However, contrary to the bi-directional cross-inhibition observed in CA1 pyramidal cells and the asymmetric cross-inhibition of I_{GABA} by glycine in spinal neurons, a cross-inhibition of I_{Gly} by GABA was detected in cortical neurons but not vise versa. This suggests a tissue-specific feature of the cross-talk machinery between GABA$_A$Rs and GlyRs.

THE POSTSYNAPTIC CHLORIDE HOMEOSTASIS

Both GABA$_A$Rs and GlyRs are predominantly Cl$^-$-permeant, therefore postsynaptic Cl$^-$ electrochemical gradient between intra- and extracellular spaces play a crucial role in shaping GABA- and glycine-mediated signaling. The cation-chloride co-transporters (CCCs) have been identified as important regulators of neuronal Cl$^-$ homeostasis. The CCC gene family consists of three broad groups: Na$^+$-Cl$^-$ co-transporters (NCCs), Na$^+$-K$^+$-2Cl$^-$ co-transporters (NKCCs) and K$^+$-Cl$^-$ co-transporters (KCCs). Other secondarily active transport proteins can also participate in overall neuronal Cl$^-$ homeostasis, including Na$^+$-dependent and Na$^+$-independent anion exchangers (NDAEs and AEs, respectively), which exchange Cl$^-$ for HCO$_3^-$ (Fig.13.5).

It has been demonstrated that neuronal specific transporter KCC2 and NKCC1 are the major Cl$^-$ extrusion and intrusion mechanisms, respectively. Furthermore, NKCC1 and KCC2 are developmentally regulated in the CNS. Neuronal expression of NKCC1 is high at birth which determines high initial levels of intracellular Cl$^-$ in immature neurons, and decreases during postnatal development. Opposite to NKCC1,

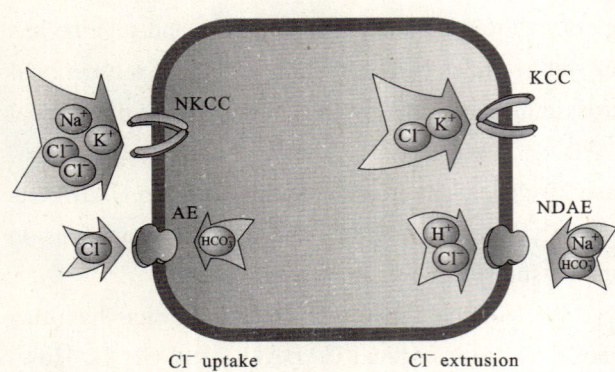

Fig.13.5 Cl⁻ transporters and their basic modes of operation. Under physiological conditions, Cl⁻ uptake is mediated by Na⁺–K⁺–2Cl⁻ co-transporters (NKCCs) and Na⁺-independent anion exchangers (AEs), whereas K⁺–Cl⁻ co-transporters (KCCs) and Na⁺-dependent anion exchangers (NDAEs) extrude Cl⁻ (Modified from Payne et al., 2003).

neuronal Cl⁻ co-transporter KCC2 expresses mini-

mally at birth and increases significantly during postnatal development. Owing to the asynchronous development of KCC2 and NKCC1, GABA and glycine-mediated responses undergo a switch from being excitatory to inhibitory during development of the CNS (Fig.13.6). In early postnatal CNS neurons, GABA and glycine evoke membrane depolarization mediated by the efflux of Cl⁻, resulting from a high intracellular Cl⁻ concentration ($[Cl^-]_i$). This depolarization activates voltage-dependent Ca^{2+} channels (VDCCs) and NMDA receptors and hence elevates intracellular Ca^{2+}. Such elevation of intracellular Ca^{2+} is likely to play a critical role in neuronal development. With neuronal maturation, in turn, $[Cl^-]_i$ becomes lower, which results in the conventional hyperpolarization actions of GABA and glycine.

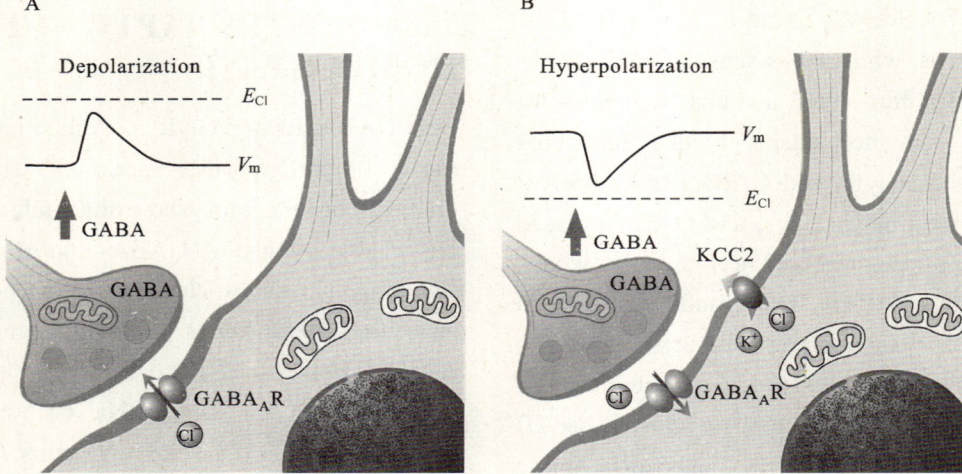

Fig.13.6 Chloride homeostasis and signaling by the inhibitory neurotransmitter GABA. A. Levels of intracellular Cl⁻ are high, and the equilibrium potential for Cl⁻, E_{Cl}, is positive relative to resting membrane potential, V_m. Opening of Cl⁻ channels by activation of the GABA$_A$R depolarizes the cell. B. Expression of the KCC2 transporter maintains a low level of intracellular Cl⁻. E_{Cl} is negative relative to V_m and activation of the GABA$_A$R hyperpolarizes the cell.

Interestingly, short- and long-term shift from hyperpolarizing to depolarizing (sometimes even excitatory) GABA$_A$-mediated responses have been observed under various experimental conditions, including tetanic stimulation, neuronal trauma, axotomy, and kindling-induced or spontaneous seizures. Thus the depolarizing or excitatory actions of GABA have been implicated in the pathogenesis of epilepsy, stroke, neuropathic pain, and cocaine addiction. Therefore, it will be important to understand: (i) regulatory

mechanisms controlling chloride homeostasis in neurons; (ii) physiological roles of the depolarizing or excitatory actions of GABA and glycine on synaptic plasticity and neural development; (iii) how dysfunction of chloride homeostasis may contribute to such neurological diseases as epilepsy, depression, neuronal injury, cerebral ischemia and Alzheimer's disease, and how these neuronal disorders can be prevented by GABAergic and glycinergic drugs.

PLASTICITY OF THE INHIBITORY TRANSMISSION

The mechanisms leading to long-term changes in synaptic strength have been extensively studied at excitatory glutamatergic synapses in the CNS. However, activity-dependent modulations of inhibitory synapses would also have important consequences in brain development and physiological functions. In the past decades, long-term changes of inhibitory synapses have been reported in several regions of the brain, including the hippocampus, cortex, cerebellum, deep cerebellar nucleus, lateral superior olive and brain stem. According to the direction in the strength change of synaptic efficacy, they are classified as potentiation and depression. Although the specific mechanisms vary among different conditions, on the whole, they are ascribed to the changes of presynaptic transmitters, postsynaptic receptors or chloride homeostasis.

With regard to transmitter release, retrograde signaling provides an efficient feedback mechanism that enables postsynaptic neurons to control their presynaptic inputs. For example, repetitive depolarization of cerebellar Purkinje or hippocampal CA1 neurons increases postsynaptic Ca^{2+}, initiating the retrograde release of endocannabinoids. These compounds then activate presynaptic CB1 receptors, suppressing the release of GABA and hence decreasing GABAergic transmission. In another case, at the interneuron-Purkinje cell (IN-PC) synapse, physiological stimuli results in postsynaptic Ca^{2+} increase and subsequent retrograde release of glutamate that diffuses to presynaptic NMDA receptors. Activation of these receptors and subsequent release of Ca^{2+} from ryanodine-sensitive presynaptic stores are then sufficient to facilitate GABA release and thus enhance GABAergic transmission.

At functional synapses, where there is a high opening probability of postsynaptic receptors, changes in synaptic efficacy can also be effectively achieved by modifying the sensitivity or the number of postsynaptic receptors. In cerebellar Purkinje cells, stimulation of the excitatory climbing fibre synapses is followed by a long-lasting (up to 75 min) potentiation of GABA$_A$R-mediated IPSCs. Besides, the response of Purkinje cells to bath-applied exogenous GABA is also enhanced after climbing fibre-stimulation with a time course similar to that of the potentiation of IPSCs. Based on these findings, it is proposed that the potentiation is caused by an upregulation of postsynaptic GABA$_A$Rs function. By using whole-cell patch-clamp recordings and nonstationary fluctuation analysis of synaptic currents, Otis *et al.* demonstrated that an increase in functional receptor number in kindled granule cells underlies an augmented GABA$_A$Rs-mediated inhibition in dentate gyrus granule cells. Similarly, combining quantal analysis of evoked IPSCs with quantitative immunogold localization, Nusser *et al.* demonstrated that the postsynaptic insertion of new GABA$_A$Rs underlies potentiation at hippocampal inhibitory synapses induced by kindling.

As noted above, chloride homeostatic mechanisms appear to play a critical role in regulating inhibitory synaptic strength. Due to the developmental changes in Cl^- co-transporters, GABAergic transmission in hippocampal neurons and glycinergic transmission in lateral superior olive neurons experienced maturational transformation from excitatory to inhibitory. Deafferentation is also reported to lead to rapid disruption of chloride homeostasis and hence to decrease inhibitory synaptic efficacy in auditory midbrain. Besides, Woodin *et al.* recently reported that in both hippocampal cultures and acute hippocampal slices, coincident pre- and postsynaptic activation led to a persistent change in synaptic strength due to a local decrease in KCC2 activity.

FUNCTIONS OF THE INHIBITORY TRANSMISSION

During early development, GABA and glycine exert important roles in the maturation of the nervous system through their excitatory effects. But here we focus on their inhibitory roles because GABA and glycine act as the main inhibitory neurotransmitters in the adult CNS.

On one hand, GABA$_A$R/GlyR-mediated inhibition has been considered the province of fast synaptic (phasic) neurotransmission. Phasic inhibition is considered to be synaptic or perisynaptic inhibition (Fig. 13.7A and B). Specific proteins, such as gephyrin, anchor synaptic GlyRs/GABA$_A$Rs. Synaptic receptors usually have specific subunit composition. Synaptic GABA$_A$Rs usually contain γ subunits, in particular γ2, while synaptic GlyRs contain β subunits. Generally, synaptic transmission is produced by high concentration of GABA or glycine that is short-lived in the synaptic cleft. The activation of synaptic GABA$_A$Rs/GlyRs produces an IPSC or IPSP. In the adult CNS, preventing overexcitation of neurons is the basic function of inhibitory system. Besides, GABAergic and glycinergic transmission-mediated phasic inhibition has more important roles, which depend crucially on synapse location and IPSC timing. Thus, GABA- and glycine-releasing interneurons play a key role in the operation of neuronal networks. They control both the number of active pyramidal cells and their firing frequency by feedforward and feedback inhibition, which is important for signal integration and output. Interneurons also control the timing of principal cell discharge and are thought to play a pivotal role in the generation of network oscillations and rhythmic activity.

On the other hand, some types of GABA$_A$Rs/GlyRs also participate in a distinct form of "tonic" inhibition produced by the continuous activation of extrasynaptic GABA$_A$Rs/GlyRs (Fig.13.7C). The tonic activation of these receptors is the result of such paracrine activity. Tonic GABA$_A$R-mediated currents were first observed in cerebellar granule cells during voltage-clamped recordings. Application of GABA$_A$R antagonists, bicuculline and SR-95531 (gabazine), could decrease the "holding" current that was required to clamp the cells at a given membrane potential, suggesting a reduction of input conductance. Subsequent studies suggest tonic inhibition exists in many other regions, such as hippocampus and cortex. Tonic

GABA$_A$Rs are localized extrasynaptically and have unusual high GABA affinity. Tonic receptors also have specific subunit composition. The tonic current in cerebellar granule cells is mediated by GABA$_A$R containing δ and α6 subunits. In dentate granule cells, the tonic current only partially depends on

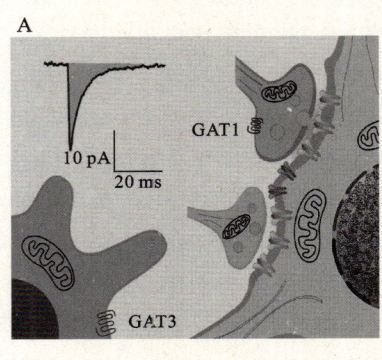

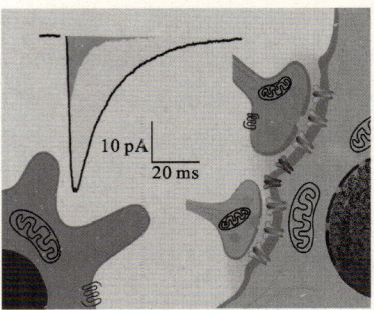

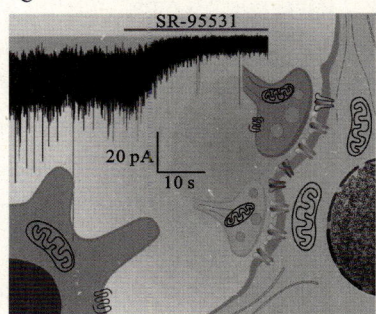

Fig.13.7 Modes of GABA$_A$R activation. A. The release of a single vesicle from a presynaptic terminal activates only those postsynaptic GABA$_A$Rs that are clustered in the membrane immediately beneath the release site. GAT, GABA transporter. B. Action potential-dependent release of multiple vesicles or evoked release from several terminals promotes GABA "spill-over", and activates both synaptic receptors and perisynaptic or extrasynaptic receptors. C. A low concentration of ambient GABA, which persists despite the activity of the neuronal and glial GABA transporters (GAT1 and GAT3), tonically activates high-affinity extrasynaptic receptors (Modified from Farrant and Nusser, 2005).

GABA$_A$R containing the δ subunit. In hippocampus, at least part of the tonic current is mediated by γ-subunit-containing receptors. The tonic GlyRs might contain α2 subunit. The charge carried by the activation of tonically active GABA$_A$Rs can be more than three times larger than that produced by phasic inhibition, even when the frequency of phasic events is large. Experimental and theoretical studies indicate that a tonic GABA conductance produces a shunt that affects excitability and gain control. Tonic activation of GABA$_A$R has one straightforward outcome: a persistent increase in the cell's input conductance. So, for a given excitatory input, the size and duration of the excitatory postsynaptic potential (EPSP) will be reduced and the temporal and spatial window over which signal integration can occur will be narrowed, making it less likely that an action potential will be generated. An increase in the slope of the input–output relationship could be observed after the blockade of the tonic conductance.

CONCLUSION

In summary, recent years have witnessed a dramatic accumulation of our knowledge about the inhibitory transmission, their pre- and postsynaptic components, chemical markers, synaptic signaling, receptor dynamics, Cl$^-$ homeostasis, short- and long-term plasticity, and physiological functions. On the other hand, when inhibitory-excitatory relations are unbalanced by excitatory overactivity, diseases may occur. Thus, a reduction in inhibition, such as might result from decreases in numbers of inhibitory neurons or decreased availability of inhibitory transmitters, loss of inhibitory synapses, and alterations in inhibitory receptors or transporters, can lead to hyperexcitability in neuronal networks and/or enhanced synchrony of neuronal firing, and may be one underlying mechanism in a variety of neurological diseases. Overbalancing in favor of the inhibitory transmission can lead to maladaptive decrement in neural activity and even coma. The roles of inhibition and disinhibition in information processing in various regions of the CNS are so complex that it appears doubtful that many useful drug therapies will come from approaches that are aimed at affecting one or another aspect of the inhibitory transmission. Currently, there are no drugs that are process and site specific. In this regard, the detailed cellular and molecular characterization that is being carried out of the inhibitory transmitters and transporters, inhibitory receptors and postsynaptic Cl$^-$ homeostasis should give rise to many opportunities for devising specific therapeutic modalities.

GENERAL CITATIONS

Barnard EA, Skolnick P, Olsen RW, Mohler H, Sieghart W, Biggio G, Braestrup C, Bateson AN, Langer S Z. 1998., International Union of Pharmacology. XV. Subtypes of gamma-aminobutyric acidA receptors: classification on the basis of subunit structure and receptor function. *Pharmacol Rev*, 50: 291-313.

Cryan JF, Kaupmann K. 2005. Don't worry 'B' happy!: a role for GABA(B) receptors in anxiety and depression. *Trends Pharmacol Sci*, 26: 36-43.

Farrant M, Nusser Z. 2005. Variations on an inhibitory theme: phasic and tonic activation of GABA(A) receptors. *Nat Rev Neurosci*, 6: 215-229.

Gaiarsa JL, Caillard O, Ben-Ari Y. 2002. Long-term plasticity at GABAergic and glycinergic synapses: mechanisms and functional significance. *Trends Neurosci*, 25: 564-570.

Legendre P. 2001. The glycinergic inhibitory synapse. *Cell Mol Life Sci*, 58: 760-793.

Lynch JW. 2004. Molecular structure and function of the glycine receptor chloride channel. *Physiol Rev*, 84: 1051-1095.

Martin DL, Olsen R W. 2000.*GABA in the Nervous System: The View at Fifty Years*. Lippincott, Williams & Wilkins, Philadelphia.

Macdonald RL, Olsen RW. 1994. GABA$_A$ receptor channels. *Annu Rev Neurosci*, 17: 569-602.

Mody I, Pearce RA. 2004. Diversity of inhibitory neurotransmission through GABA(A) receptors. *Trends Neurosci*, 27: 569-575.

Payne JA, Rivera C, Voipio J, Kaila K. 2003. Cation-chloride co-transporters in neuronal communication, development and trauma. *Trends Neurosci*, 26: 199-206.

Semyanov A, Walker MC, Kullmann DM, Silver R A. 2004. Tonically active GABA$_A$ receptors: modulating gain and maintaining the tone. *Trends Neurosci*, 27: 262-269.

Whittington MA, Traub RD. 2003. Interneuron diversity series: inhibitory interneurons and network oscillations *in vitro*. *Trends Neurosci*, 26: 676-682.

DISCOVERY CITATIONS

Ben-Ari Y. 2002. Excitatory actions of GABA during development: the nature of the nurture. *Nat Rev Neurosci*, 3: 728-739.

Coull JA, Boudreau D, Bachand K, Prescott SA, Nault F, Sik A, De Koninck P, De Koninck Y. 2003. Trans-synaptic shift in anion gradient in spinal lamina I neurons as a mechanism of neuropathic pain. *Nature*, 424: 938-942.

Duguid IC, Smart TG. 2004. Retrograde activation of presynaptic NMDA receptors enhances GABA release at cerebellar interneuron-Purkinje cell synapses. *Nat Neurosci*, 7: 525-533.

Ganguly K, Schinder AF, Wong ST, Poo M. 2001. GABA itself promotes the developmental switch of neuronal GABAergic responses from excitation to inhibition. *Cell*, 105: 521-532.

Jonas P. Bischofberger J, Sandkuhler J. 1998. Corelease of two fast neurotransmitters at a central synapse. *Science*, 281: 419-424.

Kano M, Rexhausen U, Dreessen J, Konnerth A. 1992. Synaptic excitation produces a long-lasting rebound potentiation of inhibitory synaptic signals in cerebellar Purkinje cells. *Nature*, 356: 601-604.

Li Y, Wu LJ, Legendre P, Xu TL. 2003. Asymmetric cross-inhibition between GABA$_A$ and glycine receptors in rat spinal dorsal horn neurons. *J Biol Chem*, 278: 38637-38645.

Li YF, Wu LJ, LiY, Xu L, Xu TL. 2003. Mechanisms of H$^+$ modulation of glycinergic response in rat sacral dorsal commissural neurons. *J Physiol*, 552: 73-87.

Lu H, Xu TL. 2002. The general anesthetic pentobarbital slows desensitization and deactivation of the glycine receptor in the rat spinal dorsal horn neurons. *J Biol Chem*, 277: 41369-41378.

Meyer G, Kirsch J, Betz H, Langosch D. 1995. Identification of a gephyrin binding motif on the glycine receptor beta subunit. *Neuron*, 15: 563-572.

Nabekura J, Xu TL, Rhee JS, Li JS, Akaike N. 1999. Alpha2-adrenoceptor-mediated enhancement of glycine response in rat sacral dorsal commissural neurons. *Neuro-science*, 89: 29-41.

Nusser Z, Hajos N, Somogyi P, Mody I. 1998. Increased number of synaptic GABA(A) receptors underlies potentiation at hippocampal inhibitory synapses. *Nature*. 395: 172-177.

Ohno-Shosaku T, Maejima T, Kano M. 2001. Endogenous cannabinoids mediate retrograde signals from depolarized postsynaptic neurons to presynaptic terminals. *Neuron*, 29: 729-738.

Otis TS, de Koninck Y, Mody I. 1994. Lasting potentiation of inhibition is associated with an increased number of gamma-aminobutyric acid type A receptors activated during miniature inhibitory postsynaptic currents. *Proc Natl Acad Sci USA*, 91: 7698-7702.

Rivera C, Voipio J, Payne JA, Ruusuvuori E, Lahtinen H, Lamsa K, Pirvola U, Saarma M, Kaila K. 1999. The K$^+$/Cl$^-$ co-transporter KCC2 renders GABA hyperpolarizing during neuronal maturation. *Nature*, 397: 251-255.

Roberts E, Frankel S. 1950. gamma-Aminobutyric acid in brain: its formation from glutamic acid. *J Biol Chem*, 187: 55-63.

Vale C, Schoorlemmer J, Sanes DH. 2003. Deafness disrupts chloride transporter function and inhibitory synaptic transmission. *J Neurosci*, 23: 7516-7524.

Woodin MA, Ganguly K, Poo MM. 2003. Coincident pre-and postsynaptic activity modifies GABAergic synapses by postsynaptic changes in Cl$^-$ transporter activity. *Neuron*, 39: 807-820.

Wu LJ, Li Y, Xu TL. 2002. Co-release and interaction of two inhibitory co-transmitters in rat sacral dorsal commissural neurons. *Neuroreport*, 13: 977-981.

Xu TL, Dong XP, Wang DS. 2000. *N*-methyl- D-aspartate enhancement of the glycine response in the rat sacral dorsal commissural neurons. *Eur J Neurosci*, 12: 1647-1653.

Xu TL, Li JS, Jin YH, Akaike N. 1999. Modulation of the glycine response by Ca^{2+}-permeable AMPA receptors in rat spinal neurones. *J Physiol*, 514 (Pt 3): 701-711.

Xu TL, Nabekura J, Akaike N. 1996. Protein kinase C-mediated enhancement of glycine response in rat sacral dorsal commissural neurones by serotonin. *J Physiol*, 496 (Pt 2): 491-501.

Xu TX, Gong N, Xu TL. 2005. Inhibitors of GlyT1 and GlyT2 differentially modulate inhibitory transmission. *Neuroreport*, 16: 1227-1231.

Zeilhofer HU. 2005. Synaptic modulation in pain pathways. *Rev Physiol Biochem Pharmacol*, 154: 73-100.

Plasticity of Inhibition; GABA/glycine Systems

CHAPTER 14

Yves De Koninck

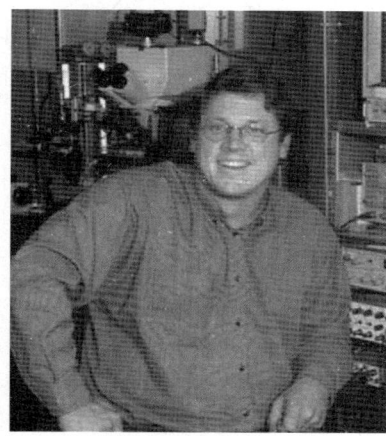

Dr. Koninck is Professor and Director, in the Division of Cellular Neurobiology, Centre de recherche Universite Laval Robert-Giffard, Quebec, Canada. He graduated from the Laval Univeristy and obtained a Ph.D. in Physiology from McGill University. He pursued postdoctoral training at Stanford University and the University of Texas Southwestern Medical Center.

MAJOR CONTRIBUTIONS

1. Chéry N, de Koninck Y. 1999. Junctional *vs.* extrajunctional glycine and GABA$_A$ receptor-mediated IPSCs in identified lamina I neurons of the adult rat spinal cord. *J Neurosci*, 19:7342-7355.

2. Keller AF, Coull JAM, Chéry N, Poisbeau P, de Koninck Y. 2001. Region-specific developmental specialization of GABA/glycine cosynapses in laminae I-II of the rat spinal dorsal horn. *J Neurosci*, 21:7871-80.

3. Prescott SA, de Koninck Y. 2003. Gain control of firing rate by shunting inhibition: roles of synaptic noise and dendritic saturation. *Proc Natl Acad Sci USA*, 100:2076-2081.

4. Coull JAM, Boudreau D, Bachand K, Prescott SA, Nault F, Sík A, de Koninck P, De Koninck Y. 2003. Transsynaptic shift in anion gradient in spinal lamina I neurons as a mechanism of neuropathic pain. *Nature*, 424: 938-942.

5. Coull JAM, Beggs S, Boudreau D, Boivin D, Tsuda M, Inoue K, Gravel C, Salter MW, de Koninck Y. 2005. BDNF from microglia mediates the shift in neuronal anion gradient that underlies neuropathic pain. *Nature*, 438:1017-1021

MAIN TOPICS

Altering GABA$_A$/glycine -mediated spinal inhibition as a means to control nociception

Organization of the GABA/glycine system

Pre-vs. postsynaptic inhibition

GABA/glycine co-synapses

Plastic change in GABA/glycine-mediated inhibition in chronic pain models

Collapse of the transmembrane anion gradient

A specific subunit of the glycine receptor responsible for inflammatory pain hypersensitivity

Plasticity of GABA-glycine synapses through development in spinal pain pathways

Change in gain

Change in polarity

Pre- vs. postsynaptic inhibition

SUMMARY

Several conditions of pathological pain involve plastic changes in GABA/glycine-mediated inhibition in the CNS which can (i) alter the gain of the response to nociceptive input (hyperalgesia), but also (ii) allow cross talk between non-nociceptive and nociceptive pathways as a substrate for aberrant pain perception to normally innocuous input (allodynia). While plasticity of the GABA/glycine system had been traditionally overlooked and poorly studied, especially in the context of the pain system, recent findings highlight a richness of mechanisms by which inhibition is modulated that open several avenues for innovative therapeutic treatment for the prevention, as well as the reversal of pathological pain. These findings include (i) evidence of highly plastic GABA/glycine co-synapses, (ii) modulation of specific receptor subclasses by endogenous agents traditionally thought to act mainly in the periphery, but which also act centrally (e.g., neurosteroids and prostaglandins) and (iii) active regulation of anion homeostasis as a means to modulate both the strength and the sign of GABA/glycine action (i.e., excitatory vs. inhibitory).

INTRODUCTION

Much focus has been placed in recent years on plasticity of excitatory transmission to explain pain hypersensitivity or central sensitization following nerve injury or inflammation. Yet, altering inhibition also critically affects pain threshold and recent compelling evidence indicate that pathological pain involves plastic changes in inhibition. Plasticity of inhibition is likely to affect network function at several levels. For example, not only can changes in inhibition mask or unmask existing inputs, it can also gate other mechanisms of plasticity (e.g., promote NMDA-receptor-mediated synaptic plasticity). Thus, alterations in inhibitory control are likely to play a pivotal role in the etiology of chronic pain.

Inhibition occurs at several levels and this Chapter will focus on local circuit inhibition mediated the inhibitory amino acids γ-aminobutyric GABA and glycine, principally at the level of the spinal cord. While GABA acting on ionotropic GABA$_A$ receptors mediates the majority of the *fast* inhibitory postsynaptic transmission in the brain, in the spinal cord and brain stem, GABA shares this task with glycine. Finally, unlike in the brain, GABA$_A$ receptors also play

an active role in presynaptic inhibition of transmitter release from sensory afferents terminals in the spinal cord and brain stem.

Descending inhibition and its modulation is covered more specifically in Chapter 25. While some descending control pathways exert their action by modulating intrinsic spinal GABA/glycine-mediated inhibition, here we will be focusing on plasticity of GABA/glycine system *per se*.

ALTERING GABA$_A$/GLYCINE-MEDIATED SPINAL INHIBITION AS A MEANS TO CONTROL NOCICEPTION

There is ample evidence indicating that altering inhibition at the spinal level affect the relay of nociceptive information to the brain. Block of spinal inhibition mediated by GABA and glycine promotes the transmission of nociceptive information and makes innocuous input apparently painful (allodynia), akin to what is observed in neuropathic and inflammatory pain (Sivilotti & Woolf, 1994; Yaksh, 1989). At the spinal level, the local inhibitory network represses a large amount of established excitatory connections and suppression of this inhibition unmasks a profound network of polysynaptic input, which has the potential for allowing inputs to be relayed through ascending pathways that do not convey these inputs in normal conditions. For example, after blockade of GABA$_A$ receptors, lamina II neurons with normally little or no low threshold input can be seen to receive considerable input from low threshold afferents (comparable in magnitude to that from high threshold afferents; Fig. 14.1.) via polysynaptic connections Blocking glycine receptors also facilitates low threshold input to lamina II neurons, but to a much smaller degree (Baba *et al.*, 2003). Nociceptive specific lamina I neurons show responses to innocuous input after depression of intrinsic GABA$_A$/glycine inhibition (Keller *et al.*, 2005) and nociceptive specific thalamic neurons display responses to innocuous input following blockade of glycine receptors at the lumbar spinal level indicating subliminal low threshold input to normally nociceptive specific output pathways (Fig.14.2) (Sherman *et al.*, 1997). Because there are normally no monosynaptic connections to Lamina I from low threshold afferents, these findings reveal that there are polysynaptic pathways (i.e., via local feed forward excitatory interneurons) that can convey low threshold input to lamina I neurons and that these pathways are normally repressed by GABA$_A$/glycine receptor-mediated transmission.

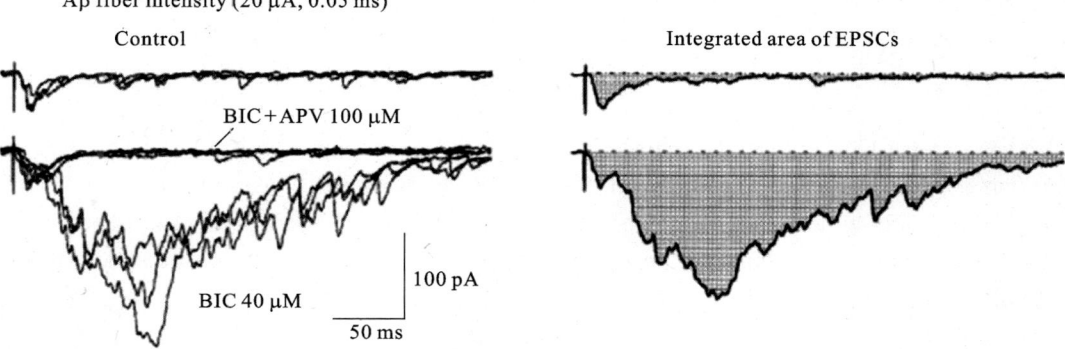

Fig.14.1   Unmasking massive polysynaptic excitatory input from sensory afferents to spinal lamina II neurons by blocking GABAA receptor-mediated inhibition (modified from Baba *et al.*, 2003).

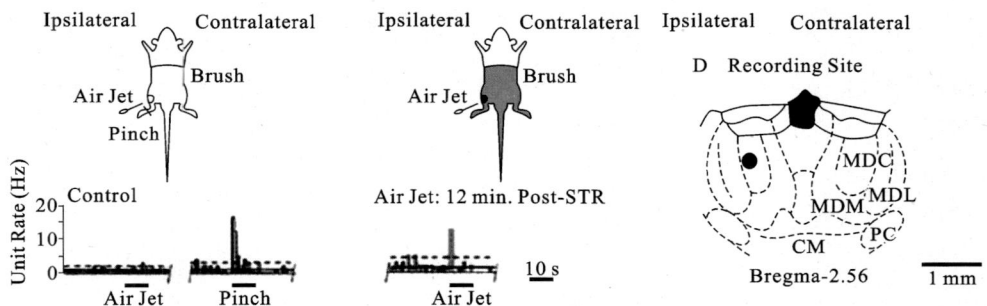

Fig.14. 2   Intrathecal injection of strychnine at the lumbar level to block spinal segmental glycine receptor-mediated inhibition unmasks low threshold input to normally nociceptive specific thalamic neuron (modified from Sherman *et al.*, 1997).

Showing that blockade of inhibition replicates symptoms characteristic of chronic pain conditions does not mean that a deficit in inhibition is necessarily a substrate of the condition. Hence a number of studies aimed at identifying plastic changes in the inhibitory system associated with experimental models of chronic pain have emerged in recent years and continue to emerge.

ORGANIZATION OF THE GABA/GLYCINE SYSTEM

Pre- vs. Postsynaptic Inhibition

Details of the structural arrangement of GABA and glycine synapses in the spinal cord are given in Chapter 23. Here we should remind the reader that GABA-Mediated inhibition can occur through very distinct mechanism.

On primary afferent nerve endings, ionotropic GABA$_A$ mediated presynaptic inhibition occurs via a depolarizing mechanism. GABA is depolarizing in primary afferents because the latter cells have a higher intracellular Cl$^-$ concentration than most other neurons in the adult CNS. This is due to the fact that primary afferents do not express the K$^+$-Cl$^-$ co-transporter KCC2 (Coull *et al.*, 2003), which normally extrudes chloride (down the potassium gradient), nor do they express CLC-2, a Cl$^-$ channel postulated to prevent Cl$^-$ accumulation in neurons (Staley *et al.*, 1996), while they express the Na$^+$-K$^+$-Cl$^-$ co-transporter NKCC1, which normally imports chloride(Ahmadi *et al.*, 2002). Inhibition of transmitter release appears to be achieved mainly through (i) membrane shunt and (ii) a depolarization-induced inactivation of voltage gated sodium and calcium channels (for reviews, see Rudomin, 1998; Willis, 1999). While inhibition of the release of excitatory transmitter from the central endings of sensory nerves in the spinal dorsal horn constitutes a first level of control of input, the majority of GABA and glycine containing terminals are presynaptic to dorsal horn neurons, not sensory nerve terminals (Todd & Spike, 1993). In fact, glycine-Mediated transmission only occurs postsynaptically. In the adult, postsynaptic glycine and $GABA_A$ receptor activation, in addition to causing a shunt of the membrane, is normally hyperpolarizing; both of these effects normally cause inhibition. Upon intense activity, however, a collapse of the chloride gradient can occur (Staley *et al.*, 1995), leading to a rebound excitation (Fig. 14.3; which may be multiplied by extracellular accumulation of K^+ in some systems (Kaila *et al.*, 1997).

Metabotropic $GABA_B$ receptors are involved at several sites, with potentially opposing net effects, which can complicate understanding the net effect of plasticity at these receptors. Indeed, they occur presynaptically on terminals of primary afferents where the mediate inhibition of excitatory transmitter release while they are also located on GABAergic terminals where they provide a negative feedback control on GABA release (i.e., causing disinhibition). Finally, they are expressed postsynaptically on dorsal horn neurons where they produce inhibition. Plasticity at $GABA_B$ receptors may thus lead to opposite effects depending on their location.

While hyperpolarization is generally considered inhibitory, it should not be overlooked that sometimes itself can also lead to rebound excitation (i.e., other than through the Cl^- accumulation mechanism mentioned above): hyperpolarization can cause deinactivation of voltage-gated channels (e.g., Na^+ or Ca^{2+}), altering action potential threshold and altering either the firing mode of the cell (e.g., bursting vs. tonic firing) or leading to rebound action potentials at the end of the hyperpolarizing event (Roy *et al.*, 1984).

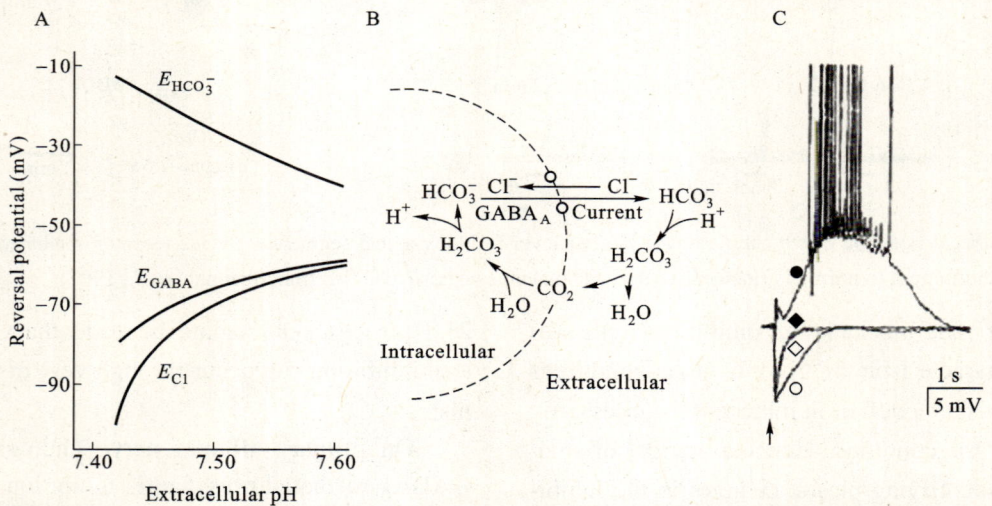

Fig.14.3 Collapse of anion gradient during sustained GABAergic activity causes a rebound excitation. A. GABAA receptor channels are permeable to both chloride and bicarbonate (in a 1 to 5 ratio). B. Massive chloride influx through GABAA channels can overwhelm chloride extrusion (e.g., via the KCC2). This is in contrast to the bicarbonate gradient, which is maintained stable because CO_2 diffusion across the membrane is not rate limited. C. The net result of a collapsed chloride gradient in response to repetitive GABAergic input is a rebound depolarization, which causes massive firing. Part of the rebound excitation involves amplification via NMDA receptor activity due to relief from Mg^{2+} block from the GABAA-mediated depolarization (modified from Staley *et al.*, 1995).

GABA/Glycine Co-synapses

In the spinal cord and brain stem, both GABA and glycine mediate inhibition and the same synapses can use both transmitters (Jonas *et al.*, 1998; O'Brien & Berger, 1999). In fact, in the superficial dorsal horn, it appears that nearly all glycine-immunoreactive cells in this area are also GABA-immunoreactive, while approximately half of GABAergic cells contain glycine (Mitchell *et al.*, 1993; Todd & Sullivan, 1990). These two transmitters are co-localized at synapses (Todd *et al.*, 1996) and appear to be co-packaged in the same synaptic vesicles (Chéry & Koninck, 1999).

These findings are puzzling since GABA and glycine both gate ionotropic receptors that have very similar properties and are both permeable to chloride (and to a lesser extend bicarbonate). This raises the question of the significance of having two transmitters co-packaged in the same vesicles, co-released and acting of very similar receptors. Two notable differences between $GABA_A$ and glycine receptors may shed some light on this question:

(i) Channel gating kinetics. The $GABA_A$ currents typically have slower off-rate kinetics; approximately 4-5 fold in the outward direction (the GABA channels gating is heavily voltage-dependent (Chéry & Koninck, 1999; Otis, 1991); the consequence is that synaptic currents with a $GABA_A$ component have a significantly greater area. The total charge carried is thus much greater and the conductance change last longer, being more amenable to temporal summation.

(ii) Allosteric binding sites. The $GABA_A$ receptor binding and channel gating properties are heavily modulated by a broad range of agents such as benzodiazepines, barbiturates, alcohol, zinc, and neurosteriods. In contrast, much fewer agents are known to bind to the glycine receptor to modulate the glycine channel (akin to the contrast between NMDA and non-NMDA ionotropic glutamate receptors). Because $GABA_A$ channels are ubiquitous in the CNS, agents active at the $GABA_A$ site broadly affect CNS function. In contrast, glycine receptors are only present in the spinal cord and brain stem; thus, agents modulating glycine receptors have the potential to produce fewer side effects. In this respect, specific modulation of glycine receptor subtypes may be promising avenue for therapeutic treatment (see below).

The $GABA_A$ and glycine receptors being differentially regulated by intracellular mechanisms (e.g. phosphorylation), they have the potential for independently shaping synaptic events. This is pertinent in the superficial dorsal horn, where switches in the contribution of $GABA_A$ receptor-mediated component at these co-synapses may represent a mechanism for gain control (see BOX 14.1). This may not be unrelated to the fact that $GABA_A$ receptors are so amenable to allosteric modulation by a variety of agents.

BOX 14.1   GABA/glycine co-synapse as a tool for plasticity.

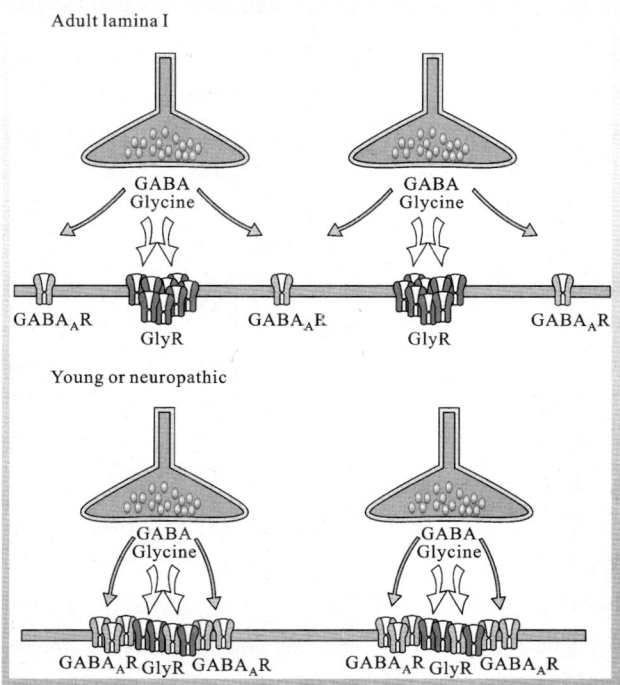

Adult lamina I

Young or neuropathic

In adult spinal lamina I neurons, quantal inhibitory synaptic currents (IPSCs) events are blocked with nanomolar concentrations of strychnine showing that they are all mediated by glycine receptors. Yet, a $GABA_A$ component to these quantal events can be unmasked in the presence of benzodiazepines (which raise the affinity of the receptor for GABA) indicating that while the two transmitters are co-released, they are not co-detected at these synaptic junctions. The rise time of the $GABA_A$ component is slow and conditions that favour spill over of GABA from the synapses, such as upon a large burst of synchronous input, also unmask the GABA component, which suggests that $GABA_A$ receptors are not located at synaptic junctions, but located peri-or extrasynaptically. This subcellular segregation of the receptors provides for distinct functional roles to inhibition mediated by these two transmitters: while glycine receptors appear to mediate most of inhibitory tone at these synapses, $GABA_A$ receptor mediated inhibition may contribute to control stronger inputs (Chery & Koninck, 1999).

Such an arrangement can also serve to control the gain of inhibition at this co-synapse. Indeed, appearance of the slow GABA$_A$ component dramatically prolongs the duration of the synaptic currents and thus total charge carried, increasing the gain of the response and the potential for temporal summation.   A switch from predominantly GABA$_A$–mediated towards pure, larger amplitude glycine-receptor mediated quantal synaptic currents occurs during development in lamina I(Keller *et al.*, 2001; Sorkin & Puig, 1996), as in other areas. Because the silent GABA$_A$ component can be unmasked at adult synapses by benzodiazepines, this tuning appears to be due to a postsynaptic change in receptor availability (Keller *et al.*, 2001; Sherman & Loomis, 1996; Sherman *et al.*, 1997) at these synapses. Return of a GABA$_A$ component to miniature IPSCs at adult lamina I synapses occurs after peripheral nerve injury, apparently recapitulating early developmental conditions and perhaps compensating for the decrease in glycinergic tone (Coull *et al.*, 2003).

Modulation of the relative contribution of the glycine and GABA$_A$ receptor-mediated components may thus be a general mechanism of gain control at this mixed synapse. This is intriguingly reminiscent of the situation at glutamatergic synapses where the AMPA vs. NMDA receptor–mediated components have respective fast and slow kinetics, comparable to that of the glycine vs. GABA$_A$ components.

PLASTIC CHANGE IN GABA/GLYCINE–MEDIATED INHIBITION IN CHRONIC PAIN MODELS

Several reports have linked the central hypersensitivity following peripheral nerve injury with selective degeneration of certain classes of neurons (Sugimoto, 1990) including inhibitory interneurons (Ibuki *et al.*, 1997; Moore *et al.*, 2002; Scholz *et al.*, 2005) in the spinal dorsal horn. It was suggested that this occurs through transsynaptic apoptosis (i.e. beyond the afferents of the injured nerve, into the dorsal horn) (Moore *et al.*, 2002; Scholz *et al.*, 2005). Consistent with this, continuous intrathecal infusion of an anti-apoptotic agent immediately following nerve injury prevents the loss of GABAergic interneurons and the reduction in inhibitory currents measured in response to stimulation of primary afferents (Scholz *et al.*, 2005). Other conflicting reports however indicate that hypersensitivity can occur without apparent loss of inhibitory interneurons neurons or other types of neurons in the dorsal horn following a similar nerve injury model(Polgar *et al.*, 2003).

Altered expression of GABA (or its synthesizing enzyme GAD) and/or GABA$_A$ receptors have also been reported following nerve injury or peripheral inflammation. The changes are often opposite between the two conditions and there appear to be differences between specific chronic pain models and animal strains. Further, in depth analysis of these structural changes are reviewed in details in Chapter 23 and will not be covered here.

While structural changes in the GABA glycine systems undoubtedly occur following injury to peripheral nerves and/or central damages, the prolonged time course of several of these changes cannot account for some of the early events involved in central sensitization. Thus, for disinhibitory mechanisms to be involved, more subtle functional changes must be taking place. Furthermore, it is often difficult to derive the impact of measured changes in transmitter and or receptor expression in functional terms. For example, the growing body of work revealing the importance of receptor translocation and diffusion to and away from synapses as a mechanism of synaptic plasticity (Choquet & Triller, 2003; Wan *et al.*, 1997) indicate that receptor expression on the membrane does not imply their functional participation at synapses. This is well illustrated by the finding that functional postsynaptic GABA$_A$ receptors are present on adult lamina I neurons, yet do not participate in quantal synaptic events and thus inhibitory tone (Chéry & Koninck, 1999) in this area (see BOX 14.1). In addition, receptor/channel properties (affinity, gating, desensitization, etc.) may be alternatively affected. Evaluating the involvement of plastic changes in GABA/glycine–mediated transmission thus requires direct assessment of functional implication.

Both nerve injury and peripheral inflammation appear to lead to loss of functional inhibition. In lamina II, a decrease in afferent evoked GABA$_A$-receptor mediated IPSCs has been reported following nerve injury models (spared nerve injury, SNI; and chronic constriction in jury, CCI) (Moore *et al.*, 2002) (experiments were conducted in the presence of strychnine, so changes in glycine receptor-mediated mechanisms was not assessed). In the same study, analysis of spontaneous synaptic activity revealed a decrease in frequency, but not amplitude of GABA$_A$ receptor-mediated miniature IPSCs, typically interpreted as indicating a presynaptic change in GABAergic transmission, consistent with the proposed loss of inhibitory interneurons (Moore *et al.*, 2002). Other compatible mechanisms can however be envisaged, such as loss of functional synapses or excitatory drive onto inhibitory interneurons. A selective disconnection of inhibitory interneurons from input as suggested in models of temporal lobe epilepsy is a possibility that deserves attention (Bekenstein & Lothman, 1993; Sloviter, 1991) Regardless of the underlying mechanisms, a loss functional GABA$_A$-mediated inhibition occurs in lamina II after peripheral nerve injury.

In spinal lamina I, where a major portion of ascending nociceptive output neurons originate, a decrease in synaptically-mediated glycinergic tone has been reported after both peripheral nerve injury (Coull *et al.*, 2003) and inflammation (Muller *et al.*, 2003). Given that glycine receptor-mediated synaptic input appears to dominate the inhibitory tone in lamina I neurons (Chéry & Koninck; 1999), these findings could suggest effective disinhibition of lamina I neurons. However, an opposite, significant upregulation of a GABAergic component to synaptic events occurred after nerve injury, (Coull *et al.*, 2003) which

should counterbalance the deficit in glycinergic input. It remains unclear what the final outcome of this plasticity is on spinal nociceptive output.

Collapse of the Transmembrane Anion Gradient

In addition to the above findings, a novel mechanism is emerging to further explain functional disinhibition at the spinal level. It involves the reduction in the expression of the K$^+$-Cl$^-$ exporter, KCC2, and the consequent disruption of anion homeostasis in neurons of lamina I of the spinal dorsal horn following peripheral nerve injury. This resulted in a shift in the anion reversal potential to more depolarized values, effectively eliminating the hyperpolarizing action of GABA and glycine. In most cases, the shift in anion reversal potential was sufficient to invert GABA/glycine-mediated hyperpolarization to depolarization (Fig. 14.4) and, in a subset of cells, it effectively converted inhibition into net excitation. Local blockade or knock-down of spinal KCC2 in intact rats markedly reduced nociceptive threshold, confirming that disruption of anion homeostasis in superficial dorsal horn neurons is sufficient to cause neuropathic pain (Coull *et al.*, 2003). This finding may significantly alter our interpretation of previous results on plasticity of inhibition. Indeed, apparent increase in GABA$_A$-or glycine receptor mediated responses can be effectively counterbalanced or even inverted by the altered anion gradient.

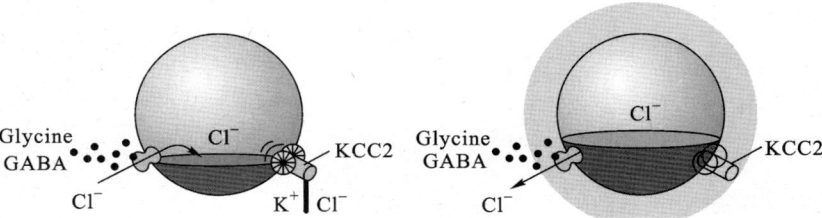

Fig.14.4 Loss of expression of KCC2 in spinal dorsal horn neurons after peripheral nerve in jury can cause accumulation of intracellular chloride — as little as 10–15mM—, which effectively inverts the polarity of the GABA$_A$/glycine receptor-mediated current (Based on Coull *et al.*, 2003; modified from Price *et al.*, 2005).

It should be noted here however that disinhibition does not imply lack of inhibition (see BOX 14.2). Indeed, in the case of GABA$_A$ and glycine receptors, elimination of postsynaptic hyperpolarizing inhibition

does not remove shunting inhibition. In the study by Coull *et al.*(2003), for example, conversion to direct GABAergic excitation (i.e. anion reversal potential being depolarized beyond action potential threshold) was only observed in 20% of the cells. Thus, overall, GABA and glycine likely continue to have a net inhibitory action on most lamina I neurons (and inhibition via primary afferent depolarization is maintained). The deficit in inhibition that results from a loss in postsynaptic hyperpolarizing action of GABA$_A$ and glycine receptors on dorsal horn neurons is however sufficient to potentiate nociceptive responsiveness and unmask low threshold input to lamina I (Keller *et al.*, 2005).

BOX 14.2 When are GABA and glycine inhibitory?

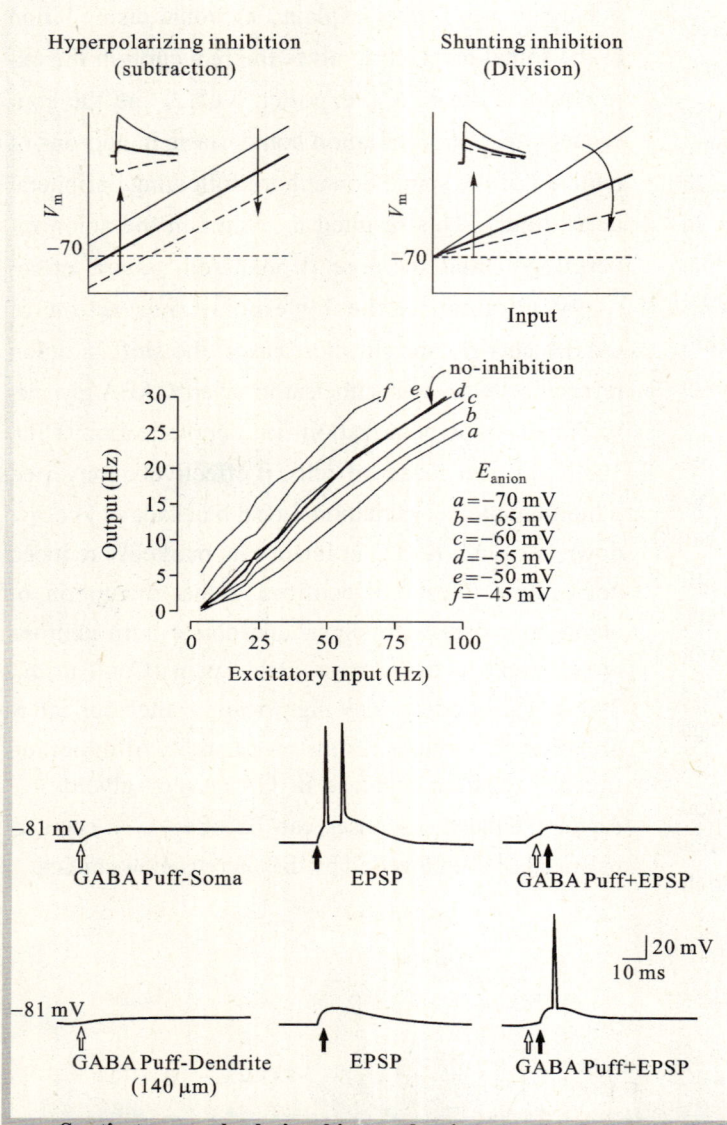

Extrapolating the net result of GABA$_A$ or glycine receptor–mediated action depends on several factors, including the site of action on the cells, polarity of ion flux and concurrence with other synaptic mechanisms.

Net excitation vs. disinhibition. While it is easy to understand that when the GABA/glycine reversal potential is above threshold for action potential, activation of their ionotropic receptors can yield direct excitation, the net effect of changing the anion (Coull *et al.*,2003)gradient is less obvious because two components of inhibition must be considered: shunt vs. hyperpolarizing inhibition. While shunting inhibition controls the gain or slope of the input-output curve (yielding multiplication/division), hyperpolarizing inhibition affects the offset of the input output curve (yielding addition/subtraction).

Thus, even though shunting inhibition remains a dominant factor at all values of anion reversal potential that fall below action potentials threshold, changing the reversal affects the offset of the input output curve. This is confirmed with simulations of inputs, using a realistic model cell bombarded by synaptic inputs comparable to that seen in the in vivo situation (see description in (Coull *et al.*, 2003)). It is obvious from the accompanying graph that a shift in anion reversal potential as small as 5 mV is sufficient to cause a significant upward shift in the input output curve. Thus, while GABA and glycine continue to have a **net inhibitory action** (compare curves *a*, *b* & *c*, to the no-inhibition curve), the shift in the input output curve reflects a **net disinhibition** with respect to the control condition and thus a greater excitability of the network.

Spatio-temporal relationship to other inputs. The site of action of GABA$_A$/glycine input on the somato-dendritic axis of the cell can critically affect the net outcome of the response. Indeed, Gulledge and Stuart (2003) showed that when GABA responses are depolarizing from rest, they can potentiate or inhibit concurrent glutamatergic input depending on their temporal and spatial relationship with the latter: dendritic GABA responses were excitatory regardless of timing, whereas somatic GABA responses were inhibitory when coincident with a glutamatergic synaptic input but excitatory at earlier times. These excitatory actions of GABA occur even though the GABA reversal potential is below action potential threshold.

Gating mechanisms for other plasticity. Even though depolarizing GABA/glycine may be insufficient to trigger action potential and cause a shunt in membrane resistance, non-linearities in membrane excitability may yield unexpected results. For example, relief from Mg^{2+} block that occurs in NMDA channels upon depolarization can override the membrane shunt to give rise to action potentials (see Fig.14.3; Staley *et al*, 1995; Ben, 2003).

In addition to the above mechanism of disinhibition, altered anion homeostasis may also play an important role in plastic changes underlying the development of pain hypersensitivity. Indeed, GABA/glycine-mediated depolarization provides an additional substrate for enabling voltage-dependent mechanisms of plasticity, such as releasing the Mg^{2+} block of NMDA receptors (see BOX 14.2) and may thus be a step upstream of plastic changes in excitatory transmission.

Modulating ion gradients as a means to control the strength of synaptic transmission provide a novel perspective on synaptic plasticity. Indeed, while changes in ion gradients, especially chloride gradients, have been well documented throughout development, little consideration had been given to the possibility that ion gradients could be actively modulated in adult tissue. A recent study by Rivera *et al.* (2002) showed that BDNF could rapidly (within minutes) affect KCC2 expression in the hippocampus. This prompted us to examine whether BDNF-mediated signaling could be involved in the collapse of the anion gradient in dorsal horn neurons following peripheral nerve injury. Local administration to spinal slices taken from normal rats mimicked the alteration in anion gradient observed with nerve injury. In addition, blocking BDNF-TrkB signaling reversed established allodynia as well as the shift in anion reversal potential in lamina I neurons following peripheral nerve injury (Fig. 14.5) (Coull *et al.*, 2005). The latter finding is important as it indicates that tonic BDNF secretion is necessary to maintain the anion reversal potential at depolarized levels. Maintenance of a specific anion gradient is thus an on-going process that can be readily modulated to control the strength of GABA/glycine-receptor mediated transmission. Further evidence reviewed in Chapter 24 indicate that it is spinal microglia, activated by ATP, that appear to release BDNF after nerve injury to cause the collapse in anion gradient in lamina I neurons. Plasticity of the anion gradient is thus a biophysical mechanism by which microglia can act on neuronal excitability. Whether the microglia-BDNF-anion gradient signaling mechanism occurs in other areas of the pain pathways remains to be investigated.

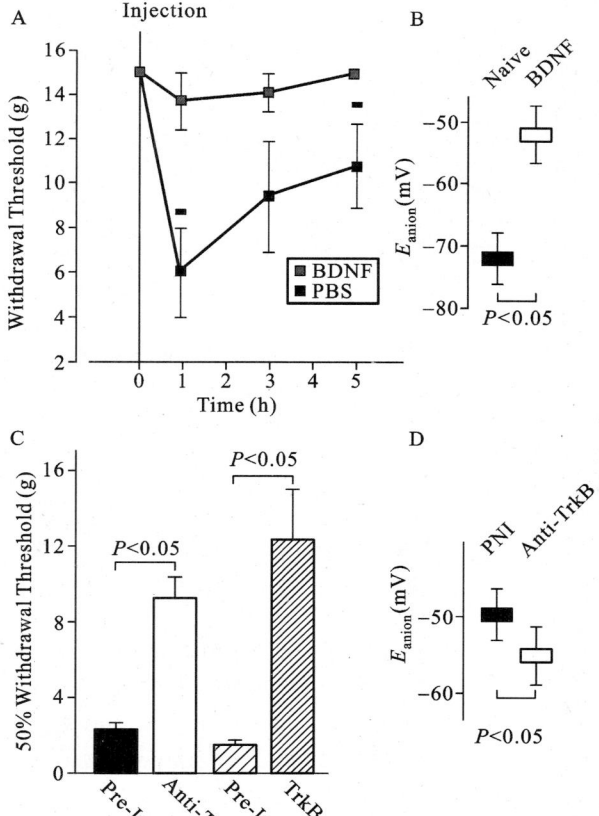

Fig.14.5 BDNF mediates pain hypersensitivity and a concurrent depolarizing shift in the anion reversal potential (E_{anion}) in dorsal horn neurons. A. Exogenous administration of BDNF causes a facilitation of the nociceptive withdrawal reflex. B. A depolarizing shift in E_{anion} in lamina I neurons in control animals. In animals that had sustained nerve injury, blocking BDNF-TrkB signalling reversed both. C. The established pain hypersensitivity. D. Collapsed anion gradient.

The intracellular second messenger pathways by which BDNF-TrkB signaling controls KCC2 expression have also been elucidated. It involves both Shc/FRS-2 (src homology 2 domain containing transforming protein/FGF receptor substrate 2) and PLCγ (phospholipase Cγ)-cAMP response element-binding protein signaling (Rivera et al., 2004). Interestingly, activation of both Shc and PLCγ cascades is required for trkB-mediated downregulation of KCC2, whereas activation of the Shc pathway in the absence of PLCγ

activation leads to an upregulation of KCC2 (Fig. 14.6). This is particularly interesting, because BDNF has been shown to play an important role in the ontogeny of chloride homeostasis by promoting the upregulation of KCC2 during the early postnatal period (Aguado et al., 2003). The bidirectional action of BDNF on KCC2 expression depending on whether both Shc and PLCγ are involved or not provides a potential mechanisms for the divergent action of BDNF in early developmental stages vs. adulthood.

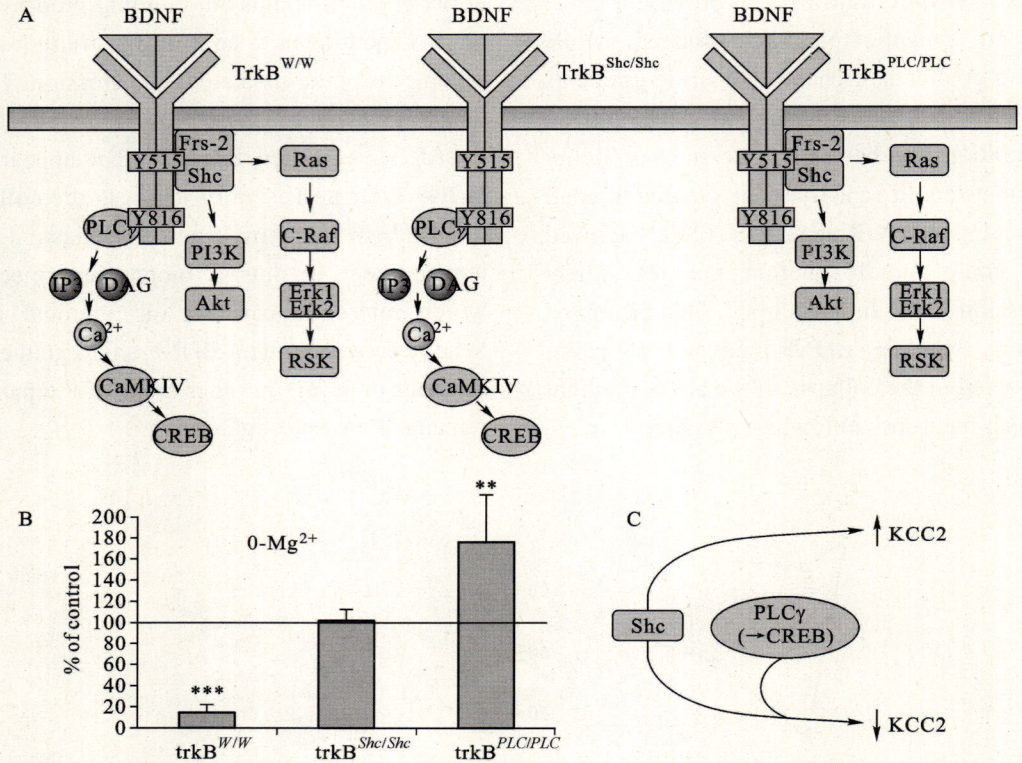

Fig.14.6 Both PLC and Shc docking sites of TrkB are required for BDNF–TrkB-mediated KCC2 downregulation, whereas the Shc site acting in isolation mediates an upregulation of KCC2. A. Schematic representation of the mutant TrkB receptors with a point mutation at either the tyrosine 515 or Shc site in the juxtamembrane region or at the tyrosine 816 or PLCγ site in the C-terminal region. B. In the trkB*PLC/PLC* and trkB*SHC/SHC* mutant receptors, tyrosine (Y816) and tyrosine (Y515) were replaced by phenylalanine (F816) and phenylalanine (F515),respectively. In the control trkB*W/W* mice, BDNF induced downregulation of KCC2 as expected. On the contrary, KCC2 was not downregulated in the trkB*SHC/SHC* mutants, indicating that the Shc/FRS-2-coupled pathway is important for KCC2 downregulation. Strikingly, KCC2 was upregulated by BDNF in the trkB*PLC/PLC* mutant mice. (means±SEM; t test; ***, P<0.001; **, P<0.01). C. Activation of both Shc and PLCγ cascades is required for trkB-mediated downregulation of KCC2, whereas activation of the Shc pathway in the absence of PLCγ activation leads to an upregulation of KCC2 (Modified from Rivera et al. 2004).

A Specific Subunit of the Glycine Receptor Responsible for Inflammatory Pain Hypersensitivity

A novel mechanism has recently been proposed to account for the decrease in spinal glycinergic inhibi-

tion following peripheral inflammation. Recent evidence has shown that the endogenous prostaglandins are synthesized not only by peripheral inflamed tissue, but also in the CNS, in particular in the spinal cord, where they sensitize dorsal horn neurons. While it was long thought that prostaglandins, in particular

PGE₂, mainly acted by potentiating glutamatergic transmission, recent evidence indicated that PGE₂ selectively blocked strychnine-sensitive glycinergic transmission in the spinal dorsal horn (Ahmadi *et al.*, 2002). More importantly, this effect was restricted to neurons that expressed glycine receptors that contain the α3 subunit and these neurons were restricted to the superficial layers of the dorsal horn. The effect involved activation of the EP₂ subtype of prostaglandin E receptors and PKA, consistent with the finding that PGE₂-induced thermal hyperalgesia was significantly diminished in mice lacking neuronal PKA (Fig. 14.7) (Malmberg *et al.*, 1997). Mice deficient in α3 subunit of the glycine receptor (and which exhibit no apparent change in nociceptive threshold) lack both (i) inhibition of glycinergic neurotransmission by PGE₂ seen in wildtype mice and (ii) a reduction in pain sensitization induced by spinal PGE₂ injection or peripheral inflammation. This finding is of particular interest because it points to a potentially very specific target for the treatment of pathological pain.

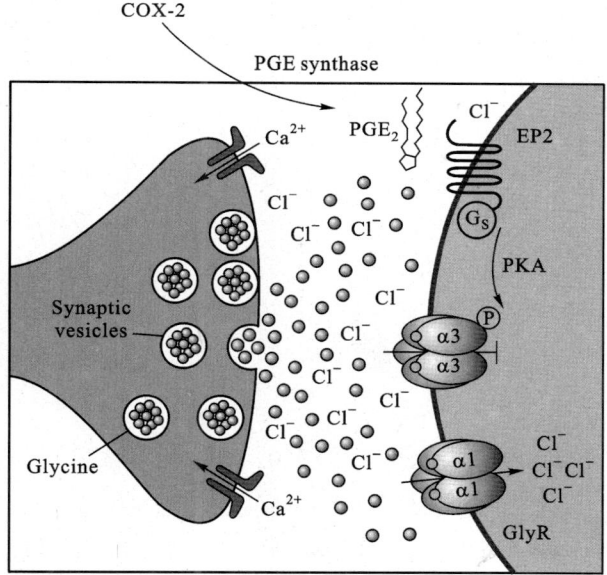

Fig.14.7 PGE₂-mediated inhibition of glycinergic neurotransmission in the superficial layers of the spinal cord dorsal horn. Peripheral inflammation induces the expression of COX-2 and microsomal prostaglandin E synthase in the spinal cord. PGE₂ produced by these two enzymes activates prostaglandin receptors of the EP₂ subtype, which activates protein kinase A (PKA) to cause phosphorylation and inhibition of glycine receptors containing the α3 subunit. (Based on Harvey *et al.*, 2004; Zeilhofer, 2005)

PLASTICITY OF GABA-GLYCINE SYNAPSES THROUGH DEVELOPMENT IN SPINAL PAIN PATHWAYS

Change in Gain

Early postnatal development involves a switch between predominantly GABAₐ-mediated towards pure, and larger amplitude glycine-receptor mediated quantal synaptic currents in lamina I (Keller *et al.*, 2001; Sorkin and Puig, 1996)(see BOX 14.1). Maturation of the glycine receptors involve a switch from α2 to α1 expression responsible for the acceleration of the kinetics of glycine receptor-mediated synaptic events with development (Malosio *et al.*, 1991a; Malosio *et al.*, 1991b; Takahashi *et al.*, 1992). Expression of the α1 subunit also appear to be an adult subunit. A four-fold acceleration of the decay kinetics of GABAₐ receptor-mediated synaptic events also occurs with maturation (Keller *et al.*, 2001). The slower kinetics of the GABAₐ component of miniature IPSCs has been attributed to the tonic production of 5α-reduced neurosteroids in the immature spinal cord (Keller *et al.*, 2004). Interestingly, promoting the synthesis of endogenous 5α-reduced neurosteroids increased the proportion of mixed GABAₐ/glycine mIPSCs in immature animals and led to the reappearance of mixed GABAₐ/glycine mIPSCs in adults. This raises the intriguing possibility that endogenous neurosteriod production may be responsible for the plastic switch observed after nerve injury (see BOX 14.1).

Change in Polarity

A developmental shift in anion gradient from depolarizing to hyperpolarizing and thus affecting the action of GABA and glycine during development has been well documented (for review see (Ban, 2002)). At early developmental stages, NKCC1 expression levels are high and KCC2 levels are low, making NKCC1 the dominant cation-chloride cotransporter. NKCC1 expression diminishes, and KCC2 expression increases during the early postnatal period, causing a negative shift in the anion reversal potential (Rivera *et al.*, 1999). Upregulation of KCC2 expression during development may not be sufficient to account for its function and thus regulation of KCC2 activity may be an important factor in the maturation of chloride homeostasis (Kelsch *et al.*, 2001). Interestingly, BDNF appears to have opposite actions on KCC2 expression at different developmental stages, stimulating its upregulation at early stages (Aguado *et al.*, 2003), while causing its downregulation in the adult brain (Rivera *et al.*, 2002). Thus, while BDNF release from spinal microglia after nerve injury in the adult spinal cord (see above and (Coull *et al.*, 2005)) may constitute a repair response, it triggers an opposite, and pain-enhancing effect on anion homeostasis to that at early developmental stages.

It is not easy to determine the net impact of the gradual hyperpolarizing shift in anion reversal potential on the strength of postsynaptic inhibition throughout development. While it had been postulated for a long time that a deficit in inhibition at the spinal level (Fitzgerald, 1985) may account for the nociceptive hypersensitivity in the new born, this idea has been questioned given the fact that GABA$_A$-induced depolarization in the newborn spinal dorsal horn remains subthreshold for action potentials (Baccei and Fitzgerald, 2004). Suprathreshold responses to GABA are however not the only mechanism by which the excitability of the network can be raised (see BOX 14.2). Yet, there is also an apparent mismatch between the behavioural hypersensitivity after birth and the maturation of the anion gradient: the developmental shift in anion reversal potential is completed within one week after birth while reflex hypersensitivity persists throughout the first two to three postnatal weeks (Baccei and Fitzgerald, 2004). Interestingly however, it appears that even though one week after birth the anion reversal potential predicts GABA$_A$- or glycine induced hyperpolarization from rest, the chloride extrusion capacity of the superficial dorsal horn neurons remains incomplete, which makes the cells more prone to rebound excitation (Fig. 14.3) upon repetitive or bursts of GABA/glycine inputs (Fig. 14.8). Thus, changes in the functionality of the chloride homeostasis may affect network activity in subtle ways and this may be revealed only in conditions where GABA/glycine system is being challenged.

Pre-vs. Postsynaptic Inhibition

NKCC1 expression in sensory afferents is maintained throughout development and into adulthood (while KCC2 expression remains lacking). Thus, contrary to postsynaptic mechanisms mediated by GABA$_A$ and glycine receptors on dorsal horn neurons, GABA$_A$ receptor activation maintains the same polarity – depolarizing - throughout development in primary sensory neurons where it presumably continuously produces presynaptic inhibition. In certain extreme conditions, however, it may be conceived that enhanced NKCC1 expression or activity may yield enhanced GABA$_A$-mediated depolarization of afferent terminals to a point that it triggers action potentials. This may be responsible for cross talk between low and high threshold afferents, a potential substrate for allodynia (Cervero and Laird, 1996; Galan and Cervero; 2005).

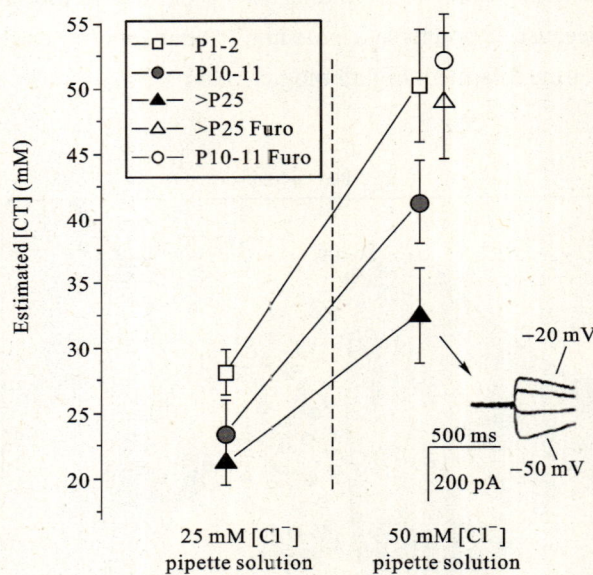

Fig.14.8 Incomplete chloride extrusion capacity until late in postnatal development. Estimated [Cl⁻]i, based on Eanion measurements in whole cell recorded neurons, with two high [Cl⁻] pipette solutions, at three developmental stages. There is a significant effect of age (*P*<0.001) and pipette [Cl⁻] (*P*<0.001) on the resulting [Cl⁻]i (two-way ANOVA analysis). In the presence of the KCC2 antagonist furosemide, the estimated [Cl⁻]i of P10-11 and adult neurons was not different from that of the pipette solution (50mM). Inset: example of responses to GABA obtained at different holding potentials (10mV apart) of an adult neuron with 50mM [Cl⁻] in the pipette. (Modified from Cordero- Erausquin *et al.*, 2005).

Expression (or function) of presynaptic GABA$_B$ receptors appears to precede postsynaptic receptors in several brain areas as well as in the spinal cord during the first week of postnatal development (Baccei and Fitzgerald, 2004; Fukuda *et al.*, 1993; Gaiarsa *et al.*, 1995). In the hippocampus, while presynaptic GABA$_B$-mediated inhibition is present at birth, homosynaptic presynaptic autoinhibition of GABA release however does not appear to be functional (Caillard *et al.*, 1998). If a similar distinction occurred in the spinal cord between homo- and heterosynaptic control of GABA release at early developmental stages, it could have significant impact on spinal nociceptive processing.

CONCLUSION

Plastic changes in the GABA/glycine system associated with pathological pain may take several forms. Beyond examining the more conventional changes in transmitter / receptor expression, it is important to assess functional changes. Indeed, altered functionality of GABA/glycine-mediated transmission occurs throughout development as well as after inflammation and peripheral nerve injury. These include switches in the respective contributions of GABA$_A$ and glycine receptors to inhibitory tone and altered intracellular chloride homeostasis.

The net effect of the switches observed at the GABA/glycine co-synapses on network excitability however remains to be elucidated. Negative regulation of the α3 containing spinal glycine-receptors by prostaglandins after inflammation suggests a specific therapeutic target for inflammatory pain. A collapse of the anion gradient in adult dorsal horn after peripheral nerve injury appears to be sufficient to explain at least some of the central sensitization underlying pain hypersensitivity in neuropathic pain. The fact that the anion gradient is maintained in a collapsed state after nerve injury by continuous secretion of BDNF from spinal microglia indicates that it may be possible to reverse the pain hypersensitivity, rather than just prevent its development, which is promising for restorative treatment. Treatments aimed at restoring normal anion homeostasis also have the potential for fewer side effects as they will simply restore endogenous GABA/glycine-mediated inhibitory control rather than causing a general depression of excitability (as with exogenous opiates for example).

The impact of the maturation of GABA/glycine system at early developmental stages remains to be elucidated and will require a detailed assessment of the balance between excitatory and inhibitory influences as well as an assessment of function under conditions that challenge inhibitory capacity.

Whether the novel mechanisms of plasticity of the GABA/glycine systems that have recently been identified in the spinal cord can be transposed to plasticity in different relay points in the pain pathways remains to be determined.

GENERAL CITATIONS

Ben Ari Y. 2002. Excitatory actions of gaba during development: the nature of the nurture. *Nat Rev Neurosci*, 3: 728-739.

Gaiarsa JL, Caillard O, Ben Ari Y. 2002. Longterm plasticity at GABAergic and glycinergic synapses: mechanisms and functional significance. *Trends Neurosci*, 25: 564-570.

Price TJ, Cervero F, de Koninck Y. 2005. Role of cation-chloride-cotransporters (CCC) in pain and hyperalgesia. *Curr Top Med Chem*, 5: 547-555.

Rudomin P. 1998. *Presynaptic Inhibition and Neural Control.* New York: Oxford University Press.

Willis W D Jr. 1999. Dorsal root potentials and dorsal root reflexes: a double-edged sword. Exp Brain Res, 124: 395-421.

Zeilhofer H U. 2005. The glycinergic control of spinal pain processing. *Cell Mol Life Sci*, 62: 2 027-2 035.

DISCOVERY CITATIONS

Aguado F, *et al.*, 2003. BDNF regulates spontaneous correlated activity at early developmental stages by increasing synaptogenesis and expression of the K$^+$/Cl$^-$ co-transporter KCC2. *Development*, 130: 1 267-1 280.

Ahmadi S, Lippross S, Neuhuber WL , Zeilhofer HU. 2002. PGE(2) selectively blocks inhibitory glycinergic neurotransmission onto rat superficial dorsal horn neurons. *Nat Neurosci*, 5: 34-40.

Alvarez-Leefmans FJ, Gamiño SM, Giradelz F, Noguerón I.

1998. Intracellular chloride regulation in amphibian dorsal root ganglion neurones studied with ion-selective micro-electrodes. *J Physiol (Lond)*, 406: 225-246.

Baba H, *et al.* 2003. Removal of GABAergic inhibition facilitates polysynaptic A fiber-mediated excitatory transmission to the superficial spinal dorsal horn. *Mol Cell Neurosci*, 24: 818-830.

Baccei ML, Fitzgerald M. 2004. Development of GABAergic and glycinergic transmission in the neonatal rat dorsal horn. *J Neurosci*, 24: 4749-4757.

Bekenstein JW, Lothman EW. 1993. Dormancy of inhibitory interneurons in a model of temporal lobe epilepsy. *Science*, 259: 97-100

Ben Ari Y. 2002. Excitatory actions of gaba during development: the nature of the nurture. *Nat Rev Neurosci*, 3: 728-739 .

Caillard O, McLean HA, Ben Ari Y, Gaiarse JL. 1998. Ontogenesis of presynaptic GABAB receptor-mediated inhibition in the CA3 region of the rat hippocampus. *J Neurophysiol*, 79: 1341-1348.

Cervero F, Laird JM. 1996. Mechanisms of touch-evoked pain (allodynia): a new model. *Pain*, 68: 13-23.

Chéry N, de Koninck Y. 1999. Junctional versus extrajunctional glycine and GABA(A) receptor-mediated IPSCs in identified lamina I neurons of the adult rat spinal cord. *J Neurosci*, 19: 7342-7355.

Choquet D, Triller A. 2003. The role of receptor diffusion in the organization of the postsynaptic membrane. *Nat Rev Neurosci*, 4: 251-265.

Cordero-Erausquin M, Coull JA, Boudreau D, Rolland M, de Koninck Y. 2005. Differential maturation of GABA action and anion reversal potential in spinal .amina I neurons; impact of chloride extrusion capacity. *Journal of Neuroscience*,. (in press)

Coull JA, *et al.* 2005. BDNF from microglia mediates the shift in neuronal anion gradient that underlies neuropathic pain. *Nature.* (in press)

Coull JA, *et al.* 2003. Trans-synaptic shift in anion gradient in spinal lamina I neurons as a mechanism of neuropathic pain. *Nature*, 424: 938-942.

Fitzgerald M. 1985. The post-natal development of cutaneous afferent fibre input and receptive field organization in the rat dorsal horn. *J Physiol*, 364: 1-18.

Fukuda A, Mody I, Prince DA. 1993. Differential ontogenesis of presynaptic and postsynaptic GABAB inhibition in rat somatosensory cortex. *J Neurophysiol*, 70: 448-452.

Gaiarsa JL, *et al.* 1995. Postnatal maturation of gamma-aminobutyric acid A and B-mediated inhibition in the CA3 hippocampal region of the rat. *J Neurobiol*, 26: 339-349.

Galan A, Cervero F. 2005. Painful stimuli induce *in vivo* phosphorylation and membrane mobilization of mouse spinal cord NKCC1 co-transporter. *Neuroscience* 133: 245-252.

Gulledge AT, Stuart GJ. 2003. Excitatory actions of GABA in the cortex. *Neuron*, 37: 299-309.

Ibuki T, Hama AT, Wang XT, Pappas GD, Sagen J. 1997. Loss of GABA-immunoreactivity in the spinal dorsal horn of rats with peripheral nerve injury and promotion of recovery by adrenal medullary grafts. *Neuroscience*, 76: 845-858.

Jonas P, Bischofberger J, Sandkuhler J.1998. Corelease of two fast neurotransmitters at a central synapse. *Science*, 281: 419-424.

Kaila K,Lamsa K, Smirnov S, Taira T, Voipio J. 1997. Long-lasting GABA-mediated depolarization evoked by high-frequency stimulation in pyramidal neurons of rat hippocampal slice is attributable to a network-driven, bicarbonate-dependent K^+ transient. *J Neurosci*, 17: 7 662-7 672.

Keller AF, Beggs S,Salter MW, de Koninck Y. 2005. Disrupting anion homeostasis in the spinal dorsal horn induces a disinhibition of lamina I projection neurons. *11th World Congress on Pain*, 136337.

Keller AF, Breton JD, Schlichter R, Poisbeau P. 2004. Production of 5alpha-reduced neurosteroids is developmentally regulated and shapes GABA(A) miniature IPSCs in lamina II of the spinal cord. *J Neurosci*, 24: 907-915.

Keller AF, Coull JA, Chery N, Poisbeau P, de Koninck Y. 2001. Region-specific developmental specialization of GABA-glycine cosynapses in laminas I-II of the rat spinal dorsal horn. *J Neurosci*, 21: 7 871-7 880.

Kelsch W, *et al.* 2001. Insulin-like growth factor 1 and a cytosolic tyrosine kinase activate chloride outward transport during maturation of hippocampal neurons, *J Neurosci*, 21: 8 339-8 347.

Malmberg AB, *et al.* 1997. Diminished inflammation and nociceptive pain with preservation of neuropathic pain in mice with a targeted mutation of the type I regulatory subunit of cAMP-dependent protein kinase. *J Neurosci*, 17: 7 462-7 470.

Malosio ML, *et al.* 1991a. Alternative splicing generates two variants of the alpha 1 subunit of the inhibitory glycine receptor, *J Biol Chem*, 266:   2 048-2 053.

Malosio M L, Marqueze-Pouey B, Kuhse J, Betz H 1991b. Widespread expression of glycine receptor subunit mRNAs in the adult and developing rat brain. *EMBO J*, 10: 2 401-2 409.

Mitchell K, Spike RC, Todd AJ. 1993 An immunocytochemical study of glycine receptor and GABA in laminae I-III of rat spinal dorsal horn. *J Neurosci*, 13: 2 371-2 381.

Moore KA, *et al.* 2002. Partial peripheral nerve injury promotes a selective loss of GABAergic inhibition in the superficial dorsal horn of the spinal cord. *J Neurosci* ,22: 6 724-6731.

Muller F, Heinke B, Sandkuhler J. 2003. Reduction of glycine receptor-mediated miniature inhibitory postsynaptic currents in rat spinal lamina I neurons after peripheral inflammation. *Neuroscience*, 122: 799-805 .

O'Brien JA, Berger AJ. 1999. Cotransmission of GABA and glycine to brain stem motoneurons. *J Neurophysiol*, 82: 1 638-1 641.

Otis TS, Staley KJ, Mody I. 1991. Perpetual inhibitory activity in mammalian brain slices generated by spontaneous GABA release. *Brain Res*, 545:142-150.

Polgar E, Gray S, Riddell JS, Todd AJ. 2004. Lack of evidence for significant neuronal loss in laminae I-III of the spinal dorsal horn of the rat in the chronic constriction injury model. *Pain*, 111: 144-150.

Polgar E, Hughes DI, Arham AZ, Todd AJ. 2005. Loss of neurons from laminas I-III of the spinal dorsal horn is not required for development of tactile allodynia in the spared nerve injury model of neuropathic pain. *J Neurosci*, 25: 6 658-6 666.

Polgar E, *et al.* 2003. Selective loss of spinal GABA-ergic or glycinergic neurons is not necessary for development of thermal hyperalgesia in the chronic constriction injury model of neuropathic pain. P*ain*, 104: 229-239.

Rivera C, *et al.* 2002. BDNF-induced TrkB activation down-regulates the K^+- Cl^- cotransporter KCC2 and impairs neuronal Cl^- extrusion, *J Cell Biol*, 159:747-752.

Rivera C, *et al.* 1999. The K^+/Cl^- co-transporter KCC2 renders GABA hyperpolarizing during neuronal maturation. *Nature*, 397: 251-255.

Rivera C, *et al.* 2004. Mechanism of activity-dependent downregulation of the neuron-specific K-Cl cotransporter KCC2. *J Neurosci*, 24: 4 683-4 691 .

Roy JP, Clercq M, Steriade M, Deschenes M. 1984. Electrophysiology of neurons of lateral thalamic nuclei in cat: mechanisms of long-lasting hyperpolarizations. *J Neurophysiol*, 51: 1 220-1 235.

Rudomin P. 1998. *Presynaptic Inhibition and Neural Control.* New York: Oxford University Press.

Scholz J, *et al.* 2005. Blocking caspase activity prevents transsynaptic neuronal apoptosis and the loss of inhibition in lamina II of the dorsal horn after peripheral nerve injury. *J Neurosci*, 25: 7 317-7 323.

Sherman SE, Loomis CW.1996. Strychnine-sensitive modulation is selective for non-noxious somatosensory input in the spinal cord of the rat. *Pain*, 66: 321-330.

Sherman SE, Loomis CW. 1994. Morphine insensitive allodynia is produced by intrathecal strychnine in the lightly anesthetized rat. *Pain*, 56:17-29.

Sherman SE, Luo L, Dostrovsky JO. 1997. Spinal strychnine alters response porperties of nociceptive-specific neurons in rat medial thalamus. *J Neurophysiol*, 78: 628-637.

Sivilotti L, Woolf CJ. 1994. The contribution of GABA$_A$ and glycine receptors to central sensitization: disinhibition and touch-evoked allodynia in the spinal cord. *J Neurophysiol*, 72: 169-179.

Sloviter RS. 1991. Permanently altered hippocampal structure, excitability, and inhibition after experimental status epilepticus in the rat: the "dormant basket cell" hypothesis and its possible relevance to temporal lobe epilepsy. *Hippocampus*, 1: 41-66 .

Sorkin LS, Puig S. 1996. Neuronal model of tactile allodynia produced by spinal strychnine: effects of excitatory amino acid receptor antagonists and a m-opiate receptor agonist. *Pain*, 68: 283-292.

Staley K, Smith R, Schaack J, Wilcox C, Jentsch TJ. 1996. Alteration of GABAA receptor function following gene transfer of the CLC-2 chloride channel. NeuYon,17: 543-551.

Staley KJ, Soldo BL, Proctor WR. 1995. Ionic mechanisms of

neuronal excitation by inhibitory GABAA receptors. *Science*, 269: 977-981.

Sugimoto T, Bennett G J, Kajander KC. 1990. Transsynaptic degeneration in the superficial dorsal horn after sciatic nerve injury: effects of a chronic constriction injury, transection, and strychnine. *Pain*, 42: 205-213.

Takahashi T, Momiyama A, Hirai K, Hishinuma F, Akagi H. 1992. Functional correlation of fetal and adult forms of glycine receptors with developmental changes in inhibitory synaptic receptor channels. *Neuron*, 9: 1 155-1 161.

Todd AJ , Spike RC. 1993. The localization of classical transmitters and neuropeptides within neurons in laminae I-III of the mammalian spinal dorsal horn. *Prog Neurobiol*, 41: 609-645.

Todd AJ, Sullivan AC. 1990. Light microscope study of the coexistence of GABA-like and glycine-like immunoreactivities in the spinal cord of the rat. *J Comp Neurol*, 296: 496-505.

Todd AJ, Watt C, Spike RC, Sieghart W. 1996. Colocalization of GABA, glycine, and their receptors at synapses in the rat spinal cord. *J Neurosci*, 16: 974-982.

Wan Q, *et al.* 1997. Recruitment of functional GABA$_A$ receptors to postsynaptic domains by insulin. *Nature*, 388: 686-690.

Willis W D Jr. 1999. Dorsal root potentials and dorsal root reflexes: a double-edged sword. *Exp Brain Res*, 124: 395-421.

Yaksh TL. 1989. Behavioral and autonomic correlates of the tactile evoked allodynia produced by spinal glycine inhibition: Effects of modulatory receptor systems and excitatory amino acid antagonists. *Pain*, 37: 111-123.

Part V Postsynaptic Signaling and Gene Regulation

Protein Kinases and Phosphatases

CHAPTER 15

Ronald A. Merrill, Stefan Strack

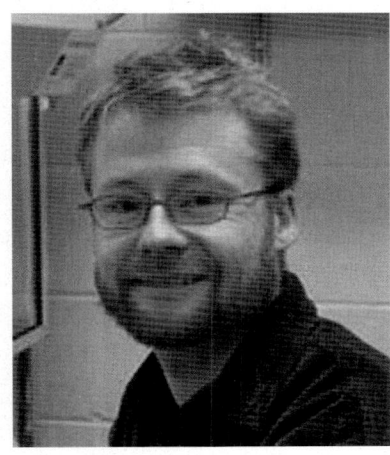

Dr. Strack is an Associate Professor in the Department of Pharmacology, University of Iowa, Iowa City, USA. He graduated from the University of Würzburg and obtained a M.S. in Computer Science at the University at Albany, State University of New York. After gaining a Ph.D. in Biology at the same institution, he pursued postdoctoral training at Vanderbilt University.

MAJOR CONTRIBUTIONS

1. Strack S, Ruediger R, Walter G, Dagda RK, Barwacz CA, Cribbs JT. 2002. Protein phosphatase 2A holoenzyme assembly. Identification of contacts between B-family regulatory and scaffolding A subunits. *J Biol Chem*, 277(23):20750-20755.
2. Strack S. 2002. Overexpression of the protein phosphatase 2A regulatory subunit B[gamma] promotes neuronal differentiation by activating the MAP kinase cascade. *J Biol Chem*, 277(44):41525-41532.
3. Dagda RK, Zaucha JA, Wadzinski BE, Strack S. 2003. A developmentally regulated, neuron-specific splice variant of the variable subunit B-beta targets protein phosphatase 2A to mitochondria and modulates apoptosis. *J Biol Chem*, 278:24976-24985.
4. Strack S, Cribbs JT, Gomez L. 2004. Critical role for protein phosphatase 2A heterotrimers in mammalian cell survival. *J Biol Chem*, 279:47732-47739.
5. Dagda RK, Barwacz CA, Cribbs JT, Strack S. 2005. Unfolding-resistant translocase targeting: a novel mechanism for outer mitochondrial membrane localization exemplified by the Bβ2 regulatory subunit of protein phosphatase 2A. *J Biol Chem*, 280:27375-27382.

MAIN TOPICS

Classification
  Kinases
  Phosphatases
Structure and catalytic mechanisms
  Kinases
  Phosphatases
Substrate specificity
Regulation
  Kinases
  Phosphatases
Phosphorylation in long-term synaptic plasticity
Kinase/phosphatase complexes in synaptic plasticity
Receptor tyrosine kinases in neuronal function and plasticity
Kinases and phosphatases in addiction

SUMMARY

Reversible protein phosphorylation is the most prominent posttranslational regulatory mechanism in eukaryotes. Protein kinases catalyze the addition of a phosphoester group to proteins while protein phosphatases oppose kinase activity by removing phosphates. The recent sequencing of numerous genomes has allowed for the identification and classification of most if not all kinases and phosphatases. Kinases represent a large group of enzymes (>500 in humans) and are classified by sequence similarity, with most kinases containing a conserved catalytic domain. Phosphatases are a smaller group (~140 in humans) and are classified by their catalytic mechanisms, as well as sequence similarity. Most kinases and phosphatases contain domains involved in intramolecular regulation of the catalytic domain. In contrast, some of the abundant Ser/Thr phosphatases form holoenzymes with a variety of regulatory subunits, which affect both localization and substrate binding.

Precise regulation of cellular responses requires the formation of large signaling complexes containing both kinases and phosphatases. In neurons, regulatory complexes containing ion channels and neurotransmitter receptors are important for basal neurotransmission and synaptic plasticity. Such microcompartmentalization of kinases and phosphatases allows for synapse–specific adjustments of synaptic strength. Recent advances in proteomics techniques have led to the identification of synaptic protein–protein interaction and phosphorylation networks, which provide a first global picture of the molecular machinery that underlies neuronal communication.

INTRODUCTION

Regulation of nearly all cellular processes, including metabolism, gene expression, cell proliferation, and apoptosis, involves the addition and removal of phosphates from proteins. The importance of reversible phosphorylation is highlighted by the sheer number of protein kinases and phosphatases, as well as by their high degree of sequence conservation across all eukaryotic organisms. Protein kinases catalyze the transfer of the γ-phosphate from ATP to specific amino acids, while protein phosphatases hydrolyze

the phosphoester bond to release the phosphate and regenerate the unmodified amino acid. Hence, the balance of kinase and phosphatase activities determines the phosphorylation state of proteins, and nature has developed intricate spatial and temporal control mechanisms for each class of enzymes.

Whereas prokaryotic proteins are commonly phosphorylated on histidine (His) and aspartate (Asp) residues, protein phosphorylation in eukaryotes occurs mainly on serine (Ser), threonine (Thr), and tyrosine (Tyr) residues. This Chapter focuses, therefore, on the structure and function of kinases and phosphatases that act on Ser, Thr, and Tyr in proteins. The role of protein kinases in pain will be discussed in Chapter 17.

At least a third of all cellular proteins are phosphorylated at any given time, and greater than 99% of this phosphorylation is on Ser and Thr residues. The relative scarcity of phospho(p)-Tyr resulted in the discovery of this modification more than two decades after the discovery of Ser/Thr phosphorylation. A phosphate adds considerable bulk and two negative charges to an amino acid and can either build or destroy interaction surfaces between proteins or between proteins and other cell constituents. More commonly, phosphorylation will induce conformational changes to alter the activity or macromolecular interactions of enzymes and ion channels.

CLASSIFICATION

In the human genome, 518 genes or 1.7%, code for protein kinases. The "kinome" is opposed by about 140 genes encoding recognizable protein phosphatase catalytic domains (Fig.15.1, see also the color plate). This imbalance is particularly pronounced for Ser/Thr modifying enzymes, where the kinases outnumber the phosphatases by 10 to 1, and may reflect a greater promiscuity of the phosphatases for their substrates. However, Ser/Thr phosphatase catalytic subunits, including PP1 and PP2A tend to associate with a large array of regulatory subunits, which contribute substrate specificity as discussed later in the Chapter.

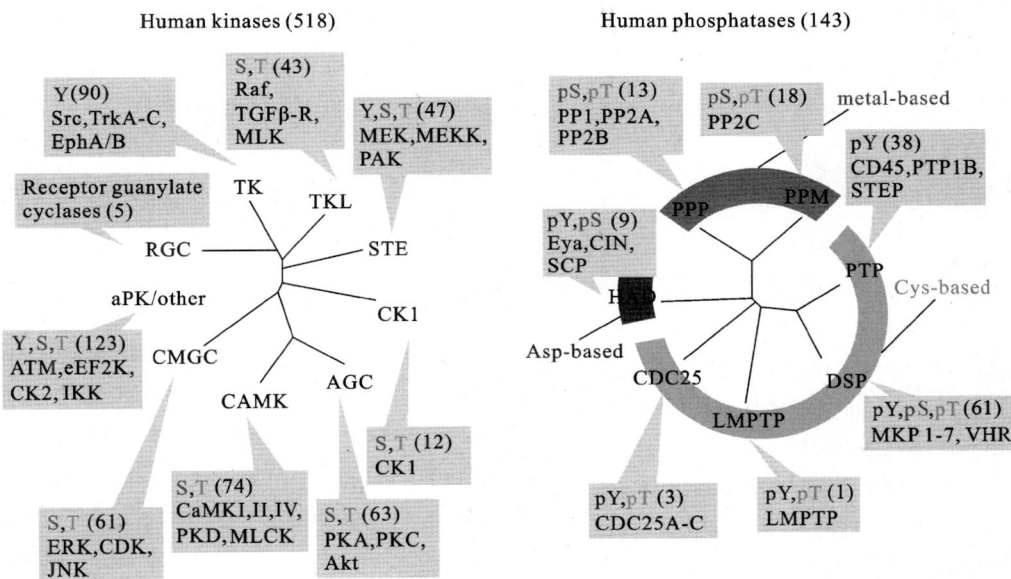

Fig.15.1 The human kinome and phosphatome. The human complement of protein kinases (left) and protein phosphatases (right) has been identified and divided into groups based on sequence similarity and catalytic mechanisms. The number of enzymes within each group, as well as a few representative members are listed. The kinomes and phosphatomes of other mammals are very similar, as was recently shown for the mouse. The 518 human protein kinases share catalytic mechanisms and belong to seven groups which phosphorylate serine (S), threonine (T), and tyrosine (Y) as indicated. The RGC group contains receptor guanylate cyclases with an inactive kinase domain that shares sequence similarity with the tyrosine kinases (TK). The large atypical protein kinase (aPK) and "other" groups contain more distantly related kinases. The number of human protein phosphatases is approximate, because the haloacid dehalogenase (HAD)-family of phosphatases has not yet been fully catalogued. Color coding indicates distinct catalytic mechanisms to dephosphorylate p-serine (pS), -threonine (pT), and -tyrosine (pY).

Kinases

Most of the 518 human protein kinases fall into the eukaryotic protein kinase (ePK) super-group, characterized by a well-conserved catalytic domain (Fig. 15.1). The remaining 8% have kinase activity, but they feature less well-conserved catalytic domains and are therefore classified as atypical protein kinases (aPK). EPKs are further subdivided into seven groups based on sequence similarity, which tends to predict substrate specificity and regulatory mechanisms.

The tyrosine kinase (TK) group includes receptor TKs (RTKs), such as the neurotrophin receptors TrkA/B/C and the eph receptors. Eph receptors have undergone an explosive gene expansion to become the largest RTK family in the vertebrate lineage, which reflects their importance in axonal pathfinding and other developmental processes. Src and related kinases make up the subgroup of non-receptor TKs.

The receptor guanylate cyclase (RGC) group includes the receptors for atrial natriuretic factor and retinal guanylate cyclase. The tyrosine kinase like domain of the RGC regulates cGMP formation, but has no phosphoryl transfer activity.

Unintuitively, the diverse group of tyrosine kinase like (TKL) kinases is composed of Ser/Thr kinases such as Raf and the type 1 and 2 TGFβ receptors. The STE group (homologs of yeast Sterile 7/11/20 kinases) contains mitogen-activated protein kinase (MAPK) cascade families including MEK and MEKK with Ser/Thr or dual (Ser/Thr/Tyr) specificity.

The remaining four groups (CK1, AGC, CAMK, CMGC) contain exclusively Ser/Thr kinases. Twelve kinases related to casein kinase 1 form the CK1 group, while the AGC group is named after three of its well-known members, PKA, PKG, and PKC. Many, but not all kinases in the CAMK group are activated by calcium/calmodulin, like its founding family, the calmodulin (CaM) kinases. Finally, the CMGC family includes the proline-directed kinases of the MAPK and cyclin-dependent kinase (CDK) families, as well as glycogen synthase kinase-3 (GSK3).

Phosphatases

The approximately 140 human protein phosphatases are classified according to catalytic mechanisms as metal-based, Cys-based, or Asp-based phosphatases. Further divisions are based on sequence and structural similarities (Fig.15.1). The metal-based phosphatases are specific for p-Ser/Thr and belong to two groups, PPP and PPM. The PPP group includes the catalytic subunits of PP1, PP2A, PP2B (or calcineurin), and PP4-7. The PPM (or PP2C) family consists of magnesium-dependent protein phosphatases with some structural similarity to PPP-class catalytic domains. PP1, PP2A, PP2B, and PP2C account for the majority of Ser/Thr phosphatase activity and are abundant proteins, particularly in brain. The more recently identified PP4 through PP7 are less abundant and may have relatively narrow substrate specificities.

Cys-based phosphatases feature a conserved catalytic motif (CX_5R) and are classified into four groups. Similar to the Tyr kinases, the protein Tyr phosphatase (PTP) group can be further divided into receptor and non-receptor PTPs. The group of dual-specificity phosphatases (DSPs) includes the MAPK phosphatases (MKPs) that dephosphorylate Tyr and Thr residues in the activation loop of the MAPKs. The LMPTP group is defined by a single member in the human genome, the low molecular weight protein Tyr phosphatase, an ancestral enzyme with homologs in bacteria. Members of the CDC25 group of dual specificity phosphatases are structurally related to rhodaneses, and they function as cell cycle regulators by dephosphorylating and activating CDKs.

The Asp-based phosphatases are related to the prokaryotic haloacid dehalogenase (HAD) superfamily of hydrolases and are characterized by a catalytic motif containing two aspartates (DXDXT). This growing group of Tyr/Ser phosphatases contains the eyes absent (Eya) transcription factors, a cofilin phosphatase, and RNA polymerase II C-terminal domain phosphatases, which contribute to neuronal-specific gene expression.

STRUCTURE AND CATALYTIC MECHANISMS

Kinases

The highly conserved ePK catalytic domain adopts a two-lobed structure containing an N-terminal and a C-terminal lobe. The smaller N-lobe and larger C-lobe bind ATP and protein substrates, respectively, to coordinate the phosphoryl transfer in the cleft between the lobes. An invariant Lys residue, which is often mutated to produce "kinase-dead" or "dominant-negative" versions of kinases, and a glycine-rich phosphate binding (P) loop form the ATP binding site.

Two regions in the C-lobe that are critical for catalysis are the catalytic loop and the activation loop. The catalytic loop contains a conserved Asp residue, which acts as the catalytic base, to deprotonate the hydroxyl group of the substrate residue for nucleophilic attack of the γ-phosphate of ATP. The orientation of the activation loop is essential for proper alignment of the γ-phosphate and the substrate residue. The activation loop is often phosphorylated as discussed below.

Kinases exist in inactive and active conformations. The structural transformation can be quite dramatic between the two states. The active confirmation for all kinases appears to be very similar, which implies that precise orientation of the catalytic pocket is necessary for efficient kinase activity. Conversely, the inactive confirmations are quite diverse. While ATP is often able to bind the inactive confirmation, the N-lobe is positioned to prevent proper alignment with the protein substrate-binding pocket.

The structure of the activation loop varies greatly between the active and inactive conformations. In the active conformation, the activation loop takes on a rigid, open conformation that facilitates proper substrate binding. In the inactive kinase, the activation loop either blocks access to the substrate binding site or is disorganized, preventing the required contacts with the substrate residue.

Phosphatases

Protein phosphatases use different mechanisms for hydrolysis of phosphoester bonds. Protein Ser/Thr phosphatases belong to a large and diverse family of metallophosphoesterase enzymes, which also include DNA polymerases and exonucleases. The catalytic domain consists of a β-α-β-α-β-α-β scaffolding structure. The most highly conserved amino acids are situated in loops between secondary structures and make contacts with two metal ions ($Fe^{2+/3+}$, Zn^{2+}, and/or Mn^{2+}). The metal ions increase the nucleophilic character of a water molecule so it can directly displace the phosphate from the phosphorylated residue. This mechanism does not require the formation of a phosphoenzyme intermediate and allows for high rates of catalysis.

The related Tyr and dual-specificity phosphatases do not require metal ions for catalysis. The structure of these Cys-based phosphatases consists of four parallel β-sheets sandwiched between α-helices. The PTP signature motif (CX_5R) provides the catalytic Cys residue and an Arg residue that interacts with the phosphate. Due to the local environment, the Cys is partially deprotonated, allowing for its nucleophilic attack on the phosphorus atom and formation of a p-Cys intermediate. An invariant Asp residue outside the signature motif is also important for catalysis, as it protonates the dephosphorylated residue. A water molecule activated by acidic amino acids subsequently hydrolyzes the p-Cys to complete the catalytic cycle. Mutation of either the invariant Cys or Asp results in "substrate trapping" phosphatases that forms stable complexes with substrates. These mutants have led to the identification of many physiological substrates of Cys-based phosphatases.

The depth of the catalytic pocket determines the preference of Cys-based phosphatases for certain phosphoamino acids. Dual-specificity phosphatases have shallower catalytic pockets than tyrosine-specific phosphatases, allowing both p-Tyr and the shorter p-Thr to reach the catalytic Cys. Hydrophobic stacking interactions between the enzyme and the p-Tyr phenyl ring further increase specificity for p-Tyr.

The recently discovered group of Asp-dependent, or HAD-domain phosphatases employ a catalytic mechanism involving a p-Asp intermediate. Similar to the catalytic Cys in Cys-dependent phosphatases, the first Asp in the HAD signature (DXDXT) engages in a nucleophilic attack on the phosphate, while the second Asp protonates the substrate leaving group.

SUBSTRATE SPECIFICITY

As discussed in the previous section, the catalytic pockets of protein kinases and phosphatases can discriminate between different phosphorylatable or phosphorylated amino acids. Substrate selection is also influenced by the interaction of residues adjacent to the phosphorylation site with residues near the catalytic site. For the major kinase groups, relatively stringent consensus phosphorylation sequences have been defined by comparing phosphorylation sites in natural substrates, as well as by *in vitro* kinase assays with synthetic substrate peptides. Kinases in the AGC and CAMK groups are collectively referred to as basophilic kinases because they prefer to phosphorylate Ser/Thr with Arg residues at the –2 and/or –3 position. The CMGC group consists of proline-directed kinases that recognize the [S/T]P consensus motif. The predictive power of scanning a primary amino acid sequence for putative phosphorylation sites is somewhat diminished by the possibility that certain sites may be buried or otherwise inaccessible. Conversely, it would have not been possible to predict some phosphorylation sites with established relevance to synaptic plasticity, e.g. the CaM kinase II phosphorylation site, Ser831, in the GluR1 subunit of the AMPA-type glutamate receptor, based on primary amino acid sequence.

Compared to protein kinases, phosphatases rely less on the amino acid residues surrounding the phosphorylation site and few consensus dephosphorylation sequences have been reported. In the case of the Ser/Thr phosphatases of the PPP group, association of the catalytic subunit with variable regulatory subunits extends the substrate interaction surface to provide specificity (BOX 15.1, see also the color plate).

Secondary kinase/phosphatase interaction sites, often located far away from the actual phosphorylation site, can also contribute to signaling specificity by increasing the local concentration of enzyme and substrate. A "common docking" (CD) domain on the C-lobe of the MAP kinases interacts with these short docking sites, which are found not only on MAP ki-

nase substrates but also on the kinases and phosphatases that regulate MAP kinase activity.

Distant docking sites are also being discovered in phosphatase substrates. Dephosphorylation of the PKA site Ser1928 in the L-type calcium channel subunit $Ca_V1.2$ by PP2A depends on a PP2A binding site at the extreme C terminus of the channel. Thus, these docking interactions help assemble ternary complexes between ion channels, kinases, and phosphatases to fine-tune neuronal excitability.

BOX 15.1 Structural basis of PP1 substrate specificity.

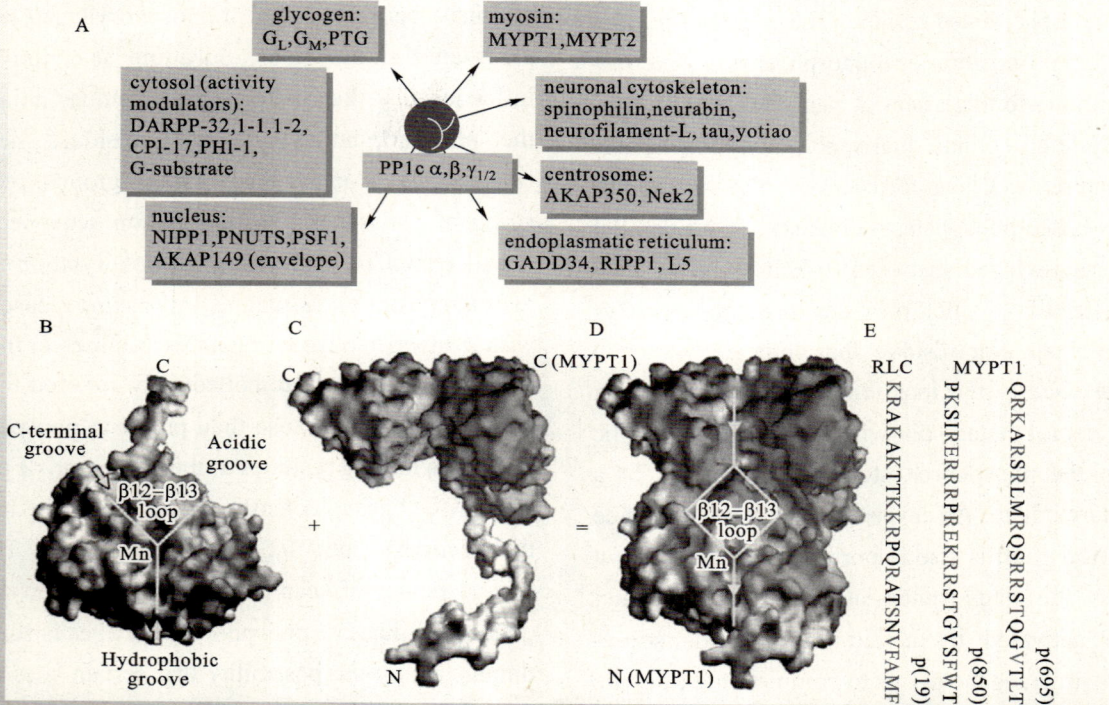

A. Four closely related PP1 catalytic subunits (PP1c α,β, γ1, γ2) associate with a growing list of anchoring and regulatory proteins to dephosphorylate proteins in a variety of cellular locations (bolded). Most PP1 regulatory proteins contain a RVxF motif that contributes to the interaction with PP1c. The crystal structure of PP1c complexed with a regulatory protein, myosin phosphatase targeting subunit 1 (MYPT1), illustrates how regulatory subunits confer substrate specificity. B. PP1c is a globular protein with a C-terminal extension. Three groves (C-terminal, acidic and hydrophobic grove) form a Y-shaped catalytic surface (yellow) with catalysis occurring in the center. C. The N-terminal fragment of MYPT1 consists of an extended, hydrophobic N terminus that includes the RVxF motif, and an ankyrin-repeat domain with numerous acidic surface charges (red). D. The PP1c-MYPT1 complex forms by insertion of the catalytic subunit's C-terminal tail between MYPT1's ankyrin repeats, and MYPT1's N-terminal tail wrapping halfway around PP1. This extends the substrate-binding surface (yellow) to include a long acidic groove on MYPT1. The acidic charges preferentially attract substrates with clustered basic residues such as myosin regulatory side chain (RLC sequence in (E)).

REGULATION

The enzymes discussed in this Chapter act as nodes in complex regulatory networks and have evolved mechanisms to integrate multiple inputs and translate them into precisely timed and localized changes in substrate phosphorylation. Kinases and phosphatases are commonly modular proteins that array a catalytic domain with various regulatory domains. These regulatory domains mediate interactions with other macromolecules and either directly or indirectly responds to second messengers to alter the conformation and activity of the catalytic domain. Smaller kinases (such as PKA) and phosphatases (such as PP1) consist of little more than the catalytic domain and have outsourced much of their regulation to separate polypeptides or regulatory subunits.

Kinases

The prototypical mechanism of kinase regulation is phosphorylation, either by the kinase itself (autophosphorylation) or by other kinases. Most kinases participate in kinase cascades, which provide signal amplification as well as opportunities for signal integration and crosstalk. The major MAP kinase cascades involve sequential kinase activation by phosphorylation of residues within the activation loop of the catalytic domain. Another common mechanism of kinase activation involves phosphorylation-dependent displacement of a pseudosubstrate sequence from the catalytic cleft. Kinase inhibition by phosphorylation can also occur in multiple ways. GSK3 prefers substrates with a +4 Ser "primed" by phosphorylation by another kinase. Inhibition of GSK3 involves phosphorylation of an N-terminal Ser that then competes with the substrate's primed Ser for binding to a site on the catalytic domain. In the case of calcium/calmodulin-dependent protein kinase II (CaMKII), calcium/ calmodulin binding to its regulatory domain induces a complex series of activating and inhibitory autophosphorylations that are critical for synaptic plasticity (BOX 15.2, see also the color plate).

A well-defined example of the influence of phosphorylation state on kinase function is illustrated by Src-family kinases, which include the brain-enriched Fyn. At the N-terminus, Src contains both a Src homology 2 (SH2) and a Src homology 3 (SH3) domain, which are both involved with protein–protein interactions. In the inactive confirmation, Src is phosphorylated at its C-terminus, Tyr527, by Csk (carboxy-terminal Src kinase), and then p-Tyr527 forms an intra-molecular interaction with the SH2 domain (Fig.15.2, see also the color plate). Additional interactions occur with the polyproline type II helix just N-terminal to the kinase domain to lock the kinase in the inactive state. Upon dephosphorylation at Tyr527, the kinase adopts an active confirmation and autophosphorylates Tyr416, which lies within the activation loop, to increase kinase activity and become fully active (Fig.15.2).

In addition to the SH2 and SH3 domains, kinases contain and are regulated by many other macromolecular interaction domains. RTKs and the Ser/Thr kinases of the TGFβ receptor family feature N-terminal extracellular ligand binding domains followed by a transmembrane helix and the cytosolic kinase domain. Generally, ligand binding induces receptor dimerization and activation by cross-phosphorylation.

Phosphatases

Protein phosphatases were once considered fairly promiscuous, constitutively active enzymes that provide the substrates for regulated kinase signaling. It has recently become clear that the activities of many protein phosphatases are as tightly controlled as kinase activities. The influence of phosphatase regulation on a hypothetical cellular response is illustrated in Fig.15.3. It is evident that reciprocal regulation of kinases and phosphatases boosts both signal amplitude and duration, which can introduce complex signal decay kinetics and even oscillatory behavior.

BOX 15.2   Regulation of postsynaptic calcium/calmodulin-dependent protein kinase II (CaMKII).

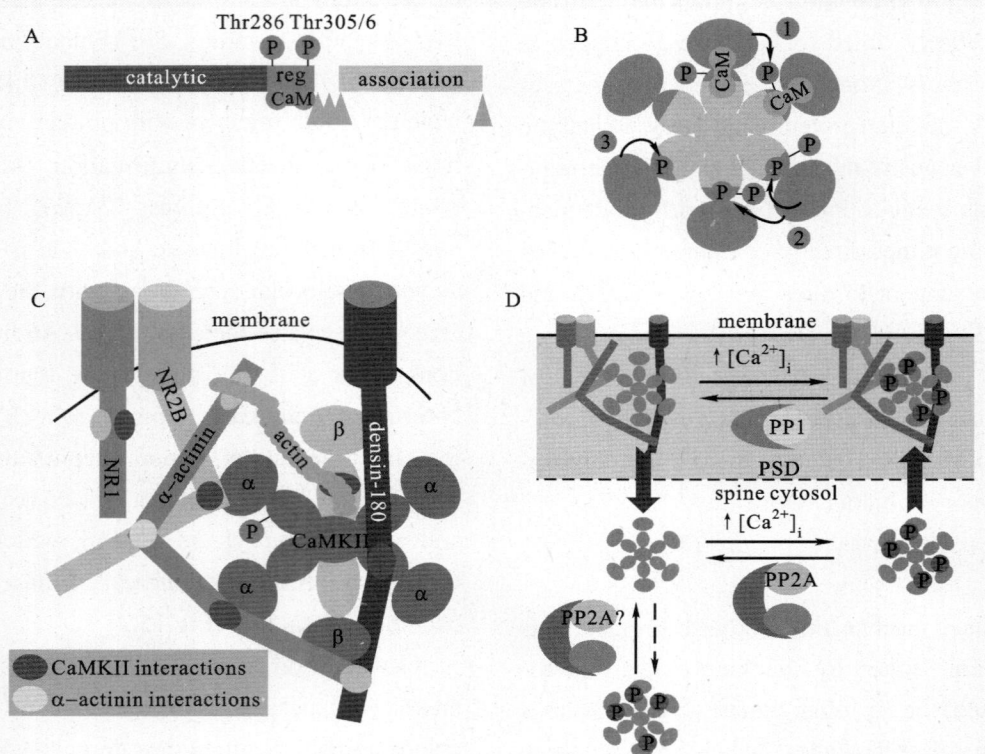

CaMKII is a family of ubiquitously expressed kinases that can integrate the amplitude and frequency of intracellular Ca^{2+} spikes into a range of activity levels. The major neuronal isoform, CaMKIIα, is particularly concentrated in the dendritic spines of mature excitatory synapses, where it serves as a critical link between NMDA receptor-dependent calcium influx and induction of long term potentiation (LTP). A. CaMKII subunits consist of an N-terminal catalytic domain, followed by a Ca^{2+}/calmodulin (CaM)-binding regulatory (reg) domain containing autophosphorylation sites. Thr286 autophosphorylation enhances Ca^{2+}/CaM binding and confers Ca^{2+}/CaM-independent activity, whereas Thr305/6 autophosphorylation prevents kinase activation by Ca^{2+}/CaM. The C terminus consists of multiple, alternatively spliced inserts and a holoenzyme association domain. B. The CaMKII holoenzyme is formed by 12–14 subunits arranged as two stacked rings of 6–7 subunits (only one ring shown). Ca^{2+}/CaM binding to two adjacent subunits is required for trans-autophosphorylation at Thr286. Upon Ca^{2+}/CaM release, intra- and inter-subunit burst autophosphorylation occurs at several residues including Thr305/306, and Ser312. In the absence of Ca^{2+}/CaM, CaMKII undergoes slow inhibitory intrasubunit autophosphorylation at Thr306. C. Four CaMKII anchoring proteins (NR2B, densin-180, α-actinin, actin/CaMKIIβ) can simultaneously interact with CaMKII holoenzymes (red ovals, interaction domains). α-actinin additionally crosslinks the other three CaMKII anchoring proteins (yellow ovals). Whereas α-actinin and NR2B bind the catalytic domains of all CaMKII isoforms, densin-180 and actin bind to α/β-isoform-specific sequences in the variable and association domain. The interaction of CaMKII with NR2B is fostered by kinase activation (Ca^{2+}/CaM binding, Thr286 autophosphorylation), while Ca^{2+}/CaM binding to CaMKII displaces actin. Thus, not all interactions occur simultaneously in the same compartment. D. A rise in dendritic Ca^{2+} levels promotes Ca^{2+}/CaM binding, dissociation from F-actin (not shown), and Thr286 autophosphorylation of CaMKII, followed by reversible translocation from the dendritic cytosol to the PSD, perhaps initiated by activity-dependent association with NR2B. Cytosolic and PSD-associated CaMKII are inactivated by two classes of phosphatases, PP2A and PP1, respectively, which are themselves regulated by synaptic activity. PP2A is thus expected to retain CaMKII in the cytosol, and PP1 holoenzymes may promote release of the kinase from the PSD. PP2A may also increase the pool of CaMKII that is competent for translocation by reversing the slow inhibitory autophosphorylation of Thr306 in the absence of Ca^{2+}. Thus, CaMKII localization and kinase activity are finely tuned by the action of two phosphatases, PP1 and PP2A.

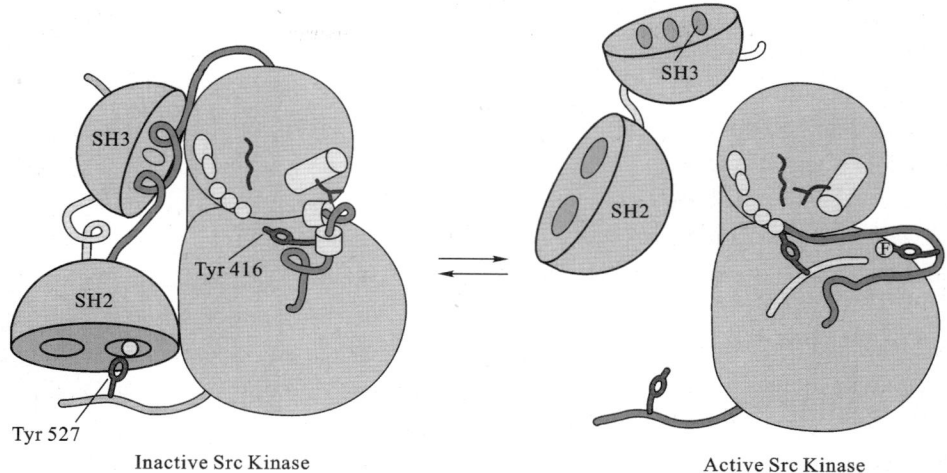

Fig.15.2 Structural basis of Src kinase activation. In the inactive form of Src, (left) intramolecular interactions, especially p-Tyr527-SH2 domain, maintain the activation loop (orange) and αC helix (purple) in improper orientation for substrate binding and kinase activity. Following dephosphorylation of p-Tyr527 and autophosphorylation of Tyr416, the activation loop and αC helix are correctly situated for substrate binding (yellow) and orientation of substrate Tyr (red) with the ATP and Src catalytic amino acids.

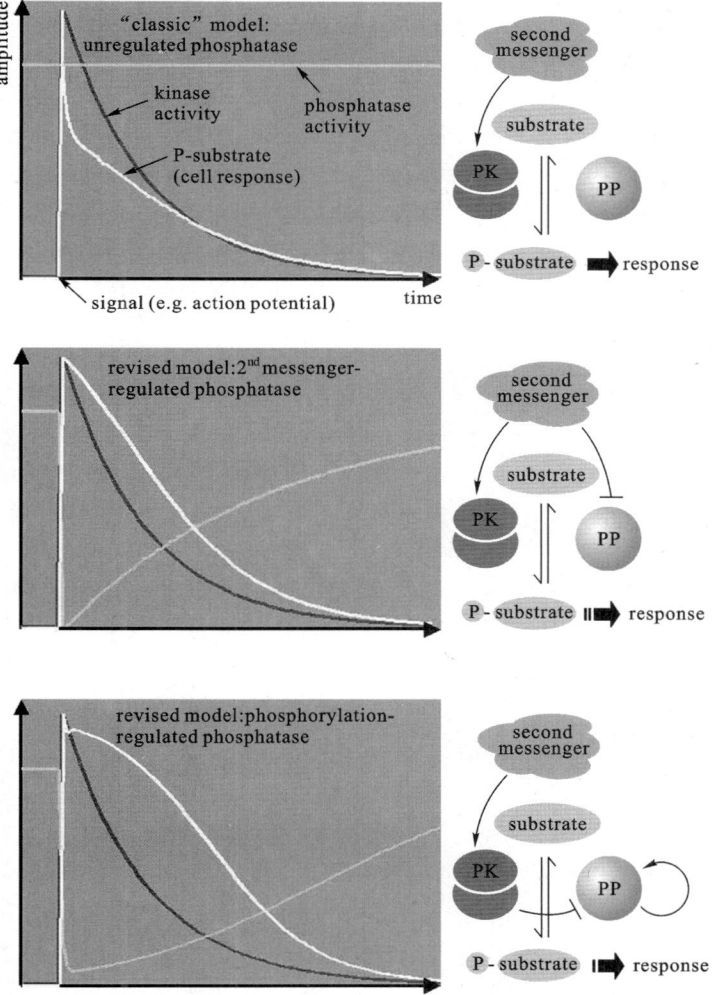

Fig.15.3 Phosphatase regulation influences signal duration. The three models show the time courses of substrate phosphorylation (yellow) as determined by transient activation of a protein kinase (PK) by a second messenger (red) and an opposing protein phosphatase (PP) activity (green). Constitutive, or unregulated phosphatase activity produces a transient phosphorylation response (top panel), while inhibition of the phosphatase by the second messenger (middle) or by kinase phosphorylation (bottom panel) sustains the response. In the bottom model, the phosphatase reactivates through autodephosphorylation.

Most Tyr and dual-specificity phosphatases have a modular domain structure. In addition to the defining catalytic domain, they may contain protein–protein and protein–lipid interacting domains (SH2, PDZ, FERM) and PEST domains, which stimulate protein degradation. The receptor PTPs are characterized by a transmembrane α-helix and N-terminal extracellular domains of variable length that may adopt immunoglobulin- or fibronectin-like folds. Several receptor PTPs have tandem PTP catalytic domains, only the N-terminal of which has catalytic activity. The inactive C-terminal catalytic domain has been suggested to nucleate signal transduction complexes, in analogy to the inactive kinase domains of certain RTKs. Just as most receptor PTP ligands remain unidentified, little is known about PTP activation mechanisms. Current models propose that dimeric receptor PTPs are inactive due to reciprocal inhibitory interactions between the juxtamembrane domain of one subunit and the catalytic domain of the other. Ligands may promote dissociation of receptor dimers to release this inhibition.

Many Tyr and dual-specificity phosphatases are modified by phosphorylation at Tyr and Ser/Thr. Commonly, phosphorylation sites are structurally situated to make autodephosphorylation unlikely, supporting the importance of a regulatory network of phosphatases. Structural studies of the tandem SH2 domain containing SHP2 revealed an intriguing mechanism of activation of this Src kinase activating phosphatase. In the absence of p-Tyr containing ligands, the N-terminal SH2 domain and the catalytic domain interact, preventing p-Tyr binding to either domain. The C-terminal SH2 domain recruits the molecule to an activated, multiple Tyr-phosphorylated receptor tyrosine kinase, thereby facilitating docking of the N-terminal SH2 domain and releasing inhibition of the catalytic domain. This switch-like mechanism presumably arose to prevent the phosphatase from dephosphorylating its own docking sites.

Even though p-Ser and p-Thr are far more abundant than p-Tyr residues in the cell, a surprisingly small number of protein phosphatases is assigned to dephosposphorylate them. Two PPP-group metallophosphatases, PP1 and PP2A, contribute at least 90% of the total Ser/Thr phosphatase activity in most cell types, including neurons. This does not mean that PP1 and PP2A are promiscuous enzymes. Both of these catalytic subunits complex with a large number of regulatory subunits, chaperones, and activity modulators. While the classification of PPP-group regulatory subunits is still in flux, it is estimated than any given cell contains several dozen PP1 and PP2A holoenzymes with distinct subcellular targeting and substrate specificities. BOX 15.1 lists some of the PP1 regulatory subunits. Of particular interest to neuroscientists are DARPP-32 (dopamine-regulated phosphoprotein of 32 kDa), an integrator of dopamine and glutamate neurotransmission, and the actin-binding proteins spinophilin and neurobin, which anchor PP1 to the postsynaptic density of dendritic spines.

The PP2A catalytic subunit is mainly found in a trimeric holoenzyme, which includes a constant scaffold subunit and a variable regulatory subunit. Three unrelated gene families encode regulatory subunits. With few exceptions (BOX 15.3, see also the color plate), little is known about how these subunits work.

Both PP1 and PP2A catalytic subunits are also subject to C-terminal phosphorylation and inhibition by various kinases. The PP2A catalytic subunit is additionally regulated by an unusual posttranslational modification. Its C-terminal Leu residue is reversibly methylated by carboxyl methyltransferase and methylesterase enzymes that display remarkable specificity for PP2A and closely related catalytic subunits. Carboxyl methylation of PP2A is necessary for association with regulatory subunits. Decreased PP2A methylation was detected in the brain of Alzheimer's disease patients, which may explain the hyperphosphorylation of Tau in this neurodegenerative disorder.

PHOSPHORYLATION IN LONG-TERM SYNAPTIC PLASTICITY

Synaptic plasticity refers to modifications of synaptic strength that can last anywhere from seconds up to the lifetime of the organism. Short-term synaptic plasticity is by definition transient and involves predominantly presynaptic mechanisms, such as synaptic vesicle depletion (short-term depression) and residual calcium buildup (short-term potentiation). Long-term synaptic plasticity, the focus of this section, is associated with pre- and postsynaptic changes that include posttranslational modification, new protein synthesis, as well as dramatic changes in synapse morphology and number. The widely held, but not completely uncontested, dogma posits that long-term synaptic plasticity is the physiological substrate of higher cognitive processes including learning and memory. Similar, if not identical, molecular and cellular changes are believed to be associated with the sensory sensiti-

zation and habituation processes that underlie pain perception. While plasticity is a universal attribute of synapses, the detailed signal transduction mechanism by which synaptic strength is dialed up or down can vary between synapses. Postsynaptic calcium influx through the NMDA-type glutamate receptor is a requirement common to most forms of long-term synaptic plasticity.

BOX 15.3 Detecting kinase/phosphatase complexes in living cells.

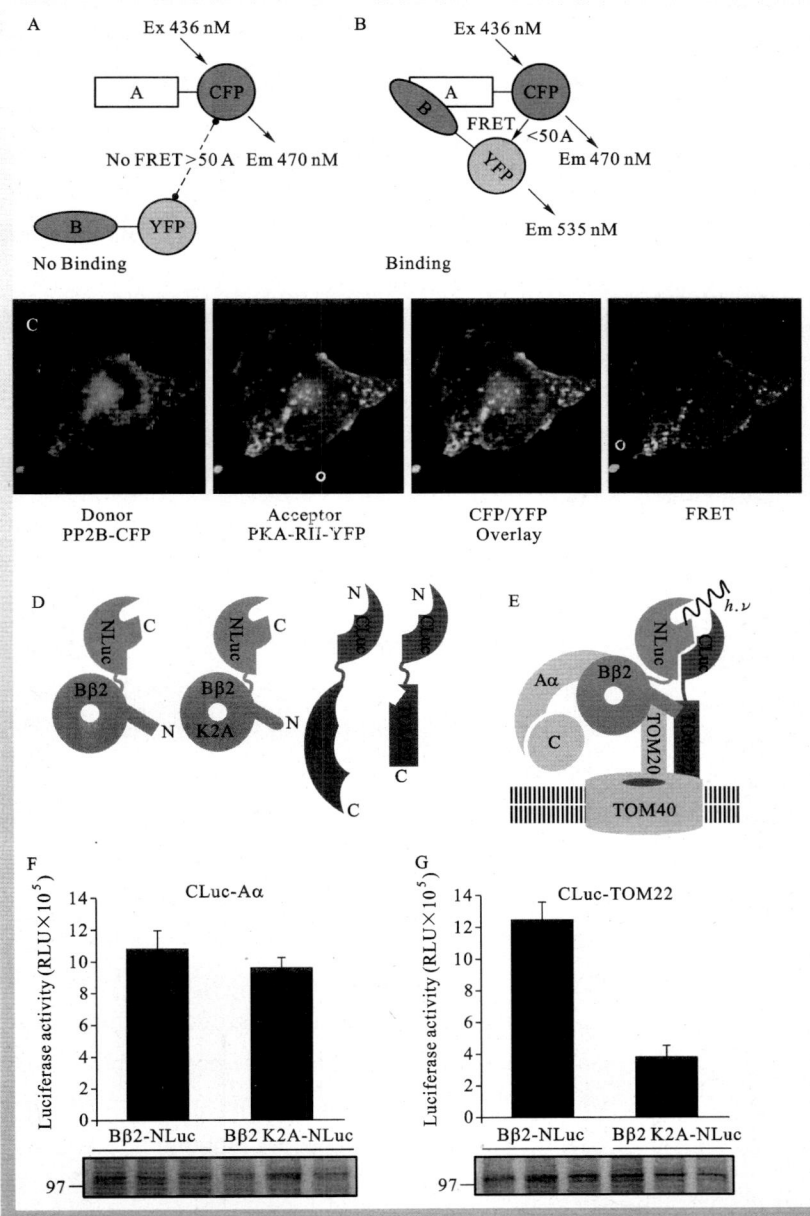

Fluorescence resonance energy transfer (FRET) and the related bioluminescence resonance energy transfer (BRET) have been used to characterize protein–protein interactions in living cells. FRET involves expressing two fusion proteins with different-color fluorescent protein tags (e.g. CFP, YFP), and then illuminating cells to specifically excite the fusion protein with the shorter excitation wavelength (CFP). If no interaction occurs, the emission spectrum will match that of CFP alone (A). If proteins under analysis interact and if their fluorophores are separated by less than 50 nm, some fluorescence energy transfers to YFP, resulting in emission in the yellow band (B). An application of FRET to study kinase/phosphatase complexes is shown in (C). A-kinase anchoring protein 79 (AKAP79) acts as a scaffold for the RII regulatory subunit of PKA and protein phosphatase 2B (PP2B or calcineurin). The left two panels show donor and acceptor fluorescence in cells coexpressing fluorescence-tagged RII and PP2B, in addition to unlabeled AKAP79. While there is only a modest degree of colocalization between the two fluorescent proteins (third panel), FRET indicates that they exist in the same molecular complex whenever they are in the same region of the cell (fourth panel). FRET requires the presence of AKAP79 with intact binding domains for both RII and PP2B.

Protein phosphatase 2A (PP2A) is most often found in a trimeric complex containing a catalytic subunit (C), a scaffolding subunit (A) and regulatory/targeting subunit. The association of a neuron-specific PP2A targeting subunit (Bβ2) with its anchoring protein, the TOM22 receptor in the mitochondrial import complex, was investigated using a biochemist's version of the FRET assay. Luciferase complementation entails coexpressing fusion proteins with complementary fragments of firefly luciferase (NLuc, CLuc) (D). Light emission from cells incubated with the luciferase substrate D-luciferin is indicative of reconstitution of a functional enzyme by interaction of the fusion proteins (E). Both wild-type and a targeting deficient Bβ2 mutant (K2A) interact equally well with the scaffold subunit (Aα) (F). Luciferase complementation with TOM22, however, depends on a functional N-terminal targeting domain in Bβ2 (G).

Depending on the sign of the change, long-term plasticity is classified as long-term potentiation (LTP) or long-term depression (LTD), with the behavioral correlates of memory acquisition (learning) and erasure (forgetting), respectively. Reversible phosphorylation plays an essential role in at least the early phases of LTP and LTD. An emerging concept is that the balance of kinase and phosphatase activities determines whether a synapse undergoes LTP or LTD. LTP in the CA1 region of the hippocampus, the best characterized form of synaptic plasticity, is associated with increased activity of several kinases and decreased activity of a number of phosphatases, while the opposite holds for LTD.

Among protein kinases, the best evidence for an important role in synaptic plasticity currently exists for CaMKII (BOX 15.2). This enzyme has been referred to as a molecular memory device, in that it is activated by the initial calcium influx through the NMDA receptor but can prolong its own activity through autophosphorylation. Mice in which the gene for the major CaMKIIα isoform has been deleted, or which express a CaMKIIα mutant that cannot phosphorylate itself (Thr286 to Ala substitution), exhibit strongly impaired LTP and spatial learning.

As for the role of protein phosphatases in LTP and LTD, the best case can be made for a phosphatase cascade involving the Ca^{2+}/calmodulin-dependent phosphatase calcineurin (PP2B) and PP1. Upon Ca^{2+} influx, PP2B relieves inhibition of PP1 by dephosphorylating a PP1-modulatory protein, inhibitor-1. Active PP1 then induces LTD or counteracts LTP by reversing CaMKII autophosphorylation and dephosphorylating plasticity substrates, such as the GluR1 subunit of the AMPA-type glutamate receptor. Inhibition of PP1 by inducible expression of constitutively active inhibitor-1 improves learning in a transgenic mouse model (BOX 15.4).

Since both LTP and LTD require postsynaptic calcium influx, how is it that LTP involves activation of a calcium-dependent kinase (CaMKII), whereas LTD involves activation of a calcium-dependent phosphatase (PP2B)? One explanation may lie in the differential affinity of the two enzymes for Ca^{2+}/calmodulin. PP2B is preferentially activated by the relatively modest increase in intracellular calcium concentration seen during the low frequency synaptic stimulation that induces LTD. In contrast, only the high frequency stimulation that elicits LTP raises dendritic Ca^{2+} concentration to a level sufficient for CaMKII activation.

What are the crucial kinase/phosphatase substrates in synaptic plasticity? LTP and LTD involve conductance changes of AMPA receptors already inserted in the postsynaptic membrane, as well as AMPA receptor delivery to and removal from the synapse. Several important phosphorylation sites were identified on subunits of the AMPA type glutamate receptor that may regulate various aspects of channel function and surface expression during LTP and LTD. Kinases and phosphatases were also shown to mediate activity-dependent AMPA receptor surface delivery through stargazin and a family of stargazin-like transmembrane AMPA receptor regulatory proteins (TARPs). Stargazer mice, which carry a spontaneous mutation in the stargazin gene, have no detectable AMPA currents in the cerebellum, where expression of the other TARPs is low. NMDA receptor-dependent calcium influx during LTP induction promotes stargazin phosphorylation by both CaMKII and PKC, whereas low frequency calcium spikes to induce LTD cause dephosphorylation of the same sites by the PP2B/PP1 phosphatase cascade. Phosphorylation and dephosphorylation of stargazin is required for LTP and LTD, respectively, as was shown by overexpression of stargazin proteins with phosphorylation sites mutated to prevent or mimic phosphorylation. The phosphorylation-dependent surface delivery of AMPA receptors by stargazin requires the binding of the C terminus of stargazin to a PDZ domain of the postsynaptic density 95 (PSD95) scaffolding protein, which also binds NR2A and NR2B receptor subunits. Reversible phosphorylation of stargazin therefore provides for bidirectional control of AMPA receptor density and synaptic plasticity by calcium influx through the NMDA receptor.

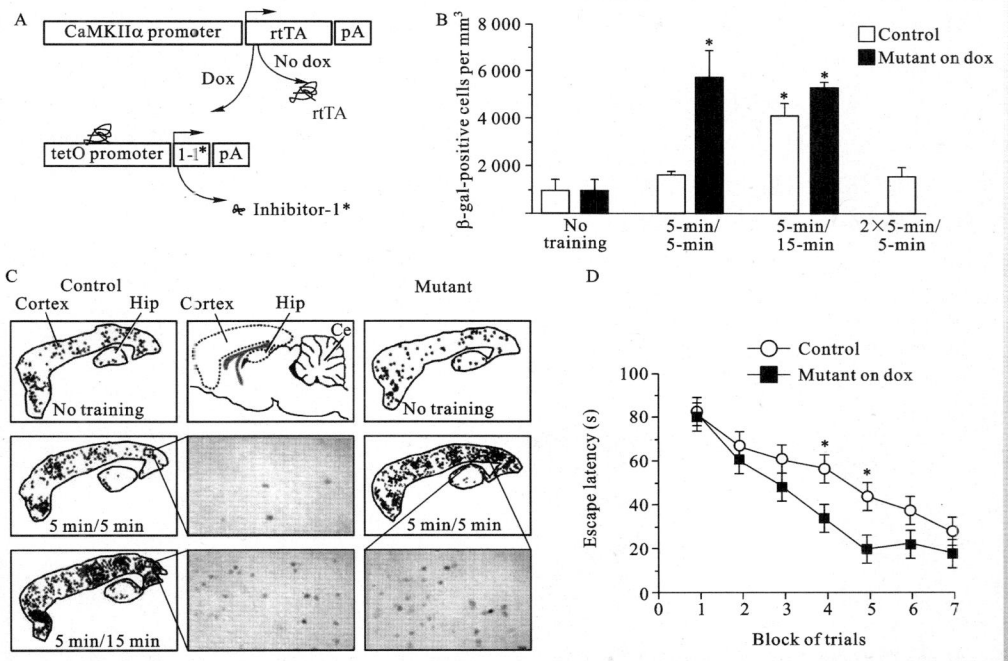

A. To inducibly inhibit PP1 in the forebrain, mice expressing the reverse tetracycline transactivator (rtTA) under the control of forebrain-specific CaMKIIα promoter were crossed with mice expressing a tetracycline-inducible, constitutively active form of a PP1 protein inhibitor, inhibitor-1 (I-1*). Feeding the offspring tetracycline or doxycycline (dox) induces the I-1* transgene and inhibits PP1 activity by 68% and 46% in the hippocampus and cortex, respectively. B. Mice learn the Morris water maze better in a spaced training protocol, where 5 min of training are separated by 15 min rest (5-min/15-min),

than in a massed training protocol with only 5 min rest (5-min/5-min). Phosphorylation of cAMP response element binding protein (CREB), a transcription factor, is counteracted by PP1 and correlates with the learning improvement. PP1 inhibition (mutant on dox) produced a significant increase in phospho-CREB staining after the suboptimal training protocol. C. Representative brains sections clearly depict the graphed data. D. Decreasing PP1 activity improves learning, as shown in a faster decline in escape latency during training in the Morris water maze.

KINASE/PHOSPHATASE COMPLEXES IN SYNAPTIC PLASTICITY

Protein complexes containing ion channels, kinases, phosphatases, and their anchoring proteins are of particular importance for synaptic plasticity, since they enable discretely localized, synapse-specific adjustment of synaptic strength. We have already discussed regulation of the Tyr-kinase Src by intermolecular interactions involving the inhibitory phosphorylation site Tyr527. Src is thought to contribute to LTP by increasing both the number and conductance of postsynaptic NMDA receptors, possibly through direct phosphoryla-

tion of the NR2A and NR2B subunits. Src and a related kinase, Fyn, are brought into proximity of the NMDA receptor through binding to the postsynaptic density 95 (PSD95) protein, a scaffold protein for many postsynaptic ion channels including the NMDA receptor. PTPα is a receptor tyrosine phosphatase with two intracellular phosphatase domains (D1 and D2), although only the D1 domain has enzymatic activity. PTPα also interacts with PSD95, thus assembling a complex of phosphatase, kinase, and the NR1 and NR2A subunits of the NMDA receptor (Fig.15.4A, B). Rather than dephosphorylating NMDA receptor subunits in the PSD95-nucleated complex, PTPα may activate Src by dephosphorylation of the inhibitory Tyr527 residue, which in turn enhances NMDA receptor function. Consistent with this model (Fig.15.4E), intracellular application of the catalytic D1 domain of PTPα enhances NMDA-receptor mediated currents (Fig.15.4C), whereas inhibition of PTPα activity by a D1-specific antibody diminishes NMDA currents (Fig.15.4D).

PSD95 and other MAGUK (membrane associated guanylate kinases) proteins recruit not only Tyr kinases and phosphatases but also their Ser/Thr-specific counterparts to glutamate receptors. PKA and PP2B are recruited via their interaction with A-kinase anchoring protein 79 (AKAP79), which binds to the SH3 and guanylate kinase (GK) domains of PSD95 and SAP97 (synapse-associated protein 97). Rather than regulating each other, PKA and PP2B act on a common set of ion channel substrates. For instance, via an interaction with SAP97, AKAP79 regulates AMPA receptor conductance by mediating phosphorylation of the GluR1 subunit at Ser845.

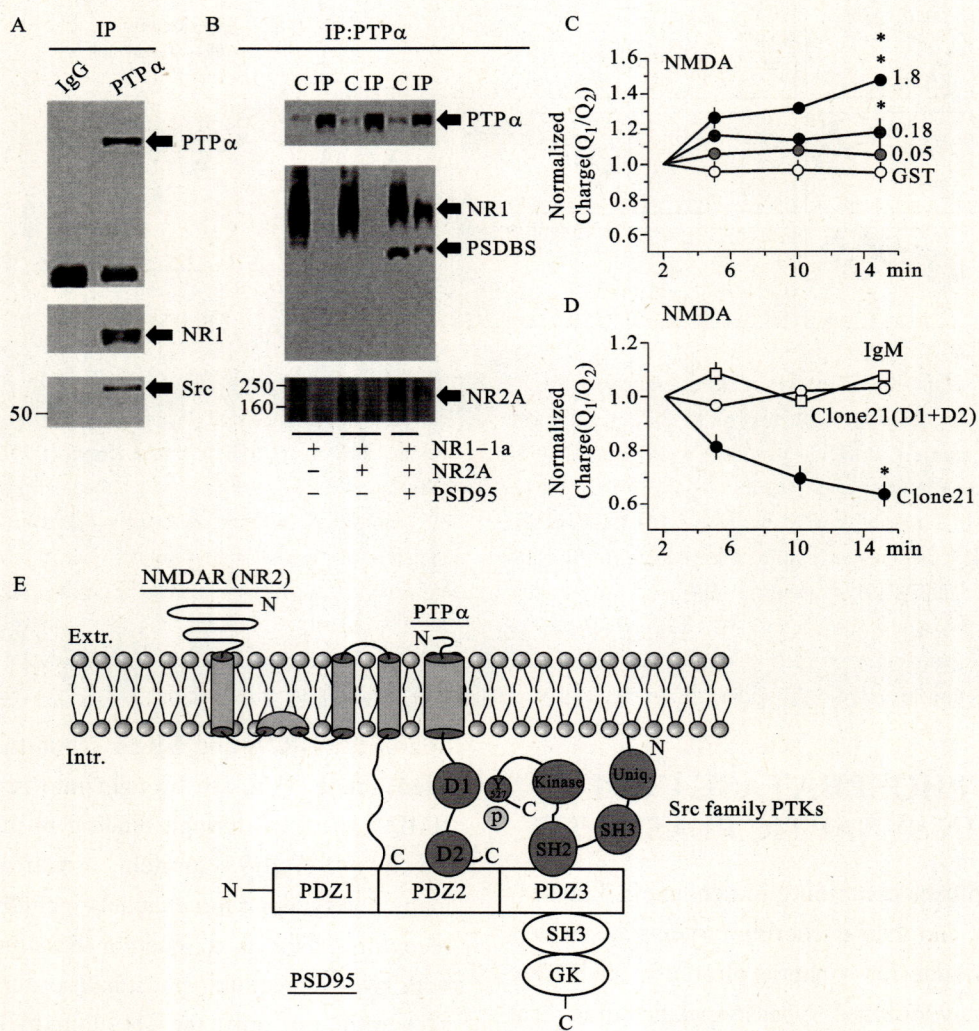

Fig.15.4 PSD95 scaffolds a regulatory complex of Src, PTPα, and the NMDA receptor. A. Immunoprecipitations from rat brain tissue demonstrating a Src, PTPα and NMDA receptor complex. B. Coimmunoprecipitation of NMDA receptor subunits using a PTPα specific antibody requires expression of PSD95 in HEK293 cells. C. An increase in NMDA specific charge is seen in cultured hippocampal neurons with increasing addition of glutathione S-transferase(GST)fused to the two Tyr phosphatase domain(D1+D2) through the recording electrodes. D. Conversely, addition of an antibody specific to the D1 phosphatase domain (clone 21) reduces the NMDA specific charge. This effect is blocked by the addition of GST-D1+D2 fusion protein. E. Model of the NMDA receptor, Src, PTPα complex bridged by PSD95.

RECEPTOR TYROSINE KINASES IN NEURONAL FUNCTION AND PLASTICITY

RTKs are transmembrane proteins with ligand-binding extracellular and catalytic intracellular domains. The Trk and Eph receptors in particular have important roles in neuronal development and function.

The neurotrophins are secreted proteins that activate the Trk family of receptor tyrosine kinase receptors. The interaction of brain-derived neurotrophic factor (BDNF) with its receptor, TrkB, has long been recognized to play a prominent role in the establishment of proper connections between forebrain neurons. Recent evidence points to an additional role of BDNF in modulating neuronal excitability. Genetic deletion of the BDNF gene in mice results in impaired LTP in the hippocampus, which can be restored by viral-mediated expression of BDNF. BDNF binding to presynaptic TrkB can enhance neurotransmitter release, while postsynaptic TrkB mediates phosphorylation of the NMDA receptor and increases its open probability. TrkB also interacts with and modulates the ion influx through the transient receptor potential channel, TrpC3, and directly gates the tetrodotoxin-insensitive sodium channel $Na_v1.9$. The neuromodulator and transmitter-like effects of BDNF and perhaps other neurotrophins may justify referring to the Trk RTKs as a third class of neurotransmitter receptors (next to ionotropic and metabotropic receptors).

The large group of Eph RTKs together with their membrane-bound ligands, the ephrins, form cell contact-mediated signaling complexes important for axon pathfinding, synapse formation and remodeling, angiogenesis, and synaptic plasticity. While the A-ephrins are attached to the cell surface via a glycosylphosphatidylinositol (GPI) anchor, B-ephrin ligands contain a cytosolic domain with no known enzymatic activity. Eph receptors are classified as EphA and EphB receptors based on their ligand specificity for A- and B-ephrins. A unique feature of the ephrin/Eph receptor complex is that it allows for bidirectional signaling across juxtaposed cell surfaces. Clustering of Eph receptors promotes autophosphorylation of multiple Tyr residues, followed by recruitment of SH2-domain containing enzymes and adaptor proteins. The intracellular domain of B-ephrins is phosphorylated by Src family kinases and recruits at least one SH2-domain containing protein. B-ephrins and most Eph receptors contain a C-terminal binding site for synaptic PDZ-containing proteins.

Ephrin-Eph receptor interactions are most often characterized as repulsive, as illustrated by growth cone collapse. However, ephrinB-ephB interactions appear to be positive and are required for dendritic spine formation. Additionally, ephrinA-ephA4 interaction may be required for stabilization of spines by glial cells. The EphB receptor, through its interaction with synaptic PDZ containing protein forms a complex with NMDA receptors, and EphB and B-ephrin knock-out mice have deficits in NMDA receptor-dependent synaptic plasticity and spatial learning. As with other plasticity modulators, EphB-ephrin-B signaling also modulates nociceptive transmission between dorsal root ganglion neurons and neurons in the dorsal horn of the spinal cord, once again emphasizing the molecular parallels between hippocampal synaptic plasticity and pain mechanisms.

KINASES AND PHOSPHATASES IN ADDICTION

Intense research efforts are focused on the role of kinases and phosphatases in mechanisms of addiction. Administration of *D*-amphetamine (*D*-amph) or cocaine leads to massive dopamine release in the ventral striatum (including nucleus accumbens), which in turn enhances overall excitability and glutamate release. In striatal medium-spiny neurons, the combination of dopamine D1 receptor (D1R)-mediated adenylate cyclase stimulation and glutamate-mediated calcium influx results in activation of PKA and ERK MAP kinase signaling cascades. PKA phosphorylates GluR1 at Ser845 to increase AMPA receptor currents, while

ERK phosphorylates transcription factors to induce expression of plasticity-related genes.

A striatum-enriched PP1 modulatory protein related to inhibitor-1, DARPP-32 is critical for boosting phosphorylation of PKA substrates as well as enabling crosstalk with NMDA receptor-dependent signaling cascades. DARPP-32 knockout mice are largely unaffected by several drugs of abuse, underscoring the importance of this protein in psychostimulant action. Several kinase and phosphatase cascades converge on DARPP-32. Thr34 phosphorylation by PKA converts DARPP-32 into a potent inhibitor of PP1. Since PKA and PP1 share many substrates, including GluR1

Ser845, concomitant PKA activation and PP1 inhibition augments both amplitude and duration of cAMP-dependent protein phosphorylation.

In addition, PP1 inhibition by p-Thr34-DARPP-32 synergizes with NMDA receptor-dependent ERK activation at two levels. First, p-Thr34-DARPP-32 acts at the level or upstream of MAPK/ERK kinase 1 (MEK1) to antagonize its inactivation by PP1. Second, PP1 inhibition promotes hyperphosphorylation and inactivation of striatal-enriched phosphatase (STEP), a Tyr-specific phosphatase with remarkable specificity for ERK (Fig.15.5C).

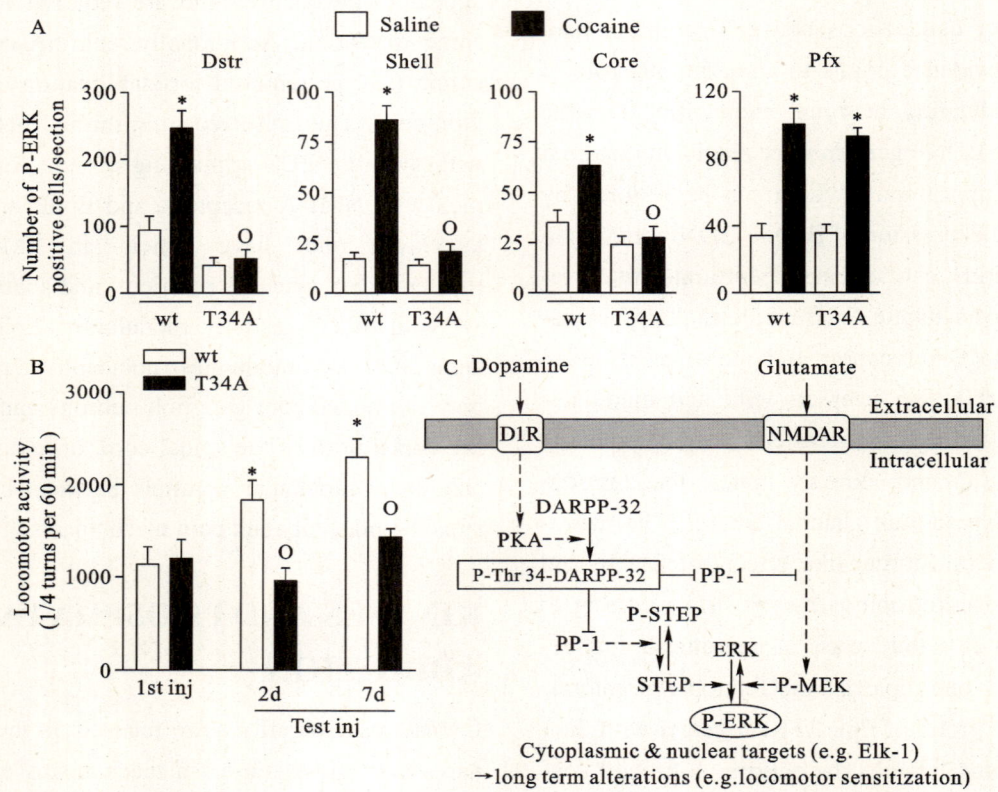

Fig.15.5 Requirement of dopamine-dependent DARPP-32 phosphorylation and NMDA receptor activity for drug-induced behavioral sensitization. Phosphorylation of dopamine-regulated phosphoprotein of 32 kDa (DARPP-32) on Thr34 by PKA converts it into a potent PP1 inhibitor. A. Cocaine induces ERK phosphorylation (P-ERK) in wild-type mice, but not in mice expressing an inactive DARPP-32 mutant (T34A). The DARPP-32 mutation blocks ERK activation in striatum (dorsal striatum, DStr; nucleus accumbens shell and core), but not in the prefrontal cortex (Pfx), which expresses predominantly a related PP1 modulator, Inhibitor-1. B. Blocking Thr34 phosphorylation of DARPP-32 (T34A knock-in mice) prevents an increase in locomotor activity following a second administration of cocaine. C. Coincident activation of dopamine D1 receptors and NMDA-type glutamate receptors activates convergent kinase/phosphatase signaling cascades to induce behavioral sensitization to drug administration. STEP (striatum-enriched phosphatase) is phosphorylated and inactive under basal conditions. Upon dephosphorylation by PP1, STEP inhibits ERK by dephosphorylating a Tyr residue in its activation loop. PP1 also inhibits MAP kinase signaling upstream of ERK.

The dependence of the drug-induced ERK activation on D1R dependent phosphorylation of Thr34-DARPP-32 appears to be specific for the medium-sized spiny neurons of the striatum, since alanine substitution of Thr34 in knock-in mice has no effect on ERK activation in prefrontal cortex (Fig.15.5A). The overall importance of DARPP-32-mediated ERK activation is apparent in behavioral sensitization experiments. Blocking ERK activation with the MEK1 inhibitor SL327 or preventing Thr34 phosphorylation in Thr34Ala-DARPP-32 knock-in animals greatly reduces locomotor activity in response to a second dose of *D*-amph or cocaine (Fig. 15.5C).

CONCLUSION AND FUTURE DIRECTIONS

Protein phosphorylation is paramount for intracellular signaling and is therefore tightly regulated. Precise control of both kinases and phosphatases is maintained through protein modification (mostly phosphorylation), subcellular localization and the formation of large signaling complexes. While the notion of phosphatase regulation is gaining acceptance, we know far more about mechanistic details of kinase regulation.

With the sequencing of genomes from a growing list of organisms, and the development of bioinformatics techniques to mine these sequences, an almost complete list of kinases and phosphatases is now available. At first glance, there appear to be many more kinases than phosphatases. Upon closer examination, however, the number of kinase and phosphatase holoenzymes may turn out to be similar, since many phosphatases form complexes with arrays of regulatory subunits.

The identification of consensus phosphorylation sides in conjunction with recent advances in (phospho)proteomics techniques has allowed us to build complex kinase-substrate networks (BOX 15.5, see also the color plate). Substrate trapping mutants have similarly aided in the identification of some abundant

tyrosine phosphatase substrates. Discovery of specific substrates for the large number of Ser/Thr phosphatase holoenzymes has been hampered by their relatively promiscuous activity *in vitro*, their apparent insensitivity to sequence context, and the lack of substrate trapping mutants.

In vivo (or intact cell) approaches are called for to identify the elusive substrates of Ser/Thr phosphatases and to assemble comprehensive regulatory networks of kinases and phosphatases. These approaches combine RNA interference of kinases/phosphatases and dominant-negative expression with mass-spectrometric identification of phosphorylated peptides in complex protein mixtures.

Microarrays of antibodies directed against different phospho-epitopes are an emerging technology designed to track the phosphorylation state of hundreds of proteins at the same time. Since many inheritable diseases and cancer result from the dysregulation of kinases and phosphatases, these arrays may help uncover disease etiologies and validate drug targets. In addition, phospho-specific antibody arrays may reveal phosphorylation signatures associated with synaptic plasticity and nociception.

GENERAL CITATIONS

Alonso A, Sasin J, Bottini N, Friedberg I, Osterman A, Godzik A, *et al*. 2004. Protein tyrosine phosphatases in the human genome. *Cell*, 117:699-711.

Biondi RM, Nebreda AR. 2003. Signalling specificity of Ser/Thr protein kinases through docking-site-mediated interactions. *Biochem J*, 372:1-13.

Blum R, Konnerth A. 2005. Neurotrophin-mediated rapid signaling in the central nervous system: mechanisms and functions. *Physiology (Bethesda)*, 20:70-78.

Colbran RJ. 2004. Protein phosphatases and calcium/calmodulin-dependent protein kinase II-dependent synaptic plasticity. *J Neurosci*, 24:8404-8409.

Gallego M, Virshup DM. 2005. Protein serine/threonine phosphatases: life, death, and sleeping. *Curr Opin Cell Biol*, 17:197-202.

BOX 15.5 A protein-protein interaction and phosphorylation network centered on the NMDA-type. glutamate receptor.

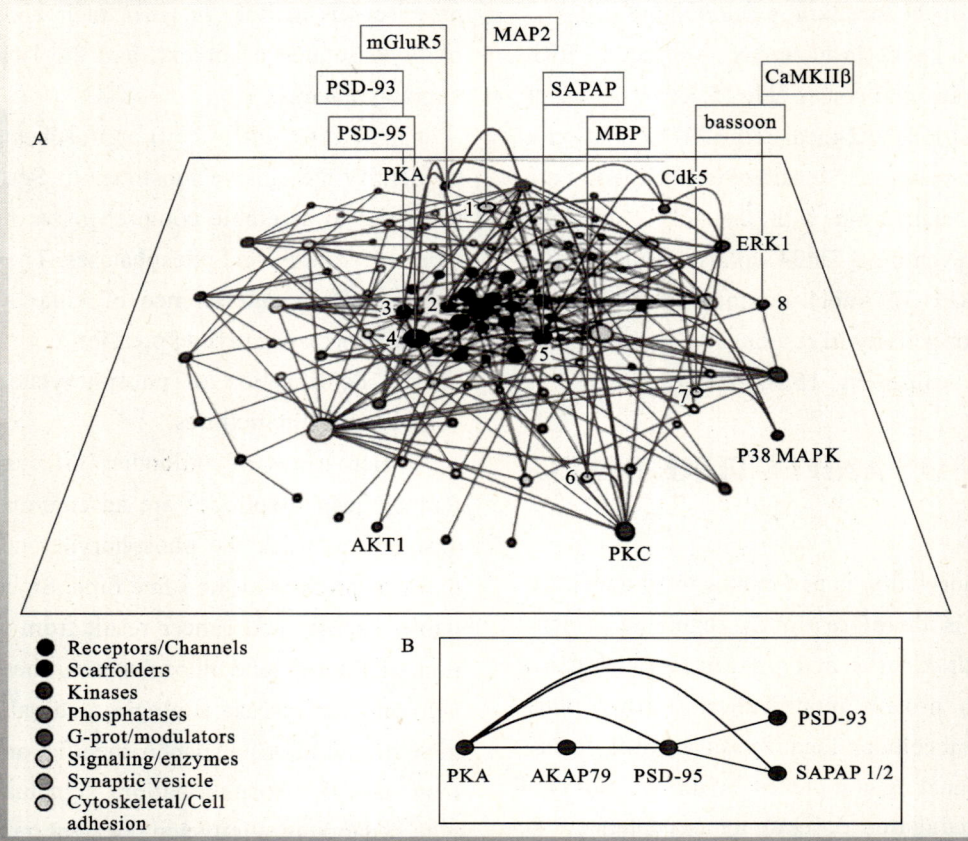

A. The planar map is a protein-protein interaction network based on 248 binary interactions centered on the NR1 subunit of the NMDA receptor; nodes are color-coded according to protein class. Phosphoproteins and specific phosphorylation sites were identified by affinity-purification of phosphopeptides derived from a synaptosomal preparation followed by mass spectroscopy. Kinase-substrate interactions (arches) were inferred based on consensus phosphorylation sequences. Red arches emanate from kinases that are part of the NMDA receptor complex; blue arches connect to kinase that perhaps only transiently associate with the complex .B. A section of the network illustrates the importance of AKAP79 for bringing PKA in close proximity to its physiological substrates, three postsynaptic scaffolding proteins. This kind of proteomic network analysis can help prioritize the functional characterization of particular kinase-substrate interactions

Huse M, Kuriyan J. 2002. The conformational plasticity of protein kinases. *Cell*, 109:275-282.

Klein R. 2004. Eph/ephrin signaling in morphogenesis, neural development and plasticity. *Curr Opin Cell Biol*, 16:580-589.

Manning G, Whyte DB, Martinez R, Hunter T, Sudarsanam S. 2002. The protein kinase complement of the human genome. *Science*, 298:1912-1934.

Munton RP, Vizi S, Mansuy IM. 2004. The role of protein phosphatase-1 in the modulation of synaptic and structural plasticity. *FEBS Lett*, 567:121-128.

Salter MW, Kalia LV. 2004. Src kinases: a hub for NMDA receptor regulation. *Nat Rev Neurosci*, 5:317-328.

DISCOVERY CITATIONS

Battaglia AA, Sehayek K, Grist J, McMahon SB, Gavazzi I. 2003. EphB receptors and ephrin-B ligands regulate spinal sensory connectivity and modulate pain processing. *Nat*

Neurosci, 6:339-340.

Blum R, Kafitz KW, Konnerth A. 2002. Neurotrophin-evoked depolarization requires the sodium channel Na(V)1.9. *Nature*, 419:687-693.

Caenepeel S, Charydczak G, Sudarsanam S, Hunter T, Manning G. 2004. The mouse kinome: discovery and comparative genomics of all mouse protein kinases. *Proc Natl Acad Sci USA*, 101:11707-11712.

Collins MO, Yu L, Coba MP, Husi H, Campuzano I, Blackstock WP, *et al.* 2005. Proteomic analysis of *in vivo* phosphorylated synaptic proteins. *J Biol Chem*, 280:5972-5982.

Davare MA, Horne MC, Hell JW. 2000. Protein phosphatase 2A is associated with class C L-type calcium channels (Cav1.2) and antagonizes channel phosphorylation by cAMP-dependent protein kinase. *J Biol Chem*, 275:39710-39717.

Davare MA, Avdonin V, Hall DD, Peden EM, Burette A, Weinberg RJ, *et al.* 2001. A beta2 adrenergic receptor signaling complex assembled with the Ca^{2+} channel Cav1.2. *Science*, 293:98-101.

Frame S, Cohen P, Biondi RM. 2001. A common phosphate binding site explains the unique substrate specificity of GSK3 and its inactivation by phosphorylation. *Mol Cell*, 7:1321-1327.

Genoux D, Haditsch U, Knobloch M, Michalon A, Storm D, Mansuy IM. 2002. Protein phosphatase 1 is a molecular constraint on learning and memory. *Nature*, 418:970-975.

Gomez LL, Alam S, Smith KE, Horne E, Dell'Acqua ML. 2002. Regulation of A-kinase anchoring protein 79/150-cAMP-dependent protein kinase postsynaptic targeting by NMDA receptor activation of calcineurin and remodeling of dendritic actin. *J Neurosci*, 22:7027-7044.

Henkemeyer M, Itkis OS, Ngo M, Hickmott PW, Ethell IM. 2003. Multiple EphB receptor tyrosine kinases shape dendritic spines in the hippocampus. *J Cell Biol*, 163:1313-1326.

Kafitz KW, Rose CR, Thoenen H, Konnerth A. 1999. Neurotrophin-evoked rapid excitation through TrkB receptors. *Nature*, 401:918-921.

Lei G, Xue S, Chery N, Liu Q, Xu J, Kwan CL, *et al.* 2002. Gain control of N-methyl-D-aspartate receptor activity by receptor-like protein tyrosine phosphatase alpha. *Embo J*, 21:2977-2989.

Li HS, Xu XZ, Montell C. 1999. Activation of a TRPC3-dependent cation current through the neurotrophin BDNF. *Neuron*, 24:261-273.

Murai KK, Nguyen LN, Irie F, Yamaguchi Y, Pasquale EB. 2003. Control of hippocampal dendritic spine morphology through ephrin-A3/EphA4 signaling. *Nat Neurosci*, 6:153-160.

Oliveria SF, Gomez LL, Dell'Acqua ML. 2003. Imaging kinase—AKAP79—phosphatase scaffold complexes at the plasma membrane in living cells using FRET microscopy. *J Cell Biol*, 160:101-112.

Sontag E, Hladik C, Montgomery L, Luangpirom A, Mudrak I, Ogris E, *et al.* 2004. Downregulation of protein phosphatase 2A carboxyl methylation and methyltransferase may contribute to Alzheimer disease pathogenesis. *J Neuropathol Exp Neurol*, 63: 1080-1091.

Svenningsson P, Tzavara ET, Carruthers R, Rachleff I, Wattler S, Nehls M, *et al.* 2003. Diverse psychotomimetics act through a common signaling pathway. *Science*, 302:1412-1415.

Tavalin SJ, Colledge M, Hell JW, Langeberg LK, Huganir RL, Scott JD. 2002. Regulation of GluR1 by the A-kinase anchoring protein 79 (AKAP79) signaling complex shares properties with long-term depression. *J Neurosci*, 22:3044-3051.

Terrak M, Kerff F, Langsetmo K, Tao T, Dominguez R. 2004. Structural basis of protein phosphatase 1 regulation. *Nature*, 429:780-784.

Tomita S, Stein V, Stocker TJ, Nicoll RA, Bredt DS. 2005. Bidirectional synaptic plasticity regulated by phosphorylation of stargazin-like TARPs. *Neuron*, 45:269-277.

Tootle TL, Silver SJ, Davies EL, Newman V, Latek RR, Mills IA, *et al.* 2003. The transcription factor Eyes absent is a protein tyrosine phosphatase. *Nature*, 426:299-302.

Vafai SB, Stock JB. 2002. Protein phosphatase 2A methylation: a link between elevated plasma homocysteine and Alzheimer's Disease. *FEBS Lett*, 518:1-4.

Valjent E, Pascoli V, Svenningsson P, Paul S, Enslen H, Corvol JC, *et al.* 2005. Regulation of a protein phosphatase cascade allows convergent dopamine and glutamate signals to activate ERK in the striatum. *Proc Natl Acad Sci USA*, 102:491-496.

Activity-dependent Gene Regulation: How Do Synapses Talk to the Nucleus and Fine-tune Neuronal Outputs?

CHAPTER 16

Haruhiko Bito, Sayaka Takemoto-Kimura, Hiroyuki Okuno

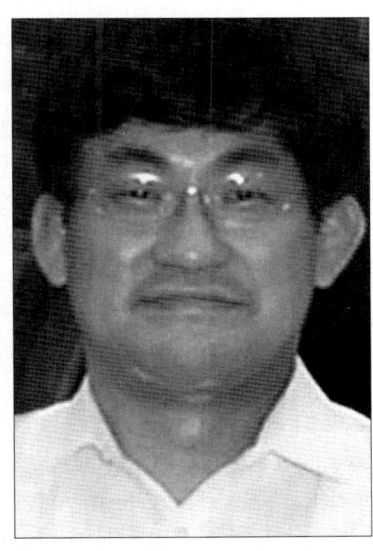

Dr. Haruhiko Bito is an Associate Professor in the Department of Neurochemistry, The University of Tokyo Graduate School of Medicine. He graduated from The University of Tokyo, gaining an M.D., followed by a Ph.D. in Biochemistry and Molecular Neurobiology. Thereafter, he pursued a postdoctoral training at Stanford University. He was an Assistant Professor and Lecturer at Kyoto University School of Medicine before establishing his new laboratory in Tokyo.
Sayaka Takemoto-Kimura, and **Hiroyuki Okuno** are Assistant Professors working in close collaboration with Dr. Bito at the Department of Neurochemistry.

MAJOR CONTRIBUTIONS

1. Bito H, Deisseroth K, Tsien RW. 1996. CREB phosphorylation and dephosphorylation: a Ca^{2+}-and stimulus duration-dependent switch for hippocampal gene expression. *Cell*, 87:1203-1214.

2. Bito H, Furuyashiki T, Ishihara H, Shibasaki Y, Ohashi K, Mizuno K, Maekawa M, Ishizaki T, Narumiya S. 2000. A critical role for a Rho-associated kinase p160ROCK in determining axon outgrowth in mammalian CNS neurons. *Neuron*, 26:431-441.

3. Furuyashiki T, Arakawa Y, Takemoto-Kimura S, Bito H, Narumiya S. 2002. Multiple spatiotemporal modes of actin reorganization by NMDA receptors and voltage-gated Ca^{2+}-channels. *Proc Nat Acad Sci USA*, 99:14458-14463.

4. Takemoto-Kimura S, Terai H, Takamoto M, Ohmae S, Kikumura S, Furuyashiki T, Arakawa Y, Narumiya S, Bito H. 2003. Molecular cloning and characterization of CLICK-III/Ca-MKIγ, a novel membrane-anchored neuronal Ca^{2+}/calmodul-in-dependent protein kinase (CaMK). *J Biol Chem*, 278: 18597-18605.

5. Nonaka M, Doi T, Fujiyoshi Y, Takemoto-Kimura S, Bito H. 2006. Essential contribution of the ligand-binding βB/β C loop of PDZ-1 and PDZ-2 in the regulation of postsynaptic clustering, scaffolding, and localization of PSD-95. *J Neurosci*, 26: 763-774.

MAIN TOPICS

Stability and plasticity of a neuronal circuit: requirement for activity-dependent gene expression to sustain a long-term adaptive response in input-output relationship

SUMMARY

A large number of molecular mechanisms contribute to ensuring that the neuronal transcriptome can be adapted in function of the various kinds of external and internal events that the neuronal network is exposed to. In recent years, activity-induced gene expression/ protein synthesis has received much attention as a potential mechanism likely to play a significant role in synaptic plasticity and long-term memory formation. The involved regulatory processes are intrinsically complex, and we still lack a detailed understanding of how specific neuronal nuclear factors are activated and modulated in concert to give rise to reliable and reproducible gene induction. In this chapter, we will consider the regulation of one of the most studied neuronal nuclear factor, the transcription factor CREB (Ca^{2+}/cAMP-response element-binding protein).

CREB structure is conserved from mollusk to rodents, and neuronal CREB mediates long-lasting forms of synaptic plasticity. Its activation was shown to be essential for higher brain functions such as learning and memory in many species. CREB usually resides in the nucleus, and is tightly bound to CRE loci, thus being ideally suited to rapidly convert cellular signaling into transcription. A large number of neuronal signaling pathways (e.g. Ca^{2+}/CaM/CaMKK/ CaMKIV, cAMP/ PKA, Ras/MAPK, CaN/PP1) are employed and converge onto the regulation of the phosphorylation state of CREB Ser-133, consistent with its presumed importance in many adaptive biological processes, including long-term neuronal plasticity and survival. The amount of information storage available in the neuronal network will soon saturate quickly, however, without built-in mechanism for reversibility and regulated extinction/erasure of plasticity. Resolving all these problems will be of an immense clinical value when addressing cases involving aberrant persistence of pain sensation or posttraumatic stress disorder.

INTRODUCTION

In order to execute a higher cognitive task in response to external and internal stimuli, the brain needs to compute an output, based upon a barrage of input information that it receives from the outside world. As our brain is able to successfully compute a correct answer above par on a continuous basis, it has been speculated that there must a particular mechanism for online storage of data about the input-output relationship of the events that have received attention (and not been neglected) from our brain. Furthermore, it is also believed that "useful" information can be consolidated within a neuronal network, thereby perhaps allowing the brain to store experience as a memory and become smarter. Such external stimuli-dependent changes in the brain have been proposed to be acquired by using mechanisms of synaptic plasticity. According to the *synaptic plasticity and memory hypothesis*, as defined by Richard Morris and colleagues, "activity-dependent synaptic plasticity is induced at appropriate synapses during memory formation and is both necessary and sufficient for the information storage underlying the type of memory mediated by the brain area in which that plasticity is observed". In recent years, both activity-induced gene expression/ protein synthesis and activity-induced changes in neuronal morphology have received much attention as potential mechanisms likely to play a significant role in synaptic plasticity and long-term memory formation. Experiments in hippocampal pyramidal excitatory neurons have shown that robust electrical activity can induce a large number of Ca^{2+}-dependent gene expression events. A crystal-clear picture of the molecular events following synaptic Ca^{2+} entry still remains missing, however, in part because the repertoire of activity-dependent transcription factors is not fully understood. Indeed, the mechanisms for their activation and their physiological significance have been elucidated for only a few of them, such as the Ca^{2+}/cAMP-response element-binding protein (CREB) or the nuclear factor of activated T-cells (NFAT). In this review, we shall overview some of the key signaling events by which the Ca^{2+}/CREB/CREB-binding protein signaling system might critically control long-term adaptive responses such as long-term synaptic plasticity.

STABILITY AND PLASTICITY OF A NEURONAL CIRCUIT: REQUIREMENT FOR ACTIVITY-DEPENDENT GENE EXPRESSION TO SUSTAIN A LONG-TERM ADAPTIVE RESPONSE IN INPUT-OUTPUT RELATIONSHIP

The central nervous system (CNS) is a complex organization consisting of 10-100 billion cells. Higher cognitive tasks and the principal information processing function of the CNS are thought to be supported in large part by the activity of excitable cells in the CNS, namely, the neurons. Each neuron receives inputs from a high number of adjacent neurons to which it physically connects to, via specialized contact domains called synapses. The number of synapses can sometimes reach over 10000, as in the case of hippocampal pyramidal neurons or cerebellar Purkinje cells. The major output axons are however relatively scarce, sometimes as few as one or two. Nonetheless, each axon can synapse onto many distinct dendritic arborizations via an array of *en passant* boutons, which can be triggered to release their neurotransmitters by the same action potential firing event with a high degree of synchrony. These features have led to the commonly believed notion that neurons are computing units that fire action potentials with accuracy and fidelity when it receives appropriate barrages of inputs within a neuronal cell assembly.

The firing features of a neuron are very reliable, to the extent that a neuron can often be defined, classified or categorized based on its temporal pattern of firing (see chapters on excitatory and inhibitory transmissions). Similarly, the spatial input-output relationship of a neuron, or more commonly called hardwiring diagram, is also strictly reproducible, as demonstrated by many anatomical tracing experiments. Remarkably, a large number of these spatial and temporal characteristics seem to be conserved across species through evolution, as critical determinants of neuron types are encoded by tightly regulated

sets of genetic programs.

Such a built-in stability of neuronal circuits is most likely to be at the foundation of the reliability and the reproducibility of sensory perception over tens of years in long-living animal species such as human. While common sensory events are usually chance events and mostly with neutral valence, certain sensory modality such as pain sensation has a special affective valence (usually negative in the case of pain), which is ethologically linked to specific patterns of emotional behavior (such as escape, cry etc.). Repeated exposure to physical stimuli that activate pain sensation may create an altered state of responsiveness (escape or coping) towards these stimuli. Similar alteration in response behavior was shown in many situations where exposure to specific and neutral sensory stimuli was associated with specific affective valence (such as in addictive state, during classical Pavlovian conditioning, or under spatial maze tasks with food reward or water escape as a reinforcer).

This experience-dependent adaptation of the behavioral output occurs entirely based on the specific patterns of the experienced incoming sensory stimuli. Many pioneering works suggest that such an adaptive responsiveness is most likely to be mediated, at least in part, by mechanisms of synaptic plasticity at the circuit level. Thus, activity-dependent synaptic plasticity (either long-term potentiation, LTP or long-term depression, LTD) is postulated to be induced at specific sets of synapses during association of sensory events with affective valence. Experimental evidence in favor of this hypothesis has been accumulated during hippocampal spatial learning and memory, fear memory, and pathological pain.

One major feature of activity-dependent synaptic plasticity is its perpetuation for sometimes more than days. The physical and molecular nature of such "memory trace" has been much debated, yet remains highly controversial. Among many hypotheses, one strong postulate that has survived intense scrutiny over dozens of years of research is the contribution of activity-induced up-regulation of novel gene products. This hypothesis posits that synaptic activity of the kind that triggers synaptic plasticity (usually a strong burst of activity or prolonged and patterned stimuli) is necessary and sufficient to give rise to an increase in new protein synthesis, which in turn allows the potentiated/depressed synaptic efficacy states to be sustained over days, if necessary.

What then are the specific sets of gene products up-regulated upon induction of synaptic plasticity? Are there common transcriptional regulatory elements and shared transcriptional machinery involved? How can synaptic activity traverse the space separating the synapses from the nucleus and yet not lose much of the specificity? We will address these few issues in the following sections.

ACTIVITY-REGULATED NEURONAL TRANSCRIPTION FACTORS: WHAT ARE THEY?

One of the immediate challenges that face any attempt for the molecular dissection of activity-dependent neuronal gene expression is the accurate understanding of how synaptic activity can be possibly and tightly coupled to activation of specific nuclear transcriptional machinery. Early work suggested that mRNA transcription was a major site of regulation, as many gene transcripts were found to be induced upon receipt of strong depolarizing stimuli such as high K^+ depolarization. Screening of various induced genes

suggested that a large number of genes up-regulated by neuronal activity contained *cis*-regulatory elements such as the cAMP-responsive element (CRE) or the serum-responsive element (SRE). Consistent with these findings, recent gene knockout experiments confirmed that the respective cognate transcription factor CREB (CRE-binding protein) and SRF (serum-responsive factor) are involved in activity-dependent gene activation in the CNS *in vivo*. Other *cis*-regulatory elements involved in neuronal activity-dependent gene expression include AP-1, NFAT, DREAM, CaRF, $NF\alpha B$, and USF. Recent evidence indicates that regulation of chromatin remodeling is also implicated in these processes as well. Clearly, activity-dependent gene regulation is likely to be a complex orchestration of these various nuclear events, triggered and modulated by many independent yet interacting cytosolic and nuclear signaling pathways(Fig.16.1).

Because of the complexity of these combined regulatory processes, and the likelihood of separate and parallel signaling pathways acting in concert, a detailed description of how each nuclear factor is activated and modulated is still missing and subject to intense ongoing research. Here, we will consider the regulation of one of the most studied neuronal nuclear factor, the transcription factor CREB.

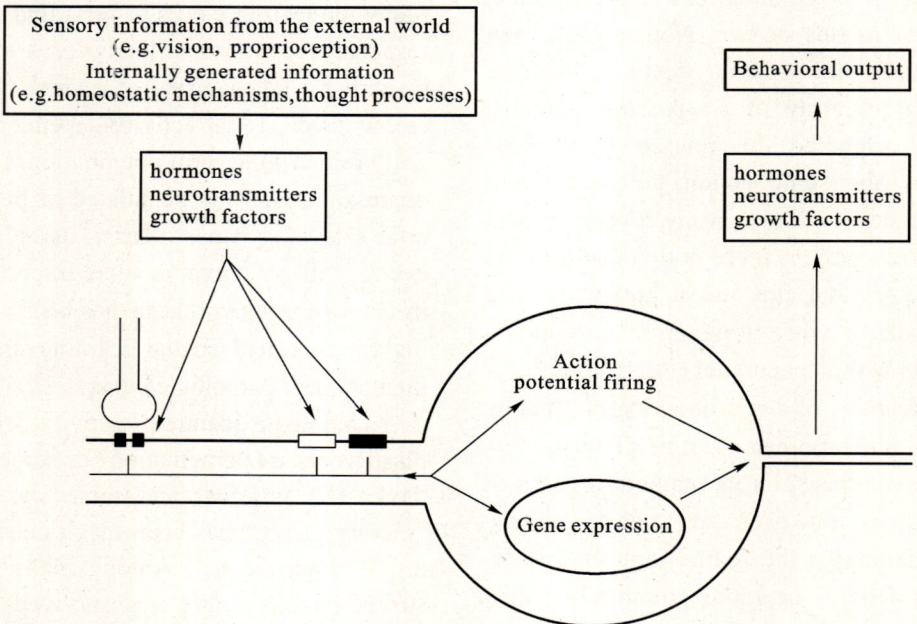

Fig.16.1 Activity-dependent gene expression critically tunes neuronal input-output function. Each neuron receives inputs from a high number of adjacent neurons via specialized contact domains called synapses. The number of synapses can sometimes reach over 10000, as in the case of hippocampal pyramidal neurons or cerebellar Purkinje cells. Each synapse is a source of EPSP that can be integrated into an axon potential in an all-or-none fashion when the summated potential exceeds the threshold to generate a sodium spike. Activity-dependent gene expression is triggered by a distinct kind of local (synapse)-to-global (nuclear) signaling with a different logic of summation.

Both gain-of-function and loss-of-function effects of CREB have been evaluated *in vivo* in various animal species including *Aplysia, Drosophila*, and mice and rats. The involvement of CREB on neuronal functions was first suggested in cultured neurons of *Aplysia*. The *Aplysia* neuronal culture, in which sensory neurons make synaptic contacts with motor neurons, shows stimulus-dependent enhancement in synaptic transmission efficiency (synaptic facilitation), which is a basis of behavioral sensitization to stimuli. Injection of CRE-containing oligonucleotide duplex into sensory neurons blocked long-term facilitation (LTF) without affecting short-term facilitation (STF). A series of following studies have demon-

strated that CREB-induced gene expression is crucial for establishment and maintenance of LTF.

A direct relationship between CREB and memory has first been shown in *Drosophila*. Transgenic flies expressing a dominant negative dCREB-2 showed impairment of long-term olfactory memory, but not short-term memory. Conversely, transgenic flies expressing a dCREB-2 activator showed enhanced performance in olfactory memory task. The phenotype of this fly line, however, remains controversial, as the dCREB-2 activator transgene contained a mutation that induced a frame-shift and a premature stop in the coding region.

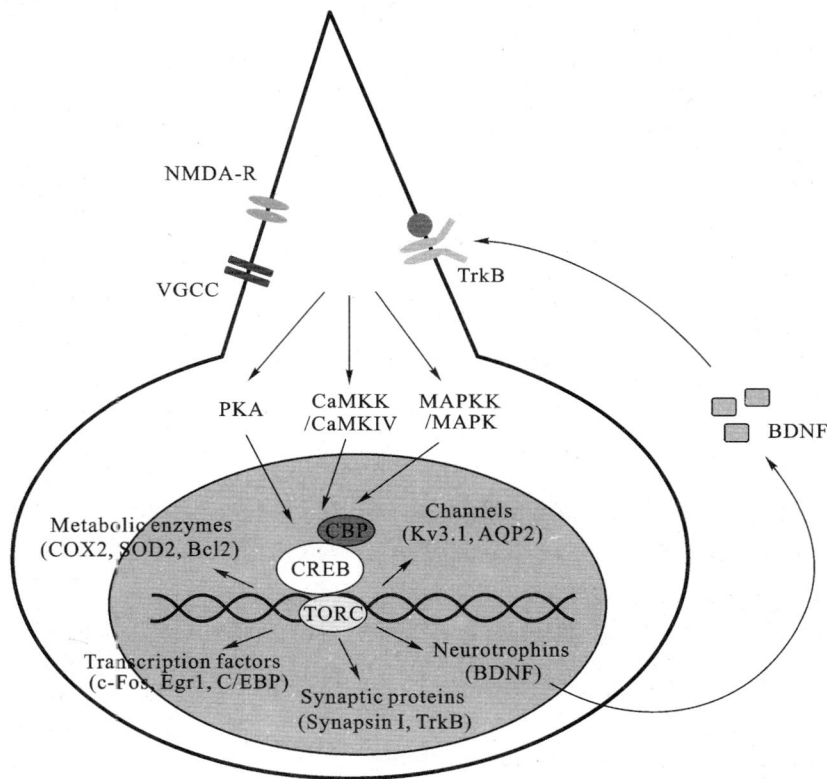

Fig.16.2   An example of signaling from synapse to nucleus: the case of CREB. CREB is a transcription factor that can be activated by many separate signaling routes that culminate in stimulating different nuclear CREB kinases. Three well described examples, the CaMKK/CaMKIV pathway, the PKA pathway and the MAPK pathway are illustrated. The activation kinetics and the resulting persistence of pCREB in the nucleus are thought to be distinctively regulated by the relative contribution of each one of these pathways, thereby accounting for the variety and diversity of the CREB-regulated transcriptome. Some of the CREB target genes such as BDNF could also participate in the late phase control of nuclear phospho-CREB amount. Such a positive feedback mechanism may critically determine the set of genes required for BDNF-dependent long-term plasticity and survival.

CREB AS A TRANSCRIPTIONAL REGULATOR

CREB is a member of the CREB/ATF family nuclear

transcription factor, which includes CREB, activating transcription factors (ATFs) and cAMP-responsive element modulator (CREM), and shares similar CRE recognition characteristics with family members. CREB homodimerizes via the leucine zipper motif at the C-terminal, and binds to the cAMP-responsive element (CRE), a specific palindromic DNA sequence, 5′-TGACGTCA-3′, often found in the 5′-upstream vicinity of transcription initiation sites of many neuronal genes. These include transcription factors (e.g., c-Fos, Egr-1, Per1, C/EBPα), cellular meta- bolic enzymes (e.g., cytochrome c, phosphorenolpyruvate carboxy kinase, cyclooxygenese-2, superoxide dismutase 2, bcl-2), growth factors and neuropeptides (e.g., somatostatin, enkephalin, brain-derived neurotrophic factor, insulin-like growth factor, fibroblast growth factor 6, vasopressin), and neuronal proteins (e.g., synapsin I, β1-and β2-adrenergic receptors, trkB). Furthermore, systematic genome-wide approaches, using comprehensive transcriptome and chromatin immunoprecipitation analyses, have confirmed the extreme complexity of CREB target gene profile, which seems to be highly cell-type and contextdependent(Fig.16.2).

CREB in a heterodimeric complex can also bind to a half-site CRE motif (5′-TGACG-3′). CREB homodimers usually reside in the nucleus, tightly bound to CRE loci, and are ideally suited to rapidly convert cellular signaling into transcription. Through regulation of CRE-dependent gene expression, CREB mediates cell growth, survival, death, proliferation and differentiation, in response to a variety of extracellular stimuli in different types of cells. CREB structure is conserved from mollusk to rodents(Fig.16.3), and neuronal CREB mediates long-lasting forms of synaptic plasticity and has been implicated in higher brain functions such as learning and memory in many species.

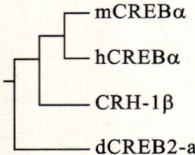

Fig.16.3 Conservation of CREB protein during evolution. The top panel shows a phylogenic tree analysis of the primary amino acid sequences of full-length CREB protein. It is likely that *D. melanogaster* CREB ortholog (dCREB2-α) has evolved separately from the mammalian CREB (mCREBα, hCREBα) gene, as the *C. elegans* full-length CREB protein (CRH-1β) has higher homology with its mammalian, rather than the fruitfly counterpart. The KID and the bZIP domains show overall a remarkable degree of conservation, as shown in the lower panels. Marked in red and green are identical and conserved amino acid residues, respectively. Ser-133 and the leucine residues forming a leucine zipper are shown with an asterisk.

KID domain

mCREBα	113	ESVDSVTDSQKRREILSRRPSYRKILNDLSSDAPGVPRIEEE	154
hCREBα	113	ESVDSVTDSQKRREILSRRPSYRKILNDLSSDAPGVPRIEEE	154
CRH-1β	9	EGGDSKDEARRRREQLNRRPSYRMILKDLETADKVMKKEPEE	50
apCREB1α	65	DLSSSDSDAKKRREILTRRPSYRKILNELSSPVSKMDDDSNS	106
dCREB2-α	211	DESLSDDDSQHHRSELTRRPSYNKIFTEISGPDMSGASLPMS	252

bZIP domain

mCREBα	280	EEAARKREVRLMKNREAARECRRKKKEYVKCLENRVAVLENQ	321
hCREBα	280	EEAARKREVRLMKNREAARECRRKKKEYVKCLENRVAVLENQ	321
CRH-1β	242	DESNRKRQVRLLKNREAAKECRRKKKEYVKCLENRVSVLENQ	283
apCREB1α	210	EEGSRKRELRLLKNREAARECRRKKKEYVKCLENRVAVLENQ	251
dCREB2-α	298	EDQTRKREIRLQKNREAARECRRKKKEYIKCLENRVAVLENQ	339

mCREBα	322	NKTLIEELKALKDLYCHKSD	341
hCREBα	322	NKTLIEELKALKDLYCHKSD	341
CRH-1β	284	NKALIEELKTLKELYCRKEKDGM	306
apCREB1α	252	NKTLIEELKALKELYCQKDA	271
dCREB2-α	340	NKALIEELKSLKELYCQTKND	360

CONTROL OF CREB ACTIVITY BY REGULATED PHOSPHORYLATION AT RESIDUE SER-133

CREB Ser-133 phosphorylation is a key switch that turns on CREB function. CREB is constitutively bound to CRE sites in the chromatin, regardless of cellular activity. However, several nuclear kinases have the potential to activate CREB via Ser-133 phosphorylation. When Ser-133 residue is phosphorylated, the kinase inducible domain (KID) which comprises this Ser-133 becomes a high-affinity binding site for the KID-interacting (KIX) domain of a general transcriptional co-activator, CREB-binding protein (CBP). Whether the high affinity of phosphorylated Ser-133 (pS133) site is sufficient in a native chromatin complex to trigger the docking and to promote the recruitment of a CBP-containing transcriptional pre-initiation complex at regions immediately adjacent and downstream to the CRE sequence remains unknown. The epigenetic state of the surrounding chromatin-DNA complexes, as well as the affinity between CREB and $TAF_{II}130$ in the TFIID complex and/or CREB-specific co-factors such as transducers of regulated CREB activity (TORCs) may also significantly contribute to this process (Fig.16.4).

In keeping with this complexity of regulation surrounding the interaction of pS133-CREB with the transcriptional pre-initiation complex, aberrance of this nuclear protein complex in the long-term appears to play a detrimental role in CNS function. Indeed, CREB/CBP-dependent transcription was shown to be repressed in several model systems of polyglutamine diseases, and this may be causative of the typical neurodegeneration associated with these diseases. Molecular or pharmacological manipulations that alleviated this transcriptional disruption significantly rescued neuronal cell death.

Although Ser133 phosphorylation of CREB was originally reported to be mediated by cAMP-dependent protein kinase (PKA), a large body of evidence now shows that the phosphorylation of this site is also achieved by a variety of kinases including protein kinase C (PKC), Rsk1-3, Msk-1, MAPKAP-K2/3, Akt, and CaMKI, II and IV. The kinases that mainly phosphorylate Ser133 of CREB may depend on types of stimuli as well as types of cells. Studies *in vitro* in cultured neurons and *in vivo* in either knockout or transgenic mice have revealed that fast Ser-133 phosphorylation triggered immediately after strongly synaptic activity is predominantly mediated by a CaMKK/CaMKIV pathway. A temporally delayed phase of phosphorylation was shown to involve a MAPK pathway as well, though the specific isoform(s) and the relevant downstream CREB kinase(s) have not been firmly elucidated (Fig.16.5).

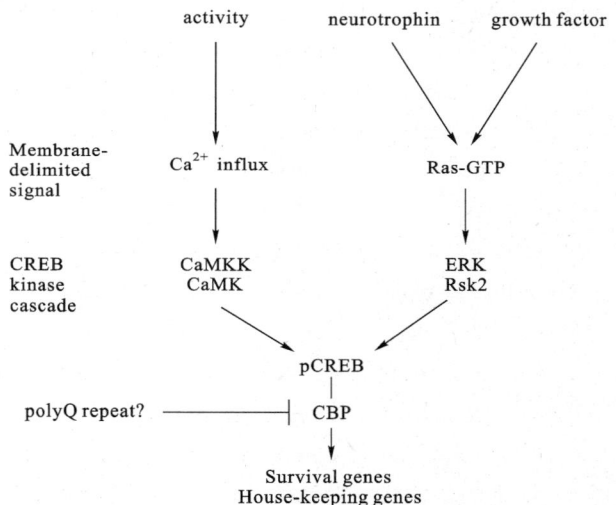

Fig.16.4   CREB/CBP complex is a biologically critical node of signal convergence and its aberrance may underlie the molecular pathology of certain polyglutamine diseases. Various kinds of neuronal signaling events implicated in neuronal activity or survival factors including neurotrophins or growth factors induce specific membrane-delimited signals that triggers and converge onto CREB phosphorylation. Phosphorylated CREB, by virtue of an increased affinity to CBP, a co-activator, can then turn on transcription of a battery of survival as well as house-keeping genes. In polyQ-diseases, the efficiency of pCREB-CBP interaction may be diminished, thus creating a deficit in the pool of CREB-dependent survival genes. This may create an increased susceptibility to insults, thereby augmenting the chance for neuronal death in the long run.

Compared to kinases, less information is available about phosphatases that dephosphorylate and thereby critically determine the decay of the nuclear amount of phospho-Ser133. Depending on the cell types, either Ser/Thr protein phosphatase 1 (PP-1) or PP-2A were shown to directly dephosphorylate CREB at Ser133 both *in vitro* and in culture cells, after phospho-CREB is unbound from CBP. Several other phosphatases such as calcineurin (PP2B), PTEN and protein tyrosine phosphatase 1B (PTP1B) were sug-

gested to be indirectly involved in dephosphorylating pS133 by suppression of upstream CREB kinases or by activation of CREB phosphotases. Together, a huge amount of neuronal signaling pathways are employed and converge onto the regulation of the phosphorylation state of pS133, consistent with its presumed importance in many adaptive biological processes, including long-term neuronal plasticity and survival.

BOX 16. 2 Gain-of-function and loss-of-function phenotypes of CREB in genetically engineered mice.

Although CREB is ubiquitously expressed in all tissues in the body, significance of CREB function has been most extensively investigated in the central and peripheral nervous systems as well as in some other systems including T-cell maturation. Also, several studies using mice expressing a dominant-negative CREB transgene have demonstrated CREB function in glucose and lipid metabolism.

In mice, disruption of the exon 2 of the CREB gene, which contains the first ATG codon, resulted in abolishment of expression of major alternative spliced isoforms (CREB alpha/delta knockout), but at the same time, unexpected upregulation of another activator CREB isoform, CREB beta, and related protein CREM in a large number of organs. These CREB hypomorphic mutant mice showed no obvious developmental abnormality in the body, in a mixed 129 x BL6 background. There were also no obvious anatomical disorders in the brain. However, when the mice were assessed with hippocampal-dependent memory tasks, the mice showed impairments in formation of long-term memory, but not short-term memory, consistent with findings reported in invertebrates (see BOX 16.1).

CREB null mutants that lack all functional activator CREB isoforms have been generated by disrupting the bZIP domain. In contrast to the CREB hypomorphic mice, the CREB null mutants were smaller than wild-type littermates and died immediately after birth from respiratory distress. The commissural fibers in the brain were dramatically reduced in the mutant mice. The mice also showed severe im-

pairments in development of T-cells of the alpha/beta lineage, but not the gamma/delta lineage.

The CREB null-mutant mice also exhibited excess apoptosis and degeneration as well as impairment in axonal growth and projections in sensory neurons, suggesting that CREB plays a role in survival and growth of peripheral neurons. Conditional forebrain-specific CREB knockout mice with a CREM null background also showed extensive neuronal apoptosis during development and progressive neurodegeneration in adult brains.

A study with transgenic mice with an inducible and reversible CREB repressor showed that CREB is crucial *in vivo* for the consolidation of long-term conditioned fear memories, but not for encoding, storage, or retrieval of these memories. In the study, it has also shown that CREB is required for the stability of reactivated conditioned fear memories.

Transgenic mice with spatially restricted and temporally regulated expression of a constitutively active CREB (VP16-CREB) have been generated to assess CREB roles in hippocampal long-term potentiation (LTP), a possible cellular basis of learning and memory. In the transgenic mice, hippocampal CA1 neurons showed facilitation of a persistent late phase of LTP (L-LTP) elicited by weak stimuli, which usually produce only an early phase long-term potentiation (E-LTP) in wild type animals. The results indicate that elevated CRE-driven gene products by VP16-CREB may be sufficient for consolidation of LTP, and support the "synaptic tag and capture" hypothesis.

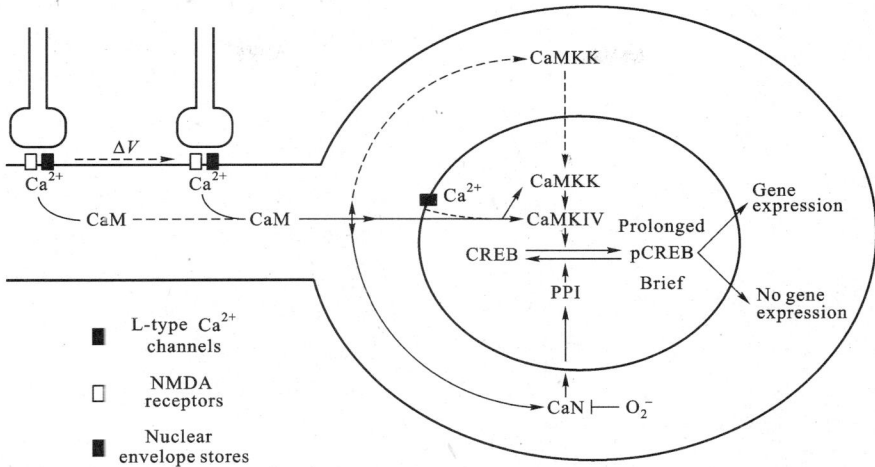

Fig.16.5 Complex control of nuclear phospho-CREB abundance by Ca^{2+}/CaM-mediated synapse-to-nucleus signaling. Patterned synaptic activity triggers robust Ca^{2+} mobilization at synaptic and perisynaptic locations via opening of NMDA-receptors and voltage-dependent Ca^{2+} channels. Calmodulin (CaM) is particular enriched at and near synapses and synaptic Ca^{2+} entry dramatically augments the amount of activated (Ca^{2+}-bound) CaM. Ca^{2+}/CaM acts as a cofactor to various neuronal enzymes including CaM kinases, calcineurin, type I adenylate cyclase, GDP/GTP-exchange factors for small GTPases such as Ras and Rac. Thus, Ca^{2+}/CaM increase could in principle participate in activation of CaMK, Ras/MAPK, and cAMP/PKA pathways. In hippocampal CA1 pyramidal neurons and in anterior cingulate cortical neurons, rapid nuclear translocation of activated CaM was shown. This is believed to account, at least in part, for the predominant role of nuclear CaMKK/CaMKIV route in CREB phosphorylation in these cell-types. In parallel to this pathway, hippocampal neurons in which Ca^{2+} was strongly mobilized generate superoxide anions, which are able to inactivate calcineurin activity. This event seems to alleviate calcineurin-mediated regulation of protein phosphatase-1-dependent dephosphorylation of pS133, thereby contributing to the persistence of pS133 amount in the neuronal nuclei.

CONCLUSION AND FUTURE DIRECTIONS

Due to limitation in our current knowledge, we were able to review only a very small subset of the nucleus-to-synapse signaling critical for long-term adaptive regulation of neuronal input-output relationship. However, there is no doubt that a far larger number of molecular mechanisms contribute to ensuring that the neuronal transcriptome can be adapted in function of the various kinds of external and internal events that the neuronal network is exposed to.

One key issue that still escapes our studies concerns the spatial distribution of the up-regulated gene products within the activated neuron. Are they just widely distributed as resources with a higher availability, or are there further specific regulations to traffic them to special locations in the neuron, such as the sites of previous strong activity? Obtaining an insight to this question will provide a clue to better understand how plastic synapses (potentiated or depressed responses triggered by predetermined sets of stimuli/sensation) could possibly coexists with the normal synapses (unchanged responses at other synapses) within the same neurons. A critical test in the future will be to determine whether these up-regulated gene products are correlated in any way (temporal or spatial) with the distribution of persistent changes in individual synaptic weights within the relevant neuronal circuit.

Another predominant issue is how a stabilized synapse could possibly be reset back to baseline value by activity. Without such a dynamic bistability, that is, the existence of regulated extinction/erasure of plasticity, the amount of information storage will soon saturate quickly. However, how stabilization of plasticity and erasure can co-exist in concert remains totally unknown. Resolving this question would also be of immense clinical value to addressing clinical cases involving aberrant persistence of pain sensation or posttraumatic stress disorder.

GENERAL CITATIONS

Bito H. 1998. The role of calcium in activity-dependent neuronal gene regulation. *Cell Calcium*, 23: 43-150.

Bito H, Takemoto-Kimura S. 2003. Ca²⁺/CREB/CB-P-dependent gene regulation: a shared mechanism critical in long-term synaptic plasticity and neuronal survival. *Cell Calcium*, 34: 425-430.

Kandel ER. 2001. The molecular biology of memory storage: a dialogue between genes and synapses. *Science*, 294:1030-1038.

Martin SJ, Grimwood PD, Morris RG. 2000. Synaptic plasticity and memory: an evaluation of the hypothesis. *Annu Rev Neurosci*, 23:649-711.

Silva AJ, Kogan JH, Frankland PW, Kida S. 1998. CREB and memory. Annu Rev Neurosci, 21:127-148.

DISCOVERY CITATIONS

Barco A, Alarcon JM, Kandel ER. 2002. Expression of constitutively active CREB protein facilitates the late phase of long-term potentiation by enhancing synaptic capture. *Cell*, 108: 689-703.

Bartsch D, Ghirardi M, Skehel PA, Karl KA, Herder SP, Chen M, *et al.* 1995. Aplysia CREB2 represses long-term facilitation: relief of repression converts transient facilitation into long-term functional and structural change. *Cell*, 83: 979-992.

Bito H, Deisseroth K, Tsien RW. 1996. CREB phosphorylation and dephosphorylation: a Ca(²⁺)-stimulus duration-dependent switch for hippocampal gene expression. *Cell*, 87: 1203-1214.

Blendy JA, Kaestner KH, Schmid W, Gass P, Schutz G. 1996. Targeting of the CREB gene leads to up-regulation of a novel CREB mRNA isoform. *Embo J*, 15: 1098-1106.

Bourtchuladze R, Frenguelli B, Blendy J, Cioffi D, Schutz G, Silva AJ. 1994. Deficient long-term memory in mice with a targeted mutation of the cAMP-responsive element-binding protein. *Cell*, 79: 59-68.

Chrivia JC, Kwok RP, Lamb N, Hagiwara M, Montminy MR, Goodman RH. 1993. Phosphorylated CREB binds specifically to the nuclear protein CBP. *Nature*, 365: 855-859.

Conkright MD, Canettieri G, Screaton R, Guzman E, Miraglia L, Hogenesch JB, *et al.* 2003. TORCs: transducers of regulated CREB activity. *Mol Cell*, 12: 413-423.

Dash PK, Hochner B, Kandel ER. 1990. Injection of the cAMP-responsive element into the nucleus of *Aplysia* sensory neurons blocks long-term facilitation. *Nature*, 345: 718-721.

Deisseroth K, Heist EK, Tsien RW. 1998. Translocation of calmodulin to the nucleus supports CREB phosphorylation in hippocampal neurons. *Nature*, 392: 198-202.

Ferreri K, Gill G, Montminy M. 1994. The cAMP-regulated transcription factor CREB interacts with a component of the TFIID complex. *Proc Natl Acad Sci USA*, 91: 1210-1213.

Ginty DD, Kornhauser JM, Thompson MA, Bading H, Mayo KE, Takahashi JS, *et al.* 1993. Regulation of CREB phosphorylation in the suprachiasmatic nucleus by light and a circadian clock. *Science*, 260: 238-241.

Gonzalez GA, Montminy MR. 1989. Cyclic AMP stimulates somatostatin gene transcription by phosphorylation of CREB at serine 133. *Cell*, 59: 675-680.

Hagiwara M, Alberts A, Brindle P, Meinkoth J, Feramisco J, Deng T, *et al.* 1992. Transcriptional attenuation following cAMP induction requires PP-1-mediated dephosphorylation of CREB. *Cell*, 70: 105-113.

Herzig S, Hedrick S, Morantte I, Koo SH, Galimi F, Montminy M. 2003. CREB controls hepatic lipid metabolism through nuclear hormone receptor PPAR-gamma. *Nature*, 426: 190-193.

Herzig S, Long F, Jhala US, Hedrick S, Quinn R, Bauer A, *et al.* 2001. CREB regulates hepatic gluconeogenesis through the coactivator PGC-1. *Nature*, 413: 179-183.

Impey S, McCorkle SR, Cha-Molstad H, Dwyer JM, Yochum GS, Boss JM, *et al.* 2004. Defining the CREB regulon: a genome-wide analysis of transcription factor regulatory regions. *Cell*, 119: 1041-1054.

Kida S, Josselyn SA, de Ortiz SP, Kogan JH, Chevere I, Masushige S, *et al.* 2002. CREB required for the stability of new and reactivated fear memories. *Nat Neurosci*, 5: 348-355.

Lonze BE, Riccio A, Cohen S, Ginty DD. 2002. Apoptosis, axonal growth defects, and degeneration of peripheral neurons in mice lacking CREB. *Neuron*, 34: 371-385.

Mantamadiotis T, Lemberger T, Bleckmann SC, Kern H, Kretz O, Martin Villalba A, *et al.* 2002. Disruption of CREB function in brain leads to neurodegeneration. *Nat Genet*, 31:

47-54.

Mayr B, Montminy M. 2001. Transcriptional regulation by the phosphorylation-dependent factor CREB. *Nat Rev Mol Cell Biol*, 2: 599-609.

Montminy MR, Bilezikjian LM. 1987. Binding of a nuclear protein to the cyclic-AMP response element of the somato-statin gene. *Nature*, 328: 175-178.

Ramanan N, Shen Y, Sarsfield S, Lemberger T, Schutz G, Lin-den DJ, *et al.* 2005. SRF mediates activity-induced gene expression and synaptic plasticity but not neuronal viability. *Nat Neurosci*, 8: 759-767.

Rudolph D, Tafuri A, Gass P, Hammerling GJ, Arnold B, Schutz G. 1998. Impaired fetal T cell development and perinatal lethality in mice lacking the cAMP response ele-ment binding protein. *Proc Natl Acad Sci USA*, 95: 4481-4486.

Sée V, Boutiller AL, Bito H, Loeffler JP. 2001. Calcium-cal-modulin dependent protein kinase type IV (CaMKIV) in-hibits apoptosis induced by potassium deprivation in cere-bellar granule cells. *FASEB J*, 15: 134-144.

Screaton RA, Conkright MD, Katoh Y, Best JL, Canettieri G, Jeffries S, *et al.* 2004 The CREB coactivator TORC2 func-tions as a calcium-and cAMP-sensitive coincidence detec-tor. *Cell*, 119: 61-74.

Shaywitz AJ, Greenberg ME. 1999. CREB: a stimulus-induced transcription factor activated by a diverse array of extra-cellular signals. *Annu Rev Biochem*, 68: 821-861.

Yin JC, Wallach JS, Del Vecchio M, Wilder EL, Zhou H, Quinn WG, *et al.* 1994. Induction of a dominant negative CREB transgene specifically blocks long-term memory in *Drosophila. Cell*, 79: 49-58.

Zhang X, Odom DT, Koo SH, Conkright MD, Canettieri G, Best J, *et al.* 2005. Genome-wide analysis of cAMP-resp-onse element binding protein occupancy, phosphorylation, and target gene activation in human tissues. *Proc Natl Acad Sci USA*, 102: 4459-4464

CHAPTER 17

Second Messenger Pathways in Pain

Kathleen A. Sluka, David A. Skyba, Marie K. Hoeger Bement, Katherine M. Audette, Rajan Radhakrishnan

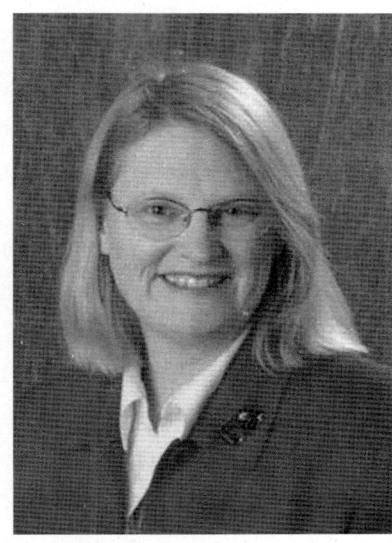

Dr. Sluka is a Professor in the Graduate Program in Physical Therapy & Rehabilitation Science, Carver College of Medicine, University of Iowa. Following her Physical Therapy degree, Georgia State University, Atlanta, she pursued a PhD in Anatomy, University of Texas Medical Branch, Galveston, Texas.

MAJOR CONTRIBUTIONS

1. Sluka KA, Rees H, Westlund KN, Willis WD. 1995. Fiber types contributing to dorsal root reflexes induced by joint inflammation in cats and monkeys. *J Neurophysiol*, 74(3): 981-989.
2. Sluka KA, Kalra A, Moore SA. 2001. Unilateral intramuscular injections of acidic saline produce a bilateral, long-lasting hyperalgesia. *Muscle Nerve*, 24(1):37-46.
3. Sluka KA. 2002. Stimulation of deep somatic tissue with capsaicin produces long-lasting mechanical allodynia and heat hypoalgesia that depends on early activation of the cAMP pathway. *J Neurosci*, 22(13):5687-5693.
4. Hoeger-Bement MK, Sluka KA. 2003. Phosphorylation of CREB and mechanical hyperalgesia is reversed by blockade of the cAMP pathway in a time-dependent manner after repeated intramuscular acid injections. *J Neurosci*, 23(13): 5437-5445.
5. Sluka KA, Price MP, Breese NM, Stucky CL, Wemmie JA, Welsh MJ. 2003. Chronic hyperalgesia induced by repeated acid injections in muscle is abolished by the loss of ASIC3, but not ASIC1. *Pain*, 106(3): 229-239.

MAIN TOPICS

Adenylate cyclase/cAMP pathway
 Peripheral role
 Spinal role
 Supraspinal role
IP3/DAG-PKC pathway
 Peripheral role
 Spinal role
 Supraspinal role
cGMP-PKG pathway
Peripheral role
Spinal role
Supraspinal role
Drug targets and therapeutic implications

SUMMARY

G protein-coupled (GPCRs) and ionotropic receptors play an important role in normal and pathological pain transmission and modulation. Activation of these receptors either directly or indirectly further activates intracellular second messenger pathways to enhance or suppress nociceptive processing. These second messenger pathways are important both in the periphery as well as in the central nervous system in mediating pain states. Major second messengers associated with GPCRs are cAMP, cGMP, inositol triphosphate (IP3), Ca^{2+} and diacylglyceride (DAG). These second messengers transmit the signals mainly by activating protein kinases, such as protein kinase A (by cAMP), protein kinase G (by cGMP), and protein kinase C (by DAG/ IP3). Ionotropic receptors also activate components of second messenger systems by increasing calcium influx. Preclinical data show that peripheral injury or inflammation activates cAMP-protein kinase A (PKA) and/ or DAG/IP3-PKC cascade in the periphery and/ or central nervous system (CNS), which leads to pain. The cyclic GMP-PKG system has been shown to either facilitate or inhibit nociception. However, the exact role of the cGMP-PKG pathway in nociception is unclear at this point, although there is sufficient evidence to show its involvement in the modulation of nociception. Experimental evidences suggest that, despite the ubiquitous distribution of these pathways throughout living cells, their selective modulation could lead to novel therapies in pain conditions.

INTRODUCTION

Activation of G-protein coupled receptors (GPCRs) by various ligands leads to either activation or inhibition of second messenger pathways, which in turn initiates or inhibits cellular events. In the periphery and central nervous system, pain is modulated by numerous ligands such as serotonin, norepinephrine, substance P, glutamate, bradykinin, histamine, prostaglandins, protons, GABA, and endogenous opioids that act on receptors or ion channels to produce their effects. Major second messengers associated with GPCRs are cAMP, cGMP, IP3, Ca^{2+} and DAG. Cyclic AMP is synthesized in the cell from ATP by

adenylate cyclase enzymes, which are inhibited or stimulated depending on the ligand that binds the GPCR. Increasing intracellular cAMP subsequently activates protein kinase A. Diacylglycerol (DAG) and inositol triphosphate (IP3) are formed by phospholipase C from phosphatidylinositol biphosphate (PIP2). DAG then activates another protein kinase, PKC, while IP3 increases intracellular calcium. Guanylate cyclase mediates the formation of cGMP from GTP and is also activated by nitric oxide. Increases in cGMP produce effects through activation of PKG.

Protein kinases mediate intracellular processes through the phosphorylation of receptors, cellular proteins, or transcription factors (Fig.17.1). Phosphorylation of intracellular receptor proteins enhances the transport of these receptors to the cell membrane thus making the cell more sensitive to ligands, whereas phosphorylation of transcription factors can initiate gene transcription and subsequently increase expression of nociception-related proteins. Ligands acting on ionotropic receptors can increase calcium influx to activate calcium/calmodulin-dependent kinases (CaMKs) and adenylate cyclases. These second messenger systems mediate a myriad of biological processes including generation and maintenance of pain. Preclinical studies utilizing a variety of persistent pain models provide evidence that modulation of the cAMP/ PKA pathway may be useful for the treatment of pain. Similarly, there is substantial evidence supporting a role for the DAG/PKC pathway in dorsal horn neurons in regulating pain hypersensitivity in a number of pain models. There is also evidence to support a role for the cGMP/PKG pathway in pain transmission; however, this data is somewhat controversial. Overall, there is ample preclinical evidence to demonstrate the role of second messenger pathways in the generation and maintenance of pain. The focus of this chapter is the role of second messenger pathways in pain modulation. In the current chapter, the role of second messengers and kinases will be discussed in relation to their site of involvement: peripheral, spinal and supraspinal.

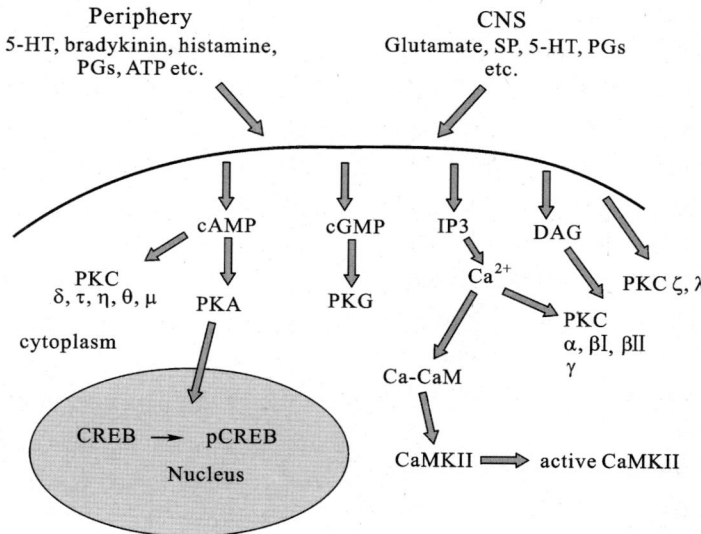

Fig.17.1   Second Messenger Systems in Pain.

ADENYLATE CYCLASE/CAMP PATHWAY

Peripheral Role

Peripheral activation of the cAMP pathway produces pain-like behavior that is decreased with inhibition of the pathway. Most studies utilize activators (forskolin or analogues of cAMP), or inhibitors of adenylate cyclase or protein kinase A to examine the role of the cAMP pathway in nociception. Intradermal administration of 8-bromo-cAMP, forskolin, or the catalytic subunit of PKA produces mechanical hyperalgesia in a dose-dependent manner (Fig.17.2), which is prolonged when phosphodiesterase inhibitors are co-injected with the forskolin. Conversely, inhibitors of PKA or adenylate cyclase administered peripherally decrease the mechanical hyperalgesia induced by an intradermal injection of epinephrine or the catalytic subunit of PKA (Fig.17.2). In the frog skin-nerve preparation, forskolin sensitizes skin nociceptors, which is inhibited by pretreatment with a PKA inhibitor, H89. Thus, pain-like behaviors are evident following activation of the cAMP pathway in the periphery.

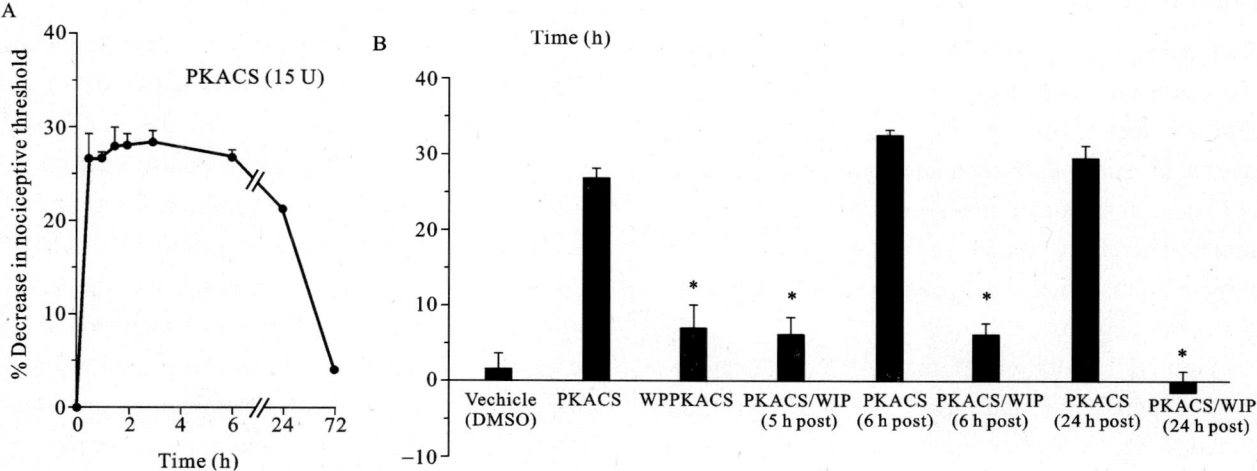

Fig.17.2   Hyperalgesia produced by local injection of PKACS (catalytic subunit of PKA) and its reversal by local administration of WIPTIDE (PKA inhibitor) (Aley KO and Levine JD, 1999, Copyright 1999 by the Society for Neuroscience).

Additional studies have examined cAMP activation in sensory ganglion neurons. Chronic compression of dorsal root ganglion neurons produces abnormal spontaneous activity, which decreases with topical application of PKA inhibitors and increases with PKA activators, *in vitro*. In cultured trigeminal ganglion neurons, capsaicin increases cAMP in a concentration dependent manner. Prostaglandin-enhanced bradykinin excitation in rat sensory neurons is inhibited when pretreated with adenylate cyclase or PKA inhibitors, whereas pretreatment with forskolin enhances the number of action potentials elicited by bradykinin in dorsal root ganglion neurons. In embryonic dorsal root ganglion neurons, prostaglandin E_2 or 8-bromo-cAMP sensitizes currents induced by capsaicin; both are suppressed with PKA inhibition. Additionally, in embryonic dorsal root ganglion neurons, prostaglandin E_2 or cAMP activation inhibits potassium currents, which is prevented by PKA inhibition. Interestingly, Oshita and colleagues demonstrated that the cannabinoid receptor agonist, HU210, significantly inhibited the forskolin-induced intracellular cAMP production in cultured rat dorsal root ganglion cells. Thus, peripheral activation of the cAMP pathway produces hyperalgesia, sensitizes nociceptors, and inhibits potassium currents *in vitro*, whereas blockade of the cAMP pathway reverses hyperalgesia and sensitization of dorsal root ganglion neurons.

Spinal Role

In the spinal cord, activation of the cAMP pathway produces a dose-dependent mechanical hyperalgesia, augments the excitatory responses of dorsal horn neurons *in vitro*, and enhances spinothalamic tract (STT) neuron responses to noxious, but not innocuous, stimuli. Therefore, spinal activation of the cAMP pathway elicits nocifensive behaviors and sensitizes nociceptive neurons.

Similarly inhibition of the cAMP pathway reverses hyperalgesia and dorsal horn sensitization. Following intradermal, intramuscular, or intraarticular capsaicin injection, or repeated intramuscular acid injections, mechanical hyperalgesia is produced that is reversed by spinal application of PKA or adenylate cyclase inhibitors (Fig.17.3). The activation of the cAMP pathway occurs in a time-dependent manner after insult to deep somatic tissue. Mechanical hyperalgesia after intramuscular acid injections or capsaicin injected into muscle or joint is reversed by blockade of PKA or adenylate cyclase in the spinal cord 24 hours, but not 1 week, after the induction of hyperalgesia(Fig.17.3). In parallel to the behavioral data, sensitization of STT neurons to intradermal capsaicin is reversed by PKA inhibition. Thus, spinal activation of the cAMP pathway produces hyperalgesia and sensitizes nociceptors, and inhibition of the cAMP pathway reverses hyperalgesia and sensitization of dorsal horn neurons.

Spinal activation of the cAMP pathway, through extracellular stimulation, may lead to increases in the phosphorylation of a number of proteins and receptors involved in pain transmission. The number of extracellular messengers that regulate the cAMP pathway is immense and includes the following: CGRP, dopamine, norepinephrine, prostaglandins, serotonin, histamine, calcium, substance P, and adenosine.

PKA modulates the NMDA and AMPA receptors through phosphorylation. Following intradermal injection of capsaicin, there is an increase in the phosphorylation of the NR1 subunit of the NMDA receptor or the GluR1 subunit of the AMPA receptor, which is prevented by blockade of PKA. The mechanisms of these increases in phosphorylation continue to be explored. Protein kinase-induced phosphorylation may increase the amplitude of glutamate-induced currents, remove the magnesium block on the NMDA receptor, increase spontaneous channel opening, or increase membrane insertion.

Previous studies have demonstrated the relationship between the NMDA receptor and the cAMP pathway. Application of 8-bromo-cAMP potentiates the NMDA responses of dorsal horn neurons in *in vitro* preparations. Furthermore, spinal administration of 8-bromo-cAMP produces mechanical hyperalgesia that is blocked by the NMDA receptor antagonist, AP5. Thus, PKA interacts with the NMDA receptor producing sensitization and hyperalgesia.

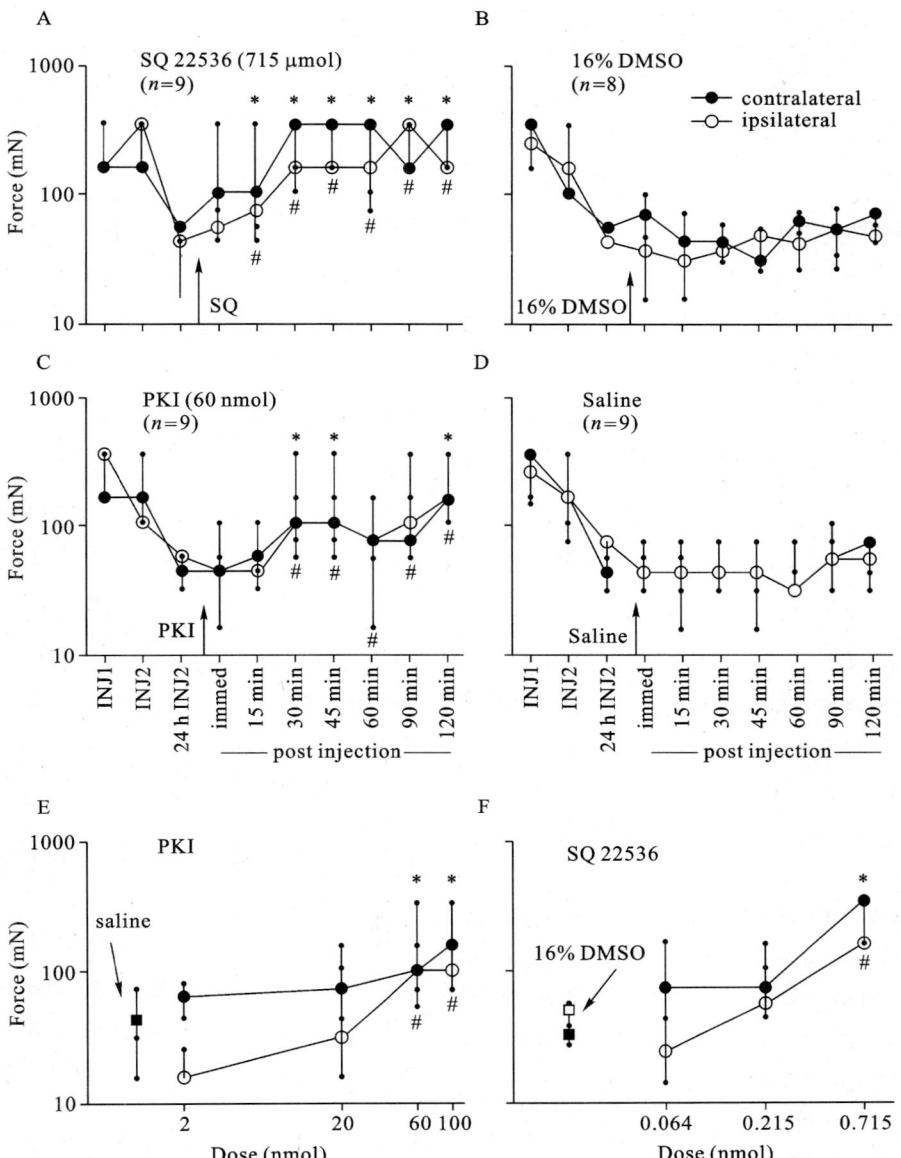

Fig.17.3 Spinal inhibition of adenylate cyclase or protein kinase A reverses mechanical hyperalgesia in an acid-induced muscle pain model (Hoeger-Bement and Sluka, 2003, Copyright 2003 by the Society for Neuroscience).

Interestingly, not all studies demonstrate an increased activation of the cAMP pathway after nociceptive stimulation. Following injection of carrageenan into the paw, cAMP decreases in the lumbar dorsal horn. One explanation is that activation of endogenous opioids could decrease intracellular cAMP. In spinal cord slices from monoarthritic rats, pretreatment with μ-and δ-opioid receptor agonists decreases cAMP concentrations. Further, forskolin-induced increases in cAMP concentrations are

prevented by activation of opioid receptors. Thus, cAMP activity may increase or decrease following tissue injury, with decreases in activity likely due to activation of endogenous opioids.

Activation of the cAMP pathway also results in phosphorylation of transcription factors. The transcription factor CREB is phosphorylated by PKA at Ser 133. An increase in phosphorylated-CREB (p-CREB) in the spinal cord is found in a number of pain models such as carrageenan paw inflammation, intradermal capsaicin injection, subcutaneous formalin, nerve growth factor, neuropathic pain, intramuscular acid injections, and sciatic nerve stimulation above C fiber threshold. In most cases, increases in p-CREB correspond to the time frame of hyperalgesia in neuropathic and inflammatory pain and are stimulus-dependent. Since a number of kinases phosphorylate CREB at the same site as PKA, increases in p-CREB may not reflect activation of the cAMP pathway. However, the increases in the spinal cord after intramuscular acid injections are PKA-dependent since blockade of adenylate cyclase reduces p-CREB. A functional role for CREB in pain modulation was demonstrated utilizing CREB antisense injected spinally to downregulate CREB following partial sciatic nerve ligation. Spinal treatment with CREB antisense significantly decreased mechanical hyperalgesia and CREB expression and prevented the increase in p-CREB expression in the dorsal horn following partial sciatic nerve lesion suggesting that CREB plays a functional role in nociceptive transmission.

Interestingly, CGRP increased the expression of the neurokinin-1 receptor and p-CREB in dissociated rat spinal neurons and co-treatment with CGRP and a PKA inhibitor inhibited the increase in CRE-dependent gene expression. Similarly, CGRP-induced hyperalgesia and sensitization of dorsal horn neurons was decreased by spinal administration of a PKA inhibitor, H89. Thus, CGRP produces pain behaviors and changes in the central nervous system that are mediated by PKA.

Supraspinal Role

In supraspinal sites such as anterior cingulate cortex, periaqueductal gray (PAG), rostral ventromedial medulla (RVM) and locus coeruleus (LC), pain modulation is mediated by various metabotropic as well as ionotropic receptors that utilize second messenger systems as intracellular effector molecules. Experimental studies indicate that supraspinal activation of the cAMP pathway is involved in pain processing. Acute treatment with opioid agonists *in vitro* inhibits

adenylate cyclase activity in the locus coeruleus (LC), dorsal raphe, frontal cortex and neostriatum. Chronic treatment with morphine *in vivo*, which produces tolerance and dependence, increases basal and forskolin-stimulated adenylate cyclase in the LC. Thus inhibition of the cAMP pathway occurs during opioid analgesia, whereas the cAMP pathway is activated when tolerance develops. On the contrary, activation of the cAMP pathway by injecting dibutyryl cAMP into the brainstem reticular formation (CRF) and periaqueductal gray (PAG), produces analgesia. Recent data show that hyperalgesia induced by paw inflammation is eliminated in adenylate cyclase 1 and 8 (AC1 and AC8) double knockout mice and restored by activation of the cAMP pathway (forskolin) in the anterior cingulate cortex (Fig.17.4). Further, the hyperalgesia following paw inflammation is reduced by blockade of PKA in the anterior cingulate cortex. Thus, activation of the cAMP pathway in the anterior cingulate cortex plays a significant role in the production of pain and hyperalgesia.

IP3/DAG-PKC PATHWAY

Peripheral Role

Tissue injury results in local release of inflammatory mediators and algogenic substances, such as epinephrine, bradykinin, histamine, ATP, and prostanoids. These proinflammatory substances sensitize primary afferent nociceptors by activation of intracellular kinases, including PKC, PKA, and extracellular signal-regulated kinases (ERKs). There is evidence to suggest that PKC mediates nociceptor sensitization and hyperalgesia induced by epinephrine and bradykinin. Application of epinephrine to cultured small diameter DRG neurons potentiates tetrodotoxin resistant sodium channel currents (TTX-R I_{Na}) that is prevented by inhibition of the intracellular mediators PKC, PKC-ε, or PKA. Similarly, intradermal injection of epinephrine produces mechanical hyperalgesia that is prevented i) by local blockade of PKC and PKA or ii) in PKC-ε knockout mice. Thus, PKC, and in particular the isozyme PKC-ε, mediate epinephrine-induced hyperalgesia in peripheral tissues.

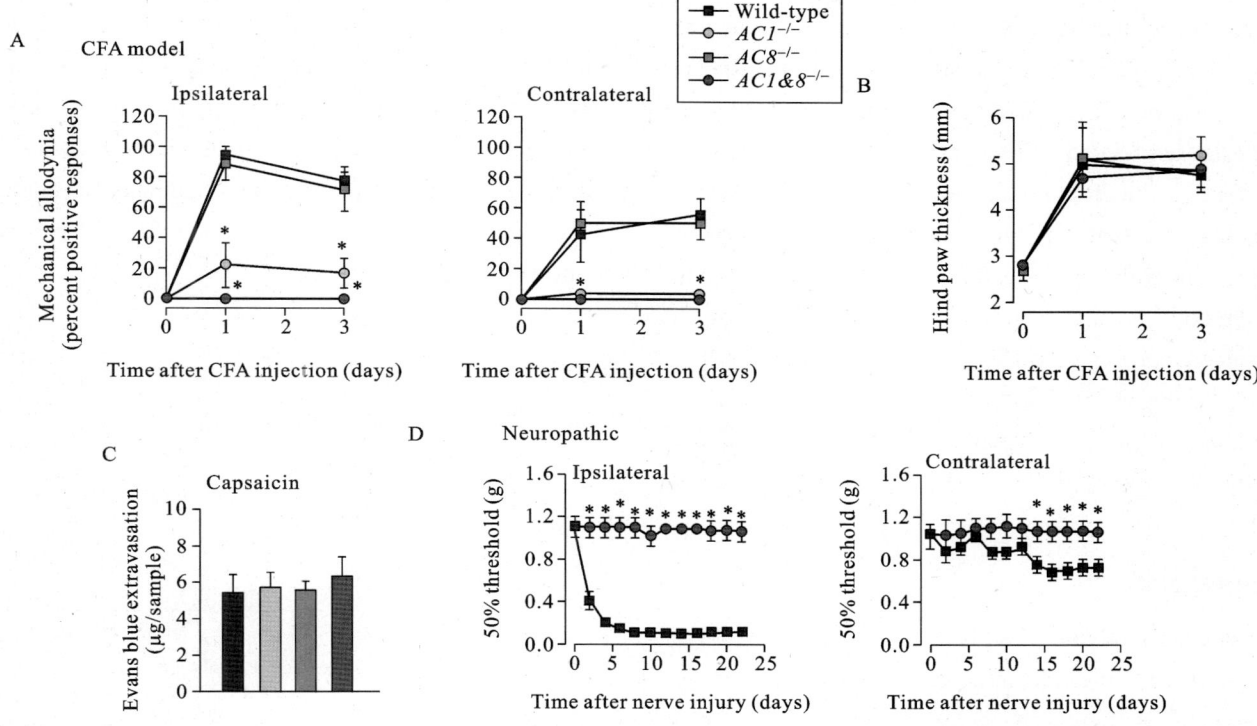

Fig.17.4   Absence of behavioral sensitization (allodynia) to CFA injection and nerve injury in AC1 & AC8 double knockout mice (Wei *et al.*, 2002, Elsevier).

Peripheral application of bradykinin (BK) produces pain and heat hyperalgesia. Bradykinin lowers the threshold temperature for heat evoked activation of the ion channel TRPV1 so that body temperature may be sufficient to activate these receptors in capsaicin sensitive DRG neurons. Sensitization of DRG neurons to heat stimuli is blocked by application of PKC inhibitors and prolonged by phosphatase inhibitors. Further, activation of the PKC pathway produces TRPV1-mediated sensitization of DRG neurons. Thus, the TRPV1 ion channel contribution to this BK-induced heat hyperalgesia is likely regulated by PKC. In particular, PKC-ε rapidly translocates to the membrane of primary afferent nociceptors in response to application of BK or the PKC activator, PMA, and inhibition of this PKC translocation attenuates BK induced sensitization of DRG neurons to heat. This TRPV1 mediated sensitization may occur through direct phosphorylation of the receptor since PKC potentiates TRPV1 function by phosphorylation of the receptor.

Development of chronic hyperalgesia after certain types of tissue injury also depends on activation of PKC. Intradermal injection of PGE2, 5-HT, or an adenosine receptor agonist produces mechanical hyperalgesia that lasts for less than four hours. However, hyperalgesia is prolonged by up to 24 hours when these substances are administered between 5 days and 3 weeks after subcutaneous carrageenan injection at the same site. Thus, the initial tissue insult mediated by carrageenan "primes" the nociceptive signal transduction system to respond more robustly to subsequent inflammatory insult. Preemptive pharmacological blockade of PKC or selective blockade of the PKC-ε isozyme prevents the prolonged phase, but not the acute phases, of PGE2induced hyperalgesia. Further, peripheral administration of a PKC-ε agonist induces hyperalgesia that lasts for up to 3 days and like carrageenan prolongs the response to PGE2 after the initial hyperalgesia subsided, both of which are blocked by pretreatment with PKC or PKC-ε inhibitors. Taken together, these findings suggest that PKC signaling, especially involving the PKC-ε isoenzyme, contributes to chronic inflammatory hyperalgesia.

PKC activation also mediates mechanical hyperalgesia associated with peripheral neuropathy. In particular, mechanical hyperalgesia in a model of alcohol consumption induced peripheral neuropathy, and neuropathy induced by the antineoplastic agent, paclitaxel, is significantly reduced by injection of a selective PKC-ε inhibitor into the area of testing. Further, peripheral inhibition of PKC-ε or PKC-δ decreases mechanical hyperalgesia in a model of diabetic neuropathy in male and female rats, respectively.

Spinal Role

As in the periphery, PKC is an important mediator of nociceptive signal transmission in the central nervous system. It is membrane bound within the cytosol of dorsal horn neurons of the spinal cord, as well as in the brain and in primary afferents. There are at least twelve isoforms of PKC. Several of these isoforms are concentrated in the superficial laminae of the dorsal horn, an anatomical indication that these PKC isoforms play a potential role in nociceptive signaling. In particular, PKCβII, PKCγ, and PKCα are found in the superficial dorsal horn, and PKC is involved in many aspects of cellular sensitization, including modulation of channel conductivity by phosphorylation and increased trafficking of receptors to the cell membrane. PKC inhibition in the spinal cord reduces the tactile allodynia caused by direct application of phorbol esters, which are PKC agonists.

Activation of PKC with phorbol esters in the spinal cord decreases heat and mechanical withdrawal thresholds and increases glutamate release in the spinal cord. Protein kinase C is involved in animal models of both neuropathic and inflammatory pain. In rats with neuropathic pain produced by spinal nerve ligation, the mechanical hyperalgesia is reversed by intrathecally administered PKC inhibitors. There is also

an increase in membrane-bound PKC and an upregulation of PKCγ and PKCβII in the spinal cord after neuropathic injury. Mechanical and heat hyperalgesia induced by nerve injury are reduced in PKCγ knockout mice when compared to wild-type mice. Similarly, spinal blockade of PKC reverses the hyperalgesia induced by subcutaneous formalin, cutaneous capsaicin, subcutaneous bee venom, intrathecal CGRP or Substance P (Fig.17.5, Fig.17.6).

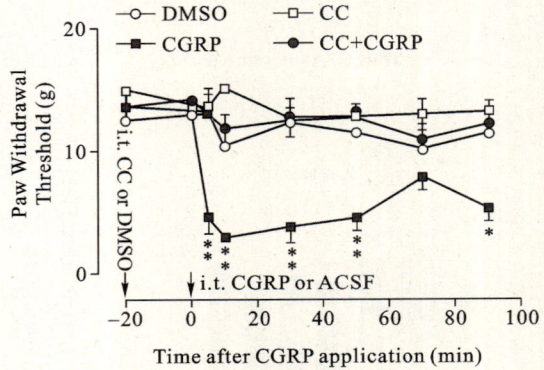

Fig.17.5 Inhibition of protein kinase C (PKC) attenuates the mechanical hyperalgesia induced by CGRP (Sun *et al.*, 2004, The American Physiological Society).

Spinothalamic tract neurons and other dorsal horn neurons sensitize after application of phorbol esters to activate PKC. Responses to innocuous and noxious mechanical stimuli and heat stimuli increase after phorbol ester application; similarly background activity also increases. Conversely, infusion of PKC inhibitors into the dorsal horn after capsaicin-induced STT cell sensitization decreases background firing activity and reverses the capsaicin-induced increase in response to brush, press, and pinch. Further, the sensitization of dorsal horn neurons induced by mustard oil does not develop in PKCγ knockout mice compared to wild-type controls.

Activation of PKC in dorsal horn neurons enhances NMDA currents on dorsal horn neurons. One mechanism could be a decrease in Mg^{2+} affinity in the NMDA receptor pore in response to PKC and increases the probability of the channel opening. Activation of PKC increases phosphorylation of the NR1 subunit of the NMDA receptor and the GluR1 subunit

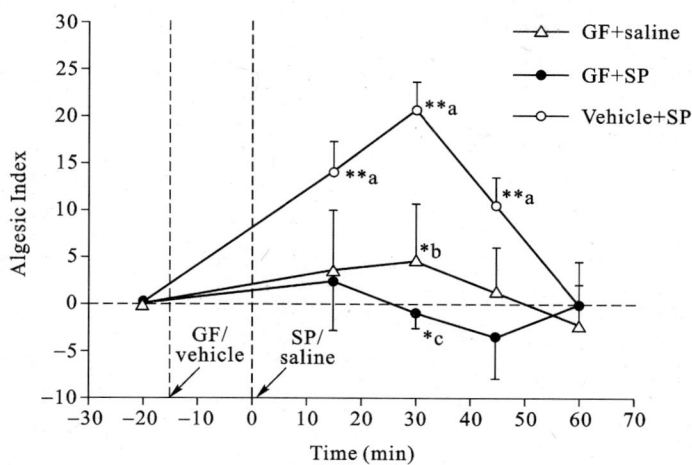

Fig.17.6 Inhibition of spinal substance P-induced thermal hyperalgesia by spinal pretreatmentwith GF109203X (PKC inhibitor) (Wajima *et al.*, 2000, Elsevier).

of the AMPA receptor likely increasing activity of the receptors. Intradermal capsaicin increases phosphorylation of Ser^{831} on the GluR1 receptor in the spinal cord that is reversed by blockade of spinal PKC. Thus, increased phosphorylation of glutamate receptors could enhance synaptic activity resulting in increased excitation of nociceptive dorsal horn neurons.

Another mechanism by which PKC produces its nociceptive effect is through decreasing efficacy of inhibitory neurotransmitters, thus increasing excitation. PKC reverses μ-opioid receptor G-protein coupled calcium channel inhibition in the spinal dorsal horn of rats leading to decreased μ-opioid receptor mediated antinociception. Intradermal injection of capsaicin reduces the inhibition of spinothalamic tract neurons normally produced by electrical stimulation of the periaqueductal gray; this loss of inhibition is prevented by spinal blockade of PKC. Thus, increased PKC activity reduces normal inhibition within the spinal cord.

Supraspinal Role

Tissue injury and inflammation produce time dependent changes in descending modulation of spinal nociceptive transmission. This is accompanied by changes in excitatory amino acid neurotransmission within the RVM, and PKC signaling appears to contribute to these changes. The expression of the AMPA subunit protein, GluR1, is significantly increased within the RVM after plantar injection of CFA. The amount of GluR1 phosphorylated at S831 in the RVM is also increased during both the early and late phases of CFA-induced inflammation. This increase in GluR1 phosphorylation is prevented by pre-administration of NMDA receptor antagonists, a PKC inhibitor, or a CaMKII inhibitor. These data would suggest that in the RVM, NMDA receptor activation and associated calcium signaling contribute to AMPA receptor phosphorylation through activation of CaMKII or PKC. Thus, enhancement of AMPA receptor mediated descending inhibition is thought to involve an increase in the number of AMPA receptors and phosphorylation mediated changes in receptor function or trafficking. Although PKC signaling may be important for enhancement of descending inhibition after tissue injury, the impact of RVM PKC blockade on spinal nociceptive transmission has not been evaluated.

cGMP-PKG PATHWAY

Peripheral Role

The role of GC/cGMP/ PKG system in the periphery has not been studied extensively in terms of nociception. However, there are a few studies showing the involvement of this second messenger system in mediating pain in the periphery. cGMP is produced by the enzyme guanylate cyclase (GC), activated by NO, and degraded by the phosphodiesterase (PDE) enzyme group. Sodium nitroprusside, a source for NO, produces analgesia when administered into the paw, in a model of PGE2-induced hyperalgesia, and the analgesic effect is blocked by a GC inhibitor, methylene blue. In the same model, a phosphodiesterase enzyme inhibitor, UK-114, 542-27, enhances the analgesia produced by a sub-effective dose of fentanyl. Nevertheless, UK-114, 542-27 alone did not cause analgesia. Further PKG-1 knockout mice show a reduction in the first and the second phase of the formalin test, suggesting both a peripheral and central role for PKG in nociceptive behaviors Therefore, it is possible that the GC/cGMP/PKG system is playing a modulatory role in pain transduction from the periphery.

Spinal Role

The cyclic GMP-PKG system has important functions in the spinal processing of pain. NMDA receptor activation is thought to activate this system through the production of nitric oxide (NO). The NO-cGMP pathway mediates tonic inhibition of spinal transmission of mechanical nociception, since spinal atropine-induced mechanical hyperalgesia is augmented by blockade of NO synthesis or inhibition of guanylate cyclase (GC) enzyme. cGMP levels increase in the dorsal spinal horn following sustained afferent nociceptive input induced by CFA injection. Spinal administration of a NO synthase inhibitor or a guanylate cyclase inhibitor decreases thermal hyperalgesia in a model of peripheral neuropathy, NMDA-induced pain behaviors. In parallel, chronic constriction injury of the sciatic nerve in rats and spinal administration of NMDA increases cGMP levels in the spinal dorsal horn. The increases in cGMP are prevented by inhibition of nitric oxide synthase (NOS) or guanylate cyclase. It may thus be postulated that activation of spinal NMDA receptors causes pain behaviors through an activation of nitric oxide and cGMP within the spinal cord.

cGMP-dependent PKGIα increases in the superficial dorsal horn of the spinal cord after injection of formalin into a hindpaw is completely blocked by inhibitors of nitric oxide synthase, guanylate cyclase, or NMDA receptors. Similarly, blockade of spinal PKGIα reduces the number of flinches and shakes in the formalin test. Thus, PKGIα may play an important role in the central mechanism of formalin-induced inflammatory hyperalgesia in the spinal cord. The upregulation of PKGIα is thought to be mediated through an NMDA-nitric oxide-cGMP signaling pathway. Some studies have shown dual effects of activating this pathway. Spinal inhibition of PKG prevents the increase in glutamate release in the dorsal horn of the spinal cord and mechanical hyperalgesia that normally occurs in response to intradermal capsaicin. Thus, the cGMP-PKG pathway is important in the spinal transmission of nociceptive input.

Supraspinal Role

Cyclic GMP pathway is involved in pain modulation at supraspinal sites in experimental studies. Activation of the cGMP pathway in the caudal brainstem reticular formation, including the RVM, is antinociceptive in acute pain tests. This antinociception is likely mediated through muscarinic receptors since the antinociception produced by a muscarinic agonist, (+)-cis-methyldioxolane, is prevented by PKG inhibitors. Morphine and carbachol produce antinociception in PGE2-induced hind paw hyperalgesia, and in tail flick test, when administered intracerebroventricularly, through the activation of activation of cGMP pathway. Thus the supraspinal activation of cGMP pathway appears to cause antinociception

DRUG TARGETS AND THERAPEUTIC IMPLICATIONS

Manipulation of second messenger pathways has been successfully utilized in therapeutic intervention in many disease conditions. In the case of pain, there is no clinically useful drug as yet, which acts on the second messenger pathways, although some promising preclinical findings have been reported. Inhibition of the cAMP pathway by pharmacological agents or genetic manipulation within the central nervous system inhibits experimental pain. It has been shown that PKA-mediated phosphorylation of glutamate receptors may enhance excitatory synaptic transmission within pain pathways after tissue injury. Also, phosphorylation of transcription factors may contribute to the maintenance of chronic pain by increasing transcription of pain-related genes. Thus, development of drugs to inhibit specific isoforms of AC or PKA could be useful for the treatment of pain conditions. Another avenue for exploration is the supraspinal cGMP pathway, the activation of which appears to inhibit pain. There are many clinically used PDEs such as sildenafil, which activate or sustain cGMP pathway signaling. There are several preclinical studies that show analgesic activity of sildenafil. These drugs could be studied for their potential analgesic effects in humans. These drugs could be studied for their potential analgesic effects. However, it should be noted that the spinal cGMP cascade mediates inflammatory pain. The major challenges for drug discovery in this area are the ubiquitous nature and functional diversity of these pathways.

CONCLUSION

There is preclinical evidence for involvement of second messenger pathways in the generation and maintenance of acute and chronic pain states. However, the ubiquitous nature and functional multiplicity of these pathways make them challenging targets for drug discovery. Also, there are a number of issues to be addressed regarding the role of second messengers in *in vivo* situations. For example, which receptors are modified by kinase-mediated phosphorylation? What genes relevant to pain are transcribed by CREB? Do these genes mediate the acute phase or the chronic phase of pain? Which specific types or isoforms of second messenger components (e.g. AC1, AC8) are important in pain? Answers to these and other similar questions will help us to move forward in delineating

the causes and discovering new targets for the treatment of pain. On a positive note, modulation of some of these pathways attenuates pain irrespective of its causes in preclinical models.

GENERAL CITATIONS

Alberts B, Bray D, Lewis J, Raff M, Roberts K, Watson D.1989. *Molecular Biology of the Cell,*(2ed). New York: Garlan Publishing.

Bennett G, Deer T, Du Pen S, Rauck R, Yaksh T, Hassenbusch SJ. 2000. Future directions in the management of pain by intraspinal drug delivery. *J Pain & Symp Manag*, 20(2): S44-50.

Greengard P. 1978. Phosphorylated proteins as physiological effectors. *Science*, 199: 146-152.

Hatt H. 1999. Modification of glutamate receptor channels: molecular mechanisms and functional consequences. *Naturwissenschaften*, 86(4): 177-186.

Wenthold RJ, Prybylowski K, Standley S, Sans N, Petralia RS. 2003. Trafficking of NMDA receptors. *Annu Rev Pharmacol Toxicol*, 43: 335-358.

Willis WD. 2001. Role of neurotransmitters in sensitization of pain responses. *Ann N Y Acad Sci*, 933: 142-56.

DISCOVERY CITATIONS

Aley KO, Levine JD. 1999. Role of protein kinase A in the maintenance of inflammatory pain. J *Neurosci*, 19(6): 2181-2186.

Aley KO, Messing RO, Mochly-Rosen D, Levine DJ. 2000. Chronic hypersensitivity for inflammatory nociceptor sensitization mediated by the e isozyme of protein kinase C. *J Neurosci*, 20(12): 4680-4685.

Anderson LE, Seybold VS. 2000. Phosphorylated cAMP response element binding protein increases in neurokinin-1 receptor immunoreactive neurons in rat spinal cord in response to formalin induced nociception. *Neurosci Lett*, 283(1): 29-32.

Baidan LV, Fertel RH, Wood JD. 1992. Effects of brain-gut related peptides on cAMP levels in myenteric ganglia of guinea-pig small intestine. *Eur J Pharmacol*, 225: 21-27.

Begon S, Pickering G, Eschalier A, Mazur A, Rayssiguier Y,

Dubay C. 2001. Role of spinal NMDA receptors, protein kinase C and nitric oxide synthase in the hyperalgesia induced by magnesium deficiency in rats. *Br J Pharm*, 134: 1227-1236.

Bhave G, Hu HJ, Glauner KS, Zhu W, Wang H, Brasier DJ, Oxford GS, Gereau RW. 2003. Protein kinase C phosphorylation sensitizes but does not activate the capsaicin receptor transient receptor potential vanilloid 1 (TRPV1). *Proc Natl Acad Sci USA*, 100(21): 12480-12485.

Brenner GJ, Ji R-R, Shaffer S, Woolf CJ. 2004. Peripheral noxious stimulation induces phosphorylation of the NMDA receptor NR1 subunit at the PKC-dependent site, serine-896, in spinal cord dorsal horn neurons. *J Neuroscience*, 20: 375-384.

Cerne R, Jaing M, Randic M. 1992. Cyclic adenosine 3′, 5′-monophosphate potentiates excitatory amino acid and synaptic responses of rat spinal dorsal horn neurons. *Brain Res*, 596: 111-123.

Cerne R, Randic M. 1992. Modulation of AMPA and NMDA responses in rat spinal dorsal horn neurons by trans-1-aminocyclopentane-1, 3-dicarboxylic acid. *Neurosci Lett*, 14: 144(1-2): 180-184.

Cerne R, Rusin KI, Randic M. 1993. Enhancement of the N-methyl-D-aspartate response in spinal dorsal horn neurons by cAMP dependent protein kinase. *Neurosci Lett*, 161: 124-128.

Cesare P, Dekker LV, Sardini A, Parker PJ, McNaughton PA. 1999. Specific involvement of PKC-ε in sensitization of the neuronal response to painful heat. *Neuron*, 23(3): 617-624.

Cesare P, McNaughton P. 1996. A Novel heat-activ- ated current in nociceptive neurons and its sensitization by bradykinin. *Proc Natl Acad Sci USA*, 93(26): 15435-15439.

Chen L, Huang L-Y M. 1992. Protein kinase C reduces Mg^{2+} block of NMDA-receptor channels as a mechanism of modulation. *Nature*, 356: 521-523.

Coderre TJ, Yashpal K. 1994. Intracellular messengers contributing to persistant nociception and hyperalgesia induced by L-glutamate and substance P in the rat formalin pain model. *Eur J Neurosci*, 6: 1328-1334.

Cui M, Nicol D. 1995. Cyclic AMP mediates the prostaglandin E_2-induced potentiation of bradykinin excitation in rat sensory neurons. *Neuroscience*, 66(2): 459-466.

Dina OA, Barletta J, Chen X, Mutero A, Martin A, Messing RO, Levine JD. 2000. Key role for the epsilon isoform of protein kinase C in painful alcoholic neuropathy in the rat. *J Neurosci*, 20(22): 8614-8619.

Dina OA, Chen X, Reichling D, Levine JD. 2001. Role of protein kinase C ε and protein kinase A in a model of paclitaxel-induced neuropathy in the rat. *Neuroscience*, 108(3): 507-515.

Dolan S, Nolan A. 2001. Biphasic modulation of nociceptive processing by the cyclic AMP protein kinase A signaling pathway in sheep spinal cord. *Neurosci Lett*, 309: 157-160.

Duarte ID, Ferreira SH. 1992. The molecular mechanism of central analgesia induced by morphine or carbachol and the L-arginine-nitric oxide-cGMP pathway. *Eur J Pharmacol*, 6: 221(1): 171-174.

Duman RS, Tallman JF, Nestler EJ. 1988. Acute and chronic opiate-regulation of adenylate cyclase in brain: specific effects in locus coeruleus. *J Pharmacol Exp Ther*, 246(3): 1033-1039

Evans AR, Vasko MR, Nicol GD. 1999. The cAMP transduction cascade mediates the PGE2 induced inhibition of potassium currents in rat sensory neurones. *J Physiol*, 516: 163-178.

Fang L, Wu J, Lin Q, Willis WD. 2003. Protein kinases regulate the phosphorylation of the GluR1 subunit of AMPA receptors of spinal cord in rats following noxious stimulation. *Mol Brain Research*, 118: 160-165.

Ferreira SH, Duarte ID, Lorenzetti BB. 1991. Molecular base of acetylcholine and morphine analgesia. *Agents Actions Suppl*, 32: 101-106.

Ferrer-Montiel A, Montal MS, Diaz-Munoz M, Montal M. 1999. Agonist-independent activation of acetylcholine receptor channels by protein kinase A phosphorylation. *Proc Natl Acad Sci USA*, 88: 10213-10217.

Garry MG, Durnett Richardson J, Hargreaves KM. 1994. Carrageenan-induced inflammation alter the content of i-cGMP and i-cAMP in the dorsal horn of the spinal cord. *Brain Res*, 646: 135-139.

Ginty DD, Bonni A, Greenberg ME. 1994. Nerve growth factor activates a ras-dependent protein kinase that stimulates c-fos transcription via phosphorylation of CREB. *Cell*, 77: 713-725.

Gold MS. Levin JD, Correa AM. 1998. Modulation of TTX-R

I_{Na} by PKC and PKA and their role in PGE$_2$- induced sensitization of rat sensory neurons *in vitro. J Neurosci*, 18(24): 10345-10355.

Gold MS, Reichling DB, Shuster MJ, Levine DJ. 1996. Hyperalgesic agents increase a tetrodotoxin-resistant Na$^+$ current in nociceptors. *Proc Natl Acad Sci USA*, 93: 1108-1112.

Gonzalez GA, Montminy MR. 1989. Cyclic AMP stimulates somatostatin gene transcription by phosphorylation of CREB at serine 133. *Cell*, 59(4): 675-680.

Granados-Soto V, Kalcheva I, Hua X, Newton A, Yaksh TL. 2000. Spinal PKC activity and expression: role in tolerance produced by continuous spinal morphine infusion. *Pain*, 85(3): 395-404.

Guan Y, Terayama R, Dubner R, Ren K. 2001. Plasticity in excitatory amino acid receptor-mediated descending pain modulation after inflammation. *JPET*, 300(2): 513-520.

Guan Y, Guo W, Zou S-P, Dubner R, Ren K. 2003. Inflammation-induced upregulation of AMPA receptor subunit expression in brain stem pain modulatory circuitry. *Pain*, 104: 401-413.

Guan Y, Guo W, Robbins MT, Dubner R, Ren K. 2004. Changes in AMPA receptor phosphorylation in the rostral ventromedial medulla after inflammatory hyperalgesia in rats. *Neuroscience Letters*, 366: 201-205.

Hoeger Bement MK, Sluka KA. 2003. Phosphorylation of CREB and mechanical hyperalgesia is reversed by blockade of the cAMP pathway in a time-dependent manner after repeated intramuscular acid injections. *J Neurosci*, 23(13): 5437-5445.

Hu JY, Zhao ZQ. 2001. Differential contribution of NMDA and non-NMDA receptors to spinal fos expression evoked by superficial tissue and muscle inflammation in the rat. *Neuroscience*, 106(4): 823-831.

Hua X, Chen P, Yaksh T. 1999. Inhibition of spinal protein kinase C reduces nerve injury-induced tactile allodynia in neuropathic rats. *Neurosci Lett*, 276: 99-102.

Hurley RW, Hammond DL. 2000. The analgesic effects of supraspinal µ and δ opioid receptor agonists are potentiated during persistent inflammation. *J Neurosci*, 20(3): 1249-1259

Igwe OJ, Chronwall BM. 2001. Hyperalgesia induced by peripheral inflammation is mediated by protein kinase C βII isozyme in the rat spinal cord. *Neuroscience*, 104(3):

875-890.

Iwamoto ET, Marion L. 1994. Pharmacological evidence that nitric oxide mediates the antinocice- ption produced by muscarinic agonists in the rostral ventral medulla of rats. *J Pharmacol Exp Ther*, 269(2): 699-708.

Jain NK, Patil CS, Singh A, Kulkarni SK. 2001. Sildenafil-induced peripheral analgesia and activation of the nitric oxide-cyclic GMP pathway. *Brain Res*, 909(1-2): 170-178.

Ji RR, Rupp F. 1997. Phosphorylation of transcription factor CREB in rat spinal cord after formalin induced hyperalgesia: relationship to c-fos induction. *J Neurosci*, 17(5): 1776-1785.

Ji RR, Brenner GJ, Schmoll R, Baba H, Woolf CJ. 2000. Phosphorylation of ERK and CREB in nociceptive neurons after noxious stimulation. *Proc. 9th World Congress on Pain*, 16: 191-198.

Joseph EK, Levine JD. 2003. Sexual dimorphism in the contribution of protein kinase C isoforms to nociception in the streptozotocin diabetic rat. *Neuroscience*, 120(4): 907-913.

Kawamata T, Omote K. 1999. Activation of spinal N-methyl-D-aspartate receptors stimulates a nitric oxide/cyclic guanosine 3,5-monophosphate/glutamate release cascade in nociceptive signaling. *Anesthesiology*, 91(5): 1415-1424.

Khasar SG, Lin Y-H, Martin A, Dadgar J, McMahon T, Wang D, Hundle B, Aley KO, Isenberg W, McCarter G, Green PG, Hodge CW, Levine JD, Messing RO. 1999. A novel nociceptor signaling pathway revealed in protein kinase C ε mutant mice. *Neuron*, 24(1): 253-260.

Khasar SG, McCarter G, Levin JD. 1999. Epinephrine produces a β-adrenergic receptor mediated mechanical hyperalgesia and *in vitro* sensitization of rat nociceptors. *J Neurophys*, 81(3): 1104-1112.

Kobayashi H, Hashimoto K, Uchida S, Sakuma J, Takami K, Tohyama M, Izumi F, Yoshida H. 1987. Calcitonin gene related peptide stimulates adenylate cyclase activity in rat striated muscle. *Experientia*, 43: 314-315.

Laufer R, Changeux J-P. 1987. Skeletal muscle: possible neurotrophic role for coexisting neuronal messenger. *EMBO J*, 6: 901-906.

Lee J-J, Hahm E-T, Min B-I, Cho Y-W. 2004. Activation of protein kinase C antagonizes the opioid inhibition of calcium current in rat spinal dorsal horn neurons. *Brain Research*, 1017: 108-119.

Levy RA, Proudfit HK, Goldstein BD. 1983. Antinociception following microinjection of dibutyryl cyclic nucleotides into the caudal reticular formation and periaqueductal gray of the rat brain. *Pharmacol Biochem Behav*, 19(1): 79-84.

Li K-C, Zheng J-H, Chen J. 2000. Involvement of spinal protein kinase C in induction and maintenance of both persisitent spontaneous flinching reflex and contralateral heat hyperalgesia induced by subcutaneous bee venom in the conscious rat. *Neurosci Lett*, 285: 103-106.

Lin Q, Wu J, Willis WD. 2002. Effects of protein kinase A activation on the responses of primate spinothalamic tract neurons to mechanical stimuli. *J Neurophysiol*, 88: 214-221.

Lin Q, Peng Y, Willis W. 1996. Possible role of protein kinase C in the sensitization of primate spinothalamic tract neurons. *J Neuroscience*, 16(9): 3026-3034.

Liu L, Oortgiesen M, Li L, Simon SA. 2001. Capsaicin inhibits activation of voltage-gated sodium currents in capsaicin-sensitive trigeminal ganglion neurons. *J Physiology*, 85: 745-758.

Lopshire JC, Nicol GD. 1998. The cAMP transduction cascade mediates the prostaglandin E_2 enhancement of the capsaicin-elicited current in rat sensory neurons: whole-cell and single-channel studies. *J Neurosci*, 18(16): 6081-6092.

Lynn B, O'Shea NR. 1998. Inhibition of forskolin-induced sensitization of frog skin nociceptors by the cyclic AMP-dependent protein kinase A antagonist H-89. *Brain Res*, 780: 360-362.

Ma W, Quirion R. 2001. Increased phosphorylation of the cyclic AMP response element binding protein (CREB) in the superficial dorsal horn neurons following partial sciatic nerve ligation. *Pain*, 93: 295-301.

Ma W, Hatzis C, Eisenach JC. 2003. Intrathecal injection of cAMP response element binding protein (CREB) antisense oligonucleotide attenuates tactile allodynia caused by partial sciatic nerve ligation. *Brain Res*, 988: 97-104.

Maegawa FA, Tonussi CR. 2003. The L-arginine/ni- tric oxide/cyclic-GMP pathway apparently mediates the peripheral antihyperalgesic action of fentanyl in rats. *Braz J Med Biol Res,* 36(12): 1701-1707.

Malmberg A, Chen C, Tonegawa S, Basbaum A. 1997. Preserved acute pain and reduced neuropathic pain in mice lacking PKCγ. *Science*, 278: 279-283.

Manning DC, Raja SN, Meyer RA, Campbell JN. 1991. Pain and hyperalgesia after intradermal injection of bradykinin in humans. *Clin Pharmacol Ther*, 50(6): 721-729.

Mao J, Mayer D, Hayes R, Price D. 1993. Spinal patterns of increased spinal cord membrane-bound protein kinase C and their relation to increases in ^{14}C-2-deoxyglucose metabolic activity in rats with painful peripheral mononeuropathy. *J Neurophy- siol*, 70(2): 469-481

Martin W, Malmberg A, Basbaum A. 2001. PKCγ contributes to a subset of the NMDA-dependent spinal circuits that underlie injury-induced persistent pain. *J Neuroscience*, 21(14): 5321-5327.

Messersmith DJ, Kim DJ, Iadarola MJ. 1998. Transcription factor regulation of prodynorphin gene expression following rat hindpaw inflammation. *Mol Brain Res*, 53: 259-269.

Miletic G, Pankratz MT, Miletic V. 2002. Increases in the phosphorylation of cyclic AMP response element binding protein (CREB) and decreases in the content of calcineurin accompany thermal hyperalgesia following chronic constriction injury in rats. *Pain*, 99: 493-500.

Miletic V, Bowen K, Miletic G. 2000. Loose ligation of the rat sciatic nerve is accompanied by changes in the subcellular content of protein kinase C beta II and gamma in the spinal dorsal horn. *Neurosci Lett*, 288: 199-202.

Ouseph AK, Khasar SG, Levine JD. 1995. Multiple second messenger systems act sequentially to mediate rolipram-induced prolongation of prostaglandin E2-induced mechanical hyperalgesia in the rat. *Neuroscience*, 64(3): 769-776.

Palecek J, Paleckova V, Willis W. 1999. The effect of phorbol esters on spinal cord amino acid concentrations and responsiveness of rats to mechanical and thermal stimuli. *Pain*, 80: 597-605.

Przewlocka B, Dziedzicka M, Lason W, Przewlocki R. 1992. Differential effects of opioid receptor agonists on nociception and cAMP level in the spinal cord of monoarthritic rats. *Life Sciences*, 50(1): 45-54.

Raymond LA, Tingley WG, Blackstone CD, Roche KW, Huganir RL. 1994. Glutamate receptor modulation by protein phosphorylation. *J Physiol Paris*, 88(3): 181-192.

Salter M, Strijbos PJ, Neale S, Duffy C, Follenfant RL,

Garthwaite J. 1996. The nitric oxide-cyclic GMP pathway is required for nociceptive signalling at specific loci within the somatosensory pathway. *Neuroscience*, 73(3): 649-655.

Seybold VS, McCarson KE, Mermelstein PG, Groth RD, Abrahams LG. 2003. Calcitonin gene related peptide regulates expression of neurokinin$_1$ receptors by rat spinal neurons. *J Neurosci*, 23(15): 1816-1824.

Siegan JB, Hama AT, Sagen J. 1996. Alterations in rat spinal cord cGMP by peripheral nerve injury and adrenal medullary transplantation. *Neurosci Lett*, 215(1): 49-52.

Skyba DA, Hoeger-Bement M, Buttjer MD, Hanfelt CR, Lander JR, Stelk CJ, Sluka KA. 2003. Spinal administration of 8-bromo-cAMP produces NMDA receptor-dependent hyperalgesia. *Neuroscience Abstract*, 383(3)

Slack S, Pezet S, McMahon S, Thompson S, Malcangio M. 2004. Brain-derived neurotrophic factor induces NMDA receptor subunit one phosphorylation via ERK and PKC in the rat spinal cord. *Eur J Neuroscience*, 20: 1769-1778.

Sluka KA. 1997. Activation of the cAMP transduction cascade contributes to the mechanical hyperalgesia and allodynia induced by intradermal injection of capsaicin. *Br J Pharmacol*, 122: 1165-1173.

Sluka KA. 2002. Stimulation of deep somatic tissue with capsaicin produces long-lasting mechanical allodynia and heat hypoalgesia that depends on early activation of the cAMP pathway. *J Neurosci*, 22(13): 5687-5693.

Sluka KA, Rees H, Chen PS, Tsuruoka M, Willis WD. 1997. Inhibitors of G-proteins and protein kinases reduce the sensitization to mechanical stimulation and the desensitization to heat of spinothalamic tract neurons induced by intradermal injection of capsaicin in the primate. *Exp Brain Res*, 115: 15-24.

Sluka KA, Rohlwing JJ, Busley RA, Eikenberry SA, Wilken JM. 2002. Chronic muscle pain induced by repeated acid injection is reversed by spinally administered μ-, and δ-, but not κ-opioid receptor agonists. *JPET*, 302: 1146-1150.

Sluka KA, Willis WD. 1998. Increased spinal release of excitatory amino acids following intradermal injection of capsaicin is reduced by a protein kinase G inhibitor. *Brain Res*, 6: 798(1-2): 281-286.

Sluka KA, Willis WD. 1997. The effects of G-protein and protein kinase inhibitors on the behavioral responses of rats to intradermal injection of capsaicin. *Pain*, 71(2): 165-178.

Sugiura T, Tominaga M, Katsuya H, Mizumura K. 2002. Bradykinin lowers the threshold temperature for heat activation of vanilloid receptor 1. *J Neurophysiol*, 88: 544-548.

Sun RQ, Tu YJ, Lawand NB, Yan JY, Lin Q, Willis WD. 2004. Calcitonin gene-related peptide receptor activation produces PKA-and PKC-dependent mechanical hyperalgesia and central sensitization. *J Neurophysiology*, 92(5): 2859-2866.

Taiwo YO, Levine JD. 1988. Characterization of the arachidonic acid metabolites mediating bradykinin and noradrenaline hyperalgesia. *Brain Res*, 458(2): 402-406.

Tao YX, Hassan A, Haddad E, Johns RA. 2000. Expression and action of cyclic GMP-dependent protein kinase Ialpha in inflammatory hyperalgesia in rat spinal cord. *Neuroscience*, 95(2): 525-533.

Taiwo YO, Bjerknes LK, Goetzl EJ, Levine JD. 1989. Mediation of primary afferent peripheral hyperalgesia by the cAMP second messenger system. *J Neurosci*, 32(3): 577-580.

Taiwo YO, Levine JD. 1991. Further confirmation of the role of adenyl cyclase and of cAMP dependent protein kinase in primary afferent hyperalgesia. *Neuroscience*, 441(1): 131-135.

Terayama R, Guan Y, Dubner R, Ren K. 2000. Activity- induced plasticity in brain stem pain modulatory circuitry after inflammation. *Neuroreport*, 11(9): 1915-1919

Tomasi V, Biondi C, Trevisani A, Martini M, Perri V. 1977. Modulation of cyclic AMP levels in the bovine superior cervical ganglion by prostaglandin E_1 and dopamine. *J Neurochem*, 28: 1289-1297.

Wajima Z, Hua XY, Yaksh TZ. 2000. Inhibition of spinal protein kinase C blocks substance P-mediated hyperalgesia. *Brain Res*, 887(2): 314-321.

Wei F, Qiu CS, Kim SJ, Muglia L, Maas JW, Pineda VV, Xu HM, Chen ZF, Storm DR, Muglia LJ, Zhuo M. 2002. Genetic elimination of behavioral sensitization in mice lacking calmodulin stimu- lated adenylyl cyclases. *Neuron*, 26: 713-726.

Wu J, Fang L, Lin Q, Willis WD. 2002. The role of nitric oxide in the phosphorylation of cyclic adenosine monophosphate-responsive element-bi- nding protein in the spinal cord after intradermal injection of capsaicin. *J Pain*, 3(3): 190-198.

Yashpal K, Fisher K, Chabot J, Coderre T. 2001. Differential effects of NMDA and group I mGluR antagonists on both nociception and spinal cord protein kinase C translocation in the formalin test and a model of neuropathic pain in rats. *Pain,* 94: 17-29.

Yashpal K, Pitcher GM, Parent A, Quirion R, Coderre TJ. 1995. Noxious thermal and chemical stimulation induce increases in 3H-phorbol 12, 13-dibutyrate binding in spinal cord dorsal horn as well as persistent pain and hyperalgesia, which is reduced by inhibition of protein kinase C. *J Neurosci,* 15(5 Pt 1): 3263-3672.

Zou X, Lin Q, Willis WD. 2000. Enhanced phosphorylation of NMDA receptor 1 subunites in spinal cord dorsal horn and spinothalamic tract neurons after intradermal injection of capsaicin in rats. *J Neurosci,* 20(18): 6989-6997.

Zou X, Lin A, Willis WD. 2002. Role of protein kinase A in phosphorylation of NMDA receptor 1 subunits in dorsal horn and spinothalamic tract neurons after intradermal injection of capsaicin in rats. *Neuroscience,* 115(3): 775-786.

Genetic Approaches for the Study of Pain

CHAPTER 18

Rohini Kuner

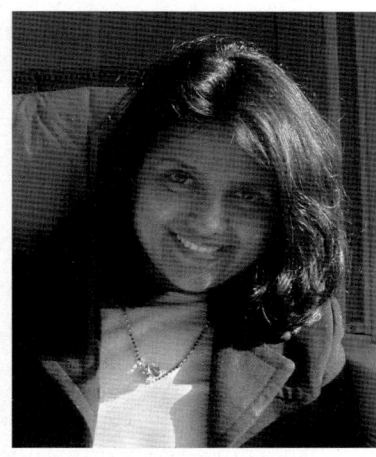

Dr. Rohini Kuner is a Principal Investigator in the Faculty of Medicine, University of Heidelberg, Germany. After graduating from the University of Bombay, she pursued a Ph.D. degree in Pharmacology and Toxicology at the College of Medicine, University of Iowa, Iowa City, USA. She continued her postdoctoral training at the University of Heidelberg and the Max-Planck-Institut for Medical Research.

MAJOR CONTRIBUTIONS

1. Kuner R, Kohr G, Grunewald S, Eisenhardt G, Bach A, Kornau H C. 1999. Role of Heteromer formation in GABA-B receptor function. *Science*, 283: 74-77.

2. Swiercz JM*, Kuner R*, Behrens J, Offermanns S. 2002. Plexin-B1 directly interacts with PDZ-RhoGEF/LARG to regu- late RhoA and growth cone morphology. *Neuron*, 35(1): 51-63. (* equal contribution)

3. Hartmann B, Ahmadi S, Heppenstall P, Zeilhofer HU, Lewin G, Schott C, Seeburg P H, Sprengel R, Kuner R. 2004. The AMPA receptor subunits, GluR-A and GluR-B reciprocally modulate spinal synaptic plasticity and inflam- matory pain. *Neuron*, 44(4): 637-50.

4. Dreyer J, Schleicher M, Tappe A, Schilling K, Kuner T, Kusumawidijaja G, Müller-Esterl W, Oess S and Kuner R 2004 (NOS)-interacting protein interacts with neuronal NOS and regulates its distribution and activity. *J Neurosci*, 24(46): 10454-10465.

5. Kuner R, Groom A, Bresink I, Kornau H C, Stefovska V, Müller G, HartmannB, Tschauner K, Waibel S, Ludolph A C, Ikonomidou C, Seeburg P H and Turski L. 2005. Late-onset motoneuron disease caused by transgenic expression of a functionally modified AMPA receptor subunit. *Proc Natl Acad Sci USA*, 102(16): 5826-5831.

MAIN TOPICS

Spatial and temporal control of gene expres- sion in mice: the art of conditional gene targeting

The Cre-loxP recombinase system

Currently available Cre-expressing mice for the study of pain

Cre expression in nociceptors

Cre expression in the forebrain

Cre expression in pain modulatory centers

The importance of appropriate controls in experiments involving knockout mice

Spatial and temporal control of gene expr- ession in mice— the use of the RNAi methodology in the study of pain

Efficacy and risks of naked siRNAs versus gene delivery systems for shRNAs

RNAi in bringing about loss-of-function in pain pathways

A comparison of Cre-loxP approach with RNAi methodology

Spatial and temporal control of gene expression in mice — overexpression of genes

Conditional overexpression of genes in transgenic mice using inducible systems

Viral-mediated gene delivery in pain pathways

SUMMARY

The development of gene technology has opened unprecedented new perspectives in the understanding as well as the treatment of medical disorders. Although molecular techniques and genetic engineering were introduced into the pain field with a significant delay, as compared with other areas in neuroscience, they are now regarded as the prime methods for addressing mechanisms which underly cellular and network changes causing chronic pain. It is now not only possible to delete or to overexpress pain-associated molecules, but also feasible to bring about these changes selectively in distinct anatomical compartments of the pain pathway. At the very forefront is the method of conditional gene deletion using the Cre-loxP system in transgenic mice. This remains by far the most robust and clean approach for selective modification of gene expression. Some limitations of the Cre-loxP system in mice are now being overcome by novel approaches such as RNA interference. Moreover, RNA- and DNA viruses are emerging as excellent tools for delivering genes or deleting them in distinct regions in the pain pathway. Not only do these methodologies offer means for rapidly testing a large number of candidate molecules for their potential functions in pain, but they also allow, for the first time, a possibility of moving gene technology out of the laboratory straight to the bedside of chronically pain-afflicted patients.

INTRODUCTION

The precise molecular events underlying physiological nociception and pathological changes thereof in chronic pain states are still very poorly understood. Plasticity of primary sensory neurons and of the synapses they make with dorsal horn neurons is an important component of the cellular basis for the development and maintenance of chronic, pathological pain. Sensitization of peripheral nociceptors and their central synapses following inflammation or nerve injury is manifest in form of dramatic phenotypic alterations such as hyperalgesia, allodynia, spontaneous pain and aberrant referral of pain. The current understanding of these phenomena has resulted from work done over decades using behavioral, physiological, pharmacological, histological and biochemical tools. Methodologies such as electrophysiology enable an understanding of the changes in the activity of nerve cells or neural networks and behavioral assays permit an analysis of how the overall response of the organism towards sensory stimuli changes in pathological pain states. However, an understanding of *how* these changes take place — that is, which molecules originally cause the cellular and network changes that lead to altered pain perception, requires the application of specific tools from molecular pharmacology. The application of molecular and genetic technology offers unprecedented scope for elucidating the molecular mechanisms underlying pathological pain. It should be stressed, however, that producing a molecular change alone does not reveal anything about a pain disorder. It is only the combination of molecular and genetic methods with analytical techniques like electrophysiology, behavior, histochemistry etc., which permit a final "cause and effect" analysis. Therefore, molecular and genetic approaches must go hand-in-hand with behavioral and electrophysiological analysis.

This chapter aims at providing an overview of exciting and novel genetic approaches, such as conditional gene targeting, RNA interference (RNAi) and viral-mediated gene delivery, which can be effectively applied for studying and, in the future, also treating pain disorders.

SPATIAL AND TEMPORAL CONTROL OF GENE EXPRESSION IN MICE: THE ART OF CONDITIONAL GENE TARGETING

Functions of neural genes can be defined in transgenic animals either by a gain-of-function produced by overexpression or by loss-of-function produced by gene ablation. Recently, the application of gene targeting technology has delivered valuable insights into several aspects of physiological nociception as well as changes in nociception in inflammatory or neuropathic conditions. However, a major limitation of studies relying on classical (or global) knockout mice is the lack of specificity of the site of gene deletion. A majority of candidate mediators for nociception or pathological pain are widely expressed in the peripheral and central nervous system. Therefore, they can not only modulate the reception, gating, and processing of noxious and nonnoxious sensory inputs, but also affect emotion, anxiety, motivation and mood. Furthermore, several behavioral pain assays involve the measurement of motor responses, such as withdrawal, to noxious sensory stimuli applied to a particular dermatome or viscerotome, thereby raising the possibility that motor defects caused by gene deletion in motor neurons are erroneously read as changes in nociception and analgesia. Moreover, many candidate genes proposed to be important in pathological pain are expressed in astrocytes and cells of the immune system, which can strongly modulate the course and outcome in pathological pain models, especially in inflammatory states. Finally, not only the site, but also the onset of gene deletion is an important factor determining the

inferences that can be made about pain and nociception in knockout mice —early gene deletion can lead to developmental defects in the nociceptive circuitry, which would cause artifacts and obfuscate the interpretation of the study. Thus, owing to the multiple limitations and liabilities of global ablation in classical mouse knock-outs, systems which enable a tightly-regulated spatial and temporal control of gene expression are required for a rigorous analysis of pain and nociception in knockout mice.

The Cre-loxP recombinase system

The Cre-loxP recombinase system is the most prominent of the binary systems available for inducible, tissue-specific gene expression, which has been successfully used for conditional expression of a multitude of genes, including several neural genes. This system utilises the activity of the enzyme, Cre recombinase (Cre) to excise or invert DNA segments flanked by Cre-recognition sequences, loxP sites (refer to BOX 18.1 for description of how the Cre-loxP system works). Thus, by flanking particular target gene sequences with loxP sites in the mouse genome and mating such mice with transgenic mice expressing Cre in a tissue-specific manner, a conditional, tissue-specific knock-out of the target gene can be achieved (Fig.18.1).

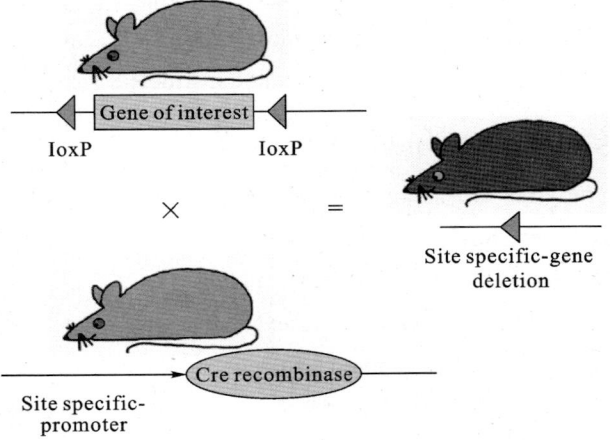

Fig.18.1   The Cre-loxP system for conditional gene deletion.

BOX 18.1 Recombinases and their uses in gene targeting ⋯

Recent advances in the Cre-loxP and Flp-FRT systems have made it possible to in(activate) genes in a conditional manner in a single gene targeting event. The site-specific recombination systems are comprised of two elements: a recombinase enzyme, such as Cre or Flp and a second element consisting of the 34 bp recognition sequences of the recombinase, such as loxP (for Cre) or Frt (for Flp). To enable conditional gene deletion, the gene to be deleted is engineered in embryonic stem cells to be flanked by two loxP sites. Then, following expression of Cre recombinase, either via a plasmid, virus or transgenic mice, the two loxP sites recombine, thereby leading to a deletion of the flanked gene sequence. Both Cre and Flp are members of the lambda integrase of site-specific recombinases which work over large distances (megabases) to produce a genetic alteration which is specific, conservative (i.e. without overall loss or gain of nucleotides), stable, heritable and functional in a wide variety of cells, both undifferentiated and post-mitotic. The two elements of the recombinase system can also be used to insert, invert or translocate DNA, depending on the design of the experiment.

CURRENTLY AVAILABLE CRE-EXPRESSING MICE FOR THE STUDY OF PAIN

The use of the Cre-LoxP system for conditional gene expression in nociceptive pathways would provide a wide scope for learning the functions of proteins, which impart specific properties to nociceptors and spinal neurons and their role in the development of aberrant pain. The bottleneck for taking full advantage of this powerful technology in pain research is the availability of mouse lines expressing Cre recombinase selectively in anatomically-and functionally-distinct components of pain pathways. However, the field is just starting to develop and a few Cre-transgenic lines have recently become available, which could be highly useful in pain research. This has been greatly facilitated by recent advances in the use of Bacterial Atrificial Chromosomes (BACs) for rapid generation of complex targeting constructs.

Cre expression in nociceptors

The first mouse line to achieve sensory neuron-specific expression of the Cre recombinase was reported by Agarwal *et al.* (2004). Using the ET-cloning technology, Cre-recombinase was targeted in a BAC containing the complete promoter elements of the mouse Nav1.8 (SNS) gene and injected targeted BACs in blastocysts to achieve several mouse lines expressing Cre in a highly specific manner (referred to as SNS-Cre mice hereafter; Fig.18.2). Cre-mediated recombination was seen in all nociceptive and thermoreceptive neurons of the dorsal root ganglia and trigeminal ganglia, in both the peptidergic as well as the non-peptidergic population. In contrast, only a very small proportion of Paravalbumin-positive, large-diameter neurons (proprioceptive neurons) express Cre in SNS-Cre mice. Cre-mediated recombination was not detectable in any regions of the brain, the spinal cord or any non-neural tissues. Importantly, expression of Cre commenced perinatally after invasion of primary afferents into the developing spinal cord, thereby enabling gene manipulations without potential undesirable effects on the development of nociceptive neurons. Thus, the SNS-Cre mice enable selective deletion of genes in subsets of sensory neurons and offer a wide scope for studying potential functions of genes in pain perception, independent of secondary effects arising from developmental defects or global gene ablation. SNS-Cre mice are now being used by several laboratories to address the potential significance of neurotransmitters, neuromediators and their signaling effectors in nociception as well as pathological pain. Another mouse line in which the genetic elements of the Nav1.8 mouse promoter were employed to express Cre recombinase was generated by Stirling *et al.* via a knock-in approach in the mouse genome. Although all the other properties of mice derived such appear to be similar to the SNS-Cre mice, they show an early onset of Cre expression, i.e. at embryonic day 14, before the development of the nociceptive circuitry is complete.

Cre expression in the forebrain

To delineate the significance of central (brain) mechanisms in pathological pain, it is very desirable to achieve conditional gene inactivation in forebrain structures. Targeting the somatosensory cortex and the thalamus is important in experiments addressing the filtering and fine-tuning of sensory information. Furthermore, limbic regions such as the anterior cingulate cortex, the hippocampus, the amygdala etc. are involved in aversive memories and emotional aspects of pain. Transgenic mouse lines expressing Cre selectively in either of these individual regions have not been reported so far. However, the Camk4cre mouse line, which uses a fragment of the promoter elements of the CamKII-alpha gene, expresses Cre selectively in principal neurons of all of the forebrain structures outlined above. These mice do not express Cre in the cerebellum, brainstem, spinal cord or the periphery, thereby enabling selective analyses of forebrain-processing of pain inputs, independently of motor defects or other phenotypes. They are therefore well suited for studying pain mechanisms such as cortical and thalamic processing of nociceptive inputs, cortical reorganization phenomena in pain models linked to amputation-induced pain (phantom limb pain), fear memories associated with pain, etc.

Cre expression in pain modulatory centers

It would be desirable to have mouse lines expressing Cre recombinase selectively in individual brain regions which process and modulate pain input, such as the Locus Ceruleus, the Nucleus Raphe Magnus, the Rostroventral Medulla, the Periaqueductal Grey, the Parabrachial Nucleus etc. To date, however, mice expressing Cre recombinase exclusively in such regions are not available. However, we have generated a transgenic mouse line expressing Cre recombinase predominantly in nonadrenergic neurons of the Locus Ceruleus, the main noradrenergic cell nucleus involved in descending modulation of nociceptive inputs. Furthermore, a mouse line has been described in which all neurons of the sympathetic nervous system express Cre recombinase under the control of the promoter of the gene encoding the enzyme, tyrosine hydroxylase, which may be helpful in addressing the sympathetic regulation of pain.

The importance of appropriate controls in experiments involving knockout mice

Like every technology, gene targeting can reveal meaningful insights only if appropriate controls are used. Therefore, it is very important to control for similarity of the genetic background between knockout mice and the controls (wildtype mice). This holds true for classical as well as conditional knockout mice. The behavioral outcome in several pain tests has been shown to be strongly influenced by the genetic background. Genetically modified mice are frequently generated in the 129 strain (129/sv or 129/svJ), which are not suitable for behavioral analysis. Mice derived such as commonly crossed back into the commonly used test strains, such as the C57Bl6 or CD1 in order to perform behavioral analysis. Crossing back 7-8 times ensures that more than 80% of the 129 genome is replaced and it is recommended to perform behavioral analysis only from the 7th or the 8th generation onwards. Furthermore, it is desirable to use wildtype littermates, originating from the same heterozygous breeding from which the knockout mice are obtained, as controls for experiments.

SPATIAL AND TEMPORAL CONTROL OF GENE EXPRESSION IN MICE—THE USE OF THE RNAi METHODOLOGY IN THE STUDY OF PAIN

RNA interference (RNAi) has emerged as a very valuable tool for specific degradation of target mRNAs. Efficiency, efficacy and cost compare so favorably with other techniques that RNAi has quickly become the method of choice for loss-of-function. This is especially true after a major hurdle was recently overcome with the use of siRNAs that seem to by-pass the defense response of the host cell (see BOX18.2 for a description of how the RNAi methodology works). Within three years of these findings, numerous studies have shown that RNAi is an impressive and reliable tool for manipulating genes in laboratory cell lines and primary cells. Furthermore, a steadily increasing number of studies is reporting the applicability of RNAi methodology in manipulating gene expression *in vivo*. However, the application of RNAi to the central nervous system remains a major challenge. Exploiting the RNAi methodology in the study of pain mechanisms and potentially as a therapeutic tool is one of the most exciting opportunities that the pain field has encountered in a long time.

BOX 18.2   How RNAi works ⋯

The RNA interference (RNAi) gene silencing technology relies on the introduction of double-stranded RNA molecules which are identical in sequence to the gene which needs to be silenced, into cells to block the translation of messenger RNAs into protein. The double-stranded RNA is cleaved into shorter fragments in the cell by an enzyme called the Dicer, resulting into degradation of the sense strand. The remaining "antisense" strand then gets incorporated into a protein complex called the RNA-induced silencing complex (RISC). The antisense strand of the RNAi-probe itself directs RISC to the target mRNA sequence to be degraded, thus effectively silencing the expression of the desired gene. Early RNAi approaches in mammalian cells relied upon the introduction of long double-stranded RNA probes (dsRNA), which triggered a defence mechanism in the host cell (the interferon response), which led to an unspecific reduction in the translation of numerous cellular proteins and ultimately to apoptosis. Key to the success of the RNAi technology was the discovery made by Thomas Tuschl and colleagues that short RNAs, ranging between 21 and 23 nucleotides, achieve selective downregulation of the desired mRNA target without evoking an interferon response in the host cell.

EFFICACY AND RISKS OF NAKED SiRNAs VERSUS GENE DELIVERY SYSTEMS FOR shRNAs

Transfected siRNAs achieve significant gene knock-down for 2-4 days before being naturally degraded. This time frame may not be enough for behavioural experiments, especially those involving chronic pain models. Another major challenge with the use of naked siRNAs *in vivo* is their delivery into target cells. Owing to the blood-brain barrier, the delivery of siRNAs to central neurons is rather difficult to achieve. Furthermore, poor delivery into the desired cells means having to administer large doses, which further increases the risk of toxicity and unspecific, "off-target" effects. Chemically synthesized and modified siRNAs show extremely low transfection efficiencies in the CNS, but are not very immunogenic. In contrast, expression vectors which stably integrate in the genome and provide a long term expression of siRNA counterparts, called short-hairpin RNAs (shRNAs), provide long-term expression but are also immunogenic. Furthermore, although such DNA vectors can be efficiently transfected into cultured neurons using lipid-based or liposomal delivery systems, efficacy of this approach has not been adequately demonstrated in the nervous system *in vivo*. In contrast, viral vectors constitute the most efficient gene transfer method to the CNS tissue and yield very high transfection efficiencies of shRNA expression, but shRNAs (and viral vectors themselves, see below) can also illicit an immune response in the brain. Recent developments in viral-based targeting systems suggest that this hurdle may be already overcome in novel, rAAV-based viral delivery systems (see below). However, it is important to stress that the ultimate choice of siRNAs versus shRNAs should depend upon the experimental goals and the design of the experiment. In either case, performing a large series of controls is inevitable.

RNAi IN BRINGING ABOUT LOSS-OF-FUNCTION IN PAIN PATHWAYS

The application of RNAi technology to pain research will allow for a large-scale screening and validation of novel drug-targets against pathological pain disorders in animal models. Furthermore, there is a possibility that RNAi may prove to be a good therapeutic approach in the treatment of pain disorders. Critical to this dream is the development and optimisation of effective, safe and, as far as possible, non-invasive delivery systems. So far, there is very little experience with the use of RNAi in the pain field. Sensory neurons in the DRG and trigeminal ganglia, the spinal dorsal horn and the forebrain will likely constitute the sites which one would want to target with RNAi. There is one study so far showing that intrathecally infused, unmodified siRNAs against the P2X3 receptor reduced chronic neuropathic pain in rats. However, infusion of unmodified siRNAs via intrathecal or intracerebroventricular routes is not likely to yield efficient delivery to target neurons due to their low penetrance and fast degradation as well as the rapid turnover of the cerebrospinal fluid. Here, viral-based delivery system may be much more promising (see below for details on the choice of viral vectors). Clearly, much work still needs to be done in terms of testing and comparing the relative merits and limitations of different modifications in siRNA-design as well as various routes of administration, in terms of penetration, efficacy and the duration of the loss of expression of the targeted gene, in order to fully exploit the potential of RNAi in pain. A further, very important aspect will be to judge for any apparent toxicity due to administration of siRNAs or virions carrying shRNAs. So far, studies using siRNAs in the nervous system have only monitored animals for hind-limb paralysis or for obvious signs of discomfort. It would be important to test for neurological functions such as motor performance, locomotion, reflexes and overall activity as well as to perform a detailed histological analysis for any signs of neuro-inflammation in the central nervous system.

A comparison of Cre-loxP approach with RNAi methodology

All methods have advantages and disadvantages. The ultimate choice of the system for a pain researcher should depend on the questions that the study is designed to ask. A concise comparison of the pros and contras of the two approaches is given in Table 18.1.

SPATIAL AND TEMPORAL CONTROL OF GENE EXPRESSION IN MICE—OVEREXPRESSION OF GENES

Conditional overexpression of genes in transgenic mice using inducible systems

Inducible expression of genes can be produced by the "tetracycline Trans-activator" (tTA) system. The system consists of two elements which are incorporated separately in transgenic animals—(i) tTA, which can be expressed in a spatially- and temporally-restricted manner, depending upon the choice of the promoter and (ii) the gene of interest, which is put under the influence of a tTA-dependent minimal promoter. By crossing animals carrying these two elements, tTA-dependent expression of the desired gene can be achieved. Upon administration of tetracycline to these animals, tTA gets sequestered, thereby blocking gene expression. On the other hand, the "reverse tTA" (rtTA) system functions to express genes only in the presence of tetracycline or its analog, doxycycline. Similar principles apply in the Estrogen receptor/Tamoxifen sytsem. Unfortunately, the CNS is a very difficult region to target with either of these inducible systems. The most successful application of the tTA system in the brain is represented by the CamKII-tTA mouse line, which can be used to drive expression of genes in principal neurons of the forebrain to address forebrain-processing of sensory inputs.

Table 18.1   Comparison of Cre-loxp approach with RNAi methodology.

Nr.	Property	Cre-loxP	siRNA/shRNA
1	Region-specificity	Limited by the availability of known region-specific promoters	High-determined by region-specific delivery
2	Time required	Takes at least a year to generate a new Cre-mouse line or a floxed gene mouse	Takes anywhere between two weeks (siRNA) to 1-2 months (shRNA)
3	Efforts	More cumbersome to make a transgenic mouse, but once lines are established, it is a simple matter of breeding	Less cumbersome approach, but every test animal has to be treated with siRNA/shRNA individually
4	Efficacy	Leads to a 100% knockout of gene expression in targeted cells; very reliable	Partial knock-down, anywhere between 30-80%, but a 100% loss rarely achieved[*]; larger variability
5	Duration of loss of expression	Permanent loss of expression of the targeted gene; immediate onset	siRNAs: short-lasting, unless siRNAs continuously supplemented shRNAs via vectors—over months In both cases, onset depends on half-life of presynthesized protein
6	Targeting the CNS	Cre recombinase works efficiently in neurons; the choice and strength of promoter determines expression levels in desired regions	siRNAs: difficult—rapidly degraded shRNAs via virions—good efficiency, but invasive methods required for expression in deeper regions
7	Safety	No harm to targeted cells	siRNAs—dose-dependent toxicity shRNAs via viral vectors—can elicit immune response (but see rAAV in text)
8	Splice variants	Targeting splice variants of genes selectively is very difficult	Can selectively knock-down splice variants
9	Multiple targets	Targeting multiple genes simultaneously is difficult; cumbersome to cross many mouse lines	Easy to deliver mixtures of siRNAs /shRNAs to target multiple target sequences simultaneously
10	Special requirements	Standard molecular biology reagents and lab; generation of floxed mice requires experience in targeting of embryonic stem cells and some special reagents & cells	Standard molecular biology reagents and lab naked siRNAs—no further requirements shRNA with viruses: simple cloning steps; generation of some virions requires a lab at biosafety level 2

Table *, This is not necessarily a disadvantage—clinically-used drugs which affect the activity of proteins rarely produce a complete inhibition. Moreover, most genetic diseases arise from heterozygous mutations, where the dosage of a particular gene is reduced or halved, but not entirely lost. Therefore, a partial knock-down is regarded by some to be more predictive of the clinical relevance of a target than a 100% loss caused by gene deletion.

Viral-mediated gene delivery in pain pathways

Of all methods tested so far for bringing foreign DNA into neurons, viral-mediated gene transfer has proved itself to be the most efficient and successful one. Viral-mediated gene delivery is brought about by cloning DNA fragments/cDNAs of interest into vectors which, although derived from wild-type viruses, do not carry elements required for replication and are thus not harmful as pathogens. Virions derived from such vectors in combination with helper viruses can infect the target cells only once and either lead to immediate, short-lasting expression (e.g. alpha viruses, see below) or integrate into the genome of the host cell and provide long-lasting expression (such as lentiviruses). Key to the success of the viral approach is not only the speed and efficiency expression, but also the ability to target anatomical specific regions without having to worry about finding appropriate promoters, as required using transgenic approaches. Furthermore, the use of viral vectors is not limited to overexpression of genes—gene deletion or known-down can be also be brought about by using viruses to efficiently deliver Cre recombinase or shRNAs, respectively, selectively in anatomically distinct compartments of the nociceptive pathway. Indeed, the combination of the RNAi technology and viral-mediated gene delivery holds great promise for clinical therapy of pain disorders in humans. Here, I will focus on outlining some major viral gene delivery systems available and list the pros and cons.

Adeno-associated virus (AAV)

The CNS is one of the most difficult of target tissues for gene manipulations due to the blood-brain barrier and the toxicity potential. Recently, recombinant adeno-associated viral (rAAV) vectors have emerged as attractive vehicles for somatic gene transfer to the CNS, due to their lack of toxicity, absence of inflammatory response and their ability to confer persisting transgene expression in neurons. AAV is a naturally occurring virus that is not associated with any disease in humans. AAV can be stable as a lytic virus or can integrate as a provirus into the host cell genome. The vectors efficiently deliver genetic information to numerous cell types, are highly stable and persist in cells for extended periods of time. Extensive work done by Matthew During and colleagues shows that chimeras of rAAV1 and rAAV2 vectors provide the best infection rates and stable expression for at least 3 months in the CNS without compromising on safety. A very peculiar and important feature of some rAAV vectors, such as those derived from AAV2, is that they appear to have a tropism for neuronal cells when injected into the CNS. It was shown in the rat brain that rAAV1/2 viral particles preferentially bind neurons and not glial cells within minutes of injection. This combination of attributes makes AAV vectors particularly useful in the analysis of molecular mechanisms underlying pathological pain. We have used chimeric AAV1/2 vectors to overexpress proteins of interest selectively

in the spinal dorsal horn via intra-parenchymal injections in mice. South et al. have demonstrated the ability to produce a spinal cord-specific knockout of the NMDA receptor subunit, NR1, by using rAAV1 to deliver Cre recombinase to the spinal cord. AAV-based delivery of genes encoding therapeutic proteins also presents an attractive alternative or complement to systemic therapy for CNS disorders, as shown by recent clinical trials.

Lentivirus

Lentivirus-based expression systems are also very well-suited for long-term expression of genes in the nervous system. One point of difference from AAV-based systems is that lentiviruses can also infect mitotic cells, such as neuronal precursors and glia, which is why they are widely used in developmental studies on cell fate mapping. One disadvantage is that, in contrast to the use of rAAV1/2-chimeric virions, generation and application of lentiviruses requires a laboratory at biosafety level 2.

Alphaviruses

Alphaviruses, such as the Sindbis virus and the Semliki Forest virus (SFV), provide rapid and high levels of expression of the desired genes (within hours), are relatively easy to generate and use (SFV at biosafety level 1) and are ideally suited for rapid, cell-culture experiments. Because they essentially work by hijacking the translational machinery of the host cell, they lead to toxicity and apoptosis of neurons within 2-3 days of infection.

Herpes Simplex Virus (HSV)

Subcutaneous inoculation of the HSV vectors can be used to transduce neurons of the dorsal root ganglion. For example gene transfer to the DRG using HSV-based vectors to produce expression of neurotrophins directly in the DRG has been shown to alleviate symptoms of cisplatin neuropathy and polyneuropathy, such as chronic regional pain, without producing any toxicity. In human trials, direct injection of replication-competent HSV into brain tumors has proven safe.

CONCLUSIONS

A variety of molecular and genetic tools, such as transgenic mice, viral vectors and the RNAi-technology are now available to produce targeted changes in the expression and functions of proteins in individual components of the pain pathway. Exploiting these techniques can provide unprec- edented scope for understanding molecular mechanisms underlying chronic pain in research studies. Moreover, it would be important to develop tools, such as viral-based gene expression and RNAi-based gene knock-down, for *in vivo* applic- ations and therapeutic approaches.

GENERAL CITATIONS

Alexandra Joyner. *Gene Targeting: A Practical Approach* (2nd ed). Oxford University Press.

Burton EA, Fink DJ, Glorioso JC. 2005. Replica- tion-defective genomic HSV gene therapy vectors: design, production and CNS applications. *Curr Opin Mol Ther*, 7(4): 326-336.

Dorsett Y, Tuschl T. 2004. siRNAs: Applications in functional genomics and potential as therapeutics. *Nat Rev Drug Discov*, 3(4): 318-329.

During M J, Young D, Baer K, Lawlor P Klugmann M.2003. Development and optimization of adeno-associated virus vector transfer into the central nervous system. *Methods Mol Med*, 76: 221-236.

Ehrengruber MU. 2002. Alphaviral vectors for gene transfer into neurons. *Mol Neurobiol*, 26(2-3): 183-201.

Janson CG, During MJ. 2001. Viral vectors as part of an integrated functional genomics program. *Genomics*, 78(1-2): 3-6.

Lariviere WR, Chesler EJ, Mogil JS. 2001. Transgenic studies of pain and analgesia: mutation or background genotype? *J Pharmacol Exp Ther*, 297(2): 467-473.

Mansuy IM, Bujard H. 2000.Tetracycline-regulated gene expression in the brain. *Curr Opin Neurobiol*, 10(5): 593-596.

Meister G, Tuschl T. 2004. Mechanisms of gene silencing by double-stranded RNA. *Nature*, 431(7006): 343-349.

Nagy A. 2000. Cre recombinase: the universal reagent for genome tailoring. *Genesis*, 26: 99-109.

DISCOVERY CITATIONS

Region-specific Cre mouse lines relevant to pain analysis:

Agarwal N, Offermanns S, Kuner R. 2004. Conditio- nal gene targeting in neurons of the dorsal root ganglia and trigeminal ganglia. *Genesis*, 38(3): 122-129

Gelman DM, Noain D, Avale ME, Otero V, Low MJ, Rubinstein M. 2003. Transgenic mice engineered to target Cre/loxP-mediated DNA recombination into catecholaminergic neurons. *Genesis*, 36(4): 196-202.

Mantamadiotis T, Lemberger T, Bleckmann SC, Kern H, Kretz O, Martin Villalba A,Tronche F, Kellendonk C, Gau D, Kapfhammer J, Otto C, Schmid W, Schutz G. 2002. Disruption of CREB function in brain leads to neurodegeneration. *Nat Genet*, 31(1): 47-54.

Stirling LC, Forlani G, Baker MD, Wood JN, Matth- ews EA, Dickenson AH, Nassar MA. 2005. Nociceptor-specific gene deletion using heterozygous NaV1.8-Cre recombinase mice. *Pain*, 113(1-2): 27-36.

Region-specific gene expression using the tTA system:

Mayford M, Bach M E, Huang Y Y, Wang L, Hawkins R D, Kandel E R. 1996. Control of memory for mation through regulated expression of a CaMK II transgene. *Science*, 274: 1678-1683.

RNAi technology (including application in pain research):

Dorn G, Patel S, Wotherspoon G, Hemmings-Mieszczak M, Barclay J, Natt FJ, Martin P, Bevan S, Fox A, Ganju P, Wishart W, Hall J. 2004. siRNA relieves chronic neuropathic pain. *Nucleic Acids Research*, 32(5): e49.

Viral-mediated gene delivery in pain research:

Eaton MJ, Blits B, Ruitenberg MJ, Verhaagen J, Oudega M.2002. Amelioration of chronic neuropathic pain after partial nerve injury by adeno-associated viral (AAV) vector-mediated over-expression of BDNF in the rat spinal cord. *Gene Therapy*, 9(20): 1387-1395.

Chattopadhyay M, Goss J, Wolfe D, Goins WC, Huang S, Glorioso JC, Mata M, Fink DJ .2004. Protective effect of herpes simplex virus-mediated neurotrophin gene transfer in cisplatin neuropathy. *Brain*, 127(Pt 4): 929-939.

South SM, Kohno T, Kaspar BK, Hegarty D, Vissel B, Drake CT, Ohata M, Jenab S, Sailer AW, Malkmus S, Masuyama T, Horner P, Bogulavsky J, Gage FH, Yaksh TL, Woolf CJ, Heinemann SF, Inturrisi C. 2003. A conditional deletion of the NR1 subunit of the NMDA receptor in adult spinal cord dorsal horn reduces NMDA currents and injury-induced pain. *J Neurosci*, 23: 5031-5040.

Part VI Peripheral Nociceptor, Amygdala and Fear

Peripheral Nociceptors

CHAPTER 19

Makoto Tominaga

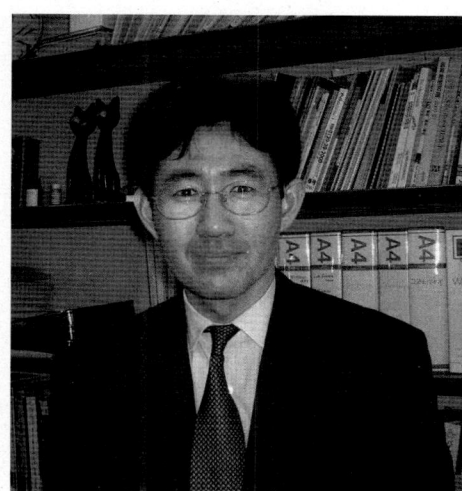

Dr. Tominaga is a Professor in the Section of Cellular Signaling, Okazaki Institute for Integrative Bioscience, Japan. He completed his Ph.D. at the Graduate School of Medicine, Kyoto University and pursued post-doctoral work at the University of California, San Francisco.

MAJOR CONTRIBUTIONS

1. Tominaga M, Wada M, Masu M. 2001. Potentiation of capsaicin receptor activity by metabotropic ATP receptors as a possible mechanism for ATP-evoked pain and hyperalgesia. *Proc Natl Acad Sci USA*, 98: 6951-6956.
2. Numazaki M, Tominaga T, Toyooka H, Tominaga M. 2002. Direct phosphorylation of capsaicin receptor VR1 by protein kinase Cepsilon and identification of two target serine residues. *J Biol Chem*, 277(16): 13375-13378.
3. Moriyama T, Iida T, Kobayashi K, Higashi T, Fukuoka T, Tsumura H, Leon C, Suzuki N, Inoue K, Gachet C, Noguchi K, Tominaga M 2003. Possible involvement of P2Y2 metabotropic receptors in ATP-induced transient receptor potential vanilloid receptor 1-mediated thermal hypersensitivity. *J Neurosci*, 23(14): 6058-6062.

4. Moriyama T, Higashi T, Togashi K, Iida T, Segi E, Sugimoto Y, Tominaga T, Narumiya S, Tominaga M. 2005. Sensitization of TRPV1 by EP_1 and IP reveals peripheral nociceptive mechanism of prostaglandins. *Molecular Pain*, 1: 3.
5. Tominaga M, Caterina MJ. 2004. Thermosensation and pain. *J Neurobiol*, 61(1): 3-12. (Review.)

MAIN TOPICS

TRP Channels
   Capsaicin Receptor TRPV1
   TRPV2
   TRPV3 and TRPV4
   TRPM8
   TRPA1
P2X receptors
Acid sensing ion channels (ASICs)
Na^+ channels
   $Na_v1.7$
   $Na_v1.8$
   $Na_v1.9$
Two-pore-domain K^+ channels

SUMMARY

Noxious stimuli excite primary afferent sensory neurons through activation of various ionotropic receptors expressed in the nerve endings, followed by action potential generation upon activation of voltage-gated Na^+ channels. Nociceptive cation channels include TRP channels, P2X receptors and acid-sensing ion channels (ASICs). On the other hand, opening of K$^+$channels causes hyperpolarization, leading to reduction in nociception. Both activity and expression of nociceptive cation channels, voltage-gated Na$^+$ channels and K$^+$channels are affected by many kinds of factors including inflammatory mediators. Thus, excitability of nociceptive neurons is regulated by dynamic balance in activities of those molecules, and clarification of molecular mechanisms in peripheral nociception would be useful for the development of novel analgesic agents.

INTRODUCTION

Pain is initiated when noxious thermal, mechanical, or chemical stimuli excite the peripheral terminals of specialized primary afferent neurons called nociceptors, most of which are small-diameter, unmyelinated

C fibers (Scholz and Woolf 2002; Wood and Perl 1999; Woolf and Salter 2000). These fibers transmit this information to the central nervous systems, leading to the sensation of pain. Activation of nociceptive pathway is subject to activity-dependent plasticity, which manifests as a progressive increase in the response to repeated stimuli. Many kinds of ionotropic and metabotropic receptors are known to be involved in the process (Caterina and Julius 1999; Julius and Basbaum 2001; McCleskey and Gold 1999). Most important function of peripheral nociceptors is action potential generation which is, then transmitted as nociceptive information. Therefore, most nociceptors are cation channels including TRP channels, P2X receptors and ASIC channels whose opening causes cation influx leading to depolarization necessary for activation of voltage-gated Na$^+$ channels (Fig.19.1).

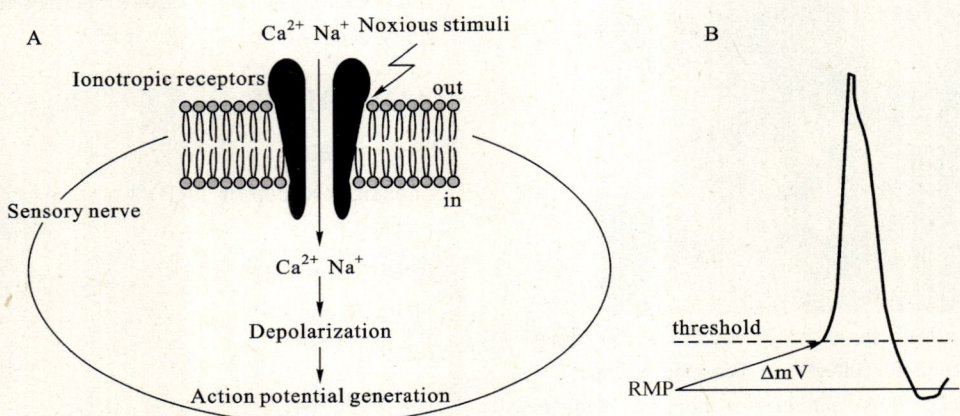

Fig.19.1   Putative mechanism of conversion of noxious stimuli to electrical signals. A. Noxious stimuli open ionotropic receptors expressed in the sensory nerve endings leading to cation influx, followed by depolarization. B. Some extent of depolarization is necessary to reach the voltage threshold for activation of voltage-gated Na$^+$ channels, followed by action potential generation. RMP, resting membrane potential.

TRP CHANNELS (Fig.19.2)

The founding member of the transient receptor potential (TRP) superfamily of cation cannels is the *Drosophila* TRP channel which was found to be deficient in a mutant exhibiting abnormal responsiveness to continuous light (Montell and Rubin 1989). TRP subunit contains six putative transmembrane domains and probably assemble as homo or hetero-tetramers to form functional cation selective channels. Based on amino acid homology, the TRP superfamily can be

devided into seven subfamilies: TRPC, TRPM, TRPV, TRPA, TRPP, TRPML, TRPN. Except for TRPN, all the other subfamilies can be found in mammals (Clapham 2003; Montell 2005).

Capsaicin Receptor TRPV1

Capsaicin is known to depolarize nociceptors and increase their cytosolic free Ca^{2+} concentration (Szallasi and Blumberg 1999). This property allowed Julius and colleagues to isolate the gene encoding the capsaicin receptor by using a Ca^{2+} imaging-based expression strategy in 1997 (Caterina et al. 1997). The cloned receptor was designated a vanilliod receptor subtype-1 (VR1) because a vanilloid moiety constitutes an essential chemical component of both capsaicin and its ultra potent analogue, resiniferatoxin (Caterina and Julius 2001). The capsaicin receptor VR1 is now called TRPV1 as a member of the TRP super family of ion channel. A functional analysis using a patch-clamp technique revealed that heterologously expressed TRPV1 exhibits membrane current activation upon capsaicin application whose properties are almost identical to those observed in native dorsal root ganglion (DRG) neurons, suggest-

ing that TRPV1 protein consists of homomeric tetramar. Upon application of capsaicin to excised membrane patches, clear single channel openings were observed, indicating that no cytosolic second messengers were necessary for TRPV1 activation by capsaicin. Furthermore, it became clear that capsaicin-activated currents showed non-selective cation permeability with an outwardly rectifying current-voltage (I-V) relationship and that Ca^{2+} was found to be about ten times more permeable than Na^+ which is effective for release of substance P or calcitoni gene-related peptide (CGRP), a phenomenon called neurogenic inflammation.

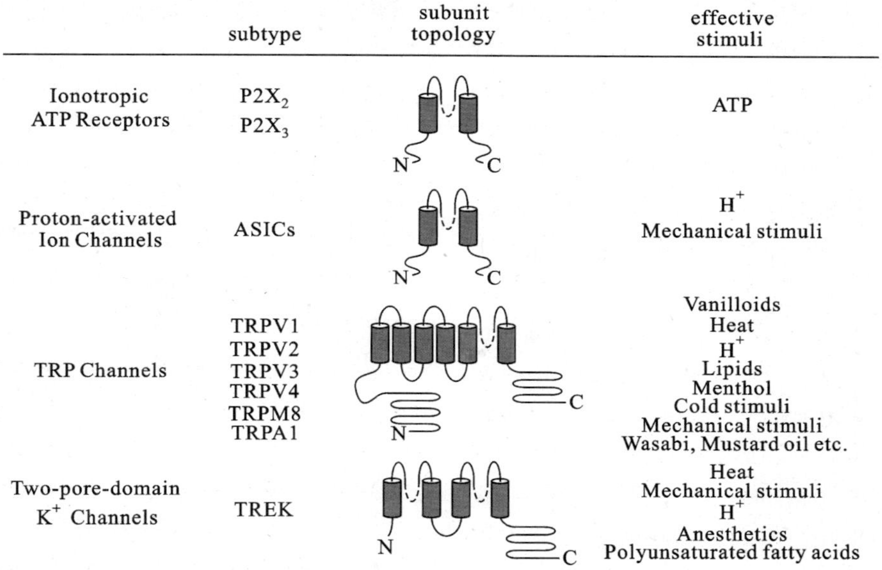

	subtype	subunit topology	effective stimuli
Ionotropic ATP Receptors	P2X$_2$ P2X$_3$		ATP
Proton-activated Ion Channels	ASICs		H$^+$ Mechanical stimuli
TRP Channels	TRPV1 TRPV2 TRPV3 TRPV4 TRPM8 TRPA1		Vanilloids Heat H$^+$ Lipids Menthol Cold stimuli Mechanical stimuli Wasabi, Mustard oil etc.
Two-pore-domain K$^+$ Channels	TREK		Heat Mechanical stimuli H$^+$ Anesthetics Polyunsaturated fatty acids

Fig.19.2 Comparison of ionotropic receptors involved in peripheral nociception. A cylinder shown in "subunit topology" indicates a transmembrane domain. Both N and C termini are located in the cytosol.

It is known that heat stimulus also induces pain sensation through the activation of polymodal nociceptors. TRPV1 was found to be activated by heat with a threshold of about 43°C, a temperature causing pain responses *in vivo*, suggesting that TRPV1 is involved in the detection of painful heat. Tissue acidification induced in inflammation and ischemia is also thought to exacerbate or cause pain. Extracellular acidification, pH 6.4~, potentiated both capsaicin- and heat-evoked TRPV1 currents by increasing agonist potency without altering efficacy (Tominaga *et al.* 1998). When proton concentration was increased to a level of pH 6.0, TRPV1 could be activated by proton

itself at room temperature. Proton concentration range activating TRPV1 is well attainable in local acidosis associated with tissue injury. Both heat- and proton-evoked TRPV1 currents were observed in excised membrane patches, indicating that the activation process does not involve cytosolic sencond messengers. Thus, TRPV1 can be activated by different stimuli causing pain *in vivo*. While capsaicin is an exogenous ligand for TRPV1, it remains possible that there exist endogenous, pain-producing, chemical regulators for this channel, other than protons. Several candidates for such endogenous ligands have been identified, including anandamide, lipoxygenase products and

N-arachidonoyl dopamine (NADA) (Huang *et al.* 2002; Hwang *et al.* 2000; Zygmunt *et al.* 1999).

Expression of TRPV1 was observed in the terminals of primary afferent neurons projecting to the superficial layers of the spinal cord dorsal horn and the trigeminal nucleus caudalis (Fig.19.3, see also the color plate) (Tominaga *et al.* 1998). TRPV1 immunoreactivity was also observed in the nucleus of the solitary tract and area postrema, which receive vagal projections from visceral organs through the nodose ganglion. These observations, plus the fact that TRPV1 protein was detected in nerve terminals, indicates that TRPV1 is expressed in both central and peripheral termini of small-diameter sensory neurons. In central nervous system, TRPV1 expression was observed in the brain (Mezey *et al.* 2000). TRPV1 function in the brain is not clear. However, the facts that NADA which is present predominantly in dopaminergic neurons in the brain can activate TRPV1 and that capsaicin or anandamide enhances neuronal excitability or influences synaptic transmission might suggest that TRPV1 is associated with synaptic plasticity in the central nervous system (Marinelli *et al.* 2003). TRPV1 is also expressed in visceral afferent neurons (Ward *et al.* 2003) and the expression has been reported to be increased in inflammatory diseases of the gastrointestinal tract and in patients with rectal hypersensitivity (Chan *et al.* 2003; Yiangou *et al.* 2001). These results suggest the involvement of TRPV1 in visceral nociception. It has been reported that inflammation or tissue injury induced increase in the number of unmyelinated C fibers expressing TRPV1 (Carlton and Coggeshall 2001). Furthermore, increase of TRPV1 expression induced by inflammation was predominantly observed in myelinated Aδ fibers compared to C fibers (Amaya *et al.* 2003). NGF induced increase of TRPV1 mRNA and release of CGRP with capsaicin treatment in primary cultured DRG neurons (Winston *et al.* 2001). Activation of p38MAPK by NGF was found to enhance the translocation of TRPV1 proteins from cell bodies in DRG to sensory nerve endings (Ji *et al.* 2002). Furthermore, p38MAPK inhibitor reduced inflammatory hyperalgesia. Thus, in addition to the phosphorylation of TRPV1 described later, increase of TRPV1 expression in the sensory nerve endings seems to be involved in the development of hyperalgesia as well.

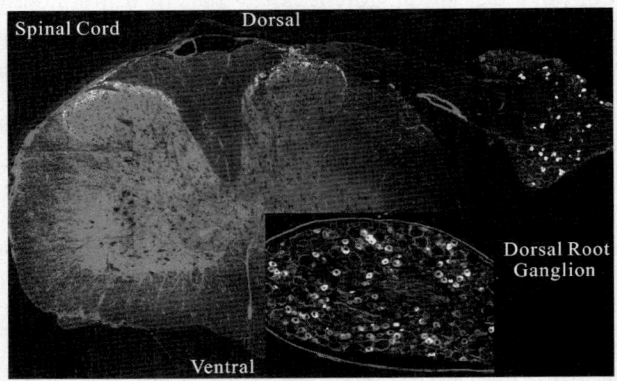

Fig.19.3 Expression of TRPV1 proteins in rat lumbar spinal cord (indicated in green) detected by anti-TRPV1 antibody. TRPV1 expression in dorsal root ganglion (DRG) neurons, superficial layers of dorsal horn and nerve fibers are observed. TRPV1 is expressed in predominantly in small-diameter neurons, probably cell bodies of unmyelinated C fibers.

Electrophysiological analysis in heterologous expression system revealed the importance of TRPV1 in detecting noxious thermal and chemical stimuli. To determine whether TRPV1 really contributes to the detection of these noxious stimuli *in vivo*, mice lacking this protein were generated and analyzed for nociceptive function (Caterina *et al.* 2000; Davis *et al.* 2000). Sensory neurons from mice lacking TRPV1 were deficient in their responses to each of the reported noxious stimuli; capsaicn, proton and heat. Consistent with this observation, behavioral responses to capsaicin were absent and responses to acute thermal stimuli were diminished in these mice. In contrast, TRPV1 knockout mice showed normal physiological and behavioral responses to noxious mechanical stimuli, implying the existence of other mechanisms for the detection of such stimuli. The most prominent feature of the knockout mouse thermosensory phenotype was a virtual absence of thermal hypersensitivity in the setting of inflammation. These findings indicate that TRPV1 is essential for selective modalities of pain sensation and for tissue injury-induced thermal hyperalgesia. Recent studies have provided further support for TRPV1 involvement in inflammatory pain and have, in addition, demonstrated that the participation of TRPV1 in pain sensation may also extend to neuropathic pain, mechanical allodynia and mechanical hyperalgesia. These conclusions are based on enhanced expression of TRPV1 in sensory neurons in the context of these conditions, as well as behavioral effects of TRPV1 antagonism with capsazepine, a competitive antagonist of TRPV1.

One important aspect of TRPV1 regulation that has received considerable attention concerns the mechanisms by which the inflammatory mediators in damaged tissues sensitize TRPV1 to its chemical and physical stimuli. The fact that one of the most impressive phenotypes observed in TRPV1-deficient mice was attenuation of thermal hyperalgesia may be related to the aspect. Whereas protons act directly on TRPV1, others influence TRPV1 indirectly such as through receptors with intrinsic Tyr kinase activity, G protein-coupled receptors or receptors coupled to JAK/STAT signaling pathway. Like other ion channels, TRPV1 can be phosphorylated by several kinases including PKA (Bhave et al. 2002; Rathee et al. 2002), PKC (Premkumar and Ahern 2000; Tominaga et al. 2001), Ca^{2+}/CaM-dependent kinase II (CaM kinase II) (Jung et al. 2004) or Src kinase (Jin et al. 2004; Zhang et al. 2005). There has been extensive work demonstrating that activation of a PKA-dependent pathway by inflammatory mediators such as prostaglandins influences capsaicin or heat-mediated actions in sensory neurons, probably by acting on TRPV1 (Distler et al. 2003; Lopshire and Nicol 1998). These results suggest that PKA plays a pivotal role in the development of hyperalgesia and inflammation by inflammatory mediators. PKC-dependent phosphorylation of TRPV1 occurs downstream of activation of Gq-coupled receptors by several inflammatory mediators including ATP, bradykinin, prostaglandins and trypsin or tryptase (Dai et al. 2004; Moriyama et al. 2005; Moriyama et al. 2003; Sugiura et al. 2002). PKC-dependent phosphorylation of TRPV1 caused not only potentiation of capsaicin or proton-evoked responses but also reduced the temperature threshold for TRPV1 activation so that normally non-painful temperatures in the range of normal body temperature were capable of activating TRPV1, thereby leading to the sensation of pain. These phenomena were also confirmed in native sensory neurons. Direct phosphorylation of TRPV1 by PKC was proven using, and two target Ser residues were identified (Numazaki et al. 2002). A reduction of direct PIP_2 (phosphatidylinositol-4, 5-bisphosphate)-mediated TRPV1 inhibition and generation of lipoxygenase derived products through PLA_2 activation are also reported to be involved in the potentiation of TRPV1 activity following Gq-coupled receptor activation (Chuang et al. 2001). Both PKC-dependent and independent potentiation mechanisms might occur at downstream of Gq-coupled receptor activation. Inhibition of calcineurin inhibits desensitization of TRPV1 (Docherty et al. 1996), indicating that a phosphorylation/dephosphorylation process is important for TRPV1 activity. Indeed, CaMKII was reported to control TRPV1 activity upon phosphorylation of TRPV1 by regulating capsaicin binding (Jung et al. 2004). Thus, phosphorylation of TRPV1 by three different kinases seems to control TRPV1 activity through the dynamic balance between the phosphorylation and dephosphorylation.

Capsaicin not only causes pain, but also seems to exhibit analgesic properties, particularly when used to treat pain associated with diabetic neuropathies or rheumatoid arthritis (Szallasi and Blumberg 1999). This paradoxical effect may relate to the ability of capsaicin to desensitize nociceptive terminals to capsaicin, as well as to other noxious stimuli following prolonged exposure. At the molecular level, an extracellular Ca^{2+}-dependent reduction of TRPV1 responsiveness upon continuous vanilloid exposure (electrophysiological desensitization) may partially underlie this phenomenon, although physical damage to the nerve terminal or depletion of CGRP or SP probably contributes to this effect as well. Ca^{2+}-and voltage-dependent desensitization of capsaicin-activated currents has also been observed in rat DRG neurons. This inactivation of nociceptive neurons by capsaicin has generated extensive research on the possible therapeutic effectiveness of capsaicin as a clinical analgesic tool. Desensitization to capsaicin is a complex process with varying kinetic components: a fast component that appears to depend on Ca^{2+} influx through TRPV1 and a slow component that does not. Calcineurin inhibitors reduce TRPV1 desensitization (the slow component), indicating the involvement of Ca^{2+}-dependent phophorylation/dephosphorylation process (Docherty et al. 1996). In addition, PKA-dependent phosphorylation of TRPV1 has been reported to mediate the slow component of TRPV1 desensitization (Bhave et al. 2002). CaM has also been reported to be involved in Ca^{2+}-dependent desensitization of TRPV1 through its binding to the cytosolic domains of TRPV1 (Numazaki et al. 2003; Rosenbaum et al. 2004).

TRPV2

TRPV2 might be a potential candidate for the receptor detecting high heat stimulus responsible for the residual high temperature-evoked nociceptive responses observed in TRPV1-deficient mice. TRPV2 with about 50% identity to TRPV1 was found to be activated by high temperatures with a threshold of ~52℃ (Caterina et al. 1999). TRPV2 currents showed similar properties to those of TRPV1 such as an outwardly rectifying I-V relationship and relatively high Ca^{2+} permeability. Intense TRPV2 immunoreactivity was observed in medium to large diameter cells in rat DRG neurons and very few of the TRPV2-positive cells stained with the isolectin IB4 or with SP antibody (Lewinter et al. 2004). However, about one-third of the TRPV2-positive cells co-stained with antibody against CGRP. Many of the TRPV2-positive neurons co-stained with a marker for myelinated neurons. Dense TRPV2 immunoreactivity in the spinal cord was found in lamina I, inner lamina II and laminae III/IV. This is consistent with the expression of TRPV2 in myelinated nociceptors that target laminae I and inner lamina II and in nonnociceptive Aβ fibers that target laminae III/IV. Aδ mechano and heat-sensitive (AMH) neurons in monkey are medium-to-large-diameter, lightly myelinated neurons that fall

into two groups: type I AMHs have a heat threshold of~53℃, and type II AMHs are activated at 43℃ (Treede et al. 1995). The TRPV2 localization data and the residual high temperature-evoked responses observed in the TRPV1-deficient mice suggest that TRPV2 expression might account for the high thermal threshold ascribed to type I AMH nociceptors. Temperatures activating TRPV2 are more harmful to our body than those activating TRPV1. Therefore, expression of TRPV2 in the myelinated sensory fibers seems reasonable because Aδ fibers can transmit the nociceptive information much faster than C fibers, which exclusively express TRPV1. The function of TRPV2 in Aβ fibers is not known. Studies using mice lacking TRPV2 will tell us how important TRPV2 is for detecting noxious thermal stimulus. TRPV2 transcript and protein were found not only in sensory neurons but also in motoneurons and in many non-neuronal tissues that are unlikely to be exposed to temperature above 50℃. These results indicate that TRPV2 undoubtedly contributes to numerous functions in addition to nociceptive processing.

TRPV3 and TRPV4

Two TRPV channels, TRPV3 and TRPV4 have been found to be activated by warm temperatures, ~34-38℃ for TRPV3 and ~27-35℃ for TRPV4, in addition to hypotonic stimulus (TRPV4) in heterologous expression systems, and to be expressed in multiple tissues, including, among others, sensory and hypothalamic neurons and keratinocytes (Guler et al. 2002; Peier et al. 2002b; Smith et al. 2002; Xu et al. 2002). Several approaches, including the knockdown of TRPV4 with gene-disruption or antisense oligonucleotides, have led to reports that this protein is involved in mechanical stimulus-and hypotonicity-induced nociception in rodents at baseline or following hypersensitivity induced by prostaglandin injection or taxol neurotoxicity (Alessandri-Haber et al. 2004; Alessandri-Haber et al. 2003; Suzuki et al. 2003). Furthermore, both TRPV3 and TRPV4 have been reported to be involved in thermosenation by keratinocytes, based on studies of wild-type and TRPV3-or

TRPV4-deficient keratinocytes. There is no physiological evidence yet that these ion channels are involved in thermal nociception although the sensitization of TRPV3 upon repeated noxious heat stimuli strongly suggests that this will be the case.

TRPM8

A distinct class of cold-sensitive fibers has been described as polymodal mociceptors, responding to noxious cold, heat and pinch (Campero *et al.* 1996), although an early study suggested a distinction between cold sensation and painful sensation (Klement and Arndt 1992). The cooling sensation of menthol, a chemical agent found in mint, is well established, and both cooling and menthol was suggested to be transduced through a non-selective cation channel in DRG neurons (Reid and Flonta 2001). Two groups independently cloned and characterized a cold receptor, TRPM8 which can be also activated by menthol (McKemy *et al.* 2002; Peier *et al.* 2002a). In heterologous expression systems, TRPM8 could be activated by menthol or by cooling, with an activation temperature of ~25-28℃. TRPM8 could alternatively be activated by other cooling compounds, such as menthone, eucalyptol and icilin.

There also appears to be interaction between effective stimuli for TRPM8, in that subthreshold concentrations of menthol increased the temperature threshold for TRPM8 activation from 25℃ to 30℃. This is reminiscent of TRPV1, whose activation temperature is reduced under mildly acidic conditions that do not open TRPV1 alone. Patch-clamp analysis revealed that TRPM8 is a non-selective cation channel with relatively high Ca^{2+} permeability and that TRPM8 shows an outwardly-rectifying *I-V* relationship like TRPV1. TRPM8 is expressed in a subset of DRG and TG neurons that can be classified as small-diameter C fiber-containing neurons. Interestingly, however, TRPM8 is not co-expressed with TRPV1, which marks a class of nociceptors. Whether TRPM8 is involved in cold nociception remains to be clarified although inflammatory mediators was found to downregulate TRPM8 via PKC-mediated phosphorylation (Premkumar *et al.* 2005).

TRPA1

TRPA1 was reported as a distantly related TRP channel which is activated by cold with a lower activation threshold as compared to TRPM8 (Story *et al.* 2003). In heterologous expression systems, TRPA1 was activated by cold stimuli with an activation temperature of about 17℃, which is close to the reported noxious cold threshold. This finding led to the suggestion that TRPA1 is involved in cold nociception. Indeed, TRPA1 has been found to be involved in cold hyperalgesia caused by inflammation or nerve injury via activation of MAP kinase (Obata *et al.* 2005). Patch-clamp analysis of TRPA1 revealed cationic permeability and an outwardly-rectifying *I-V* relationship. Whether TRPA1 is activated directly by cold remains to be elucidated. TRPA1 was also found to be activated by pungent isothiocyanate compounds such as those found in wasabi, horseradish and mustard oil, cinnamoaldehyde, a main pungent ingredient of cinnamon or allicin, a pungent ingredient of garlic (Bandell *et al.* 2004; Jordt *et al.* 2004; Macpherson *et al.* 2005). Thus, several of the thermosensitive TRP channels likely to be involved in nociception can be activated by stimuli other than temperature.

Unlike TRPM8, TRPA1 is specifically expressed in a subset of sensory neurons that express the nociceptive markers CGRP and substance P. Furthermore, TRPA1 is frequently co-expressed with TRPV1, raising the possibility that TRPA1 and TRPV1 mediate the function of a class of polymodal nociceptors. Such co-expression might also explain the paradoxical hot sensation experienced when one is exposed to a very cold stimulus.

P2X RECEPTORS (Fig.19.2)

It was reported in 1977 that ATP induced a sensation of pain when it was applied to a blister base in man (Bleehen and Keele 1977). This study has given rise to considerable interest in the notion that ATP is an important player in the initiation of noxious signals, and that its actions are mediated by receptors expressed by primary afferent nerve fibers. ATP is released from microvascular endothelial cells during hyperaemia, from nociceptive terminals after noxious stimulation (e.g. with capsaicin) and from sympathetic nerve terminal varicosities as a co-transmitter with norepinephrine and neuropeptide Y. ATP is also released from tumor cells during abrasive activity and from damaged tissues after trauma or surgery. Extracellular ATP excites the nociceptive endings of nearby sensory nerves by activating homomeric $P2X_3$ or heteromeric $P2X_{2/3}$ receptors, evoking a sensation of pain (Burnstock 2001; Chizh and Illes 2001; North 2004). It has been proposed that in tubes (e.g. ureter, salivery duct, bile duct, vigina and intestine) and sacs (e.g. urinary bladder, gall bladder and lung) nociceptive mechanosensory transduction occurs where distension releases ATP from the epithelial cells lining these organs, which then activates $P2X_3$ and/or $P2X_{2/3}$ receptors on subepithelial sensory nerve plexuses.

There are extensive studies on the actions of ATP on cell bodies of primary afferent fibers whether in nodose, trigeminal or dorsal root ganglia. Two kinds of response to ATP and α, β-methylene ATP (α, β-meATP) are observed at negative membrane potentials. The first is a rapidly rising inward current that desensitizes during a maintained application, and the second is an inward current that rises slowly and desensitizes little. Considerable evidence supports the view that the first response results from currents through P2X receptors formed as homo-oligomers of $P2X_3$ subunits because the response mirrors well in the properties of the currents observed in HEK293 cells expressing $P2X_3$ subunits (Lewis et al. 1995; North 2002), and because the response is not observed in sensory neurons from mice lacking $P2X_3$ (Cockayne et al. 2000; Souslova et al. 2000). The second response closely resembles the currents observed when $P2X_2$ and $P2X_3$ subunits are expressed together, probably currents through the $P2X_{2/3}$ hetero-oligomeric receptor (Lewis et al. 1995). The precise subunit composition of the native hetero-oligomeric channel is not known. However, the studies with co-expression of P2X subunits carrying individual cysteine substitutions indicate that the $P2X_{2/3}$ hetero-oligomeric receptor probably contains one $P2X_2$ and two $P2X_3$ subunits (Jiang et al. 2003).

Since a high level of $P2X_3$ mRNA is selectively present in a subpopulation of primary afferent neurons likely to be nociceptors, on the basis of sizes and expression of peripherin, its expression pattern in sensory ganglia has been extensively studied by immunohistochemistry at both the light microscope and electron microscope levels. In DRG, intensive $P2X_3$ immunoreactivity was found predominantly in a subset of small and medium-diameter neurons, and located in the non-peptidergic subpopulation of nociceptors that bind IB4 (Bradbury et al. 1998; Collo et al. 1996; North 2002). The subunit is present in approximately equal numbers of neurons projecting to the skin and viscera. Capsaicin-sensitive, small-sized DRG neurons have been reported to express mainly the homomeric $P2X_3$ receptor subunit, whereas the capsaicin-insensitive, medium-sized neurons have been shown to express the $P2X_{2/3}$ heteromeric receptor (Ueno et al. 1999). This $P2X_3$ expression in DRG neurons was decreased following sciatic nerve axotomy (Bradbury et al. 1998) whereas the expression was increased after chronic constriction injury to the sciatic nerve (Novakovic et al. 1999). $P2X_2$ receptor immunoreactivity is observed in many small and large DRG neurons although the level is lower than that of $P2X_3$ (Dunn et al. 2001; Vulchanova et al. 1997). Some neurons seem to contain both $P2X_2$ and $P2X_3$ immunoreactivity. In the spinal cord, immunoreactivity was observed in the entire mediolateral extent of inner lamina II of the dorsal horn where the primary afferents project (Bradbury et al. 1998; Vulchanova et al. 1997). In contrast, while $P2X_2$ immunoreactivity is prominent in lamina II, it is also seen in deeper layers (Vulchanova et al. 1997). Co-localization of $P2X_2$ and $P2X_3$ immunoreactivity was also seen in the trigeminal ganglia and the nucleus of the solitary tract.

Several kinds of tools including selective $P2X_3$ antagonists, $P2X_2$ subunit knock down with antisense oligonucleotide and gene knock out have revealed the role of P2X$_3$ subunit-containing receptors in pain sensation. Intrathecal administration of antisense oligonucleotide of P2X$_3$ caused marked reduction in chronic (but not acute) inflammation-induced thermal and mechanical hyperalgesia, and spinal nerve ligation-induced mechanical allodynia (Barclay *et al.* 2002; Honore *et al.* 2002). Two groups reported that P2X$_3$-deficient mice showed a modest reduction in hindpaw licking and lifting after intraplantar formalin injection (Cockayne *et al.* 2000; Souslova *et al.* 2000). Although P2X$_3$ receptors are not sensitive to pH, P2X$_2$ receptors have been shown to be strongly pH sensitive (Wildman *et al.* 1998) and P2X$_{2/3}$ receptors are also pH sensitive albite to a lesser extent (Stoop *et al.* 1997), suggesting that the sensitivity of nociceptive P2X$_{2/3}$ receptors might be enhanced in inflammatory conditions.

ACID SENSING ION CHANNELS (ASICs) (Fig.19.2)

High proton concentrations (pH<6) are generated during various forms of tissue injury, including infection, inflammation and ischemia. Such acidification can elicit pain or sensitize the affected area. Protons are likely to produce or exacerbate pain via their interaction with several receptors and channels on nociceptive sensory neurons, including acid sensitive ion channels (ASICs) of the degenerin family, P2X receptors and TRPV1. The major structural features of ASICs shows two transmembrane domains, a large extracellular loop, and the N and C termini facing the intracellular space, and it is believed that each subunit forms a tetramer to be a functional channel (Krishtal 2003; Waldmann and Lazdunski 1998). Now ASICs are devided into four subunits, ASIC1 to ASIC4 where both ASIC1 and ASIC2 have isoforms named ASIC1a, ASIC1b and ASIC2a and ASIC2b. Although ASIC1a, ASIC2a and ASIC2b are expressed in both central and peripheral nervous systems, ASIC1b and ASIC3 (also known as DRASIC; dorsal root ganglia-specific ASIC) are primarily expressed in sensory neurons, thereby their believed to be involved in nociception.

Although it is well accepted that ASICs can be activated by the reduction of extracellular pH, their properties are different from the native H$^+$-gated channels showing nonselective cationic permeability and high sensitivity to small changes of pH. Rapid desensitization observed in ASICs also contradicts the fact that firing of nociceptive nerve fibers demonstrates little adaptation. Despite the discrepancy, ASIC3 might explain the cardiac pain which is believed to be induced by reduction of pH in ischemic condition. Since ASIC3 co-expressed with ASIC2b shows a biphasic current with a sustained component which shows less Na$^+$ selectivity similar to that observed in native sensory neurons, and its transcript was found in the fibers innervating cardiac tissue (Lingueglia *et al.* 1997). Epithelial Na$^+$ channel super family (ENaC) to which ASICs belong are known to be activated by mechanical stimuli (Krishtal 2003). Involvement of ASIC3 in mechanosensation was clearly derived form analysis of mice lacking ASIC3 (Price *et al.* 2001). Sensitivity of noxious mechanoreceptors as well as response to acid was reduced in the mice. Although it seems to be clear that ASICs are involved in acid-induced nociception, it remains to be elucidated whether mechanical nociception involves ASICs. Involvement of ASICs in nociception was also supported by the fact that expression of ASIC is increased by the inflammatory mediators including NGF, serotonin, interleukin-1 and bradykinin (Mamet *et al.* 2002), and that non-steroidal anti-inflammatory drugs (NSAIDs) inhibit ASICs and their inflammation-induced expression (Voilley *et al.* 2001).

Na$^+$ CHANNELS (Fig.19.2)

Voltage-gated Na$^+$ channels provide a brief, regenerative inward current that underlies the action potential. Patch-clamp recordings from DRG neurons and *in situ* hybridization studies have revealed that the molecular diversity of Na$^+$ channels operating in sensory neurons (Baker and Wood 2001; Wood *et al.* 2004). Nine voltage-gated Na$^+$ channel α-subunits (Na$_v$1.1-1.9) and three associated β-subunits (β1-3) have been cloned. Among them, several α-subunits and all the β-subunits have been detected in DRG neurons. The α-subunits forms a channel pore and is associated with a β1-subunit and linked by a disulfide bridge to a β2-subunit. β-subunits function as cell adhesion molecules, and regulate channel inactivation kinetics and the level of channel protein expression on the plasma membrane. The mechanism of channel gating involves the movement of voltage sensors in response to membrane potential changes. Lysine or arginine residues found at interval of three amino acids produces a linear array of positive charges in the α-helical S4 segments, and the movement of the areas opens the sodium selective channel pore lined by short hydrophobic stretch between S5 and S6.

Tetrodotoxin (TTX), a guanidium toxin isolated in puffer fish, which binds to the ion selectivity pore of some subtypes of Na^+ channels blocks them at nanomolar concentrations. Although most sensory neurons generate TTX-sensitive Na^+ currents, TTX-resistant currents are present in a high proportion of small diameter ($<25\mu m$) DRG neurons in which micro molar TTX is necessary to block the Na^+ currents. Small-diameter sensory neurons are the apparent cell bodies of unmyelinated C-fibers or thinly myelinated Aδ fibers, many of which are nociceptors. The TTX-resistant Na^+ currents recorded in small diameter DRG neurons activated at membrane potentials more positive than -40 mV are attributable mostly to the sensory neuron-specific [SNS (PN3)] $Na_v1.8$ channel (Akopian et al. 1996) while persistent (slow kinetics) TTX-resistant Na^+ currents are probably encoded by [SNS-2 (NaN)]$Na_v1.9$ channels whose currents can be conveniently examined in DRG neurons from mice lacking $Na_v1.8$ (Cummins et al. 1999). The persistent currents activated at voltages close to the resting membrane potential is thought to play a role in thresholds activation setting and membrane potentials. On the other hand, TTX-sensitive Na^+ currents are encoded by a number of genes including $Na_v1.1$, $Na_v1.7$ and $Na_v1.6$. Local anesthetics like lidocaine mediate their useful therapeutic actions by blocking both TTX-sensitive and TTX-resistant Na^+ channels although the blocking seems to be complicated, ex-

hibiting channel state-dependent and time-dependent elements (Roy and Narahashi 1992; Scholz et al. 1998b). The volatile anesthetic halothane blocks both TTX-sensitive and TTX-resistant Na^+ currents in DRG neurons, too (Scholz et al. 1998a).

$Na_v1.7$

$Na_v1.7$ encodes a TTX-sensitive Na^+ channel found predominantly in peripheral sensory neurons and sympathetic neurons. Interestingly, this channel is located at the terminal of sensory neurons, and is regulated in its expression by inflammatory mediators such as NGF probably through a mechanism involving trafficking (Toledo-Aral et al. 1997). The fact that a chronic inflammatory dominant human disease, primary erythermalgia maps to this gene SCN10A, suggests that this channel may play an important role in inflammatory pain (Yang et al. 2004). In addition, $Na_v1.7$ channel is up-regulated in the mice lacking $Na_v1.8$ and masking the phenotype of deficient inflammatory pain (Akopian et al. 1999), further suggesting a role of $Na_v1.7$ in inflammatory pain. However, no information has been reported for the involvement of $Na_v1.7$ in neurpathic pain.

$Na_v1.8$

$Na_v1.8$ contributes a majority of the Na^+ currents underlying the depolarizing phase of the action potential in cells expressing it (Renganathan et al. 2001), and DRG neurons from $Na_v1.8$-deficient mice lose all the inactivating TTX-resistant Na^+ channel activity (Akopian et al. 1999). $Na_v1.8$ thus underlies the inactivating TTX-resistant Na^+ currents that have been found to play a critical role in many aspects of nociceptor function. In accordance with this concept, a late-onset deficits in ectopic action potential propagation has been described in mice lacking $Na_v1.8$ (Roza et al. 2003), and important roles of $Na_v1.8$ have been suggested in the studies using antisense (Lai et al. 2002). However, neuropathic pain behavior seems to be normal in the $Na_v1.8$-deficient mice (Kerr et al. 2001).

Inflammatory mediators are known to alter the TTX-resistant channel expression, and shift their threshold of activation to more negative potentials through the activation of protein kinase A (Gold *et al.* 1996). In deed, NGF has been reported to increase $Na_v1.8$ channel expression, and prostaglandin E_2, adenosine and serotonin increased the $Na_v1.8$-mediated currents, shifted its conductance-voltage relation to the hyperpolarization direction, and increased the rates of Na^+ channel activation and inactivation in small-diameter sensory neurons. These phenomena can be replicated in heterologous expression systems in which the properties of the $Na_v1.8$ channel are modulated by increasing cAMP levels. In support of a role for the $Na_v1.8$ channel in pain pathways, mice lacking $Na_v1.8$ shows deficits in inflammatory pain processing (Akopian *et al.* 1999). This channel also appears to have an important role in visceral pain. Since prostaglandin E_2 increased TTX-resistant Na^+ currents in colonic DRG neurons (Gold *et al.* 2002), and mice lacking $Na_v1.8$ had deficits in visceral pain and referred hyperalgesia (Roza *et al.* 2003).

$Na_v1.9$

As described above, $Na_v1.9$ channel with slow kinetics is involved in thresholds activation setting and membrane potentials. Its up-regulation by G- protein pathway activation, the subsequent reduction in action potential generation thresholds and the generation of spontaneous activity suggest that blockade of $Na_v1.9$ might be useful for the treatment of pain (Baker *et al.* 2003) although there is no clear evidence for the involvement of the channel in inflammatory or neuropathic pain. Conversely, it has been suggested that $Na_v1.9$ activators might alleviate pain because $Na_v1.9$ is down regulated after axotomy (Dib-Hajj *et al.* 1998), and the resultant loss of the $Na_v1.9$ persistent current and its depolarizing influence on resting membrane potential might remove resting inactivation from other sodium channels (Herzog *et al.* 2001). Further studies including one using $Na_v1.9$ null mutants will be needed to identify the precise role of this channel in nociception.

TWO-PORE-DOMAIN K^+ CHANNELS (Fig.19.2)

The class of mammalian two-pore-domain K^+ channel

subunits comprising four transmembrane segments and two pore domains in tandem, includes 15 members (Buckingham *et al.* 2005). Functional two-pore-domain K^+ channels are dimmers of subunits with heteromultimerization. Among the subfamilies of two-pore-domain K^+ channels, TREK family expressed in primary sensory neurons is thought to be involved in pain sensation. Since the channels are activated by lipid including arachidonic acid, mechanical stress, intracellular acidification or heat all of which are related to noxious stimuli (Franks and Honore 2004). Because opening of TREK-1 causes hyperpolarization of the membrane potential by efflux of K^+ ions, TREK channels might be involved in pain relief through the reduction of firing upon noxious stimulus. Alternatively, inhibition of TREK-1 by cold stimuli might lead to nociception through depolarization. In consistent with the former concept, TREK channels are known to be activated by volatile anesthetics such as halothane and chloroform (Patel *et al.* 1999), gaseous anesthetics such as nitrous oxide and xenon (Gruss *et al.* 2004), or non-volatile anesthetics, chloral hydrate and trichloroethanol (Harinath and Sikdar 2004). Further, mice lacking TREK-1 showed a marked decrease in sensitivity to the volatile agents chloroform, halothane, sevoflurane and desflurane (Heurteaux *et al.* 2004), suggesting that TREK-1 have an important role in the general anesthetic properties of volatile agents. Polyunsaturated fatty acids, activators of TREK family channels, have been reported to protect the rat brain against global ischaemia (Lauritzen *et al.* 2000). Neuroprotective effects of TREK channels have been confirmed in animal level because TREK-1-deficient mice exhibited an increased sensitivity to both ischaemia and epilepsy (Heurteaux *et al.* 2004). Together with the TREK channel sensitivity to various anesthetics, these results indicate the wider neuroprotective effects of TREK channels, reduction of nociception in the case of sensory neurons.

CONCLUSION

Many kinds of ionotropic receptors expressed in the peripheral nerve endings most of which function as non-selective cation channels are involved in nociception by causing depolarization necessary for action potential generation. Those peripheral nociceptors would definitely be useful targets for development of antinociceptive agents.

GENERAL CITATIONS

Baker MD, Wood JN. 2001. Involvement of Na^+ channels in pain pathways. *Trends Pharmacol Sci*, 22: 27-31.

Buckingham SD, Kidd JF, Law RJ, Franks CJ, Sattelle DB. 2005. Structure and function of two-pore-domain K^+ channels: contributions from genetic model organisms. *Trends Pharmacol Sci*, 26: 361-367.

Burnstock G.2001. Purine-mediated signalling in pain and visceral perception. *Trends Pharmacol Sci*, 22: 182-188.

Caterina MJ, Julius D.1999. Sense and specificity: a molecular identity for nociceptors. *Curr Opin Neurobiol*, 9: 525-530.

Caterina MJ, Julius D. 2001. The vanilloid receptor: a molecular gateway to the pain pathway. *Annu Rev Neurosci*, 24: 487-517.

Chizh BA, Illes P. 2001. P2X receptors and nociception. *Pharmacol Rev*, 53: 553-568.

Clapham DE. 2003. TRP channels as cellular sensors. *Nature*, 426: 517-524.

Dunn PM, Zhong Y and Burnstock G. 2001. P2X receptors in peripheral neurons. *Prog Neurobiol*, 65: 107-134.

Franks NP, Honore E. 2004. The TREK K2P channels and their role in general anaesthesia and neuroprotection. *Trends Pharmacol Sci*, 25: 601-608.

Julius D, Basbaum AI. 2001. Molecular mechanisms of nociception. *Nature*, 413: 203-210.

Krishtal O. 2003. The ASICs: signaling molecules? Modulators? *Trends Neurosci*, 26: 477-483.

Macpherson LJ, Geierstanger BH, Viswanath V, Bandell M, Eid SR, Hwang S and Patapoutian A. 2005. The pungency of garlic: activation of TRPA1 and TRPV1 in response to allicin. *Curr Biol*, 15: 929-934.

Reid G, Flonta ML. 2001. Physiology. Cold current in thermoreceptive neurons. *Nature*, 413: 480.

Scholz J, Woolf CJ. 2002. Can we conquer pain? *Nat Neurosci*, 5 (Suppl): 1062-1067.

Szallasi A, Blumberg PM. 1999. Vanilloid (Capsaicin) receptors and mechanisms. *Pharmacol Rev*, 51: 159-212.

Waldmann R, Lazdunski M. 1998. H(+)-gated cation channels: neuronal acid sensors in the NaC/DEG family of ion channels. *Curr Opin Neurobiol*, 8: 418-424.

Wood JN, Boorman JP, Okuse K, Baker MD. 2004. Voltage-gated sodium channels and pain pathways. *J Neurobiol*, 61: 55-71.

Wood JN, Perl ER. 1999. Pain. *Curr Opin Genet Dev*, 9: 328-332.

DISCOVERY CITATIONS

Akopian AN, Sivilotti L, Wood JN. 1996. A tetrodotoxin-resistant voltage-gated sodium channel expressed by sensory neurons. *Nature*, 379: 257-262.

Akopian AN, Souslova V, England S, Okuse K, Ogata N, Ure J, Smith A, Kerr BJ, McMahon SB, Boyce S, Hill R, Stanfa LC, Dickenson AH, Wood JN. 1999. The tetrodotoxin-resistant sodium channel SNS has a specialized function in pain pathways. *Nat Neurosci*, 2: 541-548.

Alessandri-Haber N, Dina OA, Yeh JJ, Parada CA, Reichling DB, Levine JD. 2004. Transient receptor potential vanilloid 4 is essential in chemotherapy-induced neuropathic pain in the rat. *J Neurosci*, 24: 4444-4452.

Alessandri-Haber N, Yeh JJ, Boyd AE, Parada CA, Chen X, Reichling DB, Levine JD. 2003. Hypotonicity induces TRPV4-mediated nociception in rat. *Neuron*, 39: 497-511.

Amaya F, Oh-hashi K, Naruse Y, Iijima N, Ueda M, Shimosato G, Tominaga M, Tanaka Y, Tanaka M. 2003. Local inflammation increases vanilloid receptor 1 expression within distinct subgroups of DRG neurons. *Brain Res*, 963: 190-6.

Baker MD, Chandra SY, Ding Y, Waxman SG, Wood JN. 2003. GTP-induced tetrodotoxin-resistant Na^+ current regulates excitability in mouse and rat small diameter sensory neurones. *J Physiol*, 548: 373-382.

Bandell M, Story GM, Hwang SW, Viswanath V, Eid SR, Petrus MJ, Earley TJ, Patapoutian A. 2004. Noxious cold ion channel TRPA1 is activated by pungent compounds and bradykinin. *Neuron*, 41: 849-857.

Barclay J, Patel S, Dorn G, Wotherspoon G, Moffatt S, Eunson L, Abdel'al S, Natt F, Hall J, Winter J, Bevan S, Wishart W,

Fox A, Ganju P. 2002. Functional downregulation of P2X3 receptor subunit in rat sensory neurons reveals a significant role in chronic neuropathic and inflammatory pain. *J Neurosci*, 22: 8139-8147.

Bhave G, Zhu W, Wang H, Brasier DJ, Oxford GS, Gereau RWT, 2002. cAMP-dependent protein kinase regulates desensitization of the capsaicin receptor (VR1) by direct phosphorylation. *Neuron*, 35: 721-731.

Bleehen T, Keele CA. 1977. Observations on the algogenic actions of adenosine compounds on the human blister base preparation. *Pain*, 3: 367-377.

Bradbury EJ, Burnstock G, McMahon SB. 1998. The expression of P2X3 purinoreceptors in sensory neurons: effects of axotomy and glial-derived neurotrophic factor. *Mol Cell Neurosci*, 12: 256- 268.

Campero M, Serra J, Ochoa JL. 1996. C-polymodal nociceptors activated by noxious low temperature in human skin. *J Physiol*, 497 (Pt 2): 565-572.

Carlton SM, Coggeshall RE. 2001. Peripheral capsaicin receptors increase in the inflamed rat hindpaw: a possible mechanism for peripheral sensitization. *Neurosci Lett*, 310: 53-56.

Caterina MJ, Leffler A, Malmberg AB, Martin WJ, Trafton J, Petersen-Zeitz KR, Koltzenburg M, Basbaum AI, Julius D. 2000. Impaired nociception and pain sensation in mice lacking the capsaicin receptor. *Science*, 288: 306-313.

Caterina MJ, Rosen TA, Tominaga M, Brake AJ, Julius D. 1999. A capsaicin-receptor homologue with a high threshold for noxious heat. *Nature*, 398: 436-441.

Caterina MJ, Schumacher MA, Tominaga M, Rosen TA, Levine JD, Julius D. 1997. The capsaicin receptor: a heat-activated ion channel in the pain pathway. *Nature*, 389: 816-824.

Chan CL, Facer P, Davis JB, Smith GD, Egerton J, Bountra C, Williams NS, Anand P. 2003. Sensory fibres expressing capsaicin receptor TRPV1 in patients with rectal hypersensitivity and faecal urgency. *Lancet*, 361: 385-391.

Chuang HH, Prescott ED, Kong H, Shields S, Jordt SE, Basbaum AI, Chao MV, Julius D. 2001. Bradykinin and nerve growth factor release the capsaicin receptor from PtdIns(4,5)P2-mediated inhibition. *Nature*, 411: 957-962.

Cockayne DA, Hamilton SG, Zhu QM, Dunn PM, Zhong Y, Novakovic S, Malmberg AB, Cain G, Berson A, Kassotakis L, Hedley L, Lachnit WG, Burnstock G, McMahon SB, Ford AP. 2000. Urinary bladder hyporeflexia and reduced pain-related behaviour in P2X3-deficient mice. *Nature*, 407: 1011-1015.

Collo G, North RA, Kawashima E, Merlo-Pich E, Neidhart S, Surprenant A, Buell G. 1996. Cloning of P2X5 and P2X6 receptors and the distribution and properties of an extended family of ATP-gated ion channels. *J Neurosci*, 16: 2495-2507.

Cummins TR, Dib-Hajj SD, Black JA, Akopian AN, Wood JN, Waxman SG. 1999. A novel persistent tetrodotoxin-resistant sodium current in SNS-null and wild-type small primary sensory neurons. *J Neurosci*, 19: RC43.

Dai Y, Moriyama T, Higashi T, Togashi K, Kobayashi K, Yamanaka H, Tominaga M, Noguchi K. 2004. Proteinase-activated receptor 2-mediated potentiation of transient receptor potential vanilloid subfamily 1 activity reveals a mechanism for proteinase-induced inflammatory pain. *J Neurosci*, 24: 4293-4299.

Davis JB, Gray J, Gunthorpe MJ, Hatcher JP, Davey PT, Overend P, Harries MH, Latcham J, Clapham C, Atkinson K, Hughes SA, Rance K, Grau E, Harper AJ, Pugh PL, Rogers DC, Bingham S, Randall A, Sheardown SA. 2000. Vanilloid receptor-1 is essential for inflammatory thermal hyperalgesia. *Nature*, 405: 183-187.

Dib-Hajj SD, Tyrrell L, Black JA, Waxman SG. 1998. NaN, a novel voltage-gated Na channel, is expressed preferentially in peripheral sensory neurons and down-regulated after axotomy. *Proc Natl Acad Sci USA*, 95: 8963-8968.

Distler C, Rathee PK, Lips KS, Obreja O, Neuhuber W, Kress M. 2003. Fast Ca^{2+}-induced potentiation of heat-activated ionic currents requires cAMP/ PKA signaling and functional AKAP anchoring. *J Neurophysiol*, 89: 2499-2505.

Docherty RJ, Yeats JC, Bevan S, Boddeke HW. 1996. Inhibition of calcineurin inhibits the desensitization of capsaicin-evoked currents in cultured dorsal root ganglion neurones from adult rats. *Pflugers Arch*, 431: 828-837.

Gold MS, Reichling DB, Shuster MJ, Levine JD. 1996. Hyperalgesic agents increase a tetrodotoxin- resistant Na^+ current in nociceptors. *Proc Natl Acad Sci USA*, 93: 1108-1112.

Gold MS, Zhang L, Wrigley DL, Traub RJ. 2002. Prostaglandin E(2) modulates TTX-R I(Na) in rat colonic sensory neurons. *J Neurophysiol*, 88: 1512-1522.

Gruss M, Bushell TJ, Bright DP, Lieb WR, Mathie A, Franks NP. 2004. Two-pore-domain K$^+$ channels are a novel target for the anesthetic gases xenon, nitrous oxide, and cyclopropane. *Mol Pharmacol*, 65: 443-452.

Guler AD, Lee H, Iida T, Shimizu I, Tominaga M, Caterina M.2002. Heat-evoked activation of the ion channel, TRPV4. *J Neurosci*, 22: 6408-6414.

Harinath S, Sikdar SK. 2004. Trichloroethanol enhances the activity of recombinant human TREK-1 and TRAAK channels. *Neuropharmacology*, 46: 750-760.

Herzog RI, Cummins TR, Waxman SG. 2001. Persistent TTX-resistant Na$^+$ current affects resting potential and response to depolarization in simulated spinal sensory neurons. *J Neurophysiol*. 86: 1351-1364.

Heurteaux C, Guy N, Laigle C, Blondeau N, Duprat F, Mazzuca M, Lang-Lazdunski L, Widmann C, Zanzouri M, Romey G, Lazdunski M. 2004. TREK-1, a K$^+$ channel involved in neuroprotection and general anesthesia. *Embo J*, 23: 2684- 2695.

Honore P, Mikusa J, Bianchi B, McDonald H, Cartmell J, Faltynek C, Jarvis MF. 2002. TNP-ATP, a potent P2X3 receptor antagonist, blocks acetic acid-induced abdominal constriction in mice: comparison with reference analgesics. *Pain*, 96: 99-105.

Huang SM, Bisogno T, Trevisani M, Al-Hayani A, de Petrocellis L, Fezza F, Tognetto M, Petros TJ, Krey JF, Chu CJ, Miller JD, Davies SN, Geppetti P, Walker JM, Di Marzo V. 2002. An endogenous capsaicin-like substance with high potency at recombinant and native vanilloid VR1 receptors. *Proc Natl Acad Sci USA*, 99: 8400-8405.

Hwang SW, Cho H, Kwak J, Lee SY, Kang CJ, Jung J, Cho S, Min KH, Suh YG, Kim D, Oh U. 2000. Direct activation of capsaicin receptors by products of lipoxygenases: endogenous capsaicin-like substances. *Proc Natl Acad Sci USA*, 97: 6155-6160.

Ji RR, Samad TA, Jin SX, Schmoll R, Woolf CJ. 2002. p38 MAPK activation by NGF in primary sensory neurons after inflammation increases TRPV1 levels and maintains heat hyperalgesia. *Neuron*, 36: 57-68.

Jiang LH, Kim M, Spelta V, Bo X, Surprenant A, North RA. 2003. Subunit arrangement in P2X receptors. *J Neurosci*, 23: 8903-8910.

Jin X, Morsy N, Winston J, Pasricha PJ, Garrett K, Akbarali HI.

2004. Modulation of TRPV1 by nonreceptor tyrosine kinase, c-Src kinase. *Am J Physiol Cell Physiol*, 287: C558-563.

Jordt SE, Bautista DM, Chuang HH, McKemy DD, Zygmunt PM, Hogestatt ED, Meng ID, Julius D. 2004. Mustard oils and cannabinoids excite sensory nerve fibres through the TRP channel ANKTM1. *Nature*, 427: 260-265.

Jung J, Shin JS, Lee SY, Hwang SW, Koo J, Cho H, Oh U. 2004. Phosphorylation of vanilloid receptor 1 by Ca^{2+}/calmodulin-dependent kinase II regulates its vanilloid binding. *J Biol Chem*, 279: 7048- 7054.

Kerr BJ, Souslova V, McMahon SB, Wood JN. 2001. A role for the TTX-resistant sodium channel NaV 1.8 in NGF-induced hyperalgesia, but not neuropathic pain. *Neuroreport*, 12: 3077-3080.

Klement W, Arndt JO. 1992. The role of nociceptors of cutaneous veins in the mediation of cold pain in man. *J Physiol*, 449: 73-83.

Lai J, Gold MS, Kim CS, Bian D, Ossipov MH, Hunter JC, Porreca F. 2002. Inhibition of neuropathic pain by decreased expression of the tetrodotoxin-resistant sodium channel. NaV1.8. *Pain*, 95: 143-152.

Lauritzen I, Blondeau N, Heurteaux C, Widmann C, Romey G, Lazdunski M. 2000. Polyunsaturated fatty acids are potent neuroprotectors. *Embo J*, 19: 1784-1793.

Lewinter RD, Skinner K, Julius D, Basbaum AI. 2004. Immunoreactive TRPV-2 (VRL-1), a capsaicin receptor homolog, in the spinal cord of the rat. *J Comp Neurol*, 470: 400-408.

Lewis C, Neidhart S, Holy C, North RA, Buell G, Surprenant A. 1995. Coexpression of P2X2 and P2X3 receptor subunits can account for ATP-gated currents in sensory neurons. *Nature*, 377: 432-435.

Lingueglia E, de Weille JR, Bassilana F, Heurteaux C, Sakai H, Waldmann R, Lazdunski M. 1997. A modulatory subunit of acid sensing ion channels in brain and dorsal root ganglion cells. *J Biol Chem*, 272: 29778-29783.

Lopshire JC, Nicol GD. 1998. The cAMP transduction cascade mediates the prostaglandin E2 enhancement of the capsaicin-elicited current in rat sensory neurons: whole-cell and single-channel studies. *J Neurosci*, 18: 6081-6092.

Mamet J, Baron A, Lazdunski M, Voilley N. 2002. Proinflammatory mediators, stimulators of sensory neuron excitability via the expression of acid-sensing ion channels. *J Neu-*

rosci, 22: 10662-10670.

Marinelli S, Di Marzo V, Berretta N, Matias I, Maccarrone M, Bernardi G, Mercuri NB. 2003. Presynaptic facilitation of glutamatergic synapses to dopaminergic neurons of the rat substantia nigra by endogenous stimulation of vanilloid receptors. *J Neurosci*, 23: 3136-3144.

McCleskey EW, Gold MS. 1999. Ion channels of nociception. *Annu Rev Physiol*, 61: 835-856.

McKemy DD, Neuhausser WM, Julius D. 2002. Identification of a cold receptor reveals a general role for TRP channels in thermosensation. *Nature*, 416: 52-58.

Mezey E, Toth ZE, Cortright DN, Arzubi MK, Krause JE, Elde R, Guo A, Blumberg PM, Szallasi A. 2000. Distribution of mRNA for vanilloid receptor subtype 1 (VR1), and VR1-like immunoreactivity, in the central nervous system of the rat and human. *Proc Natl Acad Sci USA*, 97: 3655-3660.

Montell C. 2005. The TRP superfamily of cation channels. *Sci STKE*, re3.

Montell C, Rubin GM. 1989. Molecular characterization of the *Drosophila* trp locus: a putative integral membrane protein required for phototransduction. *Neuron*, 2: 1313-1323.

Moriyama T, Higashi T, Togashi K, Iida T, Segi E, Sugimoto Y, Tominaga T, Narumiya S, Tominaga M. 2005. Sensitization of TRPV1 by EP1 and IP reveals peripheral nociceptive mechanism of prostaglandins. *Molecular Pain*, 1: 3-12.

Moriyama T, Iida T, Kobayashi K, Higashi T, Fukuoka T, Tsumura H, Leon C, Suzuki N, Inoue K, Gachet C, Noguchi K, Tominaga M. 2003. Possible involvement of P2Y2 metabotropic receptors in ATP-induced transient receptor potential vanilloid receptor 1-mediated thermal hypersensitivity. *J Neurosci*, 23: 6058-6062.

North RA. 2002. Molecular physiology of P2X receptors. *Physiol Rev*, 82: 1013-1067.

North RA. 2004. P2X3 receptors and peripheral pain mechanisms. *J Physiol*, 554: 301-308.

Novakovic SD, Kassotakis LC, Oglesby IB, Smith JA, Eglen RM, Ford AP, Hunter JC. 1999. Immunocytochemical localization of P2X3 purinoceptors in sensory neurons in naive rats and following neuropathic injury. *Pain*, 80: 273-282.

Numazaki M, Tominaga T, Takeuchi K, Murayama N, Toyooka H, Tominaga M. 2003. Structural determinant of TRPV1 desensitization interacts with calmodulin. *Proc Natl Acad Sci USA*, 100: 8002-8006.

Numazaki M, Tominaga T, Toyooka H, Tominaga M. 2002. Direct phosphorylation of capsaicin receptor VR1 by protein kinase Cepsilon and identification of two target serine residues. *J Biol Chem*, 277: 13375-13378.

Obata K, Katsura H, Mizushima T, Yamanaka H, Kobayashi K, Dai Y, Fukuoka T, Tokunaga A, Tominaga M, Noguchi K. 2005. TRPA1 induced in sensory neurons contributes to cold hyperalgesia after inflammation and nerve injury. *J Clin Invest*, 115: 2393-2401.

Patel AJ, Honore E, Lesage F, Fink M, Romey G, Lazdunski M. 1999. Inhalational anesthetics activate two-pore-domain background K^+ channels. *Nat Neurosci*, 2: 422-426.

Peier AM, Moqrich A, Hergarden AC, Reeve AJ, Andersson DA, Story GM, Earley TJ, Dragoni I, McIntyre P, Bevan S, Patapoutian A. 2002a. A TRP channel that senses cold stimuli and menthol. *Cell*, 108: 705-715.

Peier AM, Reeve AJ, Andersson DA, Moqrich A, Earley TJ, Hergarden AC, Story GM, Colley S, Hogenesch JB, McIntyre P, Bevan S, Patapoutian A. 2002b. A heat-sensitive TRP channel expressed in keratinocytes. *Science*, 296: 2046-2049.

Premkumar LS, Ahern GP. 2000. Induction of vanilloid receptor channel activity by protein kinase C. *Nature*, 408: 985-990.

Premkumar LS, Raisinghani M, Pingle SC, Long C, Pimentel F. 2005. Downregulation of transient receptor potential melastatin 8 by protein kinase C-mediated dephosphorylation. *J Neurosci*, 25: 11322- 11329.

Price MP, McIlwrath SL, Xie J, Cheng C, Qiao J, Tarr DE, Sluka KA, Brennan TJ, Lewin GR, Welsh MJ. 2001. The DRASIC cation channel contributes to the detection of cutaneous touch and acid stimuli in mice. *Neuron*, 32: 1071-1083.

Rathee PK, Distler C, Obreja O, Neuhuber W, Wang GK, Wang SY, Nau C, Kress M. 2002. PKA/AKAP/VR-1 module: a common link of Gs-mediated signaling to thermal hyperalgesia. *J Neurosci*, 22: 4740-4745.

Renganathan M, Cummins TR, Waxman SG.2001. Contribution of Na(v)1.8 sodium channels to action potential electrogenesis in DRG neurons. *J Neurophysiol*, 86: 629-640.

Rosenbaum T, Gordon-Shaag A, Munari M, Gordon SE. 2004. Ca^{2+}/calmodulin modulates TRPV1 activation by capsaicin.

J Gen Physiol, 123: 53-62.

Roy ML, Narahashi T. 1992. Differential properties of tetrodotoxin-sensitive and tetrodotoxin-resistant sodium channels in rat dorsal root ganglion neurons. *J Neurosci*, 12: 2104-2111.

Roza C, Laird JM, Souslova V, Wood JN, Cervero F. 2003. The tetrodotoxin-resistant Na$^+$ channel Nav 1.8 is essential for the expression of spontaneous activity in damaged sensory axons of mice. *J Physiol*, 550: 921-926.

Scholz A, Appel N, Vogel W. 1998a. Two types of TTX-resistant and one TTX-sensitive Na$^+$ channel in rat dorsal root ganglion neurons and their blockade by halothane. *Eur J Neurosci*. 10: 2547-2556.

Scholz A, Kuboyama N, Hempelmann G, Vogel W. 1998b. Complex blockade of TTX-resistant Na$^+$ currents by lidocaine and bupivacaine reduce firing frequency in DRG neurons. *J Neurophysiol*, 79: 1746-1754.

Smith GD, Gunthorpe MJ, Kelsell RE, Hayes PD, Reilly P, Facer P, Wright JE, Jerman JC, Walhin JP, Ooi L, Egerton J, Charles KJ, Smart D, Randall AD, Anand P, Davis JB. 2002. TRPV3 is a temperature-sensitive vanilloid receptor-like protein. *Nature*, 418: 186-190.

Souslova V, Cesare P, Ding Y, Akopian AN, Stanfa L, Suzuki R, Carpenter K, Dickenson A, Boyce S, Hill R, Nebenuis-Oosthuizen D, Smith AJ, Kidd EJ, Wood JN. 2000. Warm-coding deficits and aberrant inflammatory pain in mice lacking P2X3 receptors. *Nature*, 407: 1015-1017.

Stoop R, Surprenant A, North RA. 1997. Different sensitivities to pH of ATP-induced currents at four cloned P2X receptors. *J Neurophysiol*, 78: 1837- 1840.

Story GM, Peier AM, Reeve AJ, Eid SR, Mosbacher J, Hricik TR, Earley TJ, Hergarden AC, Andersson DA, Hwang SW, McIntyre P, Jegla T, Bevan S, Patapoutian A. 2003. ANKTM1, a TRP-like channel expressed in nociceptive neurons, is activated by cold temperatures. *Cell*, 112: 819-829.

Sugiura T, Tominaga M, Katsuya H, Mizumura K. 2002. Bradykinin lowers the threshold temperature for heat activation of vanilloid receptor 1. *J Neurophysiol*, 88: 544-548.

Suzuki M, Mizuno A, Kodaira K, Imai M. 2003. Impaired pressure sensation in mice lacking TRPV4. *J Biol Chem*, 278: 22664-22668.

Toledo-Aral JJ, Moss BL, He ZJ, Koszowski AG, Whisenand T, Levinson SR, Wolf JJ, Silos-Santiago I, Halegoua S, Mandel G. 1997. Identification of PN1, a predominant voltage-dependent sodium channel expressed principally in peripheral neurons. *Proc Natl Acad Sci USA*, 94: 1527-1532.

Tominaga M, Caterina MJ, Malmberg AB, Rosen TA, Gilbert H, Skinner K, Raumann BE, Basbaum AI, Julius D. 1998. The cloned capsaicin receptor integrates multiple pain-producing stimuli. *Neuron*, 21: 531-543.

Tominaga M, Wada M, Masu M. 2001. Potentiation of capsaicin receptor activity by metabotropic ATP receptors as a possible mechanism for ATP-evoked pain and hyperalgesia. *Proc Natl Acad Sci USA*, 98: 6951-6956.

Treede RD, Meyer RA, Raja SN, Campbell JN. 1995. Evidence for two different heat transduction mechanisms in nociceptive primary afferents innervating monkey skin. *J Physiol*, 483 (Pt 3): 747-758.

Ueno S, Tsuda M, Iwanaga T, Inoue K. 1999. Cell type-specific ATP-activated responses in rat dorsal root ganglion neurons. *Br J Pharmacol*, 126: 429-436.

Voilley N, de Weille J, Mamet J, Lazdunski M. 2001. Nonsteroid anti-inflammatory drugs inhibit both the activity and the inflammation-induced expression of acid-sensing ion channels in nociceptors. *J Neurosci*, 21: 8026-8033.

Vulchanova L, Riedl MS, Shuster SJ, Buell G, Surprenant A, North RA, Elde R.1997. Immunohistochemical study of the P2X2 and P2X3 receptor subunits in rat and monkey sensory neurons and their central terminals. *Neuropharmacology*, 36: 1229-1242.

Ward SM, Bayguinov J, Won KJ, Grundy D, Berthoud HR. 2003. Distribution of the vanilloid receptor (VR1) in the gastrointestinal tract. *J Comp Neurol*, 465: 121-135.

Wildman SS, King BF, Burnstock G. 1998. Zn^{2+} modulation of ATP-responses at recombinant P2X2 receptors and its dependence on extracellular pH. *Br J Pharmacol*, 123: 1214-1220.

Winston J, Toma H, Shenoy M, Pasricha PJ. 2001. Nerve growth factor regulates VR-1 mRNA levels in cultures of adult dorsal root ganglion neurons. *Pain*, 89: 181-186.

Woolf CJ, Salter MW. 2000. Neuronal plasticity: increasing the gain in pain. *Science*, 288: 1765-1769.

Xu H, Ramsey IS, Kotecha SA, Moran MM, Chong JA, Lawson D, Ge P, Lilly J, Silos-Santiago I, Xie Y, DiStefano PS,

Curtis R, Clapham DE. 2002. TRPV3 is a calcium-permeable temperature-sensitive cation channel. *Nature*, 418: 181-186.

Yang Y, Wang Y, Li S, Xu Z, Li H, Ma L, Fan J, Bu D, Liu B, Fan Z, Wu G, Jin J, Ding B, Zhu X, Shen Y. 2004. Mutations in SCN9A, encoding a sodium channel alpha subunit, in patients with primary erythermalgia. *J Med Genet*, 41: 171-174.

Yiangou Y, Facer P, Dyer NH, Chan CL, Knowles C, Williams NS, Anand P. 2001. Vanilloid receptor 1 immunoreactivity in inflamed human bowel. *Lancet*, 357: 1338-1339.

Zhang X, Huang J, McNaughton PA. 2005. NGF rapidly increases membrane expression of TRPV1 heat-gated ion channels. *Embo J*, 24: 4211-4223.

Zygmunt PM, Petersson J, Andersson DA, Chuang H, Sorgard M, Di Marzo V, Julius D, Hogestatt ED. 1999. Vanilloid receptors on sensory nerves mediate the vasodilator action of anandamide. *Nature*, 400: 452-457.

Amygdala—Pain Processing and Pain Modulation

CHAPTER 20

Volker Neugebauer

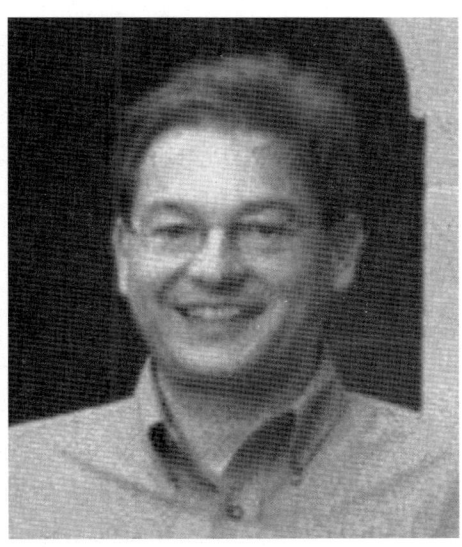

Dr. Neugebauer is an Associate Professor in the Department of Neuroscience & Cell Biology, and Associate Director, Neuroscience Graduate Program, theUniversity of Texas Medical Branch. He obtained his MD and PhD in Physiology from the University of Würzburg Medical School, Würzburg, Germany.

MAJOR CONTRIBUTIONS

1. Neugebauer V, Li W, Bird GC, Bhave G, Gereau RW. 2003. Synaptic plasticity in the amygdala in a model of arthritic pain: differential roles of metabotropic glutamate receptors 1 and 5. *J Neurosci*, 23: 52-63.
2. Neugebauer V, Li W. 2003. Differential sensitization of amygdala neurons to afferent inputs in a model of arthritic pain. *J Neurophysiol*, 89: 716-727.
3. Li, W, Neugebauer, V. 2004. Differential roles of mGluR1 and mGluR5 in brief and prolonged nociceptive processing in central amygdala neurons. *J Neurophysiol*, 91: 13-24
4. Neugebauer V, Li W, Bird GC, Han JS. 2004. The amygdala

and persistent pain. *The Neuroscientist*, 10: 221-234
5. Bird GC, Lash LL, Han JS, Zou X, Willis WD, Neugebauer, V. 2005. PKA-dependent enhanced NMDA receptor function in pain-related synaptic plasticity in amygdala neurons. *J Physiol* 564(3): 907-921
6. Han JS, Li W, Neugebauer V. 2005. Critical role of CCRP 1 receptors in the amygdala in synaptic plasticity and pain behavior. *J Neurosci*, 25: 10717-10728.

MAIN TOPICS

Nociceptive circuitry
Nociceptive processing in the amygdala
    Single cell studies
    Normal nociception
    Nociceptive plasticity
Pharmacology of nociception and plasticity
    Ionotropic glutamate receptors
    Metabotropic glutamate receptors
Pain modulation by the amygdala –behavioral data
    Pain inhibition
    Pain facilitation
Neuroimaging data

SUMMARY

As part of the limbic system the amygdala plays a key role in the emotional evaluation of sensory stimuli, emotional learning and memory, and affective states and disorders. The amygdala receives information about all sensory modalities and contains a nociceptive area, the latero-capsular part of the central nucleus (CeLC), which receives and integrates nociceptive and affect-related information. The amygdala also connects to pain modulatory systems through forebrain and brainstem connections. Electrophysiological data show pain-related sensitization and synaptic plasticity in the CeLC, which depends on presynaptic group I metabotropic glutamate receptors and postsynaptic NMDA receptors. Pain-related plasticity in the CeLC results in increased nocifensive and affective pain behavior, although the amygdala can also contribute to endogenous pain inhibition under certain circumstances. Thus, it appears that the amygdala has a dual pain-enhancing and pain-inhibiting function, which may play an important role in the state-dependent modulation and experience of pain.

INTRODUCTION

The amygdala has become one of the most systematically studied subcortical structures involved in nociceptive processing and pain modulation. As part of the limbic system the amygdala plays a key role in the emotional evaluation of sensory stimuli, emotional learning and memory, and affective states and disorders. The amygdala receives information about all sensory modalities, including nociceptive information, and has access to pain modulatory systems through forebrain and brainstem connections. Accumulating evidence suggests that the amygdala integrates nociceptive information with affective content, contributes to the emotional response to pain, and serves as a neuronal interface for the well-documented reciprocal relationship between pain and negative affect.

NOCICEPTIVE CIRCUITRY

The amygdala includes several anatomically and functionally distinct nuclei. The lateral, basolateral and central nuclei of the amygdala (LA, BLA and CeA, respectively) are of particular importance for sensory processing (see Fig.20.1A). Polymodal sensory information reaches the amygdala from thalamus (midline and posterior areas) and cortex, including insular

cortex, anterior cingulate cortex and association cortical areas. The LA serves as the major input region and initial site of sensory convergence in the amygdala. Associative learning and plasticity in the LA-BLA circuitry plays a key role in affective states and disorders such as fear and anxiety. This highly processed information with "affective" content is transmitted from the LA-BLA circuitry to the CeA, the output nucleus for major amygdala functions.

Nociceptive information reaches the CeA through polymodal pathways from thalamic and cortical areas to the LA-BLA circuitry. Importantly, the CeA also receives directly nociceptive-specific information from the brainstem (parabrachial area) and spinal cord through the spino-parabrachio-amygdaloid pain pathway and spino-amygdaloid projections, respectively. These nociceptive inputs ultimately converge onto neurons in the latero-capsular part of the CeA (Fig.20.1A), which is now defined as the "nociceptive amygdala" because of its high content of nociceptive neurons.

The CeA forms widespread connections with forebrain and brainstem areas to regulate autonomic, somatomotor, and other functions related to emotional behavior (see Fig. 20.1B). Neurons in the latero-capsular part of the CeA (CeLC) project heavily to the substantia innominata dorsalis; midline and mediodorsal thalamic nuclei and paraventricular hypothalamus via the stria terminalis. CeLC neurons also project through the ventral amygdaloid pathway (VAP) to brainstem areas such as periaqueductal gray (PAG) and parabrachial area (PB); these projections are either direct or indirect via the lateral hypothalamus.

The convergence of pain- and affect-related inputs onto the CeLC and the widespread efferent projections of the CeA to brain areas involved in emotional behavior and pain responses, suggest an important role for this particular part of the amygdala in the emotional-affective pain response and pain modulation.

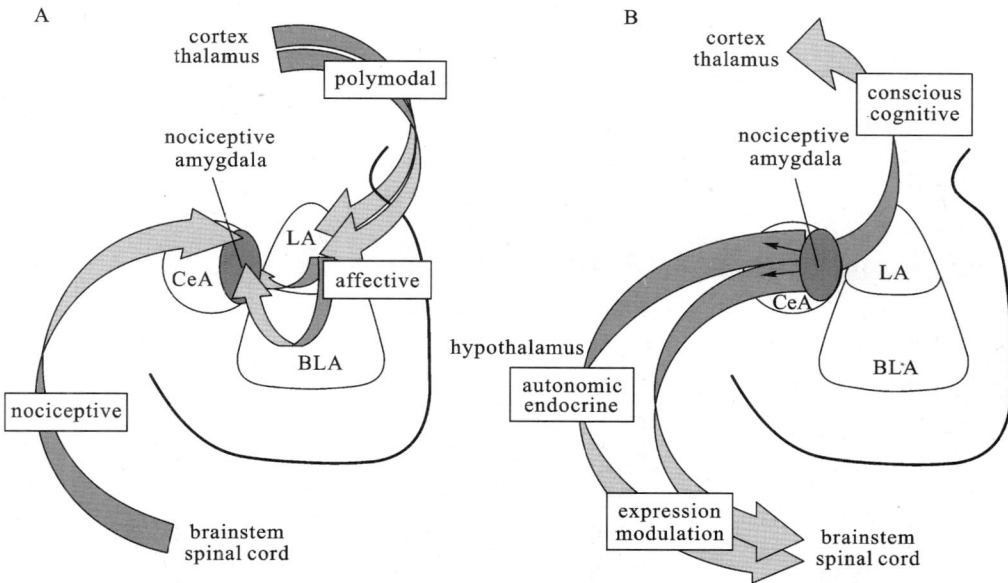

Fig.20.1   Circuitry of the nociceptive amygdala. A. Sensory and nociceptive information processing in the amygdala. The lateral nucleus of the amygdala (LA) receives and integrates polymodal information from thalamic and cortical areas. The LA represents the initial site of sensory convergence and associative plasticity in the amygdala. This highly processed information with affective content is then distributed to other amygdaloid nuclei, including the central nucleus (CeA), either directly or through the basolateral nucleus (BLA). The latero-capsular division of the CeA (CeLC) represents the "nociceptive amygdala". B. Efferent connections of the nociceptive amygdala. The CeA is the major output nucleus of the amygdala and forms widespread connections with forebrain and brainstem areas. Brainstem projections are either direct or indirect via the lateral hypothalamus; they include the parabrachial area and the periaqueductal grey matter.

NOCICEPTIVE PROCESSING IN THE AMYGDALA – SINGLE CELL STUDIES

Normal nociception

The processing of nociceptive information from superficial (skin) and deep tissue (joints and muscles) in the latero-capsular CeA has been analyzed with extracellular single-unit recordings in anesthetized animals (rats). These electrophysiological studies identified the latero-capsular CeA (CeLC) as the nociceptive amygdala. The main findings can be summarized as follows. The vast majority of CeLC neurons respond either exclusively ("nociceptive-specific" [NS] neurons) or predominantly ("multireceptive" [MR] or "wide-dynamic-range" [WDR] neurons) to noxious stimuli. More neurons are excited than inhibited by noxious stimuli. A significant number of "non-responsive" (NR) neurons (up to 20%), which do not respond to somatosensory stimuli, also exist in the

CeLC. NS and MR CeA neurons have large, mostly symmetrical bilateral receptive fields that can include the whole body; they respond to mechanical and thermal stimuli; their stimulus-response functions are not monotonically increasing linear but sigmoidal (Fig.20.2). These characteristics argue against a sensory-discriminative function of CeA neurons, such as the encoding of stimulus location and intensity. Electrical orthodromic stimulation in the pontine parabrachial nucleus evokes monosynaptic responses of NS and MR neurons in the CeLC consistent with direct input from the spino-parabrachio-amygdaloid pain pathway.

NS neurons appear to receive input exclusively from the spino-parabrachio-amygdaloid pathway whereas MR neurons integrate nociceptive-specific information with affective content from the LA-BLA circuitry. Importantly, the anatomical segregation of these two functionally distinct lines of input allows the separate analysis of transmission of nociceptive versus affective information in the in vitro brain slice preparation.

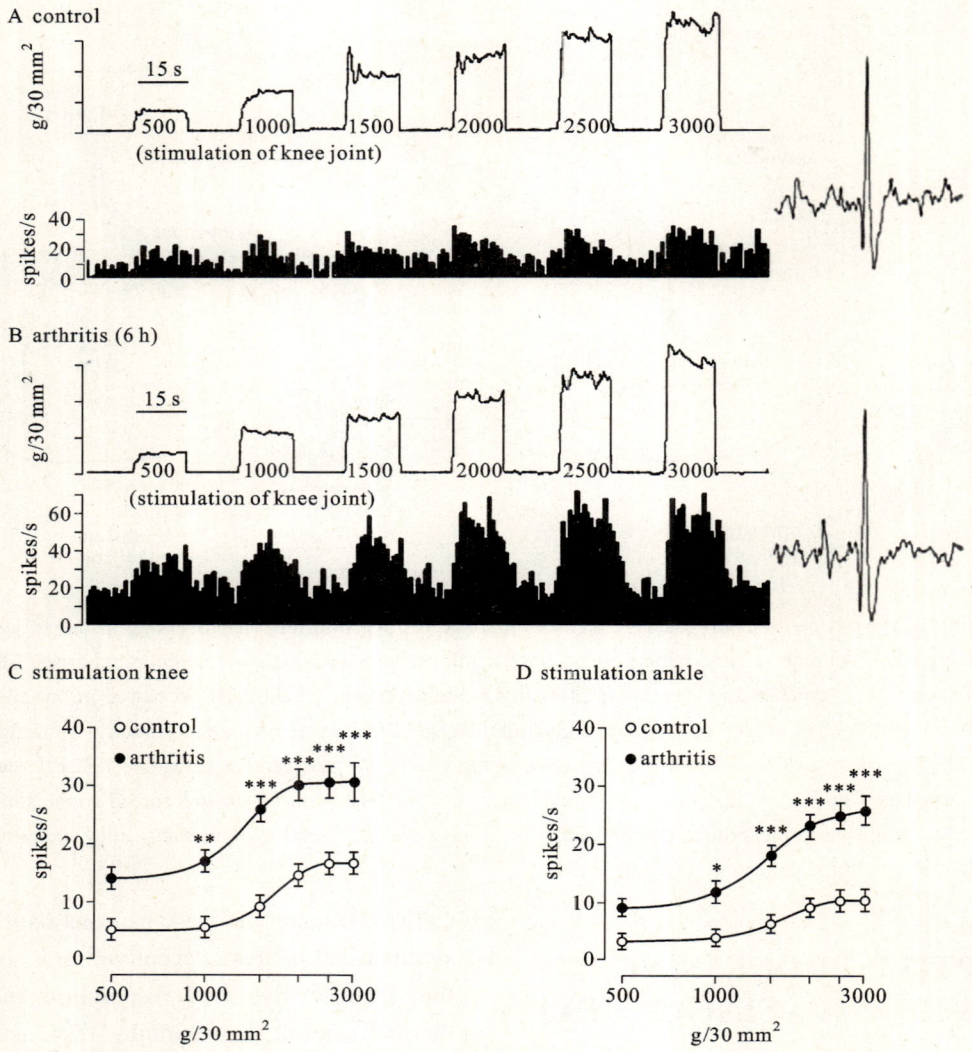

Fig.20.2   Nociceptive processing and pain-related sensitization of CeLC neurons recorded *in vivo*. Stimulus-response functions for mechanical stimulation are altered in the arthritis pain model. Extracellular recordings from an individual CeLC neuron (same neuron in A and B) show the increased responses to brief (15 s) graded mechanical stimulation of the knee joint (top traces) 6 h after induction of arthritis (B) compared to control (A). The monoarthritis was induced in one knee joint (contralateral to the recording site) by intraarticular injections of kaolin and carrageenan. Individual action potentials displayed on the right next to corresponding histograms on the left illustrate that spike configuration, shape and size remained constant throughout the experiment. Stimulus-response functions (C, D) were constructed from the averaged responses of individual CeLC neurons to graded mechanical stimuli in the innocuous (< 500g/30mm^2) and noxious range (> 1500g/30mm^2). Stimuli were applied to the arthritic knee and the non-arthritic ankle. Stimulus-response curves were best described by a sigmoidal non-linear regression model. Note the logarithmic scale. Each symbol represents the mean ± SEM. The stimulus-response relationships before and after induction of arthritis were significantly different. * $P < 0.05$, **, $P < 0.01$, *** $P < 0.001$, two-way ANOVA followed by Bonferroni post-tests (reproduced with permission from Neugebauer and Li, 2003; copyright 2003 by the American Physiological Society).

Nociceptive plasticity

Information processing in the CeA under conditions of prolonged and persistent pain was not known until recently. Our electrophysiological single-unit record

ings in anesthetized rats showed that two major subpopulations of nociceptive CeLC neurons (see above), the MR and NR neurons, but not NS neurons, become sensitized to afferent inputs in the kaolin/carrageenan-induced arthritis pain model. The arthritis pain-related sensitization of MR neurons shows the following characteristics (Fig.20.2; Neugebauer and Li, 2003): enhanced processing of mechanical, but not thermal, pain-related information as evidenced by the left- and up-ward shift of the stimulus-response functions; increased responses to stimulation of the arthritic knee as well as of non-injured tissue such as the ankle; expansion of the total size of the receptive field; and enhanced background (ongoing) activity. These changes indicate an input-specific increase of gain and activation level. Importantly, a constant input evoked by orthodromic electrical stimulation in the PB produces enhanced responses of CeLC neurons, suggesting that these neurons become in fact "sensitized" and do not just simply reflect enhanced incoming signals. Unlike changes in the peripheral nervous system and spinal cord in this arthritis model, changes of MR neurons develop with a biphasic time course. The first phase (1-3 h) may reflect changes in the spinal cord and brainstem whereas the persistent plateau phase (>5 h) is likely to involve intra-amygdala plasticity. MR neurons, which receive both nociceptive and polymodal affective inputs, are well positioned to integrate pain- and affect-related information. Recruitment of NR neurons would increase the gain of information processing and output. NS neurons would serve to distinguish nociceptive from affect-related inputs in pain-related sensitization.

Definitive proof of pain-related plasticity in the CeLC comes from electrophysiological in vitro studies using brain slices containing the amygdala. Since the brain slice is disconnected from the peripheral site of injury and from spinal nociceptive centers, any changes measured in this reduced preparation are maintained in the slice independently of continuous nociceptive input from peripheral and spinal sites. The anatomical arrangement of nociceptive-specific and polymodal-affective inputs to the CeLC (see Fig.20.1A) allows the separate analysis of transmission in these two functionally distinct pathways. Whole-cell patch-clamp recordings of CeLC neurons

were made in coronal brain slices from normal rats and from rats with a kaolin/carrageenan-induced arthritis. CeA neurons with convergent inputs from the PB and the BLA (resembling MR neurons) showed enhanced synaptic transmission and increased neuronal excitability in slices from arthritic animals compared to normal controls. Enhanced synaptic transmission (synaptic plasticity) is reflected in the increased input-output function of the PB-CeLC synapse, which provides nociceptive-specific inputs from the pontine parabrachial area, and of the BLA-CeLC synapse, which transmits polymodal-affective information (Fig.20.3). CeLC neurons recorded in slices from arthritic rats also showed increased excitability (depolarized membrane potential, reduced input resistance, increased slope conductance, and lower threshold for action potentials generated by direct intracellular current injections).

PHARMACOLOGY OF NOCICEPTION AND PLASTICITY

Ionotropic glutamate receptors

These ligand-gated ion channels include N-methyl-D-aspartate (NMDA) receptors and non-NMDA receptors of the σ-amino-3-hydroxy-5-methyl-4-isoxazolepropionic acid (AMPA) and kainate types. Administration of antagonists at the NMDA (AP5) or non-NMDA (NBQX) receptors into the CeA inhibited the extracellularly recorded responses of CeLC neurons to brief (15 s) noxious stimuli. Responses to innocuous stimuli were inhibited by block of non-NMDA, but not NMDA, receptors in the CeA. Pain-related sensitization of CeLC neurons in the kaolin/carrageenan arthritis model (6 h postinduction) was inhibited by NMDA or non-NMDA receptor antagonists suggesting the involvement of both receptor types. These data also indicate a change of NMDA receptor function in pain-related sensitization.

Accordingly, NMDA receptors play an important role in pain-related synaptic plasticity but not in normal synaptic transmission in the amygdala. Whole-cell patch-clamp recordings showed that synaptic plasticity in the arthritis pain model, but not normal synaptic transmission in control neurons, was inhibited by a selective NMDA receptor antagonist (AP5). Accordingly, an NMDA-receptor-mediated synaptic component was recorded in CeLC neurons from arthritic animals, but not in control neurons; and this synaptic component was blocked by inhibitors of PKA (KT5720) but not PKC (GF109203X). Exogenous NMDA evoked a larger inward current in neurons from arthritic animals than in control neurons, indicating a direct postsynaptic effect in CeLC neurons.

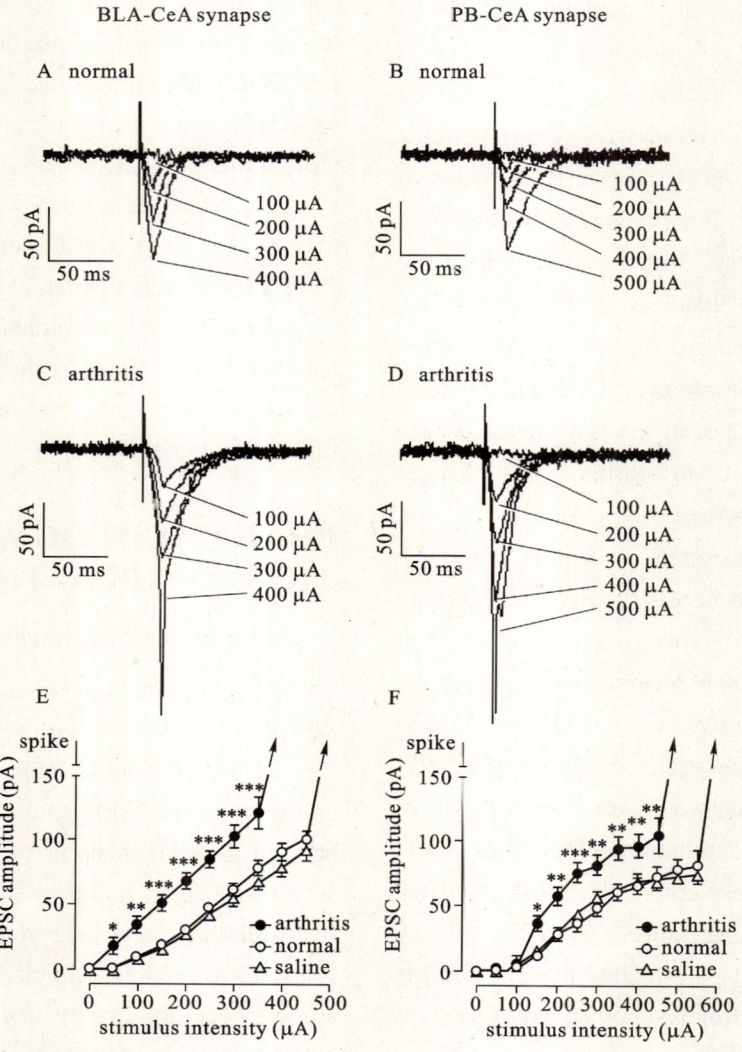

Fig.20.3 Pain-related synaptic plasticity in the CeLC recorded in vitro. Input-output functions show enhanced synaptic transmission at the nociceptive PB-CeLC and the polymodal BLA-CeLC synapses in the arthritis pain model. Whole-cell voltage-clamp recordings were made from neurons in the CeLC in brain slices from control (uninjected normal and saline-injected sham) rats and from rats with a kaolin/carrageenan-induced monoarthritis in the left knee (6-8 h post-induction). Monosynaptic excitatory postsynaptic currents (EPSCs) were evoked by electrical stimulation of afferent fibers from the basolateral amygdala (A, C; BLA-CeA synapse) and from the parabrachial area (B, D; PB-CeA synapse). Input-output relationships were obtained by increasing the stimulus intensity in 50 μA steps and measuring the peak amplitudes of evoked EPSCs. A-D, Individual examples of one CeLC neuron recorded in the brain slice from a normal rat (A, B) and another CeLC neuron from an arthritic rat (C, D). Significantly enhanced input-output relationships in neurons from arthritic animals ($n = 20$) compared to control neurons ($n = 36$; normal uninjected rats, $n = 26$; saline-injected shams, $n = 10$), suggesting enhanced synaptic transmission at the BLA-CeA (E) and the PB-CeA (F) synapses (two-way ANOVA followed by Bonferroni post-tests). * $P < 0.05$, ** $P < 0.01$, *** $P < 0.001$. Neurons were held at −60 mV (reproduced with permission from Neugebauer *et al.* 2003; copyright 2003 by the Society for Neuroscience).

Conversely, paired-pulse facilitation, a measure of presynaptic mechanisms, was not affected by AP5. Western blot analysis showed increased levels of phosphorylated NMDA-receptor 1 (pNR1) protein, but not of total NR1, in the CeA of arthritic rats compared to controls. These results suggest that pain-related synaptic plasticity in the CeLC is accompanied by protein kinase A (PKA)-mediated enhanced postsynaptic NMDA-receptor function through increased phosphorylation, but not upregulation, of NR1 subunits.

Metabotropic glutamate receptors

Metabotropic glutamate receptors (mGluRs) are G-protein coupled receptors that include group I (mGluR1 and 5), group II (mGluR2 and 3) and group III (mGluR4, 6, 7 and 8) mGluRs. Group I mGluRs can activate phospholipase C, various protein kinases (including PKC) and MAP kinases such as ERK1/2. Group II and III mGluRs couple negatively to adenylyl cyclase and inhibit cyclic AMP (cAMP) formation and cAMP-dependent protein kinase (PKA) activation.

Electrophysiological studies of CeLC neurons in anesthetized animals *in vivo* and in brain slices *in vitro* showed an important role of group I mGluRs in pain-related sensitization and synaptic plasticity in the amygdala. Presynaptic mGluR1 rather than mGluR5 subtypes appeared to be particularly important.

Extracellular single-unit recordings of CeLC neurons in anesthetized rats showed that under normal conditions, activation of mGluR1/5 in the CeA by the agonist DHPG or selective activation of mGluR5 in the CeA by CHPG enhanced the responses of CeLC neurons to brief (15 s) innocuous and noxious stimuli. This is consistent with the involvement of mGluR5 rather than mGluR1. In the kaolin/carrageenan arthritis pain model (6 h postinduction), the facilitatory effects of DHPG, but not CHPG, increased, suggesting a change in mGluR1 function. Conversely, an mGluR1 antagonist (CPCCOEt) inhibited the responses of sensitized CeLC neurons in the arthritis pain state but had no effect under normal conditions. An mGluR5 antagonist (MPEP) inhibited nociceptive responses

under normal conditions and in the arthritis pain state (Fig.20.4; Li and Neugebauer, 2004a). Agonists and antagonists were administered into the CeA by microdialysis. These data suggest a change of mGluR1 rather than mGluR5 activation and function in the CeA in pain-related sensitization.

The cellular mechanisms and site of action of group I mGluRs and their role in synaptic plasticity were determined in brain slices from normal and arthritic rats. Synaptic transmission was studied at the nociceptive PB-CeLC synapse and the polymodal-affective BLA-CeLC synapse (see Fig.20.1A). Agonists at mGluR1/5 (DHPG) and at mGluR5 (CHPG) potentiated normal synaptic transmission, thus mimicking pain-related synaptic plasticity. In slices from arthritic rats (6 h postinduction), the effects of DHPG, but not CHPG, increased, suggesting an enhanced function of mGluR1 rather than mGluR5 in pain-related synaptic plasticity in the CeLC. Importantly, these agents had no effect on membrane properties and neuronal excitability but attenuated paired-pulse facilitation, suggesting a pre-rather than post-synaptic site of action. An mGluR1 antagonist (CPCCOEt) had no effect on normal synaptic transmission but inhibited synaptic plasticity in slices from arthritic rats, whereas an mGluR5 antagonist (MPEP) inhibited normal synaptic transmission as well as synaptic plasticity (Fig.20.5; Neugebauer *et al.*, 2003). Thus, enhanced endogenous activation of presynaptic mGluR1 appears to be an important mechanism of pain-related synaptic plasticity in the CeLC.

The roles of group II and III mGluRs in nociception and pain-related plasticity in the amygdala are not clear yet. Whole-cell patch-clamp recordings of CeLC neurons in brain slices from normal and arthritic rats showed that a group III agonist (LAP4) inhibited synaptic transmission more potently in CeLC neurons from arthritic rats than in control neurons from normal animals. LAP4 had no significant effects on membrane properties but increased paired-pulse facilitation, suggesting a presynaptic site of action. Accordingly, LAP4 inhibited the frequency but not quantal size of miniature excitatory postsynaptic currents (mEPSCs).

The inhibitory effects of LAP4 were reversed by a selective group III mGluR antagonist (UBP1112). These data suggest that presynaptic group III mGluRs can modulate pain-related synaptic plasticity in the CeLC.

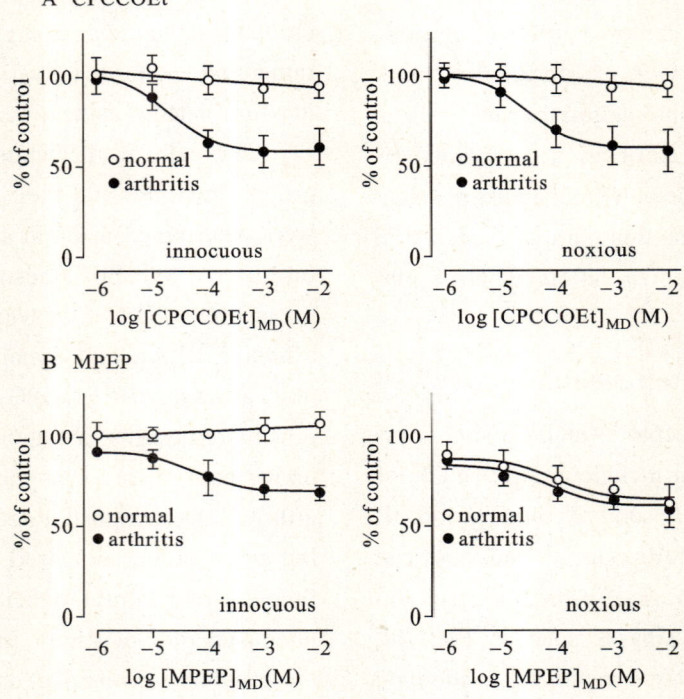

Fig.20.4 Differential changes of mGluR1 and mGluR5-mediated effects in pain-related sensitization of CeLC neurons recorded *in vivo*. A. Cumulative concentration-response relationships show that a selective mGluR1 antagonist (CPCCOEt) inhibited the enhanced responses of sensitized CeLC neurons ($n = 8$) after induction of arthritis (innocuous, 500 g/30 mm^2, $EC_{50} = 19.9 \pm 0.50$ μM; noxious, 2500 g/30 mm^2, $EC_{50} = 29.4 \pm 0.70$ μM). CPCCOEt had no significant effect under normal conditions ($P > 0.05$, linear regression analysis, $n = 12$). B, Responses of CeLC neurons to brief noxious stimuli were inhibited by a selective mGluR5 antagonist (MPEP) under normal conditions (n = 19; $EC_{50} = 93.3 \pm 10.1$ μM) and in arthritis pain-related sensitization ($n = 8$; innocuous, $EC_{50} = 57.6 \pm 1.6$ μM; noxious $EC_{50} = 62.8 \pm 5.7$ μM). There was no significant change in potency of MPEP for inhibiting brief noxious responses before and after induction of arthritis ($P > 0.05$, unpaired t-test). A and B, evoked responses were measured and expressed as spikes/s. Background activity, if present, was subtracted from the total activity during stimulus application. Responses of individual neurons to innocuous and noxious mechanical stimulation of the knee were averaged across the sample of neurons. All averaged values are given as means ± SE. Drugs were administered into the CeA by microdialysis for 15 min. Numbers refer to the concentrations in microdialysis probe (reproduced with permission from Li and Neugebauer, 2004a; copyright 2004 by the American Physiological Society).

PAIN MODULATION BY THE AMYGDALA — BEHAVIORAL DATA

The CeA, including the latero-capsular division, forms direct and indirect connections with descending pain modulating systems in the brainstem (Fig.20.1B; for review see Neugebauer *et al.*, 2004). Descending pain control systems centered on the periaqueductal gray (PAG) and rostroventral medulla (RVM) network can be inhibitory (anti-nociceptive) as well as facili-tatory (pro-nociceptive). Electrical or chemical (with D, L-homocysteic acid) activation of the CeA has been shown to excite some neurons in the PAG and inhibit others. The paradigm shift in recent years from descending pain inhibition to facilitation appears to be reflected in recent behavioral studies that link the amygdala to pro-nociceptive effects whereas earlier studies emphasized the antinociceptive role of the amygdala. Activity in the amygdala can be modified by negative and positive emotions, which in turn can enhance (anxiety and depression) or reduce (pleasant odorants and music) pain. The modulation of amygdala activity by affective state and the dual coupling of the amygdala to pain inhibition and facilitation may be an important mechanism in the modulation of pain by affective states and disorders.

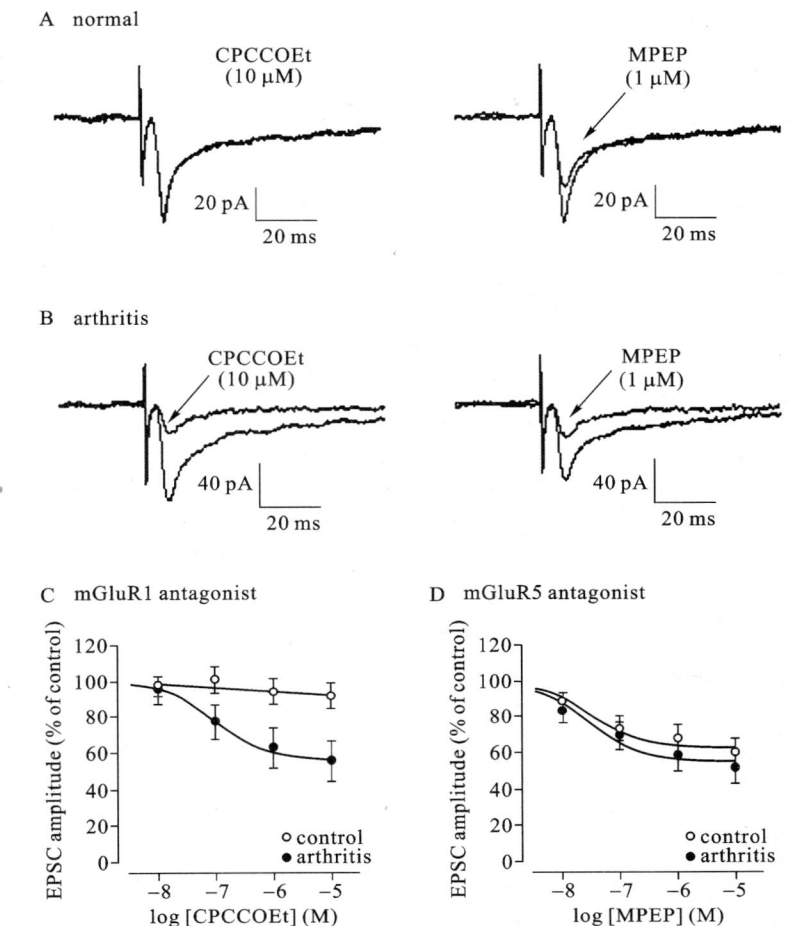

Fig. 20.5 Differential changes of mGluR1 and mGluR5-mediated effects in pain-related synaptic plasticity in the CeLC recorded *in vitro*. A. In a CeLC neuron recorded in a brain slice from a normal rat, MPEP (mGluR5 antagonist) inhibited synaptic transmission whereas CPCCOEt (mGluR1 antagonist) had no effect. B. In a CeLC neuron from an arthritic rat (6 h postinduction by intraarticular kaolin/carrageenan-injections), both CPCCOEt and MPEP inhibited synaptic transmission, suggesting a change in the endogenous activation of mGluR1 in the arthritis pain model. Each trace is the average of 8–10 monosynaptic EPSCs recorded at –60 mV. Drugs were applied by superfusion of the slice in ACSF for at least 10 min. C. CPCCOEt inhibited synaptic transmission in neurons from arthritic rats ($EC_{50} = 94$ nM, $n = 9$) but not in neurons from normal rats ($n = 11$), suggesting a change in the activation state of mGluR1 in the arthritis pain model. D. The inhibitory effects of MPEP on synaptic transmission were not significantly different in CeLC neurons from normal rats ($EC_{50} = 28.3$ nM, $n = 10$) and in CeLC neurons from arthritic rats ($EC_{50} = 27.7$ nM, $n = 9$; $P > 0.05$, two-way ANOVA) (reproduced with permission from Neugebauer *et al.*, 2003; copyright 2003 by the Society for Neuroscience).

Pain Inhibition

It is well established that the amygdala can play a role in various forms of conditioned hypoalgesia and analgesia, i.e., pain-reduction and pain-inhibition, by aversive stimuli and stressors, some of which (e.g., foot-shock) also evoke fear-related behavior. Amygdala lesions, some involving the CeA, reduced or abolished the expression of such conditioned hypoal-gesia and/or analgesia. Bilateral or unilateral amygdala lesion studies implicated the CeA, but not BLA, in the analgesic effects of systemic morphine, a μ-opioid receptor agonist, in models of tonic and phasic pain. Bilateral chemical inactivation of the CeA, but not BLA, also reduced the analgesic effects of systemic cannabinoid receptor activation in phasic and tonic pain models and the cannabinoid-induced inhibition of pain-related c-fos expression in the dorsal horn of the spinal cord. Infusions of morphine into the BLA resulted in a substantial, naloxone-reversible increase in tail flick latency, and significantly increased ongoing firing of OFF cells and depressed that of ON cells in the RVM. The antinociceptive and analgesic effects of μ-opioid receptor activation in the BLA or CeA can be inhibited by lesions or chemical inactivation of the PAG and RVM. Unilateral electrical stimulation of the amygdala, including the CeA and BLA, resulted in a reduction of phasic and tonic pain behavior. These studies suggest that the amygdala is involved in certain forms of conditioned and morphine-induced analgesia.

Pain Facilitation

More recently, it has become clear that the amygdala can also contribute to the generation and enhancement of pain responses. Unilateral excitotoxin-induced lesions of the ipsilateral CeA significantly inhibited the second, but not the first, phase of formalin-induced pain behavior. Conversely, an exciting recent study showed that activation of glucocorticoid and mineralocorticoid receptors by corticosterone administration to the CeA produced visceral hypersensitivity; importantly the pain producing effects were paralleled by increased indices of anxiety (Fig.20.6; Greenwood-van Meerveld et al., 2001). Rats with corticosterone implants spent significantly less time in the open arm of the plus maze assay than control rats, which is consistent with enhanced anxiety-like behavior. Stimulation of the CeA with corticosterone also produced increased visceromotor responses to colorectal distension (CRD) in normal rats and mimicked the visceral hypersensitivity that followed the sensitization of the colon with intracolonic acetic acid. These data suggest an important pro-nociceptive role of the amygdala, presumably the CeA, in the development of visceral hypersensitivity. They are also consistent with the hypothesis that the amygdala serves as an interface between pain and negative affect.

Subsequent studies showed that chemical activation of the amygdala can produce sensitization of spinal dorsal horn neurons through descending facilitation. In rats with elevated glucocorticoid levels in the

CeA, spinal neurons with nociceptive visceral input from the colon or the urinary bladder showed greater and longer-lasting excitatory responses to colorectal and urinary bladder distension, respectively, compared to control (cholesterol implanted) rats. Importantly, the amygdala-evoked sensitization of spinal neurons to visceral stimulation occurred in the absence of any tissue inflammation or injury, suggesting that the amygdala can increase or produce pain processing and contribute to chronic pain through central sensitization in the spinal cord. This may have important implications for so-called functional disorders, in which pain intensity and duration do not correlate with peripheral tissue pathology.

The behavioral consequence of pain-related plasticity in the amygdala (see above) is only beginning to emerge. Chemical inactivation of the CeA by agents that are now known to inhibit pain-related sensitization and synaptic plasticity in the CeLC (see above) also inhibited spinally and supraspinally organized behavioral responses in a model of arthritic pain (Fig.20.7; Han and Neugebauer, 2005). Hindlimb withdrawal thresholds (spinal reflex response) and audible and ultrasonic vocalizations (supraspinally organized behavior) evoked by mechanical stimulation of the knee were measured in awake rats before and after induction of the kaolin/carrageenan-arthritis in the knee (6 h postinduction). Audible vocalizations evoked by noxious stimuli represent a nociceptive response whereas ultrasonic vocalizations to noxious stimuli reflect a pain-related affective component. In the arthritis pain state, withdrawal thresholds were decreased and the duration of audible and ultrasonic vocalizations increased. Administration of an mGluR1 antagonist (CPCCOEt) into the CeA inhibited vocalizations during stimulation (VDS), which are organized at the brainstem level, and vocalizations that continue after stimulation (VAS; vocalization afterdischarges), which are organized in the limbic forebrain, particularly the amygdala (Fig.20.7; Han and Neugebauer, 2005). CPCCOEt in the CeA also inhibited spinally organized hindlimb withdrawal reflexes. Block of mGluR5 in the CeA with a selective antagonist (MPEP) inhibited only VAS but had no effect on

VDS and withdrawal reflexes. These findings suggest differential roles of mGluR1 .and mGluR5 in the CeA on pain behavior organized at different levels of the pain neuraxis; they also suggest different pharmacological mechanisms of pain processing in the amyg-

dala and descending pain modulation by the amygdala. The fact that mGluR1 and mGluR5 act presynaptically in the CeA may suggest that afferent inputs to the CeA play an important role in the modulation of pain behavior by the amygdala.

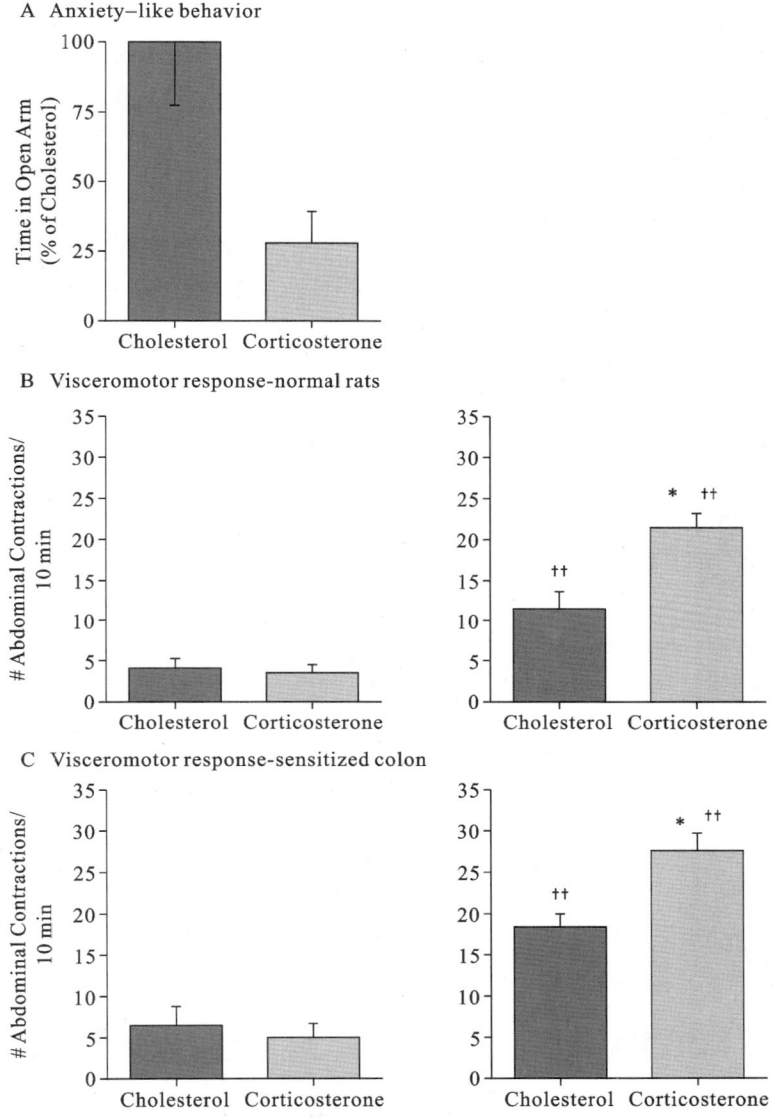

Fig.20.6   Pain and anxiety-like behavior produced by chemical activation of the amygdala. Corticosterone implants were placed on the dorsal margin of the amygdala (CeA). A. Rats with stereotaxically delivered corticosterone to the CeA spent significantly less exploration time in the open arm of the elevated plus maze than control (cholesterol implanted) rats. * $P < 0.05$. B. Effect of CeA stimulation with corticosterone on visceromotor responses in rats with normal (non-sensitized) colons. Control (cholesterol implanted) rats and corticosterone implanted rats showed no difference in the number of abdominal contractions under basal conditions (undistended colon; left), but innocuous colorectal distension with a balloon catheter (30 mmHg for 10 min; right) produced a significantly greater response in corticosterone implanted rats compared to control rats. ++ $P < 0.05$, undistended vs. distended; * $P < 0.01$, distended cholesterol vs. corticosterone. C. Effect of colon sensitization with acetic acid on the visceromotor responses of rats with corticosterone implants in the CeA and in control (cholesterol implanted) rats. Acetic acid (0.6%, 1.5 mL) was slowly infused into the colon through a silastic tube running along the balloon catheter. Colon sensitization increased the visceromotor responses of rats with corticosterone implants and of control rats but the response was greater in the group with corticosterone-stimulated CeA (right): 5.5 fold increase (corticosterone group) versus 2.6 fold increase (cholesterol group). No difference was found between corticosterone implanted rats and control rats under basal conditions (undistended, but sensitized colons; left). ++ $P < 0.05$, undistended vs. distended; * $P < 0.01$, distended cholesterol vs. corticosterone (reproduced with permission from Greenwood-van Meerveld *et al.* 2001; copyright 2001 by Elsevier).

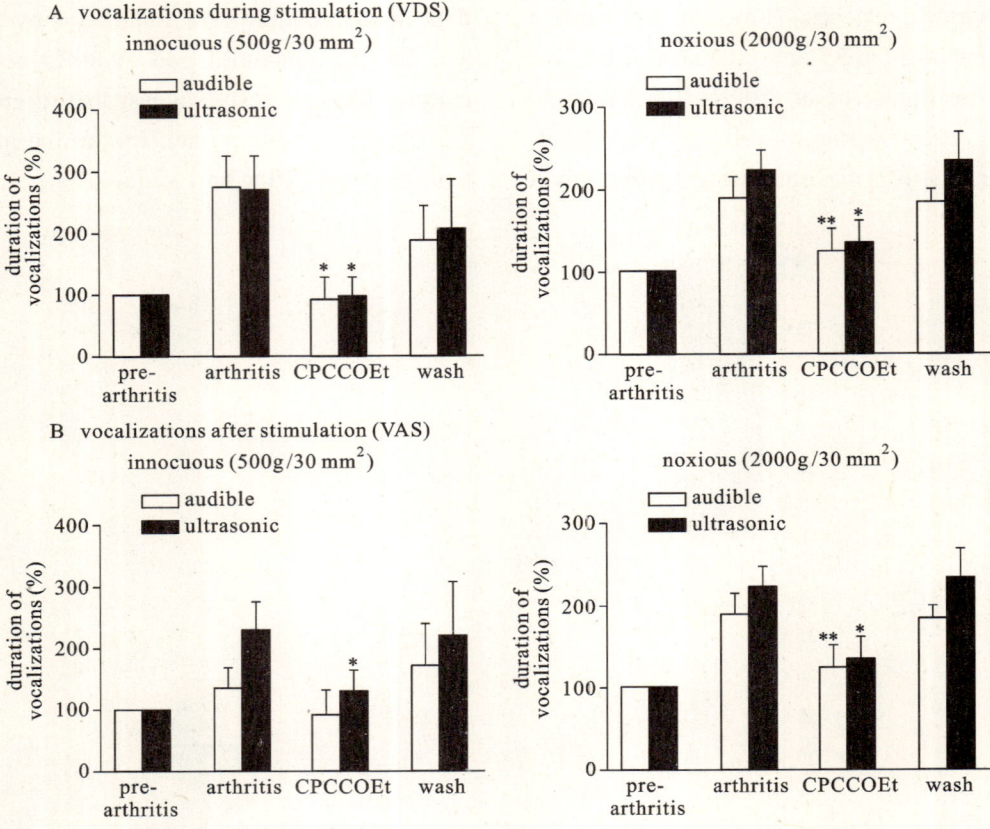

Fig.20.7 Chemical inactivation of the CeA inhibits supraspinally organized behavior in the arthritis pain model. Vocalizations during (VDS, A) and after (VAS, vocalization afterdischarges, B) mechanical stimulation of the knee increased in the arthritis pain model (6 h postinduction). A. VDS were recorded during normally innocuous (left) and noxious (right) stimulation of the knee for 15 s. Administration of an mGluR1 antagonist (CPCCOEt, 100 μM) into the CeA by microdialysis decreased the duration of audible and ultrasonic VDS ($n=9$, paired t-test; *$P<0.05$, **$P<0.01$). B. Audible and ultrasonic VAS of the same animals were also inhibited by CPCCOEt (100 μM; $n=9$). The inhibition of ultrasonic VAS following normally innocuous stimulation of the arthritic knee and of audible VAS following noxious stimuli was statistically significant ($P<0.05$; paired t-test). Durations of audible and ultrasonic VAS and VDS were expressed as percent of pre-arthritis control values (set to 100%). Washout with ACSF was for 30 min. Symbols and error bars represent mean±SE (reproduced with permission from Han and Neugebauer, 2005; copyright 2005 by The International Association for the Study of Pain, IASP).

NEUROIMAGING DATA

Neuroimaging pain studies using positron emission tomography (PET) and functional magnetic resonance imaging (fMRI), have repeatedly identified pain-related signal changes in the amygdala in animals and humans. The experimental conditions included the application of brief noxious heat stimuli to the skin of humans, vascular pain induced in humans by balloon dilatation of a dorsal foot vein, noxious colorectal stimulation in patients with irritable bowel syndrome (IBS), and mechanical allodynia in neuropathic pain patients and in a rat model of peripheral mononeu-

ropathy. In these studies activation or deactivation ("negative activation") were measured. It should also be noted that a number of previous neuroimaging pain studies were unable to detect signal changes in response to painful stimuli or in certain pain states.

CONCLUSIONS

The amygdala contains a nociceptive area, the laterocapsular part of the central nucleus (CeLC), which receives and integrates nociceptive and affect-related information. Pain-related plasticity in the nociceptive amygdala results in increased pain behavior organized at the spinal and supraspinal levels, although the amygdala can also contribute to endogenous pain inhibition under certain circumstances. Thus, it appears that the amygdala, including the CeLC, has a dual pain-enhancing and pain-inhibiting function. The bidirectional regulation of pain through the amygdala may play an important role in the reciprocal relationship between pain and negative affect, which includes pain-enhancement by some affective states (mild shock, anxiety and depression) but pain-inhibition by others (severe shock, acute stress and fear; but also pleasant odorants and music). The behavioral consequence of manipulations with known (excitatory or inhibitory) cellular and molecular effects in the amygdala needs to be further studied in models of prolonged and chronic pain to determine under which conditions the amygdala increases or inhibits pain.

GENERAL CITATIONS

Bernard J-F, Bester H, Besson JM. 1996. Involvement of the spino-parabrachio-amygdaloid and-hypothalamic pathways in the autonomic and affective emotional aspects of pain. *Prog Brain Res*, 107: 243-255.

Braz JM, Nassar MA, Wood JN, Basbaum AI. 2005. Parallel "pain" pathways arise from subpopulations of primary afferent nociceptor. *Neuron*, 47: 787-793.

Heinricher MM, McGaraughty S. 1999. Pain-modulating neurons and behavioral state. In: Lydic R, Baghdoyan HA, eds. *Handbook of Behavioral State Control*. New York: CRC Press. 487-503.

Hollmann M, Heinemann S. 1994 Cloned glutamate receptors. *Annu Rev Neurosci*, 17: 31-108.

LeDoux JE. 2000. Emotion circuits in the brain. *Annu Rev Neurosci*, 23: 155-184.

Lesage ASJ. 2004 Role of group I metabotropic glutamate receptors mGlu1 and mGlu5 in nociceptive signalling. *Current Neuropharm*, 2: 363-393.

Millan MJ. 1999. The induction of pain: an integrative review. *Progress in Neurobiology*. Elsevier Science Ltd. 1-164.

Neugebauer V. 2001. Metabotropic glutamate receptors: novel targets for pain relief. *Expert Rev Neurotherapeutics*, 1: 207-224.

Neugebauer V. 2002. Metabotropic glutamate receptors —
important modulators of nociception and pain behavior. *Pain*, 98: 1-8.

Neugebauer V, Li W, Bird GC, Han JS. 2004. The amygdala and persistent pain. *Neuroscientist*, 10: 221-234.

Price JL. 2003. Comparative aspects of amygdala connectivity. In: Shinnick-Gallagher P, Pitkanen A, Shekhar A, Cahill L, eds. *The Amygdala in Brain Function. Basic and Clinical Approaches*. New York: The New York Academy of Sciences. Vol 985: 50-58.

Rhudy JL, Meagher MW. 2001 The role of emotion in pain modulation. *Curr Opin Psychiatry*, 14: 241-245.

Suzuki R, Rygh LJ, Dickenson AH. 2004. Bad news from the brain: descending 5-HT pathways that control spinal pain processing. *Trends Pharmacol Sci*, 25: 613-617.

Vanegas H, Schaible HG. 2004. Descending control of persistent pain: inhibitory or facilitatory? *Brain Res Rev*. 46: 295-309.

Varney MA, Gereau RW. 2002. Metabotropic glutamate receptor involvement in models of acute and persistent pain: prospects for the development of novel analgesics. *Current Drug Targets*, 1: 215-225.

DISCOVERY CITATIONS

Becerra LR, Breiter HC, Stojanovic M, Fishman S, Edwards A, Comite AR, Gonzalez RG. 1999. Human brain activation under controlled thermal stimulation and habituation of noxious heat: an fMRI study. *Mag Reson in Med*, 41: 1044-1057.

Bingel U, Quante M, Knab R, Bromm B, Weiller C, Buchel C. 2002. Subcortical structures involved in pain processing: evidence from single-trial fMRI. *Pain*, 99: 313-321.

Bird GC, Lash LL, Han JS, Zou X, Willis WD, Neug-ebauer V. 2005. PKA-dependent enhanced NMDA receptor function in pain-related synaptic plasticity in amygdala neurons. *J Physiol (Lond)*, 564 (3): 907-921.

Bonaz B, Baciu M, Papillon E, Bost R, Gueddah N, Le Bas JF, Fournet J, Segebarth C. 2002. Central processing of rectal pain in patients with irritable bowel syndrome: an fMRI study. *Am J Gastroenterol*, 97: 654-661.

Bornhovd K, Quante M, Glauche V, Bromm B, Weiller C, Buchel C. 2002. Painful stimuli evoke different stimulus-response functions in the amygdala, prefrontal, insula and somatosensory cortex: a single-trial fMRI study. *Brain*, 125: 1326-1336.

Bourgeais L, Gauriau C, Bernard J-F. 2001. Projections from the nociceptive area of the central nucleus of the amygdala to the forebrain: a PHA-L study in the rat. *Eur J Neurosci*, 14: 229-255.

Burstein R, Potrebic S. 1993. Retrograde labeling of neurons in the spinal cord that project directly to the amygdala or the orbital cortex in the rat. *J Comp Neurol*, 335: 469-485.

Crown ED, King TE, Meagher MW, Grau JW. 2000. Shock-induced hyperalgesia: III. Role of the bed nucleus of the stria terminalis and amygdaloid nuclei. *Behav Neurosci*, 114: 561-573.

Da Costa Gomez TM, Behbehani MM. 1995. An electrophysiological characterization of the projection from the central nucleus of the amygdala to the periaqueductal gray of the rat: the role of opioid receptors. *Brain Res*, 689: 21-31.

Derbyshire SWG, Jones AKP, Gyulai F, Clark S, Townsend D, Firestone LL. 1997. Pain processing during three levels of noxious stimulation produces differential patterns of central activity. *Pain*, 73: 431-445.

Fox RJ, Sorenson CA. 1994. Bilateral lesions of the amygdala attenuate analgesia induced by diverse environmental challenges. *Brain Res*, 648: 215-221.

Gauriau C, Bernard J-F. 2004. A comparative reappraisal of projections from the superficial laminae of the dorsal horn in the rat: the forebrain. *J Comp Neurol*, 468: 24-56.

Gauriau C, Bernard J-F. 2002. Pain pathways and parabrachial circuits in the rat. *Exp Physiol*, 87: 251-258.

Gebhart GF. 2004. Descending modulation of pain. *Neuroscience & Biobehavioral Reviews*, 27: 729-737.

Greenwood-van Meerveld B, Gibson M, Gunder W, Shepard J, Foreman R, Myers D. 2001. Stereotaxic delivery of corticosterone to the amygdala modulates colonic sensitivity in rats. *Brain Res*, 893: 135-142.

Han JS, Bird GC, Li W, Neugebauer V. 2005. Computerized analysis of audible and ultrasonic vocalizations of rats as a standarized measure of pain-related behavior. *Neurosci Meth*, 141: 261-269.

Han JS, Bird GC, Neugebauer V. 2004. Enhanced group III mGluR-mediated inhibition of pain-related synaptic plasticity in the amygdala. *Neuropharmacology*, 46: 918-926.

Han JS, Neugebauer V. 2005. mGluR1 and mGluR5 antagonists in the amygdala inhibit different components of audible and ultrasonic vocalizations in a model of arthritic pain. *Pain*, 113: 211-222.

Helmstetter FJ. 1992. The amygdala is essential for the expression of conditional hypoalgesia. *Behav Neurosci*, 106: 518-528.

Helmstetter FJ, Bellgowan PS. 1993. Lesions of the amygdala block conditional hypoalgesia on the tail flick test. *Brain Res*, 612: 253-257.

Helmstetter FJ, Tershner SA, Poore LH, Bellgowan PSF. 1998. Antinociception following opioid stimulation of the basolateral amygdala is expressed through the periaqueductal gray and rostral ventromedial medulla. *Brain Res*, 779: 104-118.

Li W, Neugebauer V. 2004a. Differential roles of mGluR1 and mGluR5 in brief and prolonged nociceptive processing in central amygdala neurons. *J Neurophysiol*. 91: 13-24.

Li W, Neugebauer V. 2004b. Block of NMDA and non-NMDA receptor activation results in reduced background and evoked activity of central amygdala neurons in a model of arthritic pain. *Pain*, 110: 112-122.

Manning BH. 1998. A lateralized deficit in morphine antinociception after unilateral inactivation of the central amygdala. *J Neurosci*, 18: 9453-9470.

Manning BH, Martin WJ, Meng ID. 2003. The rodent amygdala contributes to the production of cannabinoid-induced antinociception. *Neuroscience*, 120: 1157-1170.

Manning BH, Mayer DJ. 1995a. The central nucleus of the amygdala contributes to the production of morphine antinociception in the formalin test. *Pain*, 63: 141-152.

Manning BH, Mayer DJ. 1995b. The central nucleus of the amygdala contributes to the production of morphine antinociception in the rat tail-flick test. *J Neurosci*, 15: 8199-8213.

McGaraughty S, Heinricher MM. 2002. Microinjection of morphine into various amygdaloid nuclei differentially affects nociceptive responsiveness and RVM neuronal activity. *Pain*, 96: 153-162.

McGaraughty S, Farr DA, Heinricher MM. 2004. Lesions of the periaqueductal gray disrupt input to the rostral ventromedial medulla following microinjections of morphine into the medial or basolateral nuclei of the amygdala. *Brain Research*, 1009: 223-227.

Mena NB, Mathur R, Nayar U. 1995. Amygdalar involvement in pain. *Indian J Physiol Pharmacol*, 39: 339-346.

Min SS, Han JS, Kim YI, Na HS, Yoon YW, Hong SK, Han HC. 2001. A novel method for convenient assessment of arthritic pain in voluntarily walking rats. *Neurosci Lett*, 308: 95-98.

Naliboff BD, Berman S, Chang L, Derbyshire SWG, Suyenobu B, Vogt BA, Mandelkern M, Mayer EA. 2003. Sex-related differences in IBS patients: central processing of visceral stimuli. *Gastroenterology*, 124: 1738-1747.

Neugebauer V, Li W. 2002. Processing of nociceptive mechanical and thermal information in central amygdala neurons with knee-joint input. *J Neurophysiol*, 87: 103-112.

Neugebauer V, Li W. 2003. Differential sensitization of amygdala neurons to afferent inputs in a model of arthritic pain. *J Neurophysiol*, 89: 716-727.

Neugebauer V, Li W, Bird GC, Bhave G, Gereau RW. 2003. Synaptic plasticity in the amygdala in a model of arthritic pain: differential roles of metabotropic glutamate receptors 1 and 5. *J Neurosci*, 23: 52-63.

Neugebauer V, Lucke T, Schaible H-G. 1993. Nmethyl-D-aspartate (NMDA) and non-NMDA receptor antagonists block the hyperexcitability of dorsal horn neurons during development of acute arthritis in rat's knee joint. *J Neurophysiol*, 70: 1365-1377.

Pare D, Quirk GJ, Ledoux JE. 2004. New vistas on amygdala networks in conditioned fear. *J Neurophysiol*, 92: 1-9.

Paulson PE, Casey KL, Morrow TJ. 2002. Long-term changes in behavior and regional cerebral blood flow associated with painful peripheral mononeuropathy in the rat. *Pain*, 95: 31-40.

Pavlovic ZW, Bodnar RJ. 1998. Opioid supraspinal analgesic synergy between the amygdala and periaqueductal gray in rats. *Brain Res*, 779: 158-169.

Petrovic P, Ingvar M, Stone-Elander S, Petersson KM, Hansson P. 1999. A PET activation study of dynamic mechanical allodynia in patients with mononeuropathy. *Pain*, 83: 447-457.

Qin C, Greenwood-van Meerveld B, Foreman RD. 2003a. Spinal neuronal responses to urinary bladder stimulation in rats with corticosterone or aldosterone onto the amygdala. *J Neurophysiol*, 90: 2180-2189.

Qin C, Greenwood-van Meerveld B, Foreman RD. 2003b. Visceromotor and spinal neuronal responses to colorectal distension in rats with aldosterone onto the amygdala. *J Neurophysiol*, 90: 2-11.

Qin C, Greenwood-van Meerveld B, Myers DA, Foreman RD. 2003c Corticosterone acts directly at the amygdala to alter spinal neuronal activity in response to colorectal distension. *J Neurophysiol*, 89: 1343-1352.

Rhudy JL, Meagher MW. 2003. Negative affect: effects on an evaluative measure of human pain. *Pain*, 104: 617-626.

Schaible H-G, Grubb B. 1993. Afferent and spinal mechanisms of joint pain. *Pain*, 55: 5-54.

Schneider F, Habel U, Holthusen H, Kessler C, Posse S, Muller-Gartner HW, Arndt JO. 2001. Subjective ratings of pain correlate with subcortical-limbic blood flow: an fMRI study. *Neuropsychobiology*, 43: 175-185.

Schoepp DD, Jane DE, Monn JA. 1999. Pharmacological agents acting at subtypes of metabotropic glutamate receptors. *Neuropharmacology*, 38: 1431-1476.

Shi C, Davis M. 1999. Pain pathways involved in fear conditioning measured with fear-potentiated startle: lesion studies. *J Neurosci*, 19: 420-430.

Stefanacci L, Amaral DG. 2000. Topographic organization of cortical inputs to the lateral nucleus of the macaque monkey amygdala: a retrograde tracing study. *J Comp Neurol*, 421: 52-79.

Tershner SA, Helmstetter FJ. 2000. Antinociceptioon produced by mu opioid receptor activation in the amygdala is partly dependent on activation of mu opioid and neurotensin receptors in the ventral periaqueductal gray. *Brain Res*, 865: 17-26.

Wang C-C, Willis WD, Westlund KN. 1999. Ascending projections from the area around the spinal cord central canal: a *phaseolus vulgaris* leucoagglutinin study in rats. *J Comp Neurol*, 415: 341-367.

Watkins LR, Wiertelak EP, McGorry M, Martinez J, Schwartz B, Sisk D, Maier SF. 1998. Neurocircuitry of conditioned inhibition of analgesia: effects of amygdala, dorsal raphe, ventral medullary, and spinal cord lesions on antianalgesia in the rat. *Behav Neurosci*, 112: 360-378.

Werka T. 1997. The effects of the medial and cortical amygdala lesions on post-stress analgesia in rats. *Behav Brain Res*, 86: 59-65.

Fear Learning

CHAPTER 21

Paul W. Frankland, Sheena A. Josselyn

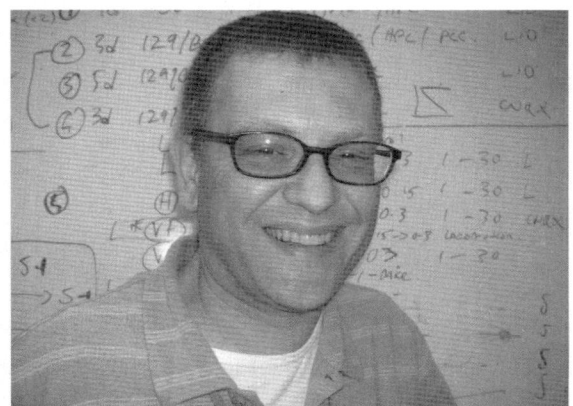

Dr. Frankland is Canadian Research Chair in Cognitive Neurobiology and Scientist in the Neuroscience and Mental Health program at The Hospital for Sick Children, Toronto, Canada. He is also an Assistant Professor in the Department of Physiology at the University of Toronto. After obtaining his PhD in Psychology/Neuroscience, he pursued postdoctoral training at Cold Spring Harbor Laboratory and UCLA.

MAJOR CONTRIBUTIONS

1. Frankland PW, Cestari V, Filipkowski RK, McDonald RJ, Silva AJ. 1998. The dorsal hippocampus is essential for context discrimination, but not for contextual conditioning. *Behavioral Neuroscience*, 112: 863-874.

2. Ohno M, Frankland PW, Chen AP, Costa RM, Silva AJ. 2001. Inducible pharmacogenetic approaches to the study of learning and memory. *Nature Neuroscience*, 4: 1238-1243.

3. Frankland PW, O'Brien C, Ohno M, Kirkwood A, Silva AJ. 2001. Alpha-CaMKII-dependent plasticity in the cortex is required for permanent memory. *Nature*, 411: 309-313.

4. Frankland PW, Bontempi B, Talton LE, Kaczmarek L, Silva, AJ. 2004. The involvement of the anterior cingulate cortex in remote contextual fear memory. *Science*, 304 (5671): 881-883.

5. Frankland PW, Bontempi B. 2005. The organization of recent and remote memory. *Nature Reviews Neuroscience*, 6: 119-130.

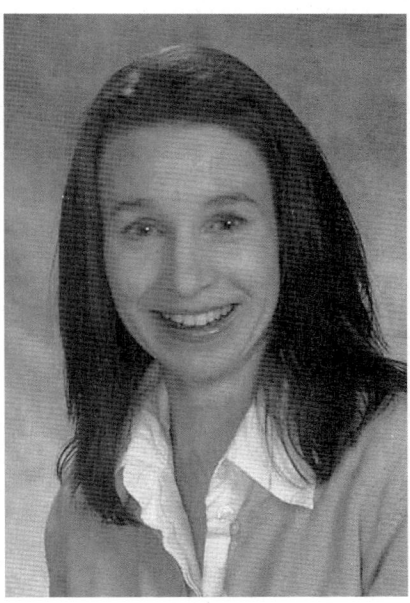

Dr. Josselyn is a Canadian Research Chair in Molecular and Cellular Cognition and an Assistant Professor at the Department of Physiology, University of Toronto, Canada. She is also a Scientist in the Neuroscience and Mental Health program at the Hospital for Sick Children, Toronto. After completing her PhD in Neuroscience/Psychology at the University of Toronto, she pursued post-doctoral training at Yale University School of Medicine.

MAJOR CONTRIBUTIONS

1. Kida S, Josselyn SA, de Ortiz SP, Kogan JH, Chevere I, Masushige S, Silva AJ. 2002.CREB required for the stability of new and reactivated fear memories. *Nat Neurosci*, 5(4): 348-355.

2. Josselyn SA, Shi C, Carlezon WA Jr, Neve RL, Nestler EJ, Davis M. 2001. Long-term memory is facilitated by cAMP response element-binding protein overexpression in the amygdala. *J Neurosci*, 21(7): 2404-2412.

3. Josselyn SA, Kida S, Silva AJ. 2004. Inducible repression of CREB function disrupts amygdala-dependent memory. *Neurobiol Learn Mem*, 82(2): 159-163. (Review).

4. Josselyn SA, Falls WA, Gewirtz JC, Pistell P, Davis M. 2005. The nucleus accumbens is not critically involved in mediating the effects of a safety signal on behavior. *Neuropsychopharmacology*, 30(1): 17-26.

5. Josselyn SA, De Cristofaro A, Vaccarino FJ. 1997. Evidence for CCK(A) receptor involvement in the acquisition of conditioned activity produced by cocaine in rats. *Brain Res*, 763(1): 93-102.

MAIN TOPICS

Pavlovian conditioning is used to study fear learning

The amygdala plays a critical role in fear learning

The LA integrates auditory and somatosensory information

Neurons in the LA respond to both auditory and somatosensory stimulation

Lesions of the LA block fear learning

Expression of conditioned fear is mediated by anatomically segregated outputs from the central nucleus of the amygdala

The cellular mechanisms of fear conditioning: Hebb's Postulate

Hebbian theory and LTP

Amygdala LTP in slice preparations

Amygdala LTP and behaving animals

Molecular machinery underlying fear learning

There are both short-term and long-term forms of fear memory

Protein synthesis is required for long-term fear memory

The transcription factor CREB is critical for long-term fear memory

SUMMARY

This chapter focuses on the biological basis of fear learning. Fear triggers an ensemble of defensive mechanisms that are critically important for survival. One way to study fear in the lab is to use Pavlovian fear conditioning. In this paradigm, an initially neutral stimulus, such as a tone, is paired with an aversive footshock. After even one pairing, subsequent presentation of the tone alone produces a range of conditioned fear responses (including freezing, fear-potentiated startle, changes in heart rate, etc.). Early on, it was recognized that the amygdala is critical for fear learning. Pioneering work in the 1980s and 1990s identified the pathways to the amygdala that transmit sensory information and pathways from the amygdala that mediate the expression of conditioned responses. Building on this anatomical foundation are experiments showing the links between fear conditioning and long-term potentiation (LTP) within the amygdala. These experiments showed that potentiation of conditioned thalamic inputs in the lateral amygdala may underlie conditioned fear. Finally, we review the molecular mechanisms whereby the amygdala encodes and stores the associations learned during conditioned fear. Long-term fear memory, like many other forms of long-term memory, critically relies on new protein synthesis. The transcription factor CREB has been shown to be particularly important in this process. These results provide important cellular and molecular insights into fear learning.

INTRODUCTION

In the previous chapter we learnt about the role of the amygdala in pain. This chapter now focuses on the role of the amygdala in learning about painful stimuli. This form of learning—commonly termed fear learning (or fear conditioning)—is adaptive since it allows us to anticipate situations associated with pain and injury. Fear learning has been studied extensively in the context of Pavlovian conditioning. Pioneering work by Joseph LeDoux, Mike Davis and others in the 1980s and 1990s led to a comprehensive description of the amygdala circuits underlying fear conditioning. While still being refined, these descriptions lay the essential foundation for more recent studies of the molecular and cellular mechanisms underlying fear learning in the amygdala. We shall first review the studies focusing on amygdala circuitry, before turning to more contemporary studies focusing on molecular and cellular mechanisms underlying fear learning.

PAVLOVIAN CONDITIONING IS USED TO STUDY FEAR LEARNING

Because survival may depend upon it, we learn about painful stimuli quickly and efficiently through a process known as Pavolvian fear conditioning. Viewed in this framework, stimuli present in the environment at the time of injury (or conditioned stimuli; CSs) are likely to become associated with the painful stimulus (or unconditioned stimulus; US). This is adaptive since when these cues are next encountered, an animal can take measures (or conditioned responses; CRs) that help to reduce the likelihood of injury.

This conceptual framework has been used to study fear learning in experimental animals, and especially in rodents. In a typical experiment, an otherwise innocuous stimulus, such as a tone or a light, is paired with an aversive stimulus, such as a mild footshock (Fig.21.1). After even a single pairing of the

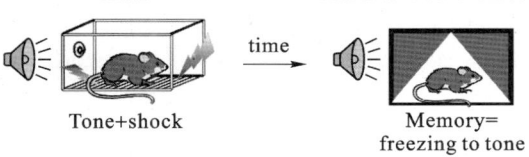

Train   Test in a novel chamber

time

Tone+shock   Memory= freezing to tone

Fig.21.1 Fear conditioning in rodents. During training in a typical fear conditioning experiment, an animal is presented with a tone followed by a brief shock. The animal is subsequently removed from the conditioning chamber and then, some time later, placed back in a different context and presented with the tone. When the tone comes on, the animal typically exhibits a wide range of conditioned fear responses (for example, changes in heart rate, breathing). The most commonly measured conditioned fear response in freezing. When an animal freezes it adopts a crouched motionless posture. It is the absence of movement during freezing that is thought to make this behavior adaptive since it reduces the likelihood of detection by a predator.

tone and shock, presentation of the tone alone is sufficient to evoke a constellation of behavioral, autonomic and endocrine changes typically associated with fear. In rodents, autonomic changes may include changes in heart rate and breathing. Endocrine

changes include the release of stress hormones (such as corticosterone). Behavioral changes include the potentiation of reflexes, as well as the development of freezing. Freezing is probably the most widely measured conditioned fear response. When an animal freezes, it adopts a crouched motionless posture. This behavior is thought to be adaptive since the absence of movement during freezing reduces the likelihood of being detected by a predator (Fig.21.2).

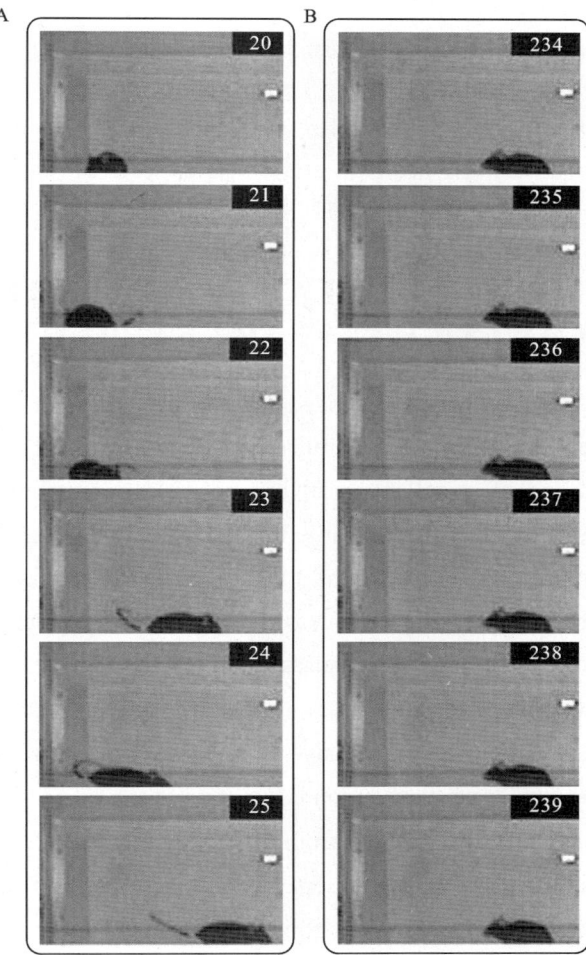

Fig.21.2 Freezing behavior in mice. Time lapse photography of a mouse (A) during training (prior to shock delivery), and, (B) during testing. During the testing phase a tone that was previously paired with shock is being played. The complete absence of movement is scored as freezing behavior.

Several features of fear conditioning have made it an attractive paradigm for studying the mechanisms of learned fear, and, more generally, the molecular and cellular bases of memory. First, the behavioral procedures are straightforward. For example, fear conditioning does not require several days of training. Rather, learning may take place in a single, discrete training session. Second, fear memories are long-lasting. For example, a single training experience produces a memory lasting at least 2 years in the rat. Not only does this make it possible to study how memories are initially formed but how memories are maintained over an animal's lifespan. Third, several conditioned fear responses may be measured using unbiased, automated procedures. For example, freezing behavior (the cessation of bodily movements) can be reliably measured using commercially available imaging software. Likewise, the downward force produced by an acoustic startle reflex can be easily measured and quantified.

THE AMYGDALA PLAYS A CRITICAL ROLE IN FEAR LEARNING

It has long been recognized that the amygdala plays a central role in emotion, and in particular, in fear. The amygdala is collection of around 12 different brain regions, located at the anterior end of the medial temporal lobe. Removal of the amygdala in monkeys produces striking changes in fear-related behaviors. For example, classic studies conducted by Kluver and Bucy more than 60 years ago showed that amygdala lesions "tamed" aggressive feral rhesus monkeys. In the last 30 years attention has shifted to the role of the amygdala in fear learning. Pioneering work by LeDoux, Davis and others has precisely defined the amygdala circuitry mediating fear learning. Using anatomical and electrophysiological approaches, these studies have established that information about CS and US converge at the level of the lateral amygdala (LA), and that the behavioral, autonomic and endocrine expression of conditioned fear is mediated via efferent connections from the central nucleus of the amygdala (Fig.21.3). These studies lay the essential foundation for more recent molecular and cellular studies of fear learning. Since the majority of studies

have used an auditory stimulus as the conditioned stimulus and we primarily focus on these below.

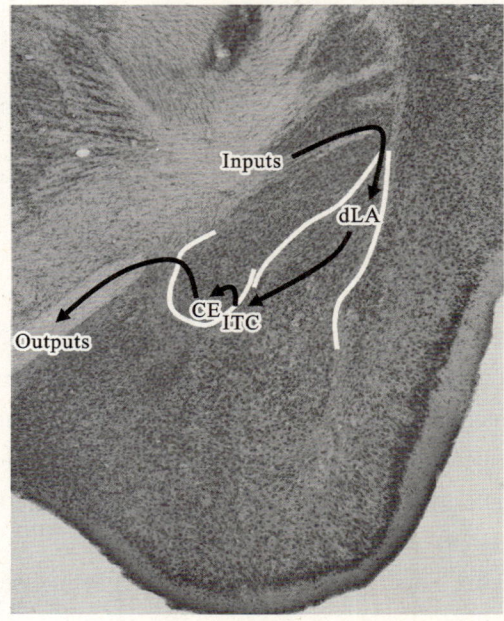

Fig.21.3 The anatomy of fear learning. Mouse brain section illustrating key brain regions involved in fear learning. Direct and indirect connections from thalamic nuclei convey information about the CS and US to the dorsal part of the lateral amygdala (dLA). The convergence of CS and US information here is thought to be critical for the formation of an associative CS-US memory. Outputs from the dLA project to the central nucleus of the amygdala (CE) via the intercalated nucleus (ITC). The expression of the behavioral, endocrine and autonomic components of conditioned fear is then thought to be mediated by anatomically segregated output pathways from the CE to various midbrain and brainstem nuclei.

THE LA INTEGRATES AUDITORY AND SOMATOSENSORY INFORMATION

Anatomical tracing studies established that the LA is ideally situated to integrate CS (tone) and US (shock) information. Information about auditory stimuli is relayed to the LA via both direct and indirect projections from the auditory thalamus. The direct projection originates in the medial geniculate nucleus (MGN) and posterior intralaminar nucleus (PIN). The indirect projection relays auditory information from auditory thalamus to the LA via the auditory association cortex (area TE3). Both these direct and indirect projections terminate predominantly in the dorsal part of the lateral amygdala (dLA). Pathways relaying US information have been less studied. However, footshock information is likely relayed via a projection that courses through the PIN and terminates in the dLA. An indirect projection relaying US information may also reach the dLA via the insular cortex.

NEURONS IN THE LA RESPOND TO BOTH AUDITORY AND SOMATOSENSORY STIMULATION

Consistent with the anatomical studies, neurons in the dLA respond to both auditory stimuli (CS) and painful stimuli (US, such as shocks). Such convergence establishes the dLA as an ideal site for plasticity underlying the formation of a CS-US associative memory. For example, Romanski and colleagues recorded from single units in the LA in anesthetized rats during the presentation of auditory (clicks) and somatosensory (footshock) stimuli. They found that neurons in the dLA showed short latency responses to both auditory and somatosensory stimulation, whereas neurons in the ventrolateral LA responded only to somatosensory stimulation.

LESIONS OF THE LA BLOCK FEAR LEARNING

Experimentally-induced brain damage is a useful tool for defining a role of a particular structure in learning. Such approaches have been extensively applied to amygdala. Early studies showed that relatively large pre-training lesions of the amygdala prevent fear learning. More restricted lesions of the LA have similar effects, consistent with the idea that the LA is important for the formation of fear memories. Consistent with these studies, temporarily disrupting activity in the LA during learning using either lidocaine, GABA receptor agonists or glutamate receptor antagonists

also prevents fear learning. To examine whether the amygdala plays a permanent role in the storage of these memories, the effects of post-training lesions of the amygdala have also been examined. Regardless of the delay between training and testing, lesioning the amygdala abolishes previously learned fear memories, suggesting that fear memories are permanently stored in the amygdala. However, an alternative interpretation is that amygdala lesions interfere with the ability of the animal to show a conditioned response—in most cases, freezing behavior. Several studies suggest that this is not the case. For example, amygdala-lesioned animals still exhibit freezing behavior when (i) exposed to predator odors or (ii) following extensive "over-training".

EXPRESSION OF CONDITIONED FEAR IS MEDIATED BY ANATOMICALLY SEGREGATED OUTPUTS FROM THE CENTRAL NUCLEUS OF THE AMYGDALA

Conditioned fear behavior is mediated via connections from the LA to the central nucleus of the amygdala (CE). The dLA does not appear to project directly to the CE. Rather, more recent studies have established that this connection is indirect, via neurons in the intercalated nucleus (ITC) of the amygdala. The expression of the behavioral, endocrine and autonomic components of conditioned fear is then thought to be mediated by anatomically segregated output pathways from the CE to various midbrain and brainstem nuclei (Fig.21.3). For example, changes in blood pressure are mediated via connections to the lateral hypothalamus, while the production of freezing behavior depends on projections to the central gray (Fig.21.4). Consistent with this organization, lesions of the lateral hypothalamus disrupt conditioned changes in arterial blood pressure without affecting freezing behavior. Conversely, lesions of the central gray block the expression of conditioned freezing without affecting changes in blood pressure.

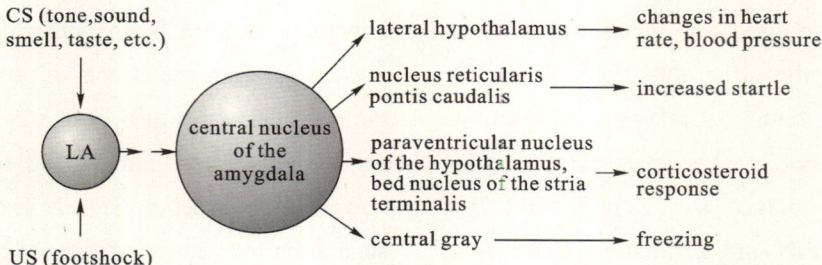

Fig.21.4   The organization of conditioned fear responses. Behavioral, endocrine and autonomic conditioned fear responses are mediated by anatomically-desegregated outputs from the central nucleus of the amygdala (CE) to various midbrain and brainstem nuclei.

THE CELLULAR MECHANISMS OF FEAR CONDITIONING: HEBB'S POSTULATE

Pioneering work in the 1980s and 1990s delineated the anatomical substrate of fear conditioning. More recent work has used this information to examine the cellular and molecular mechanisms of fear conditioning. The examination of the cellular basis of fear learning has largely been guided by the theory proposed by Donald Hebb that memory is stored in patterns of synaptic connections established during learning. Specifically, in 1949, Hebb postulated that "When an axon of cell A is near enough to excite B and repeatedly or persistently takes part in firing it, some growth process or metabolic change takes place in one or both cells such that A's efficiency, as one of the cells firing B, is increased" (p. 62). That is, modifications in the synaptic transmission efficacy are driven by correlations in the firing activity of pre- and post-synaptic neurons (or neurons that fire together wire together).

HEBBIAN THEORY AND LTP

More than 20 years after Hebb published his theory, experimental evidence was found for long-lasting increases in synaptic efficacy that were produced by correlated activity. In 1973, Bliss & Lomo showed that high-frequency stimulation of the hippocampal dentate gyrus produced an increase in excitatory post-synaptic potential (EPSP; a measure of synaptic strength). This persistent increase in synaptic strength is referred to as long-term potentiation (LTP). LTP exhibits several characteristics that make it an attractive cellular model of learning and memory; LTP is long-lasting, shows co-operativity, input specificity and reversibility. Importantly, LTP was also shown to embody the associative principle postulated by Hebb. Although numerous reviews have drawn attention to the difficulties strictly linking LTP to hippocampal-based memory, LTP remains the strongest cellular model of learning-related plasticity in the mammalian nervous system. LTP has been most extensively studied in the hippocampus, but, LTP may occur at many synapses in the brain.

Fear conditioning can be viewed as following the general rules of Hebbian-plasticity. Viewed in this way, CS inputs to the amygdala can be regarded as relatively weak and not initially capable of driving post-synaptic amygdala neurons. In contrast, inputs from the US are relatively strong and capable of activating the post-synaptic cell. During fear conditioning, both the CS pathway and US pathway are active, thereby potentiating the CS input so that it becomes capable of independently driving the post-synaptic cell. But does Hebbian-plasticity and LTP in the amygdala mediate fear learning?

AMYGDALA LTP IN SLICE PREPARATIONS

As discussed above, CS and US inputs converge onto individual neurons in the LA. Furthermore, neurons in the LA respond to both the CS (auditory tones or clicks) and US (shocks) commonly used in fear conditioning experiments. These findings provide a substrate for the Hebbian process described above. In slice preparations of the amygdala, tetanic stimulation of auditory inputs (from either the cortex or auditory thalamus) to the LA induces LTP. In addition, LTP in the LA may also be produced using a pairing protocol in which a weak, subthreshold pre-synaptic stimulation of amygdala inputs (mimicking the effects of the CS) is paired with a strong post-synaptic depolarization (mimicking the effects of the US). This pairing protocol may more closely mimic fear conditioning *in vivo*.

AMYGDALA LTP AND BEHAVING ANIMALS

In addition to the *in vitro* data showing that LTP is readily induced in the LA are data showing amygdala LTP *in vivo*. For instance, the field potentials in the LA evoked by auditory stimuli (CS) are potentiated following experimental induction of LTP (tetanically stimulating thalamic or cortical inputs to the LA) or fear conditioning training (pairing a tone with a shock in behaving animals). Importantly, this potentiation was not observed in rats trained with unpaired presentations of the CS and US. Furthermore, fear conditioning training occludes the induction of amygdala LTP in slices from the rats, suggesting that these processes share a common synaptic mechanism. Together, these findings provide compelling evidence that both fear conditioning-induced neuronal plasticity and LTP share common Hebbian mechanisms.

MOLECULAR MACHINERY UNDERLYING FEAR LEARNING

During the last few years, researchers have made substantial progress in mapping the molecular processes involved in fear memory formation. This research was facilitated by the development of technological breakthroughs in molecular genetics that allowed researchers to study the effects of disrupting the function of certain genes on fear memory. Molecular genetic manipulations that alter gene function include functional

deletions of genes (knockouts), gene replacements with mutant alleles (knockins), overexpression of wild-type or mutated genes (transgenics) and viral vectors. These techniques, along with traditional pharmacological approaches, have allowed researchers to begin to understand the molecular basis of fear memory.

THERE ARE BOTH SHORT-TERM AND LONG-TERM FORMS OF FEAR MEMORY

As with other memories, fear conditioning appears to have short-term and long-term phases of consolidation. Short-term memory for conditioned fear generally lasts for less than 2 hours while long-term memory generally lasts longer than 24 hours post-training. Using a combination of techniques, the initial cellular events that occur following the coincident activation of CS and US pathways have been shown to involve an influx of calcium though the N-methyl-D-aspartate (NMDA) receptor. NMDA receptors respond to concurrent activation of pre- and post-synaptic activation (via CS and US activation), and, in this way, are thought to function as Hebbian-like coincident detectors. In addition, voltage-sensitive calcium channels, neurotransmitters such as norepinephrine and growth factors such as brain-derived neurotrophic factor (BDNF) have been implicated in the formation of short-term memory for fear conditioning.

PROTEIN SYNTHESIS IS REQUIRED FOR LONG-TERM FEAR MEMORY

The transition from short-term to long-term fear memory requires mRNAs and protein synthesis. Intra-amygdala infusion of the protein synthesis inhibitor anisomycin, before or immediately after training, blocks long-term memory but not short-term memory for conditioned fear. For a protein to be produced, a stretch of DNA inside the neuron's nucleus must be transcribed into RNA and then translated into protein. The question then arises as to which transcription factors mediate the formation of long-term fear memories?

THE TRANSCRIPTION FACTOR CREB IS CRITICAL FOR LONG-TERM FEAR MEMORY

One attractive candidate for coupling neuronal activation that occurs during fear learning with the gene expression required for long-term memory is CREB [cAMP (cyclic adenosine 3',5'-monophosphate) responsive element binding protein]. CREB is a family of transcription factors that modulates the transcription of genes that contain cAMP responsive elements (CRE) in their promoter regions. A wealth of evidence from studies using invertebrate species shows that the CREB family of genes is important for long-term memory. Similar to many intracellular molecules, there is no specific pharmacological inhibitor of CREB. Therefore, the potential role of CREB in fear memory has been studied using a combination of molecular genetic techniques. Each of these methods alters the function of CREB in a distinct way and, when combined, the results from these studies provide substantive and convincing evidence for a key role of CREB in fear memory.

A complete knockout of CREB is homozygous lethal. However, CREB mutant mice have been generated by inserting a neomycin-resistance cassette (neo) into exon 2 of the CREB gene. The resulting mutant mice are viable, lack the two main isoforms of CREB α and δ) and have dramatically reduced levels of CREB protein in the brain. These CREB$^{\alpha\delta}$ mice show normal cued fear conditioning as assessed by both freezing and fear-potentiated startle when tested shortly (<1 h) after training, but severely disrupted fear conditioning memory tested 24 hours after training. This finding suggests a critical role for CREB in the consolidation of long-term fear memory.

One of the limitations of traditional knockout approaches such as this is that the target protein is deleted throughout development and in all tissues. Therefore, the interpretation of this memory deficit may not be clear-cut. To overcome these potential

limitations in temporal and spatial specificity of gene disruption, several approaches have been used. To address the limitation in temporal specificity, a transgenic line of mice was developed by Kida, Josselyn and colleagues that inducibly express a CREB repressor (α CREB^{S133A}) in forebrain regions. The inducibility of the system is produced by fusing the CREB repressor to a ligand-binding domain (LBD) of a human estrogen receptor with a G521R mutation (LBD^{G521R}). The activity of this mutated LBD is regulated not by estrogen but by the synthetic ligand, tamoxifen. In the absence of tamoxifen, the LBD^{G521R}-CREB^{S133A} fusion protein is bound to heat shock proteins and is inactive. However, administration of tamoxifen activates this inducible CREB repressor (CREB^{IR}) fusion protein, allowing it to compete with endogenous CREB and disrupt CRE-mediated transcription. In these transgenic mice, CREB function could be inducibly and reversibly "turned off" in forebrain neurons of an adult mouse. Using this technique it was possible to dissect the role of CREB in potentially dissociable fear memory processes. By administering tamoxifen to activate the repressor in CREB^{IR} transgenic mice at key time points in a cued fear conditioning protocol, the effects of acutely disrupting CREB function on (i) encoding or short-term memory, (ii) consolidation into long-term memory, (iii) storage or maintenance, (iv) retrieval were assessed. The results from this study show that CREB is crucial for the consolidation of long-term conditioned fear memories, but not for encoding, storage or retrieval of these memories (Fig.21.5). Although the temporal resolution offered by this approach is good (CREB activity is decreased within 6 hours of tamoxifen administration), the transgene is expressed in many forebrain regions, thus limiting the spatial resolution.

A second approach used viral vector-mediated gene transfer technology to manipulate CREB levels in specific brain regions and thus gain spatial specificity. Josselyn and colleagues used herpes simplex viral (HSV) vector-mediated gene transfer technology to specifically increase CREB expression in the

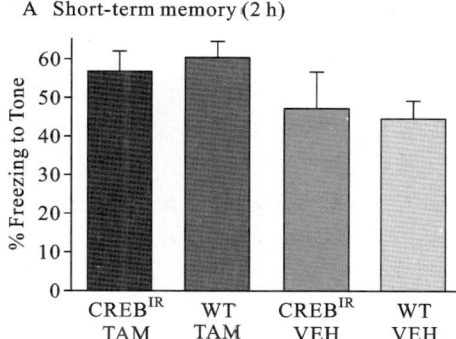

A Short-term memory (2 h)

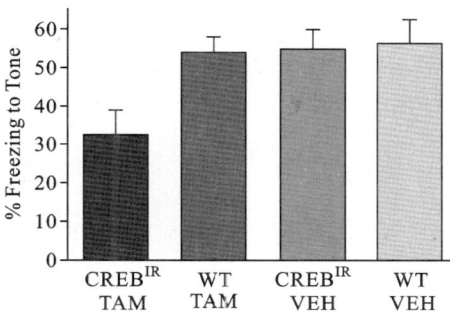

B Long-term memory (24 h)

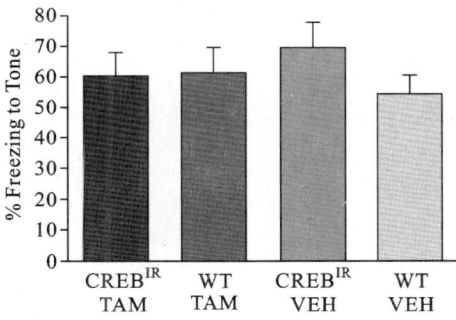

C Memory retrieval

Fig.21.5 The effects of acutely disrupting CREB function using CREB[IR] transgenic mice on different phases of tone fear memory. Activating the CREB repressor in CREB[IR] transgenic mice [by treating mice with tamoxifen (TAM)] does not disrupt short-term memory (A) or memory retrieval (B) but does disrupt long-term memory (C). Importantly the CREB[IR] transgenic mice show normal memory at all phases when treated with vehicle (VEH) and wild-type (WT) mice show no disruption of memory when treated with TAM.

amygdala of rats. This method exploits the natural ability of the HSV to insert DNA into neurons within a specific brain region. Rats were trained with a light CS, using a massed training protocol in which the four light-shocks pairings were presented with only a minimal inter-trial interval. This protocol typically produces robust short term memory but no or weak long-term memory in the fear-potentiated startle paradigm. However, rats that received HSV-CREB infusions targeted to the LA/basolateral amygdala (BLA) two days prior to training showed robust long-term memory, similar to levels produced by spaced training in which the same four the same four light-shock pairings were presented with a longer inter-trial interval (Fig.21.6). Thus, acutely increasing CREB levels and function in the amygdala enhances the acquisition of fear memory, a finding consistent with results in *Drosophila* and *Aplysia*. Together, these data provide convincing evidence that CREB and protein synthesis in the amygdala are important in the consolidation of long-term fear memory. Although CREB is perhaps the most studied transcription factor in terms of long term fear memory, it is likely that other transcription factors (such as zif268, Elk-1, etc.) play important roles.

Similar approaches have been employed to dissect the signal transduction cascades that link the initial events at the cell membrane to the transcriptional response necessary for long-term fear memory in the amygdala. These studies show that the influx of calcium in the post-synaptic neuron activates a number of intracellular factors including kinases and phosphatases [e.g., alpha calcium calmodulin kinase type II (CaM-KII), protein kinase A (PKA), MAP kinase (MAPK)]. This cascade of events is thought to culminate in the activation of nuclear transcription factors (Fig.21.7).

CONCLUSIONS

The circuitry underlying fear learning has been especially well-described, making it an ideal system in which to study the molecular and cellular basis of long-term memory formation. In particular, anatomical and electrophysiological studies have described the circuitry almost in its entirety—from sensory inputs to behavioral, endocrine and autonomic outputs. The most well studied form of fear learning is auditory fear conditioning. Auditory and somatosensory information converge at the level of the dLA, and conditioned responses are then mediated via anatomically-segregated outputs to midbrain and brain stem nuclei via the CE. The studies of amygdala plasticity underlying fear learning provide evidence that an LTP like mechanism mediates the formation of fear memories in the dLA. For example, these studies have shown that auditory-evoked field responses in the dLA are potentiated following fear conditioning training. Pharmacological approaches have established that the formation of long-term fear memories (those lasting >24 h) require *de novo* protein synthesis. Molecular-genetic studies have established that the synthesis of new proteins for long-term memory is mediated in part by the transcription factor CREB. For example, disrupting CREB function blocks the forma-

tion of fear memories, whereas over-expression of CREB facilitates the formation of fear memories. Together, these studies provide important details of how fear memories are formed in the amygdala. More broadly, because the formation and maintenance of fear memories is implicated in a number of psychiatric disorders (e.g., post-traumatic stress, panic and anxiety-related disorders), these studies are relevant in the clinic.

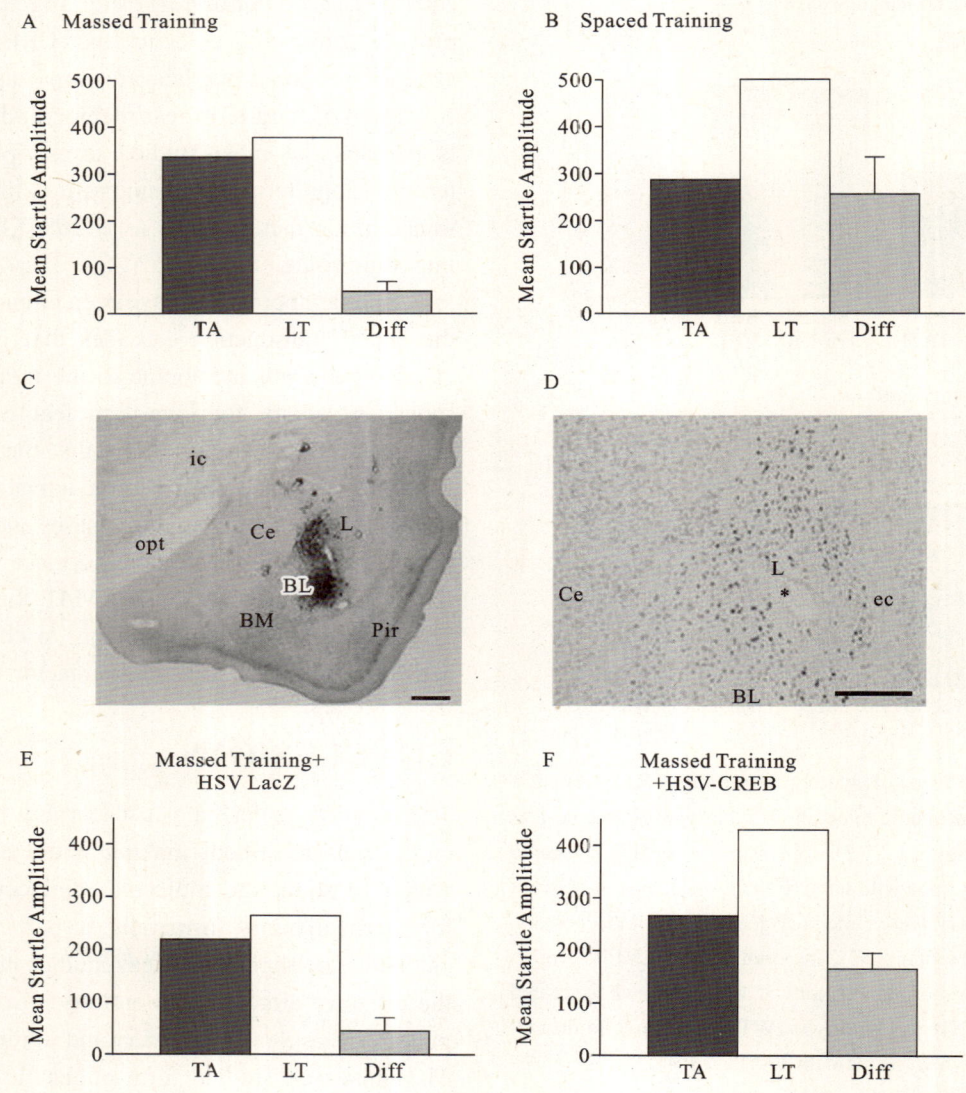

Fig.21.6 Effects of CREB over-expression in the amygdala on fear-potentiated startle. A. Massed training produces weak long term memory (LTM), as assessed by mean fear-potentiated startle difference scores (difference between mean startle amplitude on light-tone (LT) trials and tone-alone (TA) trials). B. The same number of trials presented in a spaced fashion produces robust LTM. C. Infusion of herpes simplex viral vectors encoding LacZ (HSV-LacZ) into the lateral(L) and basolateral (BL) amygdala produces high expression of β-galactosidase that is restricted to the basolateral amygdala. D. A high-power image of the amygdala following infusion of HSV-CREB showing over-expression of CREB that is restricted to the lateral nucleus of the amygdala. E. Infusion of HSV-LacZ into the amygdala does not change the weak LTM normally induced by massed training. F. Infusion of HSV-CREB into the amygdala prior to massed training enhances LTM.

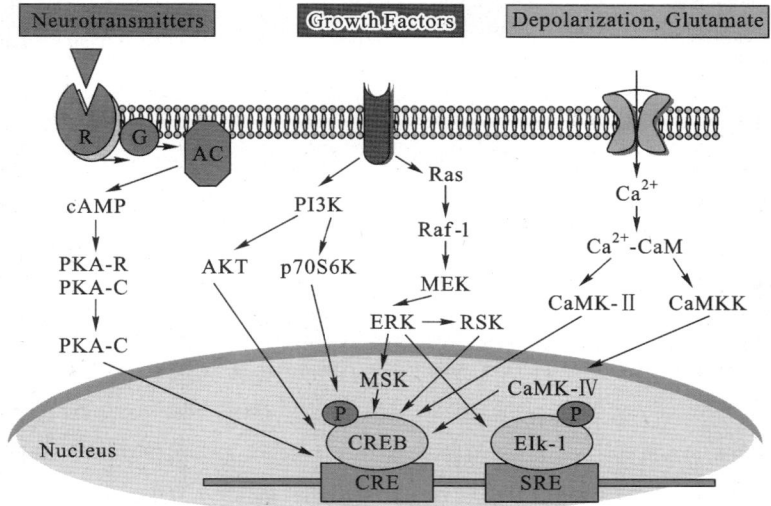

Fig.21.7   Molecular mechanisms of fear memory. This is a simplified schematic depicting the signal transduction cascades implicated in fear learning. In the first pathway, a neurotransmitter may bind to a receptor (R) that is linked to a G-protein (G), which leads to the increases in the second messenger cAMP via activation of adenylate cyclase (AC). Rising in levels of cAMP leads to the activation of protein kinase A (PKA) by dissociating the regulatory (R) from the catalytic (C) subunits. The C subunits of PKA passively translocate to the nucleus where they may phosphorylate CREB at Ser133. In the second pathway growth factors (such as NGF or BDNF) bind to and activate a Trk receptor. This, in turn, activates Ras and the downstream kinases Raf, MEK and ERK. Activated ERKs stimulate the activity of MSKs and RSKs which may then phosphorylate CREB at Ser133. In the third pathway, intracellular increases in Ca^{2+} binds to calmodulin (CaM) which activates CaM kinases (CaMKII, CaMKIV, CaMKK) which may also phosphorylate CREB at Ser133.

GENERAL READINGS

Bliss TV, Collingridge GL. 1993. A synaptic model of memory: long-term potentiation in the hippocampus. *Nature*, 361: 31-39.

Davis M. 1992. The role of the amygdala in fear and anxiety. *Annu Rev Neurosci*, 15: 353-375.

Dityatev AE, Bolshakov VY. 2005. Amygdala, long-term potentiation, and fear conditioning. *Neuroscientist*, 11: 75-88.

LeDoux JE. 2000. Emotion circuits in the brain. *Annu Rev Neurosci*, 23: 155-184.

Pare D, Quirk GJ, LeDoux JE. 2004. New vistas on amygdala networks in conditioned fear. *J Neurophysiol*, 92: 1-9.

Rodrigues SM, Schafe GE, LeDoux JE. 2004. Molecular mechanisms underlying emotional learning and memory in the lateral amygdala. *Neuron*, 44: 75-91.

DISCOVERY CITATIONS

Bauer EP, LeDoux JE, Nader K. 2001. Fear conditioning and LTP in the lateral amygdala are sensitive to the same stimulus contingencies. *Nat Neurosci*, 4: 687-688.

Bourtchuladze R, Frenguelli B, Blendy J, Cioffi D, Schutz G, Silva AJ. 1994. Deficient long-term memory in mice with a targeted mutation of the cAMP-responsive element-binding protein. *Cell*, 79: 59-68.

Huang YY, Kandel ER. 1998. Postsynaptic induction and PKA-dependent expression of LTP in the lateral amygdala. *Neuron*, 21: 169-178.

Josselyn SA, Shi C, Carlezon WA, Jr, Neve RL, Nestler EJ, Davis M. 2001. Long-term memory is facilitated by cAMP response element-binding protein overexpression in the amygdala. *J Neurosci*: 21: 2404-2412.

Kida S, Josselyn SA, de Ortiz SP, Kogan JH, Chevere I, Masushige S, Silva AJ. 2002. CREB required for the stability of new and reactivated fear memories. *Nat Neurosci*, 5: 348-355.

LeDoux JE, Cicchetti P, Xagoraris A, Romanski LM. 1990. The lateral amygdaloid nucleus: sensory interface of the amygdala in fear conditioning. *J Neurosci*, 10: 1062-1069.

LeDoux JE, Iwata J, Cicchetti P, Reis DJ. 1988. Different projections of the central amygdaloid nucleus mediate autonomic and behavioral correlates of conditioned fear. *J Neurosci*, 8: 2517-2529.

McKernan MG, Shinnick-Gallagher P. 1997. Fear conditioning induces a lasting potentiation of synaptic currents *in vitro*. *Nature*, 390: 607-611.

Miserendino MJ, Sananes CB, Melia KR, Davis M. 1990. Blocking of acquisition but not expression of conditioned fear-potentiated startle by NMDA antagonists in the amygdala. *Nature*, 345: 716-718.

Pitkanen A, Stefanacci L, Farb CR, Go GG, LeDoux JE, Amaral DG. 1995. Intrinsic connections of the rat amygdaloid complex: projections originating in the lateral nucleus. *J Comp Neurol*, 356: 288-310.

Quirk GJ, Repa C, LeDoux JE. 1995. Fear conditioning enhances short-latency auditory responses of lateral amygdala neurons: parallel recordings in the freely behaving rat. *Neuron*, 15: 1029-1039.

Rogan MT, Staubli UV, LeDoux JE. 1997. Fear conditioning induces associative long-term potentiation in the amygdala. *Nature*, 390: 604-607.

Romanski LM, Clugnet MC, Bordi F, LeDoux JE. 1993. Somatosensory and auditory convergence in the lateral nucleus of the amygdala. *Behav Neurosci*, 107: 444-450.

Schafe GE, Nader K, Blair HT, LeDoux JE. 2001. Memory consolidation of Pavlovian fear conditioning: a cellular and molecular perspective. *Trends Neurosci*, 24: 540-546.

Tsvetkov E, Carlezon WA, Benes FM, Kandel ER, Bolshakov VY. 2002. Fear conditioning occludes LTP-induced presynaptic enhancement of synaptic transmission in the cortical pathway to the lateral amygdala. *Neuron*, 34: 289-300.

Wilensky AE, Schafe GE, LeDoux JE. 1999. Functional inactivation of the amygdala before but not after auditory fear conditioning prevents memory formation. *J Neurosci*, 19: RC48.

Part VII   Spinal Plasticity, Reorganization and Chronic Pain

Silent Glutamatergic Synapses and Long-term Facilitation in Spinal Dorsal Horn Neurons

CHAPTER 22

Min Zhuo[*]

MAJOR CONTRIBUTIONS

1. Li P, Zhuo M. 1998. Silent glutamatergic synapses and nociception in mammalian spinal cord. *Nature*, 393: 695-698.
2. Li P, Calejesan AA, Zhuo M. 1998. ATP P_{2X} receptors and sensory transmission between primary afferent fibers and spinal dorsal horn neurons in rats. *J Neurophysiol*, 80:3356-3360.
3. Li P, Kerchner GA, Sala C, Wei F, Huettner JE, Sheng M, Zhuo M. 1999. AMPA receptor-PDZ protein interaction mediate synaptic plasticity in spinal cord. *Nature Neuroscience*, 2:972-977.
4. Zhuo M. 2000. Silent glutamatergic synapses and long-term facilitation in spinal dorsal horn neurons. *Progress in Brain Research*, 129:101-113. (Review)
5. Wang G-D, Zhuo M. 2002. Synergistic enhancement of glutamate-mediated responses by serotonin and forskolin in adult mouse spinal dorsal horn neurons. *J Neurophysiol*, 87:732-739.

MAIN TOPICS

Silent glutamatergic synapses

Old evidence from the spinal cord

New evidence from the Hippocampus

Spill-over theory: alternative hypothesis for silent synapses

Silent glutamatergic synapses in the spinal cord dorsal horn

Possible developmental regulation of silent glutamatergic synapses

Comparison between silent synaptic transmission and silent glutamatergic synapses

Recruitment of silent synapses by two different mechanisms

PKC activity and 5-HT induced facilitation

AMPA receptor and protein interactions

Coactivation of cAMP signaling pathways in facilitation of adult sensory synapses

Implications of silent synapses in pathological pain/ descending modulation

SUMMARY

Neurons in the superficial dorsal horn of the spinal cord are important for conveying sensory information from the periphery to the central nervous system. It has been proposed that some synapses between primary afferent fibers and spinal dorsal horn neurons are inefficient or silent. Ineffective sensory transmission could result from a small postsynaptic current that fails to depolarize the cell to threshold for an action potential or a cell with a normal postsynaptic current but an increased threshold for action potentials. One possible mechanism for ineffective synapses is the existent of silent glutamatergic synapses. In silent synapses, postsynaptic dorsal horn neurons lack functional AMPA/KA receptors and no synaptic responses are detected even when glutamate is released from

---

[*] The introduction of Dr. Zhuo, please refer to Chapter 8.

presynaptic sensory afferent fibers. Serotonin (5-HT), a major neurotransmitter of the raphe-spinal projecting pathway, transforms silent glutamatergic synapses into functional ones by recruiting postsynaptic functional AMPA receptors. AMPA receptor interaction with PDZ-containing proteins is critical for 5-HT induced recruitment. Silent synapses, as well as their recruitment mechanisms, are developmentally regulated and can still be found in adult synapses. However, they are "functional" and contribute to some sensory transmission. The recruitment of AMPA receptors into pure NMDA receptor containing sensory synapses requires coactivation of 5-HT and postsynaptic adenylyl cyclases. The recruitment of silent glutamatergic synapses provides a synaptic mechanism for spinal senstization in pathological pain, including possible pheonotype switching of dorsal horn neurons. These results suggest that the transformation of silent glutamatergic synapses may serve as a cellular mechanism for central plasticity in the spinal cord.

INTRODUCTION

Primary afferent fibers form synapses with dorsal horn sensory neurons in the spinal cord. Some of these dorsal horn neurons send ascending projecting fibers that synapse with neurons located at supraspinal sites, such as the thalamic nuclei. These ascending pathways are important for conveying sensory information from the periphery to the brain. Dorsal horn sensory synapses receive descending modulation from supraspinal structures. Most of these descending modulatory influences relay at brainstem nuclei including the rostroventral medulla (RVM). Activation of these modulatory systems could facilitate or inhibit spinal nociceptive transmission and behavioral reflexive responses to noxious stimulation, depending on the stimulation parameters used. Thus, the fine regulation of dorsal horn sensory synaptic transmission not only affects the amount of information entering the brain, but also influences behavioral responses to such stimuli.

Glutamate is a major neurotransmitter between primary afferent fibers and dorsal horn neurons. Postsynaptic sensory responses are mainly mediated by glutamate AMPA/kainate and NMDA receptors. Glutamatergic synapses are heterogeneous in the spinal dorsal horn. At least three different types of glutamatergic synapses are found. (i) Silent synapses: in some synapses, only functional NMDA receptors are found. Neither AMPA nor kainate receptors are present or functional in these synapses; (ii) AMPA receptor containing synapses: at sensory synapses that receive low-threshold inputs, only AMPA receptors are found and no functional kainate receptors exists; (iii) Kainate/AMPA receptor mixed synapses: at synapses receiving high-threshold inputs, both AMPA and kainate receptors are found. In both (ii) and (iii), NMDA receptors are always detected.

Besides being reliable and fast, glutamatergic synaptic transmission in the spinal cord is dynamic and plastic. Recent progress in molecular and cellular aspects of glutamate receptors show that postsynaptic glutamate receptors are put into the place through a family of proteins containing PDZ domains. Furthermore, these postsynaptic protein–protein interactions are very dynamic and may be involved in the clustering, removal or insertion of postsynaptic receptors, providing a novel and efficient way to regulate synaptic strength. This type of interaction could switch the phenotype of dorsal horn sensory synapses, i.e. changing silent synapses into functional synapses. In this chapter, I will first review the recent discovery of silent glutamatergic synapses in spinal dorsal horn neurons and explore possible physiological functions of these synapses in spinal nociception.

SILENT GLUTAMATERGIC SYNAPSES

Old Evidence from the Spinal Cord

The existence of ineffective, or silent, sensory synapses in the spinal cord dorsal horn was first proposed by Wall PD (1977). However, it was unclear whether ineffective sensory transmission might reflect the failure of a small postsynaptic current to depolarize a neuron to action potential threshold or rather an increased threshold in a neuron with normal synaptic responses. Further indirect evidence for silent synapses comes from intracellular recordings of synaptic responses to stimulation of a single group Ia afferents in cat spinal motor neurons. Examination of the size fluctuations of excitatory postsynaptic potentials (EPSPs), application of 4-AP or tetanization of the afferent, lead to the discovery that some previously "silent" synapses became active following stimulation. Although there are certain limitations of recording techniques, these studies provide strong evidence for the existence of silent synapses in the central nervous system (CNS). Considering the difficulty of the spinal cord preparations, however, only a few studies have followed up on these initial findings.

New Evidence from the Hippocampus

The well-defined anatomy and the hypothesized role of the hippocampus in learning and memory make hippocampal slice preparations a popular model for neuroscientists. The idea that the conversion of silent synapses to functional ones may contribute to LTP is gaining support due to direct experimental approaches using whole-cell patch-clamp recordings in young hippocampal neurons. In the CA1 region of the hippocampus, LTP induced by different protocols is NMDA receptor-dependent. Using voltage-shift in patch-clamped hippocampal neurons, it is possible to "inactivate" NMDA receptors by holding them at a negative membrane potential. At most excitatory synapses in the mammalian brain, AMPA and NMDA receptors are colocalized and respond to the release of glutamate. Investigators were able to detect pure NMDA receptor containing synapses in some cases, indicating the existence of silent glutamatergic synapses. Furthermore, after the application of different conditioning protocols, silent synapses become active or functional. These results support the hypothesis that the recruitment of silent synapses contribute to LTP.

Spill-over Theory: Alternative Hypothesis for Silent Synapses

An alternative hypothesis concerning silent synapses is that the spillover of glutamate helps to generate pure NMDA receptor mediated responses. In this case, glutamate is not limited to the synaptic cleft from which it is released but it also diffuses to adjacent synapses. Due to the different sensitivity of NMDA and AMPA receptors to glutamate, it becomes possible for glutamate to activate NMDA receptors but not AMPA receptors.

Silent Glutamatergic Synapses in the Spinal Cord Dorsal Horn

Using whole-cell patch-clamp recording techniques in brain slices, silent glutamatergic synapses are reported in various regions of the CNS including the hippocampus, neocortex, spinal cord dorsal horn and ventral horn motor neurons. In silent synapses, no effective AMPA/kainate receptors are available to detect the release of glutamate from presynaptic terminals. Consequently, these synapses do not conduct synaptic transmission at the resting membrane potential. The existence of such synapses between sensory fibers and dorsal horn neurons was shown in the lumbar spinal cord. We recorded from sensory neurons in the superficial dorsal horn of spinal cord slices using whole-cell patch-clamp recording techniques and tested for the possible existence of silent glutamatergic synapses (Fig.22.1). Fast monosynaptic, excitatory postsynaptic currents (EPSCs) were induced when cells were held at −70 mV in postnatal rats (P2-4). In order to detect silent synapses, the intensity of stimulation was decreased so that no fast EPSC was detected at −70 mV. The holding potential was then changed to +40 mV to detect NMDA receptor mediated EPSCs. In about 59% of the dorsal horn neurons tested, synaptic responses were found at +40 mV but not at −70 mV. Synaptic responses at +40 mV were abolished by the selective NMDA receptor antagonist AP-5 (50 μM). The sensitivity to AP-5 and the voltage-dependence of channel activation indicates that synaptic responses measured at +40 mV were NMDA receptor mediated. The intensity of stimulation used in these experiments was low and it is likely that only low-threshold afferent fibers were activated. Lastly, it is possible that silent synapses may exist in other neurons in the spinal cord, including spinal ventral horn neurons.

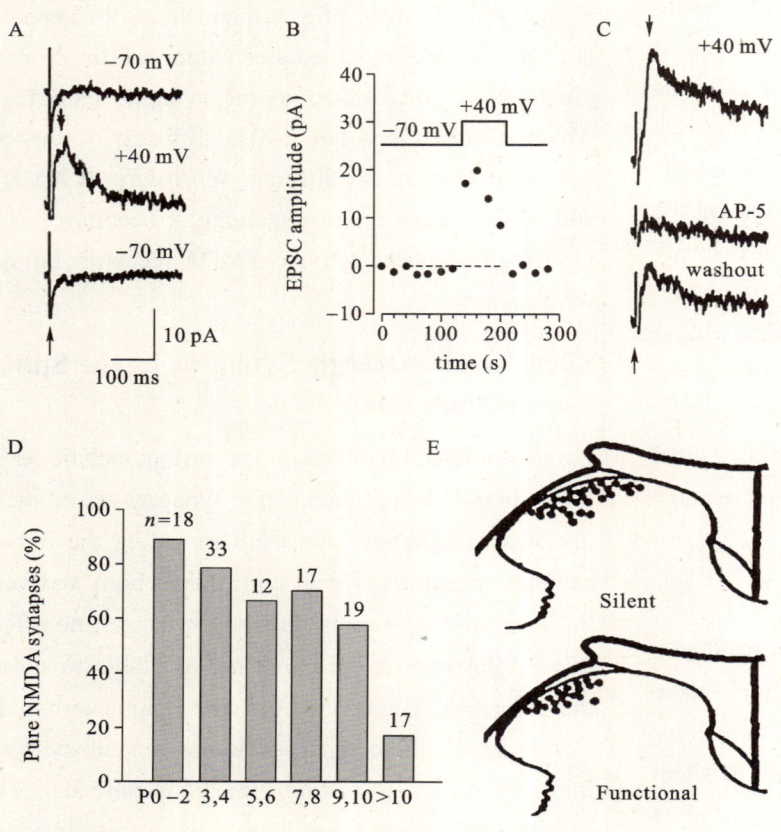

Fig.22.1 Silent glutamatergic synapses in the lumbar spinal cord. A. Examples of responses (the average of three continuous traces) at −70 or +40 mV holding potential. B. Time course of the experiment shown in A. C. Responses at +40 mV were reversibly inhibited by 50 μM AP-5. Upward arrows indicate the time of stimulation. Downward arrow indicates the peak currents measured. D. Developmentally related distribution of silent synapses in the spinal cord. The percentage of silent synapses is in the superficial dorsal horn of the lumbar spinal cord at P2-17. The numbers of cells tested are indicated above the bars. E. Distribution of labeled spinal neurons.

Possible Developmental Regulation of Silent Glutamatergic Synapses

It is also important to note that silent synapses may exist in spinal sensory neurons in adult animals. Although whole-cell patch-clamp recordings in slices and whole-animal preparations from adult rats have been reported, we found that space clamp is difficult in adult neurons. This is not surprising if we consider the complex neuritic structures formed within the spinal cord and brain by these neurons, which send ascending projections all the way to the thalamus and other supraspinal structures. For this reason, it may not be possible to identify silent synapses in sensory neurons using the same approaches. Better molecular biology techniques combined with modern electronic microscopy may serve as alternative tools to investigate this question in the near future.

Comparison Between Silent Synaptic Transmission and Silent Glutamatergic Synapses

It is important to point out that silent synapses should not be confused with potential "silent synaptic transmission". The term "silent synapses" refers to a condition where the postsynaptic cell is clamped at −70 mV and NMDA receptors are abundantly located. In an unclamped cell, these NMDA receptors may contribute to sensory synaptic transmission, for example, in the case of high intensity sensory fiber activity induced by tissue injury. These results consistently suggest that different types of glutamatergic synapses exist in spinal sensory connections between primary afferent fibers and dorsal horn neurons (Fig.22.1).

RECRUITMENT OF SILENT SYN-APSES BY TWO DIFFERENT MEC-HANISMS

Sensory transmission in the spinal cord receives descending modulation from supraspinal structures including the RVM. 5-HT-containing neurons in the RVM send descending projection fibers to targets in the spinal cord, like the superficial dorsal horn. Activation of these descending pathways can facilitate or inhibit spinal nociceptive transmission. Previous studies of this descending modulation focused on behavioral, pharmacological and electrophysiological recordings of spike firing from dorsal horn neurons. It is important to show that these modulatory effects are due to changes in spinal sensory synaptic transmission and not due to the modulation of pre-motor spinal interneurons or spinal local inhibitory synapses.

Consistent with the biphasic modulatory effect of 5-HT on spinal nociceptive transmission and behavioral reflexes, we found that 5-HT produced biphasic modulation of excitatory synaptic responses in spinal slices. 5-HT at high doses produced inhibition of AMPA receptor mediated EPSCs, while a low dose of 5-HT or a selective $5-HT_2$ receptor agonist induced facilitation of fast EPSCs in the lumbar spinal cord. 5-HT at low doses could facilitate fast EPSCs in the presence of a NMDA receptor antagonist AP-5 (50 μM), indicating that the facilitatory effect is NMDA receptor independent. Furthermore, the facilitatory effect induced by 5-HT at low doses persisted during washout of 5-HT. While activation of 5-HT receptors is important for the induction of facilitation, continuous activation of these receptors is not necessary for the expression of facilitation. Application of methysergide after the serotonergic receptor agonist DOI failed to reverse the facilitatory effect(Fig.22.2). One synaptic mechanism for the 5-HT produced facilitation is due to the recruitment of silent glutamatergic synapses. Application of 5-HT (5 μM) caused typical fast EPSCs to appear at synapses initially lacking AMPA/ kainate receptor-mediated responses (Fig.22. 3). 5-HT may affect spinal sensory transmission by acting on presynaptic or postsynaptic receptors. Post

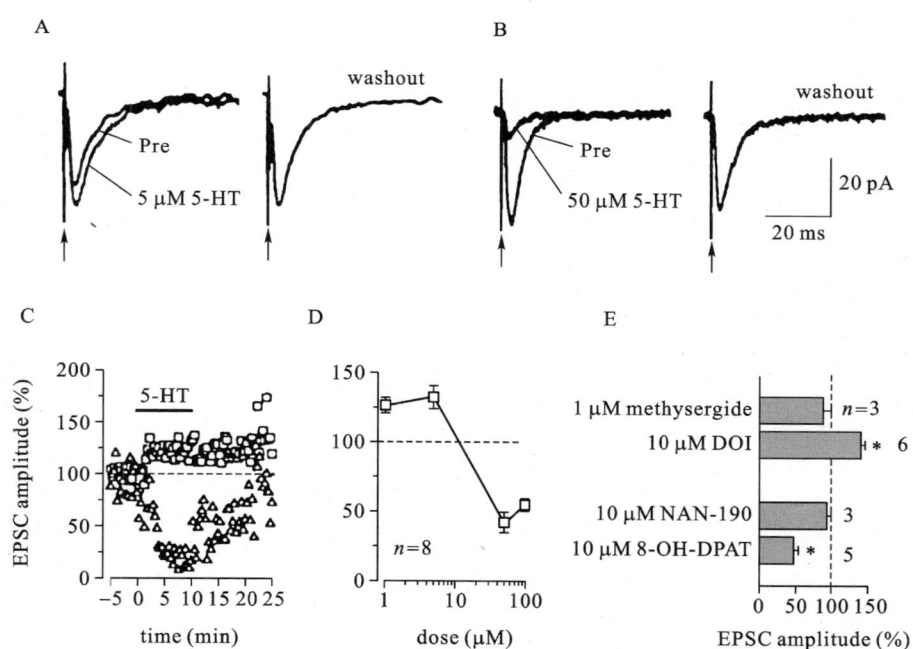

Fig.22.2 Biphasic modulation induced by 5-HT. A and B. Examples of 5-HT experiments at two doses. Upward arrows indicate the time of stimulation. C. The effect of 5-HT on amplitudes of EPSCs in experiments shown in A (squares) and B (triangles). D. Summary data of 5-HT at four different doses (*n*=8 for each dose). E. Different effects of $5-HT_{1A}$ (8-OH- DPAT) and $5-HT_2$ (DOI) receptor agonists. The effects were blocked by their receptor antagonists NAN-190 ($5-HT_{1A}$) and methysergide respectively. * $P<0.05$.

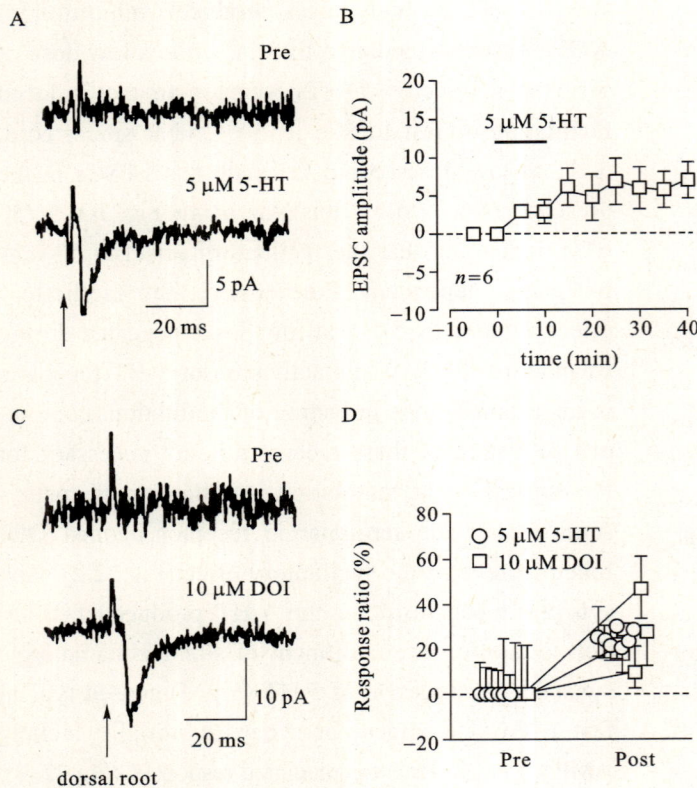

Fig.22.3 Transformation of silent synapses into functional synapses by 5-HT or DOI. A. The average of 15 continuous responses (collected at 0.05 Hz) before and 15 min after the end of 5-HT application. B. Summary data of 5-HT. C. Responses before and 15 min after DOI application using dorsal root nerve stimulation. D. Summary of response ratios before and after 5-HT or DOI application. Symbols for a given cell are connected; symbols and errors show response ratio (=the number of stimuli with responses/total number of stimuli×100) and the calculated 95% confidence intervals.

synaptic application of G protein inhibitors, introduced through the recording pipette, abolished the effect of 5-HT on synaptic transmission, suggesting that postsynaptic 5-HT receptors are critical for this effect. In support of this notion, postsynaptic Ca^{2+}-dependent processes were shown to be required for 5-HT-induced facilitation. In experiments with BAPTA (1,2-bis- (o-aminophenoxy) ethane-N,N,N', N'-tetracetic acid) in the pipette solution, the facilitatory effect of 5-HT was abolished, demonstrating the requirement for an increase in postsynaptic Ca^{2+}. Additional evidence arguing against a mechanism of 5-HT-induced synaptic facilitation involving modulation of presynaptic glutamate release comes from the observation that while 5-HT application clearly caused AMPA receptor mediated EPSCs, NMDA receptor mediated EPSCs were significantly decreased by 5-HT in the same neurons. This result suggests that postsynaptic enhancement of AMPA receptor mediated currents by 5-HT is selective.

PKC Activity and 5-HT Induced Facilitation

In central glutamatergic synapses, PKC plays an important role in long-lasting synaptic enhancement. Application of the PKC activator phorbol 12,

13-dibutyrate (PDBu) produced long-lasting enhancement of AMPA receptor mediated responses in hippocampal neurons, and inhibition of PKC prevented the induction of long-term potentiation induced by tetanic stimulation. In dorsal horn neurons of the spinal cord, the excitatory effect of PKC on spinal nociceptive transmission has been reported. Activation of PKC enhances sensory synaptic transmission in the dorsal horn, sensitizing the responses of ascending projection neurons to noxious peripheral stimuli. Mice lacking PKCγ show reduced pain behaviors following nerve injury. Because PKC acts downstream of 5-HT$_2$ receptors and these receptors are critical for the facilitatory effect of low-doses of 5-HT, we tested if postsynaptic PKC may mediate the facilitatory effect of 5-HT in spinal dorsal horn neurons. When the PKC peptide inhibitor PKCI (19-36) was present in the patch pipette, application of 5-HT failed to cause any synaptic facilitation. Consistently, bath application of the PKC activator PDBu caused enhancement of postsynaptic responses in spinal dorsal horn neurons. The effect of PDBu persisted during the washout of the drug and was independent of NMDA receptors. In a similar manner as 5-HT, the facilitatory effect induced by PKC involved the recruitment of silent glutamatergic synapses.

AMPA Receptor and Protein Interactions

One possible mechanism for the recruitment of silent synapses is through the interaction of glutamate AMPA receptors and proteins containing postsynaptic density-95/Discs large/zona occludens-1 (PDZ) domains. GluR2/3 are widely expressed in sensory neurons in the superficial dorsal horn of the spinal cord. Unlike GluR1 which is mainly expressed in spinal interneurons, GluR2/3 are mainly expressed in non-local inhibitory neurons. Glutamate receptor-interacting protein (GRIP), a protein with 7 PDZ domains that binds specifically to the C-terminus of GluR2/3, is also expressed in spinal dorsal horn neurons. In many dorsal horn neurons, GluR2/3 and GRIP coexist. Long-term overexpression of the C-terminus of GluR2 in hippocampal neurons reduces the number of synaptic AMPA receptor clusters, suggesting that the interaction between GluR2/3 and PDZ proteins is involved in the postsynaptic targeting of AMPA recep-

tors. To examine the functional significance of GluR 2/3-PDZ interactions in sensory synaptic transmission, we made a synthetic peptide corresponding to the last 10 amino acids of GluR2 ("GluR2-SVKI": NVYGI-ESVKI) which disrupts binding of GluR2 to GRIP. As expected, GluR2-SVKI peptide blocked the facilitatory effect of 5-HT. The effect of GluR2-SVKI on synaptic facilitation is rather selective, as the baseline level of evoked EPSCs and currents evoked by glutamate application did not change over time in these neurons. Experiments with different control peptides consistently indicate that the interaction between the c-terminus of GluR2/3 and GRIP/ABP (or called GRIP1 and GRIP2) is important for 5-HT induced facilitation. Furthermore, synaptic facilitation induced by PDBu is also blocked by GluR2-SVKI, suggesting that synaptic facilitation mediated by PKC activation is similar to that produced by 5-HT in its dependence on GluR2/3 C-terminal interactions. A working model for the 5-HT-induced recruitment of silent synapses is shown in BOX22.1.

BOX22.1   A model pathways explains how activation of 5-HT receptors may recruit silent synapses in spinal dorsal horn neurons.

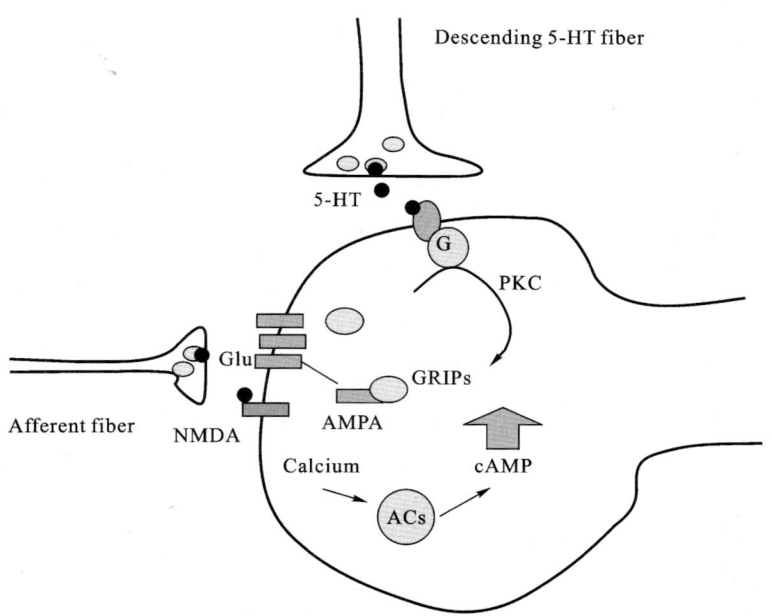

5-HT released from descending projection fibers activates postsynaptic PKC through G protein receptors. PKC activa-tion and subsequent AMPA receptor and GRIP interactions cause the recruitment of AMPA receptors to the synapse.

Coactivation of cAMP Signaling Pathways in Facilitation of Adult Sensory Synapses

cAMP signaling pathways are implicated in the function of spinal dorsal horn neurons. Activation of several receptors for sensory transmitters such as glutamate and calcitonin gene related peptide (CGRP) are reported to raise cAMP levels. In a recent study, application of forskolin did not significantly affect synaptic responses induced by dorsal root stimulation in slices of adult mice. However, co-application of 5-HT and forskolin produced long-lasting facilitation of synaptic responses(Fig.22.4). Possible contributors to the increase in cAMP levels are calcium-sensitive adenylyl cyclases (AC). We found that the facilitatory effect induced by 5-HT and forskolin was completely blocked in mice lacking AC1 or AC8, demonstrating the importance of calcium-sensitive ACs. Our results show that in adult sensory synapses, cAMP signaling pathways determine whether activation of 5-HT receptors causes facilitatory or inhibitory effects on synaptic responses. This finding provides a possible explanation for the regulation of two different signaling pathways under physiological or pathological conditions. Postsynaptic increases in cAMP levels by sensory transmitters may favor 5-HT-induced facilitation. The interaction between cAMP and 5-HT may provide an associative heterosynaptic form of central plasticity in the spinal dorsal horn to allow sensory inputs from the periphery to act synergistically with central modulatory influences descending from the brainstem RVM.

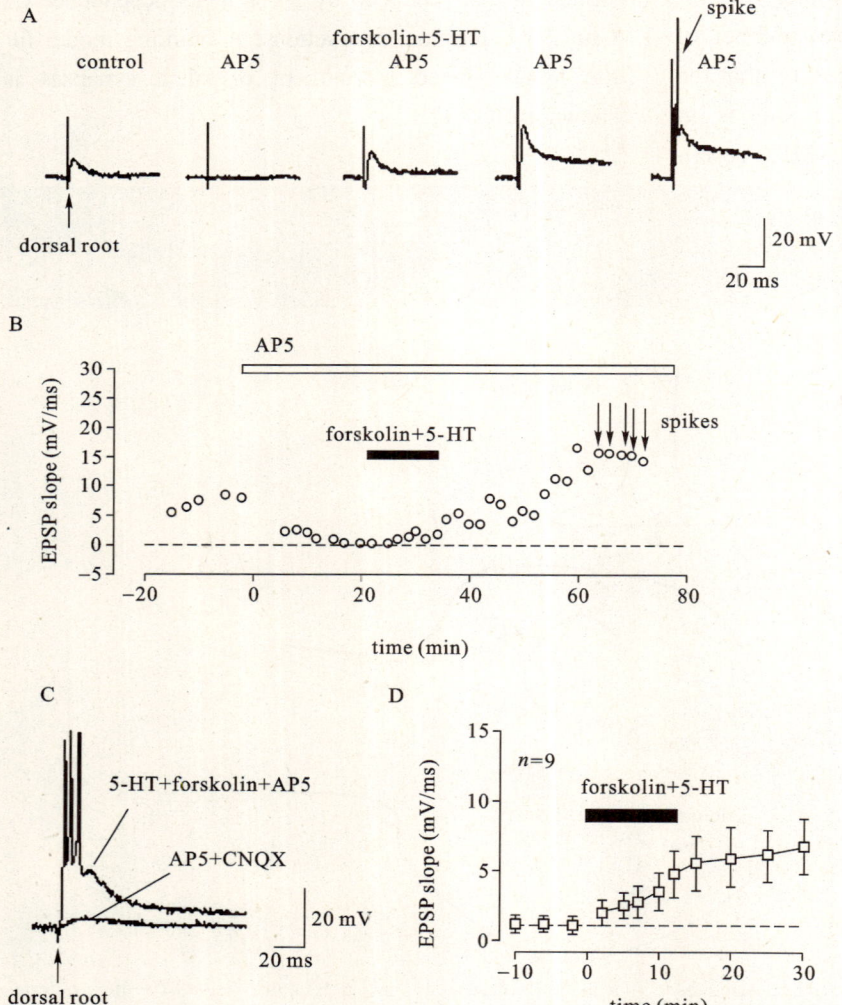

Fig.22.4 Synergistic recruitment of AMPA/kainate receptor mediated responses at pure NMDA synapses. A. Examples of EPSPs showing synaptic responses before, during, and after co-application of 5 μM 5-HT and 10 μM forskolin in the presence of 100 μM AP5. B. The effect of 5-HT and forskolin on the EPSP slopes in the experiment shown in A. Spike responses to stimulation of the dorsal root nerves at the subthreshold intensity were observed during the washout (indicated by arrows). C. In a separate experiment, 20 μM CNQX completely blocked both EPSPs and action potentials induced by 5 μM 5-HT and 10 μM forskolin in the presence of AP5. D. Summary data of 5 μM 5-HT and 10 μM forskolin. Data contain two sets of experiments: pure NMDA synapses ($n=3$) and mixed AMPA/kainate and NMDA synapses ($n=6$). In both cases, significant enhancement was observed and data were pooled together.

IMPLICATIONS FOR SILENT SYNAPSES IN PATHOLOGICAL PAIN/DESCENDING MODULATION

One potential function of silent synapses is to contribute to the formation of a descending modulatory network within the spinal cord. Most 5-HT-containing nerve fibers in the spinal cord originate from the RVM. 5-HT-induced recruitment of silent synapses could strengthen spinal sensory synapses receiving innervation from descending 5-HT projecting fibers. Through an activity-dependent mechanism, the effect of 5-HT could make those receiving innervation more likely to compete and survive in adult animals.

Silent synapses may also be involved in pathological conditions like persistent pain. As suggested by Wall (1977), the recruitment of silent or ineffective synapses could significantly enhance spinal sensory

BOX22.2   Models showing a hypothetical mechanism of silent synapse activation in two types of nociceptive sensory neurons and a possible role for this activation in hyperalgesia and allodynia.

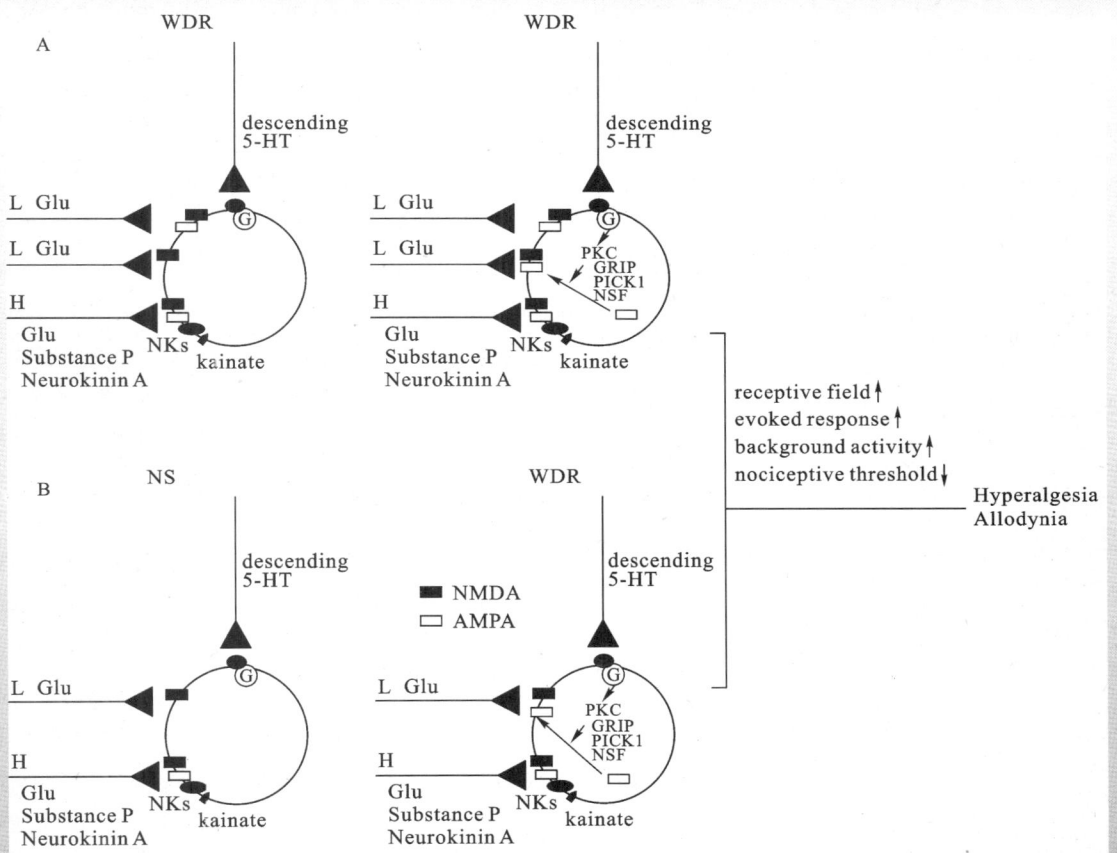

A. In a wide-dynamic range (WDR) cell, some synapses receiving low-threshold input (indicated by L) are silent (indicated by a dotted line). Release of 5-HT from descending projection fibers converts silent synapses into functional ones.

B. In a nociceptive specific (NS) cell, synapses receiving low-threshold input are all silent. Activation of these synapses renders the cell responsive to low-threshold stimulation, effectively converting it into a WDR cell. The conversion of silent synapses to functional synapses in either WDR or NS cells alters the electrophysiological properties of these neurons, thereby potentially increasing their receptive fields, enhancing their responses to sensory (noxious and non-noxious) stimuli, increasing background firing frequencies, and decreasing their nociceptive threshold. These changes, each of which is indeed observed in recordings from dorsal horn neurons in whole animals experiencing chronic pain, could contribute to both hyperalgesia and allodynia.

transmission, including nociceptive transmission. AMPA receptors are expressed in dorsal horn neurons at synapses receiving high-and low-threshold inputs. Activation of silent synapses with low-threshold afferents might cause dorsal horn neurons to exhibit an increased firing rate in response to non-noxious stimuli. Increases in postsynaptic AMPA receptor density and activation of silent synapses could contribute to plastic changes in the electrophysiological properties of dorsal horn sensory neurons, including ascending spinothalamic tract projecting neurons. These include increased receptive fields, enhanced responses to noxious and non-noxious stimuli, decreased firing thresholds, and increased background activity.

Two pieces of evidence indirectly support the notion that alterations of descending serotonergic influences and spinal glutamate AMPA receptors may contribute to persistent pain. First, descending serotonergic systems from the RVM to the spinal cord have been implicated in different types of hyperalgesia after tissue injury. Formalin-induced inflammation causes increased activity in 5-HT containing neurons in the RVM for up to two hours. Second, changes have been reported in the expression of AMPA receptors on spinal dorsal horn neurons after tissue injury. Therefore, activation of silent synapses could serve as an important cellular mechanism underlying two features of chronic pain: hyperalgesia, where the intensity of responses to noxious stimuli is increased over baseline; and allodynia, where the nociceptive threshold is decreased and a normally non-noxious stimulus, such a gentle touch, can induce pain.

CONCLUSIONS AND FUTURE PERSPECTIVES

In the dorsal horn of the lumber spinal cord, glutamate serves as a fast, excitatory neurotransmitter between primary afferent fibers and dorsal horn neurons. Activation of primary afferent fibers could activate different populations of glutamate receptors in dorsal horn neurons, depending on the intensity of stimula-

tion. At low intensities of stimulation which are likely to activate non-nociceptive fibers, synaptic responses are mainly mediated through AMPA receptors; while at high intensities of stimulation which activate nociceptive A_δ and C fibers, synaptic responses are mediated by both AMPA and kainate receptors. At some synapses receiving low-threshold afferent inputs, no effective postsynaptic AMPA receptor is available to respond to glutamate released from the central terminals of primary afferent fibers. These silent synapses are plastic and can be recruited by 5-HT, a neurotransmitter from descending projection fibers. 5-HT acts through postsynaptic PKC and requires an interaction between PDZ proteins and the C-terminus of GluR2/3 to effect synaptic facilitation. One possible step, which has not been directly tested, is that 5-HT could cause a GRIP-mediated insertion of GluR2/3 into the postsynaptic membrane. The effect of 5-HT is probably not due to the regulation of glutamate release from presynaptic terminals. The facilitatory effect of 5-HT is selective for AMPA receptors, as both postsynaptic NMDA receptors and kainate receptors are not significantly affected in the same cells. One obvious task for future studies is to elucidate the processes regulating GluR2/3 C-terminal interactions, the trafficking and membrane insertion of AMPA receptors, and PKC-mediated intracellular signaling pathways. Secondly, it is equally important to identify possible ways to silence already activated synapses. Understanding these signaling pathways will serve both to prevent sensory sensitization before it is induced, i.e., pre-emptive analgesia, as well as to decrease sensitization after its establishment. Progress in these areas will provide opportunities to design better drugs to control chronic pain in patients.

GENERAL CITATIONS

Bliss TVP and Collingridge GL. 1993. A synaptic model of memory: long-term potentiation in the hippocampus. *Nature*, 361: 31-39.

Fields HL, Heinricher MM and Mason P. 1991 Neurotransmitters in nociceptive modulatory circuits. *Annu Rev Neurosci*, 14: 219-245.

Garner CC, Nash J and Huganir RL. 2000. PDZ domains in synapse assembly and signaling. *Trends Cell Biol*, 10: 274-280.

Hollmann M and Heinemann S. 1994. Cloned glutamate receptors. *Annu Rev Neurosci*, 17: 31-108.

Lisman J. 1989. A mechanism for the Hebb and the anti-Hebb processes underlying learning and memory. *Proc Natl Acad Sci USA*, 86: 9574-9578.

Zhuo M. 2000. Silent glutamatergic synapses and long-term facilitation in spinal dorsal horn neurons. *Prog Brain Res*, 129:101-113.

Zhuo M. 2002. Glutamate receptors and persistent pain: targeting forebrain NR2B subunits. *Drug Discov Today*, 7:259-267.

Zhuo M. 2004. Central plasticity in pathological pain. *The Novaris Foundation Symposium, Pathological pain: from molecular to clinical aspects*. Chichester: Wiley. 132-148.

DISCOVERY CITATIONS

Baba H, Doubell TP, Moore KA and Woolf CJ. 2000. Silent NMDA receptor-mediated synapses are developmentally regulated in the dorsal horn the rat spinal cord. *J Neurophysiol*, 83: 955-962.

Bardoni R, Magherini PC and MacDermott AB. 1998. NMDA EPSCs at glutamatergic synapses in the spinal cord dorsal horn of the postnatal rat. *J Neurosci*, 18: 6558-6567.

Bardoni R, Magherini PC and MacDermott AB. 2000. Activation of NMDA receptors drives action potentials in superficial dorsal horn from neonatal rats. *NeuroReport*, 11:1721-1727.

Bowker RM and Abbott LC. 1990. Quantitative re-evaluation of descending serotonergic and non-serotonergic projections from the medulla of the rodent: evidence for extensive co-existence of serotonin and peptides in the same spinally projecting neurons, but not from the nucleus raphe magnus. *Brain Res*, 512:15-25.

Cerne R, Jinag M and Randic M. 1992. Cyclic adenosine 3',5'-monophosphate potentiates excitatory amino acid synaptic responses of rat spinal dorsal horn neurons. *Brain Res*, 596:111-123.

Chavez-Noriega LE and Stevens CF. 1992. Modulation of synaptic efficacy in field CA1 of the rat hippocampus by forskolin. *Brain Res*, 574:85-92.

Durand GM, Kovalchuk Y and Konnerth A. 1996. Long-term potentiation and functional synapse induction in developing hippocampus. *Nature*, 381: 71-75.

Gil Z and Amitai Y. 1996. Adult thalamocortical transmission involves both NMDA and non- NMDA receptors. *J Neurophysiol*, 76:2547- 2554.

Gomperts SN, Rao A, Craig AM, Malenka RC and Nicoll RA.1998. Postsynaptically silent synapses in signle neuron cultures. *Neuron*, 21:1443-1451.

Gu JG, Albuquerque C, Lee CJ and MacDermott AB. 1996. Synaptic strengthing through activation of Ca^{2+}-permeable AMPA receptors. *Nature*, 381: 793-796.

Haber LH, Martin RF, Chung JM and Willis WD. 1990. Inhibition and excitation of primate spinothalamic tract neurons by stimulation in region of nucleus reticularis gigantocellularis. *J Neurophysiol*, 43:1578-1593.

Hayashi Y, Shi SH, Esteban JA, Piccini A, Poncer JC and Malinow R. 2000. Driving AMPA receptors into synapses by LTP and CaMKII: requirement for GluR1 and PDZ domain interaction. *Science*, 287:2262- 2267.

Hori Y, Endo K and Takahashi T. 1996. Long-lasting synaptic facilitation induced by serotonin in superficial dorsal horn neurones of the rat spinal cord. *J Physiol (Lond)*, 492: 867-876.

Isaac JTR, Crair MC, Nicoll RA and Malenka RC. 1997. Silent synapses during development of thalamocortical inputs. *Neuron*, 18: 269-280.

Isaac JTR, Nicoll RA and Malenka RC. 1995. Evidence for silent synapses: implications for the expression of LTP. *Neuron*, 15: 427-434.

Lee HK, Barbarosie M, Kameyama K, Bear MF and Huganir RL. 2000. Regulation of distinct AMPA receptor phosphrylation sites during bi-directional synaptic plasticity. *Nature*, 405:955-959.

Li P and Zhuo M. 1998. Silent glutamatergic synapses and nociception in mammalian spinal cord. *Nature*, 393: 695-698.

Li P and Zhuo M. 2001. Cholinergic, noradrenergic, and serotonergic inhibition of fast synaptic transmission in spinal lumbar dorsal horn of rat. *Brain Res Bull*, 54:639-647.

Li P, Kerchner GA, Sala C, Wei F, Huettner JE, Sheng M and Zhuo M. 1999. AMPA receptor-PDZ interactions in facilitation of spinal sensory synapses. *Nature Neurosci*, 2:972-977.

Liao D, Hessler NA and Malinow R. 1995. Activation of postsynaptically silent synapses during pairing-induced LTP in CA1 region of hippocampal slice. *Nature*, 375: 400-404.

Liao D, Zhang X, O'Brien R, Ehlers M and Hugnir RL. 1999. Regulation of morphological postsynaptic silent synapses in developing hippocampal neurons. *Nature Neurosci*, 2:37-43.

Light AR, Trevino DL and Perl ER. 1979. Morphological features of functionally defined neurons in the marginal zone and substantia gelatinosa of the spinal dorsal horn. *J Comp Neurol*, 186:151-171.

Light AR, Casale EJ and Menetrey DM. 1986. The effects of focal stimulation in nucleus raphe magnus and periaqueductal gray on intracellularly recorded neurons in spinal laminae I and II. *J Neurophysiol*, 56:555-571.

Lopez-Garcia JA and King AE. 1996. Pre-and post-synaptic actions of 5-hydroxytryptamine in the rat lumbar dorsal horn *in vitro*: implications for somatosensory transmission. *Eur J Neurosci*, 8: 2188-2197.

Malenka RC and Nicoll RA. 1997. Silent synapses speak up. *Neuron*, 19:473-476.

Malenka RC and Nicoll RA. 2000. Long-term potentiation—a decade of progress? *Science*, 285: 1870- 1874.

Malinow R, Mainen ZF and Hayashi Y. 2000. LTP mechanisms: from silence to four-lane traffic. *Curr Opin Neurobiol*, 10:352-357.

McCreery DB, Bloedel JR and Hames EG. 1979. Effects of stimulating in raphe nuclei and in reticular formation on response of spinothalamic neurons to mechanical stimuli. *J Neurophysiol*, 42:166-182.

Petralia RS, Estban JA, Wang YX, Partridge JG, Zhao HM, Wenthold RJ and Malinow R. 1999. Selective acquisition of AMPA receptors over postnatal development suggests a molecular basis for silent synapses. *Nature Neurosci*, 2: 31-36.

Rumpel S, Hatt H and Gottmann K. 1998. Silent synapses in the developing rat visual cortex: evidence for postsynaptic expression of synaptic plasticity. *J Neurosci*, 18:

8863-8874.

Sah P, Hestrin S and Nicoll RA. 1989. Tonic activation of NMDA receptors by ambient glutamate enhances excitability of neurons. *Science*, 246: 815-818.

Schiller J, Major G, Koester HJ and Schiller Y. 2000. NMDA spikes in basal dendrites of cortical pyramidal neurons. *Nature*, 404:285-289.

Schoppa NE, Kinzie JM, Sahara Y, Segerson TP and Westbrook GL. 1998. Dendrodendritic inhibition in the olfactory bulb is driven by NMDA receptors. *J Neurosci*, 8:6790-6802.

Seeburg PH. 1993. The molecular biology of mammalian glutamate receptor channels. *Trends Neurosci*, 16: 359-365.

Solomon RE and Gebhart GF. 1988. Mechanisms of effects of intrathecal serotonin on nociception and blood pressure in rats. *J Pharmacol Exp Ther*, 245:905-912.

Sorkin LS, McAdoo DJ and Willis WD. 1993. Raphe magnus stimulation-induced antinociception in the cat is associated with release of amino acids as well as serotonin in the lumbar dorsal horn. *Brain Res*, 618:95-108.

Tan HJ and Miletic V. 1990. Electrophysiological properties of frog spinal dorsal horn neurons and their responses to serotonin: an intracellular study in the isolated hemisected spinal cord. *Brain Res*, 528:344-348.

Wall PD. 1977. The presence of ineffective synapses and the circumstances which unmask them. *Phil Trans R Soc Lond. B.*, 278: 361-372.

Wall PD. 1988. Recruitment of ineffective synapses after injury. In: *Advances in Neurology*. Vol. 47. Waxman SG, ed. New York: Raven Press. 387-400.

Weisskopf MG, Castillo PE, Zalutsky RA and Nicoll RA. 1994. Mediation of hippocampal mossy fiber longterm potentiation by cyclic AMP. *Science*, 265:1878-1882.

Willis WD. 1982. Control of nociceptive transmission in the spinal cord. In: *Progress in Sensory Physiology*. Vol. 3. Ottoson D, ed. Berlin: Springer-Verlag. 1-159.

Wu GY, Malinow R and Cline HT. 1996. Maturation of a central glutamatergic synapse. *Science*, 274: 972-976.

Xia Z and Storm DR. 1997. Calmodulin-regulated adenylyl cyclases and neuromodulation. *Current Opinion in Neurobiology*, 7: 391-396.

Yoshimura M and Jessell TM. 1989. Primary afferent-evoked synaptic responses and slow potential generation in rat substantia gelitinosa neurons *in vitro. J Neurophysiol*, 62: 96-108.

Yoshimura M and Jessell TM. 1990. Amino acid- mediated EPSPs at primary afferent synapses with substantia gelatinosa neurones in the rat spinal cord. *J Physiol (Lond)*, 430:315-335.

Zemlan FP, Kow LM and Pfaff DW. 1983. Spinal serotonin (5-HT) receptor subtypes and nociception. *J Pharmacol Exp Ther*, 226:477-485.

Zhuo M and Gebhart GF. 1990. Characterization of descending inhibition and facilitation from the nuclei reticularis gigantocellularis and gigantocellularis pars alpha in the rat. *Pain*, 42:337-350.

Zhuo M and Gebhart GF. 1991. Spinal serotonin receptors mediate descending inhibition and facilitation from the nuclei reticularis gigantocellularis and gigantocellularis pars alpha in the rat. *Brain Res*, 550:35-48.

Zhuo M and Gebhart GF. 1992. Characterization of descending facilitation and inhibition of spinal nociceptive transmission from the nuclei reticularis gigantocellularis and gigantocellularis pars alpha in the rat. *J Neurophysiol*, 67:1599-1614.

Zhuo M and Gebhart GF. 1997. Biphasic modulation of spinal nociceptive transmission from the medullary raphe nuclei in the rat. *J Neurophysiol*, 78: 746-758.

Anatomical Changes in the Spinal Dorsal Horn after Peripheral Nerve Injury

CHAPTER 23

Andrew J. Todd, Alfredo Ribeiro-da-Silva

Dr. Todd is currently Professor of Neuroscience at the Glasgow University. He received his MB, BS and PhD from the University of London.

MAJOR CONTRIBUTIONS

1. Todd AJ and Koerber HR. 2005. Neuroanatomical substrates of spinal nociception. In: *Wall and Melzack's Textbook of Pain* (5th Edition). McMahons and Koltzenburg M eds. Elsevier. 73-90.

2. Polgár E, Hughes DI, Arham AZ and Todd AJ. 2005. Loss of neurons from laminae I–III of the spinal dorsal horn is not required for development of tactile allodynia in the spared nerve injury model of neuropathic pain. *J Neurosci*, 25: 6658-6666.

3. Nagy GG, Al-Ayyan M, Andrew D, Fukaya M, Watanabe M and Todd AJ. 2004. Widespread expression of the AMPA receptor GluR2 subunit at glutamatergic synapses in the rat spinal cord and phosphorylation of GluR1 in response to noxious stimulation revealed with an antigen unmasking method. *J Neurosci*, 24: 5766-5777.

4. Hughes DI, Scott DT, Todd AJ and Riddell JS. 2003. Lack of evidence for sprouting of Aβ afferents into the superficial laminae of the spinal cord dorsal horn following nerve section. *J Neurosci*, 23: 9491- 9499.

5. Todd AJ, Puskár Z, Spike RC, Hughes C, Watt C and Forrest L. 2002. Projection neurons in lamina I of rat spinal cord with the neurokinin 1 receptor are selectively innervated by substance P-containing afferents and respond to noxious stimulation. *J Neurosci*, 22: 4103-4113.

Dr. Ribeiro-da-Silva obtained an MD from the University of Porto (Portugal), and a PhD in Normal Morphology, from the same University. He is currently Professor of Pharmacology & Therapeutics and Anatomy & Cell Biology at McGill University in Montreal.

MAJOR CONTRIBUTIONS

1. Todd AJ, Ribeiro-da-Silva A. 2005. Molecular architecture of the dorsal horn. In: *Neurobiology of Pain* Hunt SP and Koltzenburg M, eds. Oxford: Oxford University Press. 65-94.

2. Ribeiro-da-Silva A. 2004. Substantia gelatinosa of the spinal cord. In: *The Rat Nervous System*. Paxinos G, ed. San Diego: Elsevier Academic Press. 129-148.

3. Ruocco I, Cuello AC, Ribeiro-da-Silva A. 2000. Peripheral nerve injury leads to the establishment of a novel pattern of sympathetic fibre innervation in the rat skin. *J Comp Neurol*, 422: 287-296.

4. Grelik C, Bennett GJ, Ribeiro-da-Silva A. 2005. Autonomic fiber sprouting and changes in nociceptive sensory innervation in the rat lower lip skin following chronic constriction injury. *Eur J Neurosci*, 21: 2475-2487.

5. Bailey AL, Ribeiro-da-Silva A. 2006. Transient loss of terminals from non-peptidergic nociceptive fibres in the substantia gelatinosa of spinal cord following chronic constriction injury of the sciatic nerve. *Neuroscience*, 138: 675-690.

6. Yen L, Bennett GJ, Ribeiro-da-Silva A. 2006. Sympathetic sprouting and changes in nociceptive sensory innervation in the glabrous skin of the rat hind paw following partial peripheral nerve injury. *J Comp Neurol*, 495: 679-690.

MAIN TOPICS

Animal models of neuropathic pain

Do central terminals of primary afferents sprout

following nerve injury?

Ultrastructural changes affecting the central terminals of primary afferents after nerve injury

Neurochemical changes involving primary afferents

Changes involving inhibitory interneurons

Alternations involving AMPA receptors in the dorsal horn

Other neurochemical changes involving spinal neurons

Changes in the neuroglia

SUMMARY

Damage to peripheral nerves can lead to neuropathic pain, and several animal models of nerve injury have been developed to allow investigation of the underlying mechanisms. However, despite intensive research efforts, we still have rather a limited understanding of the pathophysiology of neuropathic pain states. It had been suggested that anatomical reorganisation (sprouting) of low-threshold cutaneous primary afferent arborisations in the dorsal horn could lead to a mis-coding of non-noxious information that could be partly responsible for allodynia, but the extent and significance of such a reorganisation is at present controversial and may be minimal. A loss of dorsal horn inhibitory mechanisms is known to occur and was initially thought to be caused by excitotoxic death of inhibitory interneurons. However, recent evidence indicates that the disinhibition is not a result of death of inhibitory neurons, and likely occurs through other mechanisms such as loss of inhibitory synapses and/or changes in their properties. Several other changes, including loss of synaptic connections formed by some types of primary afferent, alterations in the neurochemistry of primary afferents and dorsal horn neurons, up-regulation of receptors and glial activation are known to occur. However, it is not yet clear how much each of these phenomena contributes to neuropathic pain. Further studies are required for a proper understanding of what causes and maintains the pain that follows nerve damage. These new studies should focus, among other issues, on phenotypic and connectivity changes in both the dorsal horn and the periphery in different animal models of neuropathic pain.

INTRODUCTION

Neuropathic pain has been defined as "Pain initiated or caused by a primary lesion or dysfunction in the nervous system" (Merskey and Bogduk, 1994). Here we will focus on one major category of neuropathic pain, that which occurs following lesions of peripheral nerves, caused either by trauma or disease. Most of our current knowledge derives from studies on animals models of neuropathic pain (see below). Unfortunately, our understanding of changes in the organisation and physiology of the dorsal horn in nerve injury models, and of how these changes contribute to neuropathic pain, is still very limited. Some of the initial changes that follow nerve injury and contribute to the early phase of neuropathic pain are likely to be purely "functional" (i.e. without detectable morphological alteration), while morphological changes may occur later and underlie maintenance of the pain state (Woolf and Salter, 2000). Although there are undoubtedly many morphological changes in the dorsal horn after nerve injury, it is often difficult to demonstrate the extent to which these actually contribute to neuropathic pain.

Functional changes prevail in the initial stages of both peripheral and central sensitization, and include alterations involving membrane transporters and ion channels, as well as phosphorylation of the receptors for neurotransmitters and translocation of these receptors into the cell membrane (Woolf and Salter, 2000; Coull et al., 2003; Tsuda et al., 2003). These are beyond the scope of this review. There is also evidence that some morphological changes occur outside the CNS, including sprouting of sympathetic fibres around dorsal root ganglion neurons (McLachlan et al., 1993; Lee et al., 1998) and in the skin (Ruocco et al., 2000; Grelik et al., 2005; Yen et al., 2005). As these changes occur outside the CNS, they will not be discussed here either.

The dorsal horn of the spinal cord has a complex

neuronal organisation and contains the central terminals of primary afferent axons (which terminate with a modality-specific pattern), intrinsic interneurons with axons that remain in the spinal cord, projection cells that convey information to the brain, and descending axons that originate in several brain regions and modulate the transmission of sensory information through spinal circuits. For descriptive purposes, the dorsal horn is divided into a series of 6 parallel laminae (Rexed, 1952), of which laminae I–II make up the superficial dorsal horn (an area dominated by input from nociceptive afferents) and laminae III-VI the deep part of the dorsal horn. For more detailed descriptions of the normal anatomical organisation of the dorsal horn the reader is referred to other recent reviews (Ribeiro-da-Silva, 2004; Todd and Ribeiro-da-Silva, 2005; Todd and Koerber, 2005).

ANIMAL MODELS OF NEUROPATHIC PAIN

Several animal models have been developed in an attempt to mimic human neuropathic pain conditions. The mostly widely used models are those involving segmental spinal nerve ligation (SNL) (Kim and Chung, 1992), chronic constriction injury (CCI) (Bennett and Xie, 1988), partial sciatic nerve ligation injury (PSL) (Seltzer et al., 1990) and spared nerve injury (SNI) (Decosterd and Woolf, 2000). In the SNL model the L5 and L6 spinal nerves (or only the L5 spinal nerve) are tightly ligated unilaterally, leading to complete loss of nerve fibres distal to the ligation, with no subsequent recovery (Kim and Chung, 1992). In the CCI model, four loose chromic catgut ligatures are placed unilaterally around the sciatic nerve proximal to its trifurcation, leading to oedema and subsequent self-strangulation of the nerve (Bennett and Xie, 1988). Ultrastructural studies of the sciatic nerve distal to the ligation in this model have shown a loss of large myelinated fibres of up to 90% and a loss of thinly myelinated and unmyelinated afferents of up to 40%–50% at 10 and 14 days post-lesion (Munger et

al., 1992; Basbaum et al., 1991). Although regrowth of fibres beyond the ligatures with re-innervation of targets in the periphery is thought to occur at later stages in this model, as far as we are aware its extent has never been studied. Variations of the CCI model involve application of either 2–4 polyethylene cuffs (Mosconi and Kruger, 1996) or a single cuff around the sciatic nerve (Pitcher et al., 1999). Unfortunately, a critical comparison of the original CCI model and the variants that use polyethylene cuffs has never been performed. The PSL model (Seltzer et al., 1990) involves tight ligation of approximately half of the sciatic nerve at the high thigh level. Lastly, the SNI model consists of transection of two of the three terminal branches of the sciatic nerve (the tibial and common peroneal nerves) leaving the sural nerve intact (Decosterd and Woolf, 2000).

All of the above models can produce signs of neuropathic pain, although with different time-courses and with some variation in the pattern of neuropathic signs (e.g. thermal hyperalgesia vs tactile allodynia). The most profound morphological changes in both the CNS and the periphery seem to occur after the SNL model. The CCI models allow the partial recovery of the lesioned nerves, and there is likely to be both collateral sprouting of undamaged axons and regenerative sprouting of damaged fibres in the periphery, whereas in the other models peripheral re-innervation occurs only through collateral sprouting of fibres which were not cut or from adjacent territories.

Other models of neuropathic pain, such as the complete transection or crushing of a peripheral nerve, have also been used. However, these models have important drawbacks. For instance, transection of the sciatic nerve at mid-thigh level leads to complete loss of fibres in the nerve, with partial re-innervation of their peripheral territories from adjacent nerves. Because of the profound loss of peripheral innervation, the animals have an initial anaesthesia of the denervated territory, which makes behavioural testing difficult. In addition, crush lesions are difficult to standardize. Other clinically-relevant models have also been developed, such as the rat model of diabetic neuropathy following the injection of streptozotocin, and models involving the use of anti-cancer drugs (vincristine and paclitaxel) (Polomano *et al.*, 2001; Flatters and Bennett, 2004) and the anti-retroviral agents used in the treatment of AIDS (didanosine, ddI) (Joseph *et al.*, 2004).

DO CENTRAL TERMINALS OF PRIMARY AFFERENTS SPROUT FOLLOWING NERVE INJURY?

The central terminations of primary afferents axons in the dorsal horn have been studied with a variety of methods, including intra-axonal labelling of individual afferents, bulk-labelling of populations of afferents with tracers injected into peripheral nerves, and indirect approaches based on the use of specific neurochemical markers. Central terminals of large myelinated (Aβ) afferents, most of which are associated with tactile receptors or hair follicles, normally occupy an area extending from the ventral (inner) part of lamina II (lamina IIi) to lamina V. In contrast, fine myelinated (Aδ) and unmyelinated (C) fibres (many of which are nociceptors) terminate more dorsally (laminae I–III). Within this region, Aδ nociceptors end mainly in lamina I, while the central terminals of Aδ afferents that innervate hair-follicles arborise in laminae IIi and III. Central arborisations of C fibres occupy the whole of laminae I–II, with some also terminating in deeper laminae. Those belonging to C fibres that express neuropeptides are located more dorsally (lamina I and the outer part of lamina II, IIo) and those belonging to C fibres that appear to lack peptides ("non-peptidergic C fibres") are found mainly in the ventral part of lamina II (for a recent review see Todd and Ribeiro-da-Silva, 2005).

Woolf *et al.* (1992) proposed that following damage to a peripheral nerve, Aβ cutaneous afferents "sprouted" dorsally, so that their central terminals could enter lamina IIo and even extend into lamina I. Since this region is normally dominated by primary afferent input from nociceptors, and since lamina I

contains many neurons that send axons to the brain (projection neurons), this sprouting was thought to provide a mechanism that could result in "mis-coding" of information that was transmitted to the brain, with tactile input being conveyed by pathways that normally dealt with noxious information. Although the original observations were made on axotomised primary afferents, which had lost their connection to the periphery, it was believed that these abnormal central connections could be maintained after the distal part of the axon had regenerated and re-innervated peripheral tissues. This mechanism could therefore contribute to neuropathic pain following re-innervation. The evidence for sprouting was based on results obtained with two different experimental approaches, bulk-labelling with cholera toxin B subunit (CTb) and intra-axonal labelling of individual axotomised Aβ afferents. CTb binds selectively to the GM1 ganglioside, which is normally expressed only by myelinated primary afferents in cutaneous nerves. When injected into an intact peripheral nerve, CTb is transported through the dorsal root ganglion, to the central terminals of the myelinated afferents, and labelling is consequently seen in a band extending from lamina IIi-V (Aδ hair-follicle and Aβ afferents) and also in lamina I (Aδ nociceptors). Labelling is absent from lamina IIo, which receives very few terminals belonging to myelinated afferents. Woolf *et al.* (1992) found that when CTb was injected into a nerve that had been damaged two weeks previously, labelling extended throughout the dorsal horn, including lamina IIo. They also reported that whereas the central arbors of individual Aβ hair-follicle afferents (HFAs) labelled by intra-axonal injection normally occupied lamina III with some entering lamina IIi, chronically axotomised Aβ afferents that resembled HFAs could extend as far dorsally as lamina I.

The first evidence against sprouting of Aβ afferents came from studies by Tong *et al.* (1999) and Bao *et al.* (2002), who showed that after nerve injury, CTb was no longer taken up exclusively by myelinated afferents. Their results suggested that damaged C fibres up-regulated the GM1 ganglioside, so that CTb could be transported to their cell bodies and central terminals. This was therefore likely to account for

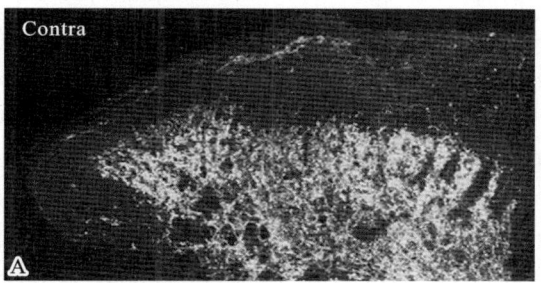

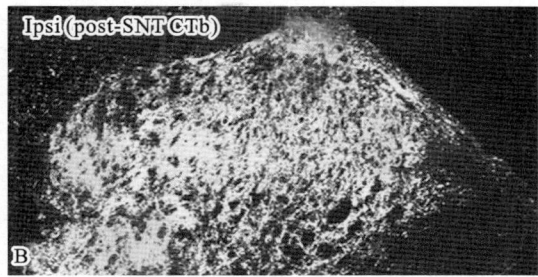

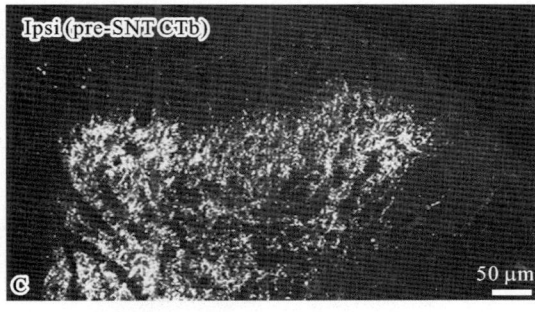

Fig.23.1 Different patterns of central labelling with CTb seen after injection of the tracer into the sciatic nerve in animals that had undergone sciatic nerve transection. A. This image shows the normal appearance of CTb labelling in the dorsal horn after the tracer was injected into the intact contralateral (Contra) sciatic nerve. CTb is seen throughout the deep dorsal horn and to a small extent in lamina I, but is absent from much of lamina II. This reflects the distribution of terminals belonging to myelinated primary afferents. B. When CTb is injected into a sciatic nerve that had been sectioned 14 days previously (Ipsi), the labelling now extends throughout the depth of dorsal horn, including lamina II. C. However, if CTb is injected into a sciatic nerve 4 days before the nerve is transected, and there is a further 14 day survival period, the distribution of central labelling is similar to that seen after injection into an intact nerve. This indicates that the CTb in lamina II seen in B. is likely to result from transport by damaged C fibres rather than from sprouting of myelinated axons into lamina II (modified and reproduced with permission from Bao *et al.*, 2002).

much of the increased labelling in the superficial dorsal horn seen when the tracer was injected into a damaged nerve. They also found that if CTb was injected into the sciatic nerve prior to transection of the nerve, the pattern of central labelling was very similar to that seen after injection into an intact nerve (Fig.23.1). Hughes *et al.* (2003) carried out intra-axonal labelling of Aβ afferents in the rat and compared the central arbors of axons in intact sciatic nerves with those in sciatic nerves that had been transected between 7 and 10 weeks previously. They found no difference in the proportion of intact and axotomised HFA-type Aβ afferents that entered lamina IIi (9 out of 27 and 5 out of 15, respectively). None of the injected afferents in either population had arbors that extended into lamina IIo or lamina I. These studies therefore do not support the suggestion that low-threshold Aβ myelinated afferents sprout dorsally following nerve injury.

More recently, Hu *et al.* (2004) have reported that the central branches of intact fine-diameter (Aδ and C) afferents, which can be labelled by injection of wheat-germ agglutinin (WGA) into a peripheral nerve, can sprout into the denervated region of the spinal dorsal horn following ligation of a spinal nerve.

ULTRASTRUCTURAL CHANGES AFFECTING THE CENTRAL TERMINALS OF PRIMARY AFFERENTS AFTER NERVE INJURY

Ultrastructural studies have revealed that the central terminations of different types of primary afferent differ considerably in terms of their normal synaptic arrangements. For instance, the central terminals of non-peptidergic nociceptive C fibres end mostly as the central boutons of complex synaptic arrangements called glomeruli, and are often postsynaptic to GABAergic axons or vesicle-containing dendrites. These glomeruli are both multiplier and modulatory devices. In contrast, at least in rodents, peptidergic nociceptive fibres generally terminate as simple boutons, establishing axodendritic synapses (for recent reviews see Ribeiro-da-Silva, 2004; Todd and Ribeiro-da-Silva, 2005). This difference is important, because it suggests that while non-peptidergic nociceptive C fibres undergo presynaptic inhibition mediated by ionotropic (GABA$_A$) receptors, both peptidergic and non-peptidergic populations are under the influence of slow, G protein-coupled receptor-mediated presynaptic inhibition (e.g., through opioid and/or GABA$_B$ receptors).

Relatively little is known concerning the fate of the central terminals of primary sensory fibres following nerve injury. Electron microscopic studies have shown that transection of a peripheral nerve leads to a transganglionic "degenerative atrophy" of virtually all of the central terminals of the synaptic glomeruli that belong to non-peptidergic C fibres, with consequent loss of their synapses (Knyihár and Csillik, 1976; Castro-Lopes et al., 1990). These central terminals can normally be identified at the light microscopic level by their capacity to bind the lectin IB4 (derived from *Bandeiraea simplicifolia*). IB4-binding in the corresponding part of the dorsal horn is substantially reduced after nerve injury (Molander et al., 1996) (Fig.23.2A, see also the color plate), and this presumably results from the transganglionic degeneration of the central boutons of the non-peptidergic C afferents. However, IB4 binding partially recovers after either transection or crush of the sciatic nerve (Molander et al., 1996), and this suggests that there may be regeneration of the central terminals of the axotomised C fibres. Direct evidence for this has been provided by Bailey and Ribeiro-da-Silva (2005), who showed that in the polyethylene cuff version of the CCI model, IB4-binding progressively diminished over the first 10 post-operative days and then returned to normal by day 15 (Fig.23.3A-C, see also the color plate). Ultrastructural studies showed a parallel loss followed by reappearance of the central axons of synaptic glomeruli that originate from the non-peptidergic C fibres (Fig.23.3D-F). Taken together, these observations suggest that nerve injury can lead to degeneration of most or all of the boutons belonging to these non-peptidergic C fibres,

depending on the type of injury, but that new boutons can subsequently form, probably from local axonal branches, and that these develop new synaptic connections.

It is much more difficult to investigate changes in central terminals of peptidergic primary afferents, partly because these do not have a characteristic ultrastructural appearance that allows them to be recognised unequivocally, and partly because of alterations in the levels of the various peptides that they contain (see below). For example, the loss of calcitonin gene-related peptide (CGRP) from boutons of peptidergic afferents in the dorsal horn that is seen after nerve injury could result from either degeneration of these boutons or from down-regulation of the peptide within individual boutons. However, there is some evidence that the changes to central axons of peptidergic afferents are less severe than those involving non-peptidergic C fibres. Thus, Zhang et al. (1995) reported that two weeks after sciatic nerve section, galanin-immunoreactive boutons that were assumed to belong to axotomised primary afferents, retained their synaptic connections even though there were significant alterations to their ultrastructural

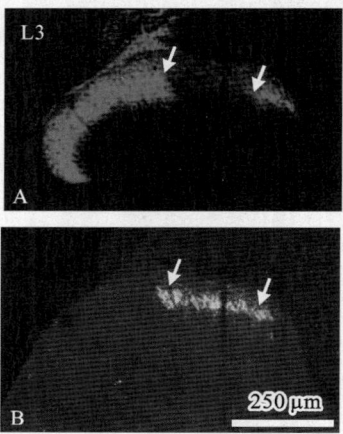

Fig.23.2 Alterations to C fibres after peripheral axotomy. These images show binding of the lectin IB4 (A) and VIP-immunoreactivity (B) in a section from the L3 segment of a rat that had the ipsilateral femoral nerve transected 2 weeks previously. There is loss of IB4 binding from superficial dorsal horn in the territory of the femoral nerve (between arrows) and a corresponding up-regulation of VIP, which is normally not present in significant amounts at this segmental level (reproduced with permission from Shehab et al., 2004 J Comp Neurol, 474: 427-437).

appearance. Primary afferents of another type, those that innervate the follicles of down-hairs (D-hair afferents), can be recognised in electron microscopic studies as they form the central axons of a different type of synaptic glomerulus. These glomeruli remain mostly intact following transection of the sciatic nerve (Popratiloff *et al.*, 1998), and therefore the central boutons of D-hair afferents presumably survive peripheral axotomy. The study by Bailey and Ribeiro-da-Silva (2005) supports this view, since the central boutons of this type of glomerulus were not affected following the application of a cuff to the sciatic nerve (Fig.23.3G). This indicates that central terminals of different types of primary afferent show markedly different responses to nerve injury. It can be speculated that these differences result from different dependency on neurotrophic factor support.

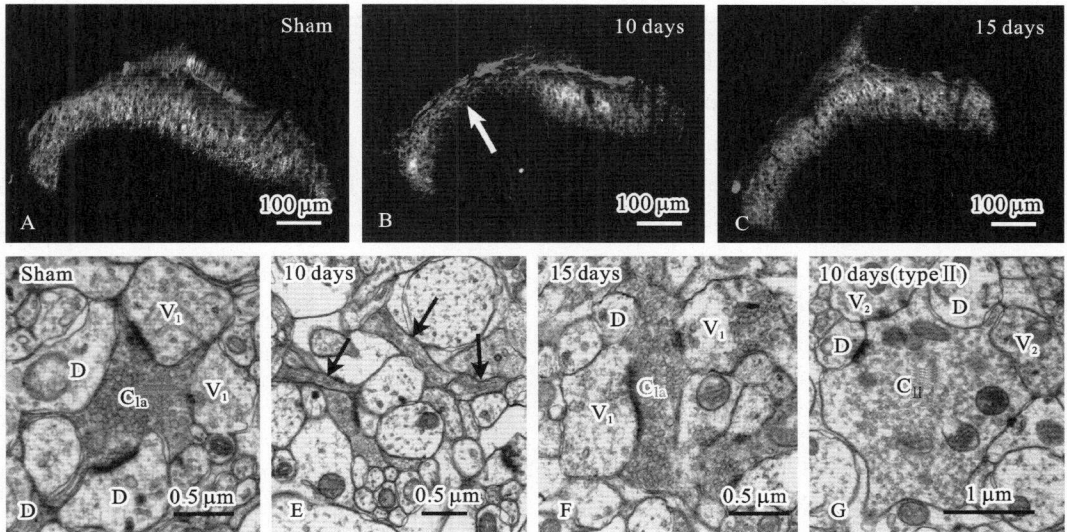

Fig.23.3 Transient loss of non-peptidergic nociceptive C afferents following the application of a polyethylene cuff to the sciatic nerve of the rat. A, B and C represent confocal images from single optical sections of the spinal dorsal horn from sham-operated (10 days post-surgery), and lesioned animals 10 and 15 days after surgery, respectively. Material was processed for the demonstration of CGRP immunoreactivity (in red) and binding of the lectin IB4 (in green). Note in B the loss of IB4 staining in the region indicated with an arrow, with recovery by 15 days (C). CGRP immunostaining was not affected by the lesion. D, E, F and G represent electron micrographs from inner lamina II of sham-operated (D) and lesioned animals (E-G). In D, note a normal type Ia glomerulus. The central boutons (C_{Ia}) of these glomeruli bind the lectin IB4 and represent the central termination of the non-peptidergic C afferents. Note that 10 days after the lesion, many dense axons were observed (arrows in E); however, true C_{Ia} boutons were sparse, as most had degenerated or lost their synaptic connections. By 15 days post-lesion (F), most C_{Ia} boutons had reappeared, as their number was back to sham-operated levels, and they had re-established synaptic connections with surrounding profiles. The central boutons of type II glomeruli (C_{II}), which represent myelinated non-nociceptive (likely D-hair) afferents, did not seem to be affected by the lesion (G). V_1, presynaptic dendrites; V_2, peripheral axons in glomeruli, likely from inhibitory interneurons; D, dendrites (original figure from data collected for study by Bailey and Ribeiro-da-Silva, 2005).

NEUROCHEMICAL CHANGES INVOLVING PRIMARY AFFERENTS

Analysis of the neurochemical changes involving central axons of primary afferents within the dorsal horn that occur after nerve injury is complicated by the fact that some of the boutons belonging to these afferents degenerate after peripheral axotomy, and that the extent of this degeneration varies considerably for different types of afferent (see above).

Nonetheless, it is clear that there are dramatic alterations in the expression of neuropeptides in the central terminals of the damaged afferents within the dorsal horn (for review see Hökfelt *et al.*, 1994). Several peptides that are normally present in fine-diameter afferents, such as substance P, CGRP, somatostatin and endomorphin 2, are largely depleted from their central terminals after nerve transection, while galanin is up-regulated. Two further peptides, which are either not expressed by intact primary afferents or are present only in a small number, appear *de novo* after nerve injury: these are vasoactive intestinal polypeptide (VIP) which is found in terminals of fine-diameter afferents in laminae I and II (Fig.23.2B), and neuropeptide Y (NPY) which is up-regulated in low-threshold cutaneous myelinated afferents that terminate in laminae III-IV. A complication in interpreting changes in the levels of peptides in damaged primary afferents in the dorsal horn is that in most cases these peptides are also present in the axons of some spinal neurons, and these may undergo alterations as well (see below).

There have been reports that substance P, which is normally expressed by few (if any) Aβ afferents, is upregulated in many afferents of this class following sciatic nerve transection (Noguchi *et al.*, 1994). In contrast, Malcangio *et al.* (2000) reported that following spinal nerve lesions substance P could be released from spinal cord slices by electrical stimulation of Aβ-fibres, but that this effect was not seen after sciatic nerve transection. The conclusions from both of these papers were that axotomy could cause a phenotypic switch, such that Aβ afferents could synthesise and release substance P. The study by Malcangio *et al.* (2000) suggested this was more likely to occur with lesions close to the dorsal root ganglion, where the cell bodies are located. Since the great majority of cutaneous Aβ afferents normally function as low-threshold mechanoreceptors, the appearance of substance P in these axons might contribute to abnormal pain sensation. However, although substance P immunoreactivity was seen in large axons in the dorsal roots by Noguchi *et al.* (1994), it has apparently not been possible to demonstrate that the peptide is present in the central terminals of Aβ afferents after

nerve injury. Further evidence for a phenotypic switch has been provided in a recent physiological study by Pitcher and Henry (2004). These authors reported that peripheral nerve stimulation at a frequency that normally excites only myelinated afferents produced a characteristic afterdischarge in dorsal horn neurons that was blocked by a substance P receptor antagonist in rats with neuropathy induced by the polyethylene cuff model, but not in controls. Therefore, further studies are required to determine whether substance P is expressed by larger diameter afferents following peripheral nerve injury.

Other neurochemical changes affecting central terminals of primary afferents include an alteration in the levels of brain-derived neurotrophic factor (BDNF) that is dependent on the nature of the peripheral injury (Cho *et al.*, 1998) and down-regulation of the vesicular glutamate transporter 1 (VGLUT1) in terminals of low-threshold myelinated afferents (Hughes *et al.*, 2004).

CHANGES INVOLVING INHIBITORY INTERNEURONS

There are several lines of evidence which suggest that loss of inhibition in the dorsal horn is at least partially responsible for symptoms of neuropathic pain. The main inhibitory transmitters in the dorsal horn are GABA and glycine, and intrathecal administration of bicuculline or strychnine (GABA$_A$ and glycine receptor antagonists, respectively) to naïve animals produces tactile allodynia, similar to that seen in neuropathic pain (Yaksh, 1989). In addition, intrathecal administration of GABA$_A$ agonists can alleviate allodynia in neuropathic models (Hwang and Yaksh, 1997). Following nerve injury, reduced levels of GABA and its synthetic enzyme glutamatic acid decarboxylase (GAD) have been found in the dorsal horn (Castro-Lopes *et al.*, 1993; Moore *et al.*, 2002). Direct evidence for loss of inhibition has been provided by Moore *et al.* (2002), who observed a substantial reduction in primary afferent-evoked IPSCs in lamina II neurons in both CCI and SNI models. Ap-

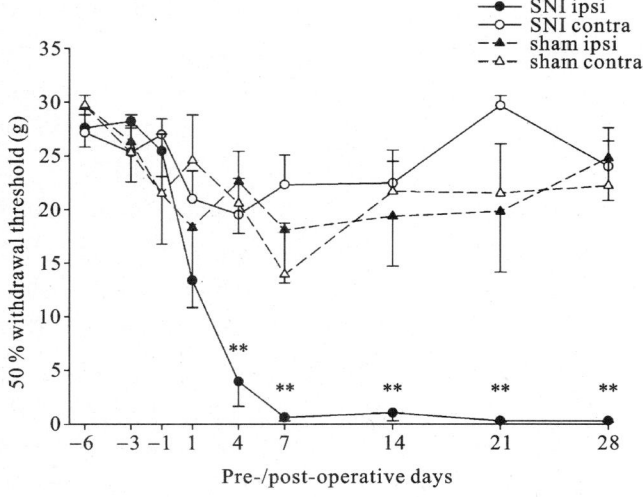

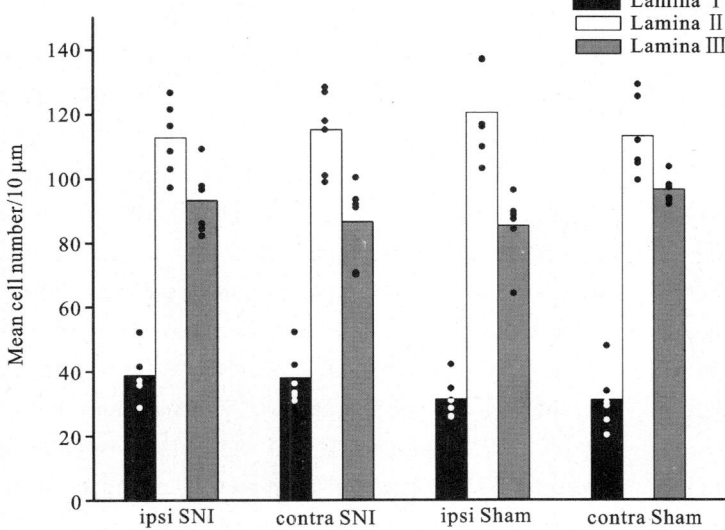

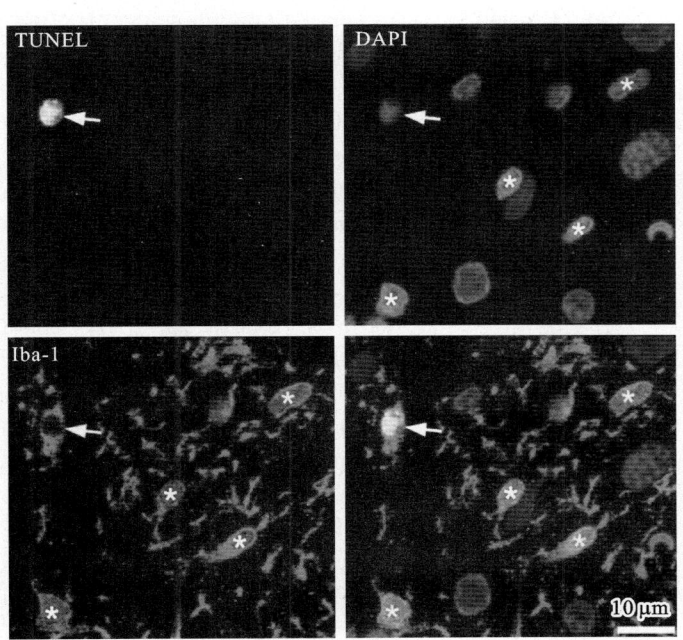

Fig.23.4 Evidence that loss of neurons from the superficial dorsal horn is not required for development of tactile allodynia in the spared nerve injury (SNI) model. The top panel shows the development of tactile allodynia, indicated by reduction in 50% withdrawal threshold of the hindpaw to application of von Frey hairs. Note the dramatic reduction in threshold on the ipsilateral side in the SNI animals, indicating tactile allodynia, which was first detected on the 4th post-operative day. The middle panel shows the mean numbers of neurons counted with a stereological method in laminae I–III on the ipsilateral (ipsi) and contralateral (contra) sides in SNI (n=6) and sham-operated (n=6) animals that had survived 4 weeks after operation. Individual results are shown as circles. There is no significant difference in the density of neurons per 10μm length of spinal cord between either side of either group, indicating that there was no detectable loss of neurons. Apoptotic cells (detected with the TUNEL method) were detected in the spinal cord of SNI animals in this study, but the great majority of these (87/93, 94%) were identified as microglia by the presence of Iba-1 (a specific marker for microglia) in their cytoplasm. An example is shown in the lower panel (reproduced with permission from Polgár *et al.*, 2005).

plication of bicuculline to spinal cord slices leads to enhanced excitatory synaptic transmission in the superficial laminae, with many cells responding polysynaptically to stimulation of Aβ afferents (Baba *et al.*, 2003), and a similar phenomenon is observed after peripheral nerve injury in the absence of bicuculline (Okamoto *et al.*, 2001). Bicuculline has a much smaller effect on the excitability of lamina II neurons following nerve injury, and this is consistent with a reduced level of GABAergic inhibition in this situation (Baba *et al.*, 2003). A significant proportion of lamina I neurons project to the brain, and under normal circumstances most of the neurons in this lamina respond to noxious, but not tactile stimuli. However, both nerve injury (Catheline *et al.*, 1999) and blockade of GABA$_A$ receptors with bicuculline (Baba *et al.*, 2003) enable low-threshold afferents to activate cells in lamina I. It is therefore likely that the mis-coding of low-threshold input by these cells plays an important part in the tactile allodynia seen in neuropathic pain.

It has been proposed that disinhibition in the dorsal horn is caused by apoptotic death of inhibitory interneurons, which make up between 30 and 45% of the neuronal population in laminae I-III. This suggestion is based on the finding of "dark" neurons (which are assumed to be undergoing degeneration) (Sugimoto *et al.*, 1990), and TUNEL-positive (apoptotic) nuclei (Moore *et al.*, 2002; Azkue *et al.*, 1998; White-

side and Munglani, 2001) in laminae I-III of the dorsal horn after various types of nerve injury. However, stereological counts of the neuronal packing density in laminae I-III of the spinal cord from rats that had undergone CCI or SNI show no reduction in the numbers of neurons in these laminae, despite behavioural signs of neuropathic pain (Polgár *et al.*, 2004, 2005) (Fig.23.4). In addition, the proportion of neurons in laminae I-III that are GABA-immunoreactive is not altered in the CCI model (Polgár *et al.*, 2003) (Fig.23.5). Furthermore, it has been reported that the TUNEL-positive cells seen in the spinal cord after transection of the sciatic nerve (Gehrmann and Banati, 1995) and in the SNI model (Polgár *et al.*, 2005) are microglia (Fig.23.4, see also the color plate). Taken together, these findings do not support the suggestion that there is a significant degree of neuronal death in the dorsal horn after nerve injury. Alternative explanations for the disinhibition include reduced activity of inhibitory interneurons (for example due to a reduced primary afferent input), loss of synapses formed by axons of the inhibitory interneurons, depletion of GABA (and/or glycine) from the presynaptic boutons at these synapses, or loss of GABA$_A$ (and/or glycine) receptors from these synapses. A recent study (Coull *et al.*, 2003) has shown that the potassium-chloride exporter KCC2 is down-regulated in dorsal horn neurons after nerve injury, which would result in GABA and glycine having a depolarising (excitatory) action.

ipsilateral contralateral

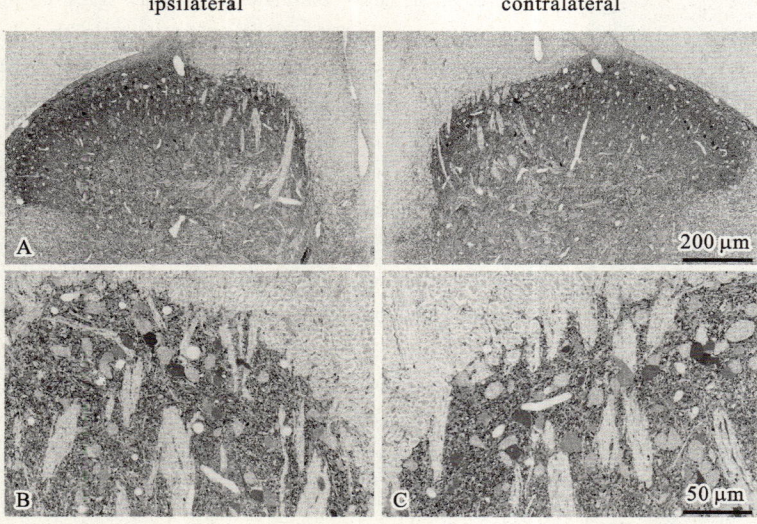

Fig.23.5 GABA-immunostaining in a semithin section from the L4 segment of a rat that had undergone chronic constriction injury of the left sciatic nerve two weeks previously. A shows a low magnification view through the dorsal horn on both sides, while B and C show higher magnification views of the medial parts of the ipsilateral (left) and contralateral (right) dorsal horns, respectively. Numerous immunoreactive and non-immunoreactive cell bodies can be seen in the dorsal horn on each side, and there is no detectable difference between the two sides. Stereological analysis showed that the proportion of cells in each of laminae I, II and III that were GABA-immunoreactive did not differ between ipsilateral and contralateral sides (reproduced from with permission Polgár *et al.*, 2003).

ALTERNATIONS INVOLVING AMPA RECEPTORS IN THE DORSAL HORN

One of the changes that is thought to contribute to neuropathic pain is an increase in the efficacy of excitatory synapses on dorsal horn neurons, known as central sensitization (Ji *et al.*, 2003). This form of synaptic plasticity has certain features in common with long-term potentiation (LTP) in the hippocampus. One of the main mechanisms underlying hippocampal LTP is an increase in the effectiveness of AMPA receptors at glutamatergic synapses, brought about initially by receptor phosphorylation, and subsequently by insertion of new AMPA receptors. Phosphorylation of AMPA receptor subunits and insertion of new receptors into synapses might therefore occur following nerve injury, and play a role in neuropathic pain (Ji *et al.*, 2003; Garry and Fleetwood-Walker, 2004). Consistent with this suggestion, it has been reported that tactile allodynia and thermal hyperalgesia in the CCI model are both attenuated by intrathecal administration of AMPA receptors antagonists (Garry *et al.*, 2003). There are several reports of an up-regulation of AMPA receptor subunits and their mRNAs in the dorsal horn following nerve injury (Harris *et al.*, 1996; Garry *et al.*, 2003). However, identifying AMPA receptors at synapses is technically difficult, because the high protein content of the postsynaptic density and synaptic cleft dramatically reduces access of antibodies in immunocytochemical studies (Nagy *et al.*, 2004). In one study that used a post-embedding immunogold method to avoid this problem, it was reported that there was a significant increase in the density of AMPA receptors at synapses formed by one class of primary afferent (Aδ D-hair afferents) (Popratiloff *et al.*, 1998) following peripheral nerve transection. It is not yet known whether there is an alteration in AMPA receptor density at synapses formed by those primary afferents that remain intact following a nerve injury. This would obviously be important as it

could contribute to allodynia and hyperalgesia.

OTHER NEUROCHEMICAL CHANGES INVOLVING SPINAL NEURONS

Substance P acts on the neurokinin 1 (NK1) receptor, which is expressed by many dorsal horn neurons, including most of those in laminae I–III that project to the brain. NK1 receptor-immunoreactivity in the dorsal horn has been found to increase following transection of the sciatic nerve and in neuropathic pain models (Abbadie *et al.*, 1996; Goff *et al.*, 1998; Honoré *et al.*, 2000) (Fig.23.6). It is not known whether these increases are the result of up-regulation by neurons that normally express the receptor, or of *de novo* expression by other neurons, although some reports would suggest the former. Interestingly, Allen *et al.* (1999) reported that following nerve injury, electrical stimulation of primary afferents at Aβ strength did not evoke internalisation of the receptor, and this finding does not support the suggestion that substance P is up-regulated in axotomised Aβ primary afferents (Noguchi *et al.*, 1996) (see above). Immunostaining for the μ-opioid receptor (MOR-1) was increased in the ipsilateral dorsal horn in the CCI model, but reduced following sciatic nerve transection (Goff *et al.*, 1998). However, interpretation of this finding is complicated, since MOR-1 is present on both nociceptive primary afferent terminals and intrinsic interneurons in the superficial part of the dorsal horn.

One neuronal population that has been implicated in neuropathic pain consists of neurons that express the γ isoform of protein kinase C (PKCγ). This population of excitatory interneurons has a very specific distribution in the dorsal horn, being largely restricted to the inner half of lamina II. It has been shown that PKCγ is moderately upregulated following peripheral nerve injury and, remarkably, mice which lack PKCγ have substantially reduced neuropathic pain following peri pheral nerve injury (Malmberg *et al.*, 1997; Martin *et al.*, 2001). The synaptic circuitry involved is at present unclear, although it has been suggested that PKCγ mediates the transition from short-to long-term hyperexcitability of lamina V wide dynamic range neurons (Martin *et al.*, 2001). The opioid peptide dynorphin is thought to play a role in neuropathic pain, and is expressed by neurons in both superficial and deep parts of the dorsal horn. Studies using immunocytochemistry and *in situ* hybridisation have demonstrated an up-regulation of dynorphin and the mRNA for its precursor, preprodynorphin, in the ipsilateral dorsal horn after nerve injury (Draisci *et al.*, 1991; Honoré *et al.*, 2000). The neuronal isoform of nitric oxide synthase (bNOS) is found in many dorsal horn neurons, most of which are GABAergic, and is down-regulated after tight ligation of the sciatic nerve and in the CCI model (Goff *et al.*, 1998).

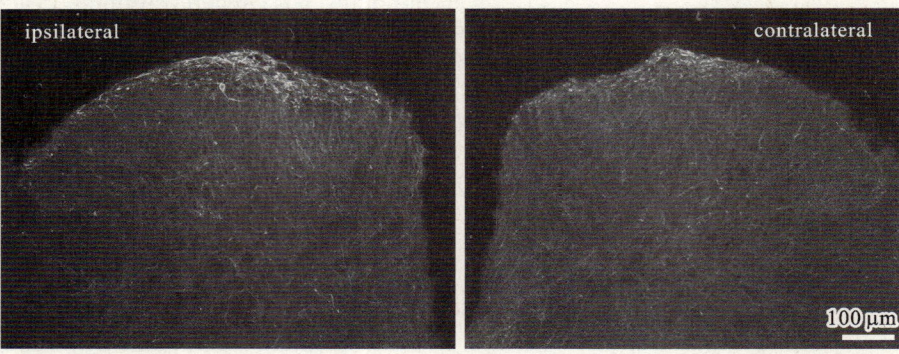

Fig.23.6 Immunostaining for the NK1 receptor in the dorsal horn of the L4 segment from a rat that had undergone chronic constriction injury of the left sciatic nerve two weeks previously. NK1 receptor-immunoreactivity is concentrated in the superficial dorsal horn (lamina I) on both sides, but the staining is considerably stronger on the ipsilateral side, compared to that on the contralateral side.

CHANGES IN THE NEUROGLIA

Following lesions of peripheral nerves, there is a transient activation of astrocytes, as shown by increased levels of glial fibrillary acidic protein (GFAP) after spinal nerve ligation (Madiai *et al.*, 2003). This is also likely to occur after other types of peripheral nerve injury. However, the activation of microglia, which had been reported already over a decade ago, has received considerable attention lately (Eriksson *et al.*, 1993). This is because in a recent study, rats with a spinal nerve ligation were shown to have tactile allodynia mediated by purinergic P2X4 receptors induced in activated microglia (Tsuda *et al.*, 2003). This issue is covered at length in the chapter "Glia and neuropathic pain".

CONCLUSIONS

The main conclusion from this review of the morphological and neurochemical changes in the spinal dorsal horn that follow nerve injury is that the available data is clearly insufficient for a proper understanding of the pathophysiology of neuropathic pain. Several animal models have been used, but they have not all been fully characterised, and it is likely that there are subtle but significant differences between versions of the same model used in different laboratories. Furthermore, some changes have been studied only in specific models, and may not be the same in other models. Lastly, a correlation between the time-course of the few morphological/neurochemical changes which have been well studied, and the development and maintenance of the neuropathic pain state is often not obvious. The current situation is most likely due to the incomplete knowledge and understanding of the morphological and neurochemical changes. Because it is thought that chronic neuropathic pain conditions can be maintained by a "rewiring" in the CNS, the understanding of such rewiring and how to prevent it is particularly critical. However, substantial further research will be required to achieve this goal.

GENERAL CITATIONS

Hökfelt T, Zhang X, Wiesenfeld-Hallin Z. 1994. Messenger plasticity in primary sensory neurons following axotomy and its functional implications. *Trends Neurosci*, 17: 22-30.

Ji RR, Kohno T, Moore KA, Woolf CJ. 2003. Central sensitization and LTP: do pain and memory share similar mechanisms? *Trends Neurosci*, 26: 696-705.

Merskey H, Bogduk N. 1994. *Classification of Chronic Pain*: *Descriptions of Chronic Pain Syndromes and Definitions of Pain Terms*. Seattle: IASP Press.

Ribeiro-da-Silva A. 2004. Substantia gelatinosa of the spinal cord. In: *The Rat Nervous System*. Paxinos G, ed. San Diego: Elsevier Academic Press. 129-148.

Todd AJ, Koerber HR. 2005. Anatomical substrates of spinal nociception. In: *Wall and Melzack's Textbook of Pain*. McMahon SB and Koltzenburg M, eds. Churchill Livingstone. 73-90.

Todd AJ, Ribeiro-da-Silva A. 2005. Molecular architecture of the dorsal horn. In: *Neurobiology of Pain*. Hunt SP and Koltzenburg M, eds. Oxford: Oxford University Press. 65-94.

Woolf CJ, Salter MW. 2000. Neuronal plasticity: increasing the gain in pain. *Science*, 288: 1765-1768.

DISCOVERY CITATIONS

Abbadie C, Brown JL, Mantyh PW, Basbaum AI. 1996. Spinal cord substance P receptor immunoreactivity increases in both inflammatory and nerve injury models of persistent pain. *Neuroscience*, 70: 201-209.

Allen BJ, Li J, Menning PM, Rogers SD, Ghilardi J, Mantyh PW, Simone DA. 1999. Primary afferent fibers that contribute to increased substance P receptor internalization in the spinal cord after injury. *J Neurophysiol*, 81: 1379-1390.

Azkue JJ, Zimmermann M, Hsieh TF, Herdegen T. 1998. Peripheral nerve insult induces NMDA receptor-mediated, delayed degeneration in spinal neurons. *Eur J Neurosci*, 10: 2204-2206.

Baba H, Ji RR, Kohno T, Moore KA, Ataka T, Wakai A,

Okamoto M, Woolf CJ. 2003. Removal of GABAergic inhibition facilitates polysynaptic A fiber-mediated excitatory transmission to the superficial spinal dorsal horn. *Mol Cell Neurosci*, 24: 818-830.

Bailey AL, Ribeiro-da-Silva A. 2006. Transient loss of terminals from non-peptidergic nociceptive fibres in the substantia gelatinosa of spinal cord following chronic constriction injury of the sciatic nerve. *Neuroscience*, 138: 675-690.

Bao L, Wang HF, Cai HJ, Tong YG, Jin SX, Lu YJ, Grant G, Hökfelt T, Zhang X. 2002. Peripheral axotomy induces only very limited sprouting of coarse myelinated afferents into inner lamina II of rat spinal cord. *Eur J Neurosci*, 16: 175-185.

Basbaum AI, Gautron M, Jazat F, Mayes M, Guilbaud G. 1991. The spectrum of fiber loss in a model of neuropathic pain in the rat: an electron microscopic study. *Pain*, 47: 359-367.

Bennett GJ, Xie Y-K. 1988. A peripheral mononeuropathy in rat that produces disorders of pain sensation like those seen in man. *Pain*, 33: 87-107.

Castro-Lopes JM, Coimbra A, Grant G, Arvidsson J. 1990. Ultrastructural changes of the central scalloped (C1) primary afferent endings of synaptic glomeruli in the substantia gelatinosa Rolandi of the rat after peripheral neurotomy. *J Neurocytol*, 19: 329-337.

Castro-Lopes JM, Tavares I, Coimbra A. 1993. GABA decreases in the spinal cord dorsal horn after peripheral neurectomy. *Brain Res*, 620: 287-291.

Catheline G, Le GS, Honoré P, Besson JM. 1999. Are there long-term changes in the basal or evoked Fos expression in the dorsal horn of the spinal cord of the mononeuropathic rat? *Pain*, 80: 347-357.

Cho HJ, Kim JK, Park HC, Kim JK, Kim DS, Ha SO, Hong HS. 1998. Changes in brain-derived neurotrophic factor immunoreactivity in rat dorsal root ganglia, spinal cord, and gracile nuclei following cut or crush injuries. *Exp Neurol*, 154: 224-230.

Coull JA, Boudreau D, Bachand K, Prescott SA, Nault F, Sik A, De Koninck P, De Koninck Y. 2003. Trans-synaptic shift in anion gradient in spinal lamina I neurons as a mechanism of neuropathic pain. *Nature*, 424: 938-942.

Decosterd I, Woolf CJ. 2000. Spared nerve injury: an animal

model of persistent peripheral neuropathic pain. *Pain*, 87: 149-158.

Draisci G, Kajander KC, Dubner R, Bennett GJ, Iadarola MJ. 1991. Up-regulation of opioid gene expression in spinal cord evoked by experimental nerve injuries and inflammation. *Brain Res*, 560: 186-192.

Eriksson NP, Persson JK, Svensson M, Arvidsson J, Molander C, Aldskogius H. 1993. A quantitative analysis of the microglial cell reaction in central primary sensory projection territories following peripheral nerve injury in the adult rat. *Exp Brain Res*, 96: 19-27.

Flatters SJ, Bennett GJ. 2004. Ethosuximide reverses paclitaxel-and vincristine-induced painful peripheral neuropathy. *Pain*, 109: 150-161.

Garry EM, Fleetwood-Walker SM. 2004. A new view on how AMPA receptors and their interacting proteins mediate neuropathic pain. *Pain*, 109: 210-213.

Garry EM, Moss A, Rosie R, Delaney A, Mitchell R, Fleetwood-Walker SM. 2003. Specific involvement in neuropathic pain of AMPA receptors and adapter proteins for the GluR2 subunit. *Mol Cell Neurosci*, 24: 10-22.

Gehrmann J, Banati RB. 1995. Microglial turnover in the injured CNS: activated microglia undergo delayed DNA fragmentation following peripheral nerve injury. *J Neuropathol Exp Neurol*, 54: 680-688.

Goff JR, Burkey AR, Goff DJ, Jasmin L. 1998. Reorganization of the spinal dorsal horn in models of chronic pain: Correlation with behaviour. *Neuroscience*, 82: 559-574.

Grelik C, Bennett GJ, Ribeiro-da-Silva A. 2005. Autonomic fiber sprouting and changes in nociceptive sensory innervation in the rat lower lip skin following chronic constriction injury. *Eur J Neurosci*, 21: 2475-2487.

Harris JA, Corsi M, Quartaroli M, Arban R, Bentivoglio M. 1996. Upregulation of spinal glutamate receptors in chronic pain. *Neuroscience*, 74: 7-12.

Honoré P, Rogers SD, Schwei MJ, Salak-Johnson JL, Luger NM, Sabino MC, Clohisy DR, Mantyh PW. 2000. Murine models of inflammatory, neuropathic and cancer pain each generates a unique set of neurochemical changes in the spinal cord and sensory neurons. *Neuroscience*, 98: 585-598.

Hu J, Mata M, Hao S, Zhang G, Fink DJ. 2004. Central sprouting of uninjured small fiber afferents in the adult rat spinal cord following spinal nerve ligation. *Eur J Neurosci*, 20: 1705-1712.

Hughes DI, Polgar E, Shehab SA, Todd AJ. 2004. Peripheral axotomy induces depletion of the vesicular glutamate transporter VGLUT1 in central terminals of myelinated afferent fibres in the rat spinal cord. *Brain Res*, 1017: 69-76.

Hughes DI, Scott DT, Todd AJ, Riddell JS. 2003. Lack of evidence for sprouting of Abeta afferents into the superficial laminas of the spinal cord dorsal horn after nerve section. *J Neurosci*, 23: 9491-9499.

Hwang JH, Yaksh TL. 1997. The effect of spinal GABA receptor agonists on tactile allodynia in a surgically-induced neuropathic pain model in the rat. *Pain*, 70: 15-22.

Joseph EK, Chen X, Khasar SG, Levine JD. 2004. Novel mechanism of enhanced nociception in a model of AIDS therapy-induced painful peripheral neuropathy in the rat. *Pain*, 107: 147-158.

Kim SH, Chung JM. 1992. An experimental model for peripheral neuropathy produced by segmental spinal nerve ligation in the rat. *Pain*, 50: 355-363.

Knyihár E, Csillik B. 1976. Effect of peripheral axotomy on the fine structure and histochemistry of the Rolando substance: degenerative atrophy of central processes of pseudounipolar cells. *Exp Brain Res*, 26: 73-87.

Lee BH, Yoon YW, Chung KS, Chung JM. 1998. Comparison of sympathetic sprouting in sensory ganglia in three animal models of neuropathic pain. *Exp Brain Res*, 120: 432-438.

Madiai F, Hussain SR, Goettl VM, Burry RW, Stephens RL Jr, Hackshaw KV. 2003. Upregulation of FGF-2 in reactive spinal cord astrocytes following unilateral lumbar spinal nerve ligation. *Exp Brain Res*, 148: 366-376.

Malcangio M, Ramer MS, Jones MG, McMahon SB. 2000. Abnormal substance P release from the spinal cord following injury to primary sensory neurons. *Eur J Neurosci*, 12: 397-399.

Malmberg AB, Chen C, Tonegawa S, Basbaum AI. 1997. Preserved acute pain and reduced neuropathic pain in mice lacking PKCgamma. *Science*, 278: 279-283.

Martin WJ, Malmberg AB, Basbaum AI. 2001. PKCgamma contributes to a subset of the NMDA-dependent spinal circuits that underlie injury-induced persistent pain. *J Neurosci*, 21: 5321-5327.

McLachlan EM, Jänig W, Devor M, Michaelis M. 1993. Peripheral nerve injury triggers noradrenergic sprouting within dorsal root ganglia. *Nature*, 363: 543-546.

Moore KA, Kohno T, Karchewski LA, Scholz J, Baba H, Woolf CJ. 2002. Partial peripheral nerve injury promotes a selective loss of GABAergic inhibition in the superficial dorsal horn of the spinal cord. *J Neurosci*, 22: 6724-6731.

Mosconi T, Kruger L. 1996. Fixed-diameter polyethylene cuffs applied to the rat sciatic nerve induce a painful neuropathy: ultrastructural morphometric analysis of axonal alterations. *Pain*, 64: 37-57.

Munger BL, Bennett GJ, Kajander KC. 1992. An experimental painful peripheral neuropathy due to nerve constriction. I. Axonal pathology in the sciatic nerve. *Exp Neurol*, 118: 204-214.

Nagy GG, Al-Ayyan M, Andrew D, Fukaya M, Watanabe M, Todd AJ. 2004. Widespread expression of the AMPA receptor GluR2 subunit at glutamatergic synapses in the rat spinal cord and phosphorylation of GluR1 in response to noxious stimulation revealed with an antigen-unmasking method. *J Neurosci*, 24: 5766-5777.

Noguchi K, Dubner R, de Leon M, Senba E, Ruda MA. 1994. Axotomy induces preprotachykinin gene expression in a subpopulation of dorsal root ganglion neurons. *J Neurosci Res*, 37: 596-603.

Noguchi K, Kawai Y, Fukuoka T, Senba E, Miki K. 1995. Substance P induced by peripheral nerve injury in primary afferent sensory neurons and its effect on dorsal column nucleus neurons. *J Neurosci*, 15: 7633-7643.

Okamoto M, Baba H, Goldstein PA, Higashi H, Shimoji K, Yoshimura M. 2001. Functional reorganization of sensory pathways in the rat spinal dorsal horn following peripheral nerve injury. *J Physiol*, 532: 241-250.

Pitcher GM, Henry JL. 2004. Nociceptive response to innocuous mechanical stimulation is mediated via myelinated afferents and NK-1 receptor activation in a rat model of neuropathic pain. *Exp Neurol*, 186: 173-197.

Pitcher GM, Ritchie J, Henry JL. 1999. Nerve constriction in the rat: model of neuropathic, surgical and central pain. *Pain*, 83: 37-46.

Polgár E, Gray S, Riddell JS, Todd AJ. 2004. Lack of evidence for significant neuronal loss in laminae I-III of the spinal dorsal horn of the rat in the chronic constriction injury model. *Pain*, 111: 144-150.

Polgár E, Hughes DI, Arham AZ, Todd AJ. 2005. Loss of neurons from laminae I-III of the spinal dorsal horn is not required for development of tactile allodynia in the spared nerve injury model of neuropathic pain. *J Neurosci*, 25:6648-6666.

Polgár E, Hughes DI, Riddell JS, Maxwell DJ, Puskar Z, Todd AJ. 2003. Selective loss of spinal GABAergic or glycinergic neurons is not necessary for development of thermal hyperalgesia in the chronic constriction injury model of neuropathic pain. *Pain*, 104: 229-239.

Polomano RC, Mannes AJ, Clark US, Bennett GJ. 2001. A painful peripheral neuropathy in the rat produced by the chemotherapeutic drug, paclitaxel. *Pain*, 94: 293-304.

Popratiloff A, Weinberg RJ, Rustioni A. 1998. AMPA receptors at primary afferent synapses in substantia gelatinosa after sciatic nerve section. *Eur J Neurosci*, 10: 3220-3230.

Rexed B. 1952. The cytoarchitectonic organization of the spinal cord in the cat. *J Comp Neurol*, 96: 415-495.

Ruocco I, Cuello AC, Ribeiro-da-Silva A. 2000. Peripheral nerve injury leads to the establishment of a novel pattern of sympathetic fibre innervation in the rat skin. *J Comp Neurol*, 422: 287-296.

Seltzer Z, Dubner R, Shirabe S. 1990. A novel behavioral model of neuropathic pain disorders produced in rats by partial sciatic nerve injury. *Pain*, 43: 205-218.

Sugimoto T, Bennett GJ, Kajander KC. 1990. Transsynaptic degeneration in the superficial dorsal horn after sciatic nerve injury—effects of a chronic constriction cnjury, transection, and strychnine. *Pain*, 42: 205-213.

Todd AJ, Ribeiro-da-Silva A. 2005. Molecular architecture of the dorsal horn. In: *Neurobiology of Pain*. Hunt SP and Koltzenburg M, eds. Oxford: Oxford University Press. 65-94.

Tong YG, Wang HF, Ju G, Grant G, Hökfelt T, Zhang X. 1999. Increased uptake and transport of cholera toxin B-subunit in dorsal root ganglion neurons after peripheral axotomy: possible implications for sensory sprouting. *J Comp Neurol*, 404: 143-158.

Tsuda M, Shigemoto-Mogami Y, Koizumi S, Mizokoshi A, Kohsaka S, Salter MW, Inoue K. 2003. P2X$_4$ receptors induced in spinal microglia gate tactile allodynia after nerve injury. *Nature*, 424: 778-783.

Whiteside GT, Munglani R. 2001. Cell death in the superficial dorsal horn in a model of neuropathic pain. *J Neurosci Res*, 64: 168-173.

Woolf CJ, Shortland P, Coggeshall RE. 1992. Peripheral nerve injury triggers central sprouting of myelinated afferents. *Nature*, 355: 75-78.

Yaksh TL. 1989. Behavioral and autonomic correlates of the tactile evoked allodynia produced by spinal glycine inhibition: effects of modulatory receptor systems and excitatory amino acid antagonists. *Pain*, 37: 111-123.

Yen L, Bennett GJ, Ribeiro-da-Silva A. 2006. Sympathetic sprouting and changes in nociceptive sensory innervation in the glabrous skin of the rat hind paw following partial peripheral nerve injury. *J Comp Neurol*, 495: 679-690.

Spinal Microglia in Neuropathic Pain Plasticity

CHAPTER 24

Michael W. Salter

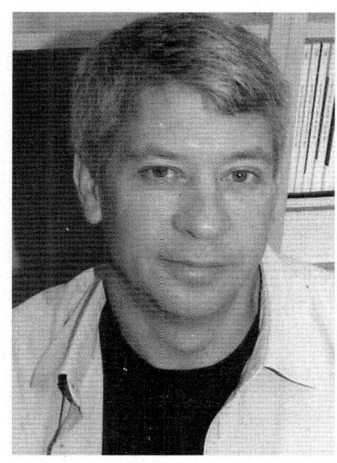

Dr. Salter is a Professor and Senior Scientist in the University of Toronto, Centre for the Study of Pain, Canada. He received his MD degree from the University of Western Ontario and continued on to a PhD at McGill University. He pursued postdoctoral research at the Toronto Hospital and Mount Sinai Hospital, Toronto, Canada.

MAJOR CONTRIBUTIONS

1. Lu YM, Roder JC, Davidow J, Salter MW. 1998. Src activation in the induction of long-term potentiation in CA1 hippocampal neurons. *Science*, 279: 1363-1368.

2. Woolf CJ and Salter M. 2000. Neuronal plasticity — increasing the gain in pain. *Science*, 288:1765-1768.

3. Cheng H-Y M, Pitcher, GM, Laviolette SR, Whishaw IQ, Tong KI, Kockeritz L, Goncalves J, Wada Y, Sarosi I, Joza NA, Woodgett J, Ikura M, van der Kooy D, Salter MW, Penninger JM. 2002. Identification of DREAM as a critical transcription repressor for pain modulation. *Cell*, 108: 31-43.

4. Kalia LV and Salter MW. 2004. Src kinases: a hub of synaptic regulation. *Nature Reviews Neuroscience*, 5: 317-328.

5. Coull JAM, Beggs S, Boudreau D, Boivin D, Tsuda M, Inoue K, Salter MW, DeKoninck Y. 2005. BDNF from microglia mediates the shift in neuronal anion gradient that underliesneuropathic pain. *Nature*, 438: 1017-1021.

MAIN TOPICS

Plasticity in the dorsal horn nociceptive processing network

Microglial activation after peripheral nerve injury

Spinal microglia are intermediaries of pain plasticity

How are microglia activated following peripheral nerve injury?

Mechanism of microglia-to-neuron signaling in the dorsal horn

SUMMARY

Neuropathic pain affects a growing number of people worldwide, arising from a diversity of causes including traumatic nerve injury, neurotoxic chemicals or diseases that affect peripheral nerves, such as diabetes, HIV/AIDS and cancer. Despite these varying causes, it is clear that a principal cause of neuropathic pain is pathological alterations in the balance of excitation and inhibition in dorsal horn of the spinal cord resulting in hyperexcitability and enhanced activity in central nociceptive networks. It is the neuropathology that must be targeted for effective therapy of which there is none presently available. The focus of understanding of neuropathic pain mechanisms has been on neuronal processes that produce lasting enhancement of excitation or suppression of inhibition. There is, however, growing evidence that critical cellular processes are not restricted to neurons in the dorsal horn. Rather recent findings demonstrate involvement of glia, and of glia-neuronal signaling, in initiating and sustaining enhancement of nociceptive transmission. In particular, a role has emerged for microglia in pain hypersensitivity following nerve injury. Thus, an expanded understanding of cellular and molecular signalling mechanisms in the dorsal horn that will provide a basis of creating new types of strategies for management, and also for diagnosis, of neuropathic pain needs to include both neurons and glia.

INTRODUCTION

As is discussed in detail in other chapters, pain exists in three mechanistically distinct types—nociceptive, inflammatory and neuropathic. Nociceptive pain is a crucial defensive mechanism that warns an individual of recent or imminent damage to the body, and is produced as the physiological consequence of normally functioning of peripheral and central nervous systems. Inflammatory or neuropathic pain, by contrast, are reflections of aberrant functioning of peripheral or central nervous systems that have been pathologically modified. Typically, these persistent pains are not directly related to tissue damage, and may persist long after any tissue damage, which may have initiated nociceptive pain, has subsided. Recognition that the pathological alterations underlying and amplifying chronic pain occur in the peripheral nervous system or numerous sites within the central nervous system has led to the emerging concept that chronic pain is a disorder of the nervous system. More precisely, chronic pain should be considered a group of mechanistically separable nervous system disorders produced and maintained by one or more abnormal cellular signalling processes.

PLASTICITY IN THE DORSAL HORN NOCICEPTIVE PROCESSING NETWORK

In the dorsal horn of the spinal cord is located a complex nociceptive processing network through which inputs from the periphery are transduced and modulated (Fig.24.1). The network includes local, as well as descending, inhibitory control mechanisms, and the output of this network is transmitted to other areas of the CNS involved in sensory, emotional, autonomic and motor processing. Normally this network reliably transduces inputs from nociceptive primary afferents such that the output, which of course serves as the input to these brain areas, is well-matched to the degree of peripheral tissue damage – nociceptive pain (Fig.24.1A). By contrast, a prominent feature of persistent pain is aberrant activation of intracellular signaling pathways, the ultimate effect of which is alteration of the normally finely tuned balance of excitation and inhibition in dorsal horn nociceptive processing network such that the output of this network, for a given input, is increased (Fig.24.1B). This increased output may arise from alteration of the intrinsic voltage-dependent or – independent currents in dorsal horn neurons, enhancement of excitatory inputs or depression of inhibitory control mechanisms, or a combination of these. The diverse mechanisms have been subject to several recent reviews and are described in other chapters. Here I focus on the role of glia cells, and of neuronal-glial-neuronal signalling, in nerve injury-induced pain.

MICROGLIAL ACTIVATION AFTER PERIPHERAL NERVE INJURY

Although outnumbering neurons by approximately 10 : 1 glial cells have traditionally been viewed as cells that serve primarily housekeeping roles, this has changed dramatically over the past decade. Glia are known to play key roles in regulating synaptic transmission and participating in synaptic plasticity.

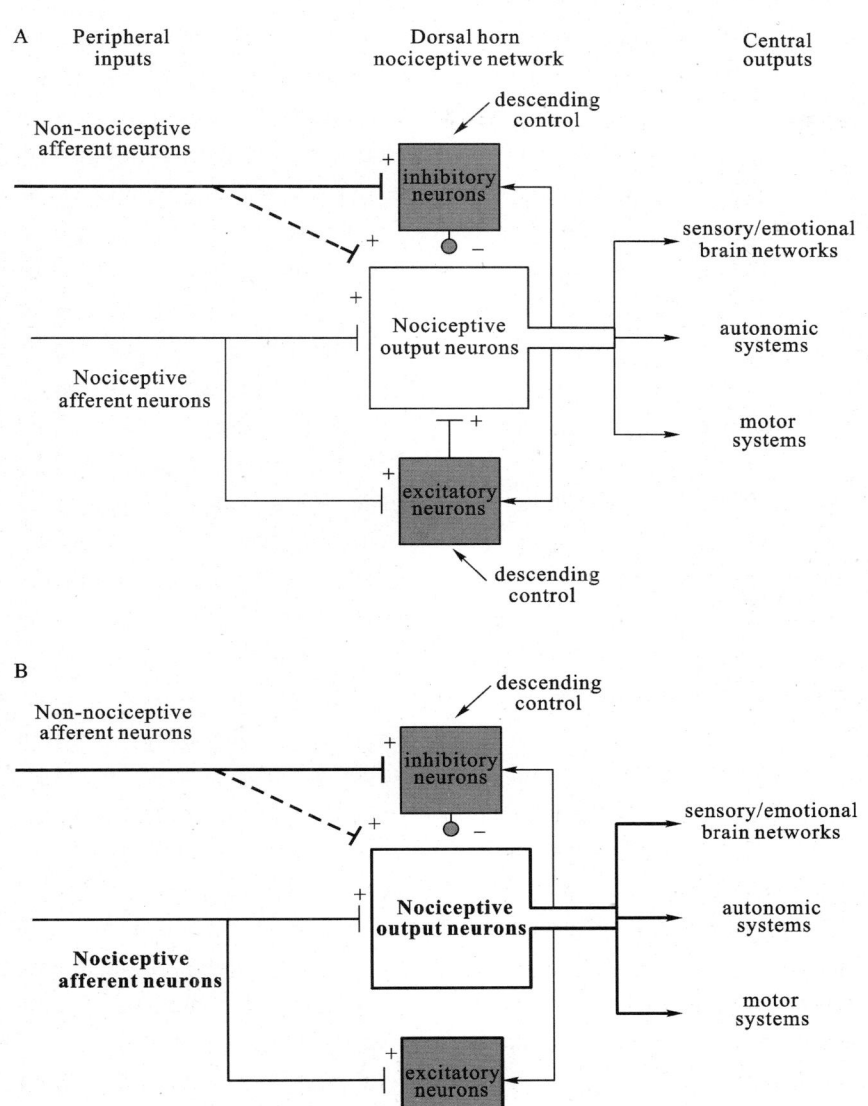

A   Peripheral inputs

Dorsal horn nociceptive network

Central outputs

Fig.24.1 Schematic illustration of the peripheral input, local processing and output of the dorsal horn nociceptive network. The basal functioning of the network, underlying nociceptive pain, is shown in (A). The dashed line from non-nociceptive primary afferents to the nociceptive output neurons signifies that some, but not all, nociceptive output neurons receive non-nociceptive input and this might be direct or indirect. In (B) mechanisms for enhancing the output of the nociceptive processing network, underlying some forms of persistent pain, are indicated by the highlighted lines and boldface type. These mechanisms include: increased activity of primary afferent nociceptors and enhancement of transmission onto nociceptive output neurons; enhanced activity or transmission of excitatory interneurons; depressed number, activity or transmission of inhibitory interneurons; or alteration of the intrinsic membrane properties of the nociceptive output neurons.

In particular for pain resulting from peripheral nerve injury, there is a abundant evidence indicating that hyperalgesia, allodynia and ongoing pain involve active participation of glia in the spinal dorsal horn. The CNS contains three types of glia—astrocytes, oligodendrocytes and microglia. It is the microglia, which comprise 5%-10% of the total glial population in the CNS, that have emerged as a central character in enhanced pain behaviours after peripheral nerve-injury.

Under normal conditions microglia are in a so-called "resting" state, which is now known to be an active surveillance mode in which these cells continuously and vigorously monitor the local environment. Even in the "resting" state, microglia show re-

sponses within minutes to neural damage. In addition, a wide variety of stimuli that threaten physiological homeostasis evoke a program of changes in morphology, gene expression, function and number in microglia. As defined by responses following neuroinflammatory stimulation there are four cardinal signs of microglial activation: (i) hypertrophy and shape change, (ii) proliferation, (iii) immunophenotypic change, and (iv) change in secretory molecules produced. Activated microglia change their morphology from a resting, ramified shape progressively to retract small secondary and tertiary processes. The main processes become engorged and ultimately the activated microglia take on an amoeboid shape. Such fully activated microglia are capable of performing phagocytosis, giving rise to the view that these cells are resident macrophages of the CNS. Not only do microglia undergo dramatic morphological changes they also proliferate generating new cells capable of local action. Indeed microglia are the only non-stem in the CNS that is capable of division. In addition to shape changes and proliferation, during activation these cells dramatically alter the repertoire of molecules expressed on the cell surface. These molecules include CD11b/CD18 [also known as complement receptor 3 (CR3) or Mac-1; comprised of integrin subunits αM (CD11b) and $\beta 2$ (CD18) and recognized by the widely-used antibody OX-42]. Activated microglia also show enhanced express immunomolecules such as major histocompatibility complex (MHC) class II which play a role in antigen presentation to T-lymphocytes. Activated microglia produce and release various chemical mediators, including proinflammatory cytokines, which can produce immunological actions and can also act on neurons to alter their function.

Activation is not uniform however – different responses are evoked by different types of stimulation and also different responses to the same stimulation occur in different regions of the CNS. Therefore, the response state of microglia needs to be investigated based on the CNS region and the stimulus producing activation. Within the spinal cord dorsal horn the four cardinal signs of microglial activation develop in a stereotyped fashion following injury to a peripheral nerve (Fig.24.2, see also the color plate). Evidence for microglial activation following injury to sensory nerves goes back more than 25 years. Subsequently the state of microglia in the spinal cord has been examined in a variety of models: compression, ligation or transaction of sciatic nerve, spinal nerves or peripheral branches of the sciatic nerve. Common to these models, a feature that is often considered to be clinically relevant, is that after the nerve injury withdrawal behaviours are evoked by stimuli that are innocuous, like gentle mechanical stimulation. The potential clinical relevance of the behaviour change is that allodynia is a common, and often very severe, component of neuropathic pain in humans. Following peripheral nerve injury there is series of changes in microglia within spinal dorsal horn, although there may be some variability between the models in terms of the extent and time course of the changes. Within hours after peripheral nerve injury, signs of microglia activation are observed with the small soma becoming hypertrophic and the long and thin processes withdrawing. Subsequently, microglia proliferate, with this peaking about 3 days after nerve injury. After peripheral nerve injury the microglia in the dorsal horn show an increased level of a number of activation "marker" proteins including CD11b/CD18, toll-like receptor 4 (TLR4), cluster determinant14 (CD14), CD4 and MHC class II protein.

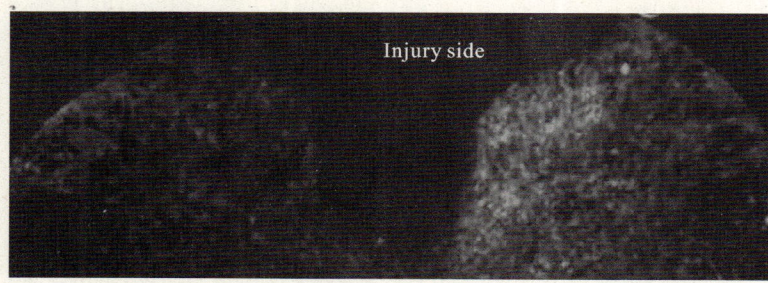

Fig.24.2 Activation of microglia in the spinal cord ipsilateral to the side of peripheral nerve injury. The bright indicates immunofluorescence of OX-42.

SPINAL MICROGLIA ARE INTERMEDIARIES OF PAIN PLASTICITY

While many reports have shown a correlation between activation of microglia and signs of pain hypersensitivity, only recently was it established that microglia have a causal role in these nerve injury-evoked pain behaviours in studies implicating $P2X_4$ receptors and p38 MAP kinase.

$P2X_4$ receptors are a subtype of the P2X family

of ligand-gated ion channels that are activated by ATP. It has been found that mechanical allodynia following spinal nerve ligation is acutely reversed by means of intrathecally administering a P2X$_4$ antagonist. However, P2X$_4$ receptors are found neither in neurons nor astrocytes the dorsal horn, but these receptors are expressed in microglia. The expression is low in the naïve spinal cord but increases progressively in the days following nerve injury paralleling the development of mechanical allodynia. Inhibiting the rise in P2X$_4$ expression prevents the development of allodynia. Thus, microglial P2X$_4$ receptors are required for mechanical allodynia after nerve injury. Moreover, it has been found that in otherwise naïve animals, mechanical allodynia develops after administering microglia in which P2X$_4$ receptors are stimulated *in vitro*. By contrast, unstimulated microglia do not cause allodynia. Thus, stimulating P2X$_4$ receptors in activated microglia appears to be sufficient as well as required for causing mechanical allodynia.

Like blockade of P2X$_4$ receptors, inhibiting p38 MAP kinase pharmacologically, by means of an inhibitor administered intrathecally, reverses mechanical allodynia following spinal nerve ligation. Infusing the p38 inhibitor beginning prior to the nerve injury prevented allodynia from developing. The nerve lesion leads to persistent activation of p38 MAP kinase, as judged by labeling for phospho-p38 MAP kinase, which is restricted to microglia. Thus, these two proteins, p38 P2X4 receptors and MAP kinase, and by inference activated microglia themselves, are critical for maintaining mechanical allodynia after peripheral nerve injury. These findings thereby provide open the question of whether agents that inhibit function or expression of these proteins may cause reduction of neuropathic pain in humans.

HOW ARE MICROGLIA ACTIVATED FOLLOWING PERIPHERAL NERVE INJURY?

One key mechanistic issue is to determine how microglia in the spinal cord become activated after nerve injury in the periphery (Fig.24.3). A large number of molecules are known to be capable of activating microglia and thus there is a large list of candidates for the signaling molecules most proximal to these cells. Very recently it has been reported that mice lacking TLR4, a member of the interleukin 1/toll-like receptor superfamily, show markedly reduced mechanical allodynia following peripheral-nerve injury compared to wild type controls. Moreover, it was found that

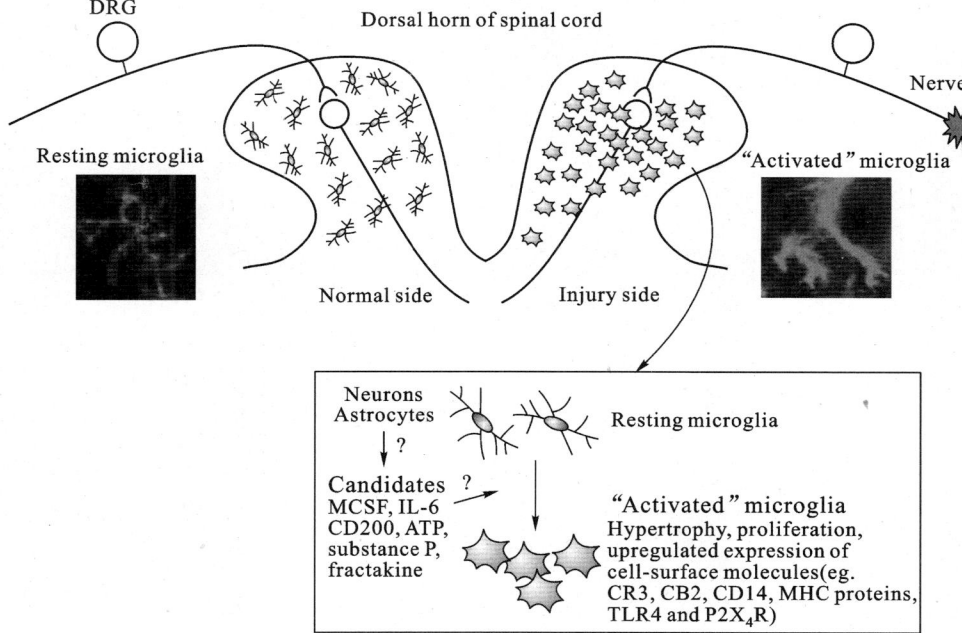

Fig.24.3 Possible mechanisms for activation of dorsal horn microglia after peripheral nerve injury.

suppressing TLR4 expression in the spinal cord by antisense oligonucleotides administered daily suppressed the development of allodynia. Not only was the allodynia suppressed but the activation of the microglia, as judged by expression of CR3 and other molecular markers was also markedly blunted. Thus, TLR4 in spinal microglia appears to be a key mediator of microglial activation after peripheral nerve injury. One minor caveat is that intrathecally administered antisense oligonucleotides may be able reach the dorsal root ganglia and therefore it is possible that depressed expression of TLR4 there is involved. Nevertheless, this report opens up the important question of what is the identity of the endogenous ligand for TLR4 and which cells are producing it? Also, because neither the allodynia nor the microglia activation was completely prevented in either the knockouts or by the antisense oligonucleotides, there must be additional molecules and signaling pathways that participate in the response to peripheral nerve injury. Identifying these additional pathways is a crucial goal for the future.

MECHANISM OF MICROGLIA-TO-NEURON SIGNALING IN THE DORSAL HORN

The other key issue is to determine how microglia signal to neurons in the dorsal horn nociceptive network in order to effect an increase in network output. There are a number of possibilities to consider because microglia could conceivably interact with neurons through direct contact factors, through release of diffusible chemical mediators, or even by phagocytosis of neuroactive molecules in the local environment (Fig.24.4). Moreover, the effect of the microglia signaling on the dorsal horn neurons could be via facilitation of excitatory synaptic transmission or the activity of local excitatory neurons, suppression of inhibition or inhibitory neuron activity, alteration of the intrinsic membrane properties of the dorsal horn nociceptive output neurons, or a combination of these.

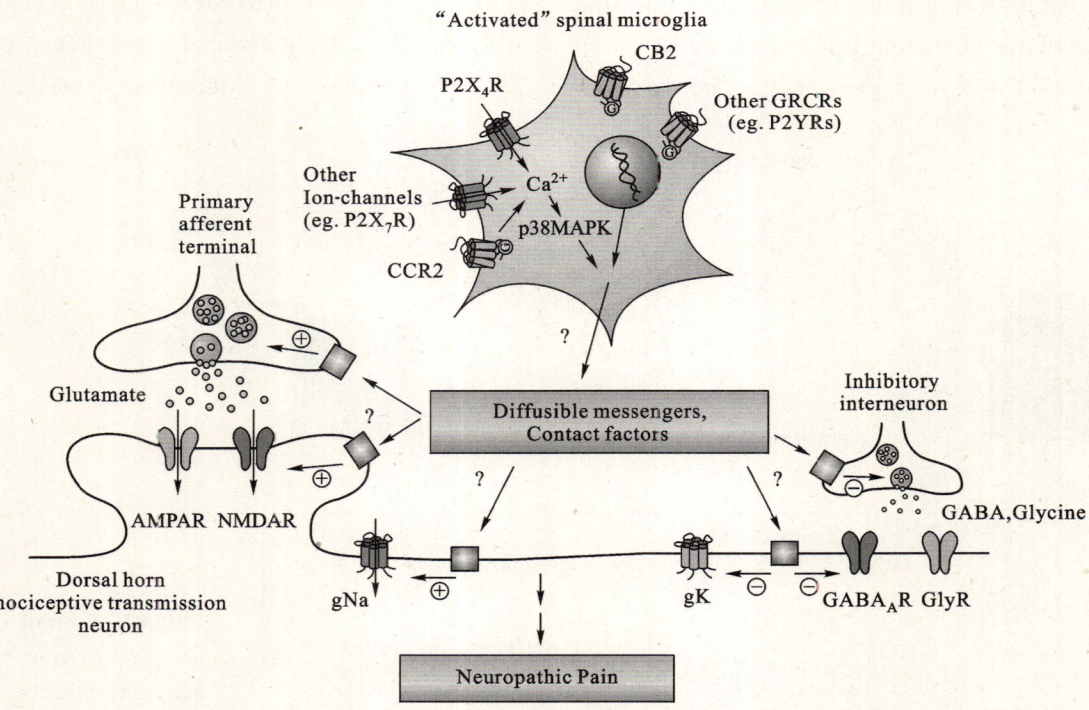

Fig.24.4 Potential effects of microglia on excitatory or inhibitory synaptic transmission, or on intrinsic membrane conductances in spinal dorsal horn nociceptive network output neurons.

Recently, the effect of microglia on spinal neurons in lamina I of the dorsal horn has been investigated. These neurons are one of the major outputs of the dorsal horn nociceptive network, and a rise in their intracellular chloride concentration, which causes disinhibition, is a key mechanism for mechanical allodynia following peripheral nerve injury, as is described in the chapter on spinal inhibitory mechanisms. It has been discovered that administering ATP-stimulated microglia intrathecally in naïve rats causes accumulation of the anion chloride in lamina I neurons in the dorsal horn. Moreover, acute pharmacological blockade of P2X receptors in the dorsal horn reverses the increase in chloride in lamina I neurons observed following peripheral nerve injury. In addition, it was found that microglia produce this increase chloride via releasing brain-derived neurotrophic factor (BDNF) which acts on its cognate receptor, trkB, on lamina I neurons. These findings thereby define a cellular signaling pathway from microglia to neurons that has a major role in mechanical allodynia following experimental nerve injury (Fig.24.5). The extent to which this pathway is activated in humans with neuropathic pain, and contributes to this pain, is now open for investigation.

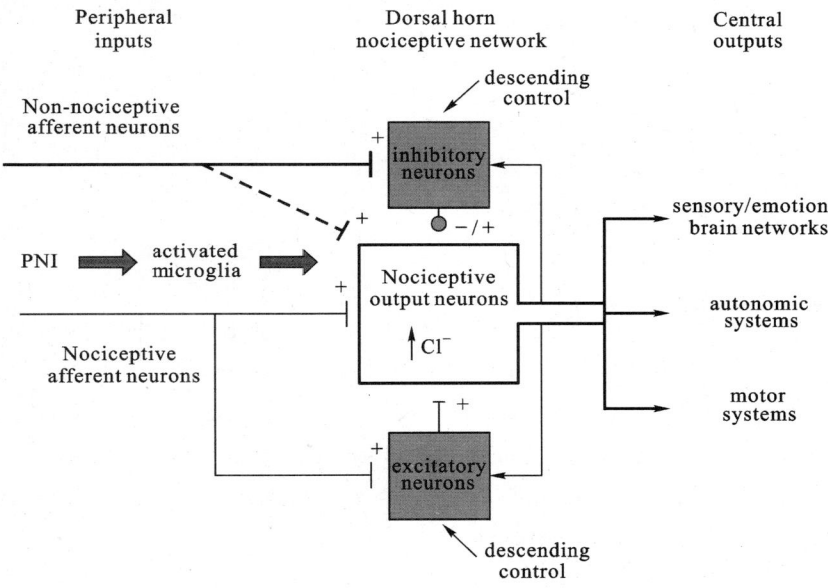

Fig.24.5   Role for microglia activation and microglia-neuron signaling following peripheral nerve injury (PNI). Microglia become activated after PNI and signal to dorsal horn output nociceptive neurons causing an increase in intracellular chloride (Cl⁻) concentration that results in disinhibition (−/+) and enhanced output of the network.

GENERAL CITATIONS

Carson MJ, Thrash JC, Lo D. 2004. Analysis of microglial gene expression: identifying targets for CNS neurodegenerative and autoimmune disease. *Am J Pharmacogenomics*, 4:321-330.

Ji RR, Strichartz G. 2004. Cell signaling and the genesis of neuropathic pain. *Sci STKE*, 2004: reE14.

Marchand F, Perretti M, McMahon SB. 2005. Role of the immune system in chronic pain. *Nat Rev Neurosci*, 6: 521-532.

Salter MW. 2005. Cellular signalling pathways of spinal pain neuroplasticity as targets for analgesic development. *Curr Top Med Chem*, 5:557-567.

Stoll G, Jander S. 1999. The role of microglia and macrophages in the pathophysiology of the CNS. *Prog Neurobiol*, 58: 233-247.

Streit WJ, Walter SA, Pennell NA. 1999. Reactive microgliosis. *Prog Neurobiol*, 57:563-581.

Tsuda M, Inoue K, Salter MW. 2005. Neuropathic pain and spinal microglia: a big problem from molecules in "small" glia. *Trends Neurosci*, 28: 101-107.

Watkins LR, Milligan ED, Maier SF. 2001. Glial activation: a driving force for pathological pain. *Trends Neurosci*, 24: 450-455.

Woolf CJ, Salter MW. 2006. State dependent plasticity. In: *The Textbook of Pain*, 5th ed. Koltzenburg M and McMahon

SB, eds. 91-106.

DISCOVERY CITATIONS

Abbadie C, Lindia JA, Cumiskey AM, Peterson LB, Mudgett JS, Bayne EK, DeMartino JA, MacIntyre DE, Forrest MJ. 2003. Impaired neuropathic pain responses in mice lacking the chemokine receptor CCR2. *Proc Natl Acad Sci USA*, 100: 7947-7952.

Colburn RW, DeLeo JA, Rickman AJ, Yeager MP, Kwon P, Hickey WF. 1997. Dissociation of microglial activation and neuropathic pain behaviors following peripheral nerve injury in the rat. *J Neuroimmunol*, 79: 163-175.

Coull JA, Boudreau D, Bachand K, Prescott SA, Nault F, Sik A, De Koninck P, De Koninck Y. 2003. Trans-synaptic shift in anion gradient in spinal lamina I neurons as a mechanism of neuropathic pain. *Nature*, 424:938-942.

Cova JL, Aldskogius H, Arvidsson J, Molander C. 1988. Changes in microglial cell numbers in the spinal cord dorsal horn following brachial plexus transection in the adult rat. *Exp Brain Res*, 73: 61-68.

Coyle DE. 1998. Partial peripheral nerve injury leads to activation of astroglia and microglia which parallels the development of allodynic behavior. *Glia*, 23: 75-83.

Ehlers MR. 2000. CR3: a general purpose adhesion-recognition receptor essential for innate immunity. *Microbes Infect*, 2: 289-294.

Eriksson NP, Persson JK, Svensson M, Arvidsson J, Molander C, Aldskogius H. 1993. A quantitative analysis of the microglial cell reaction in central primary sensory projection territories following peripheral nerve injury in the adult rat. *Exp Brain Res*, 96: 19-27.

Jin SX, Zhuang ZY, Woolf CJ, Ji RR. 2003. p38 mitogen-activated protein kinase is activated after a spinal nerve ligation in spinal cord microglia and dorsal root ganglion neurons and contributes to the generation of neuropathic pain. *J Neurosci*, 23: 4 017-4 022.

Ledeboer A, Sloane EM, Milligan ED, Frank MG, Mahony JH, Maier SF, Watkins LR. 2005. Minocycline attenuates mechanical allodynia and proinflammatory cytokine expression in rat models of pain facilitation. *Pain*, 115: 71-83.

Lindia JA, McGowan E, Jochnowitz N, Abbadie C. 2005. Induction of CX3CL1 expression in astrocytes and CX3CR1 in microglia in the spinal cord of a rat model of neuropathic pain. *J Pain*, 6: 434-438.

Ling EA. 1979. Evidence for a haematogenous origin of some of the macrophages appearing in the spinal cord of the rat after dorsal rhizotomy. *J Anat*, 128: 143-154.

Liu L, Tornqvist E, Mattsson P, Eriksson NP, Persson JK, Morgan BP, Aldskogius H, Svensson M. 1995. Complement and clusterin in the spinal cord dorsal horn and gracile nucleus following sciatic nerve injury in the adult rat. *Neuroscience*, 68: 167-179.

Milligan ED, Zapata V, Chacur M, Schoeniger D, Biedenkapp J, O'Connor KA, Verge GM, Chapman G, Green P, Foster AC, Naeve GS, Maier SF, Watkins LR. 2004. Evidence that exogenous and endogenous fractalkine can induce spinal nociceptive facilitation in rats. *Eur J Neurosci*, 20: 2 294-2 302.

Raghavendra V, Tanga F, DeLeo JA. 2003. Inhibition of microglial activation attenuates the development but not existing hypersensitivity in a rat model of neuropathy. *J Pharmacol Exp Ther*, 306: 624-630.

Sweitzer SM, Colburn RW, Rutkowski M, DeLeo JA. 1999. Acute peripheral inflammation induces moderate glial activation and spinal IL-1beta expression that correlates with pain behavior in the rat. *Brain Res*, 829: 209-221.

Sweitzer SM, White KA, Dutta C, DeLeo JA. 2002. The differential role of spinal MHC class II and cellular adhesion molecules in peripheral inflammatory versus neuropathic pain in rodents. *J Neuroimmunol*, 125: 82-93.

Tanga FY, Nutile-McMenemy N, DeLeo JA. 2005. The CNS role of Toll-like receptor 4 in innate neuroimmunity and painful neuropathy. *Proc Natl Acad Sci USA*, 102: 5 856-5 861.

Tanga FY, Raghavendra V, DeLeo JA. 2004. Quantitative real-time RT-PCR assessment of spinal microglial and astrocytic activation markers in a rat model of neuropathic pain. *Neurochem Int*, 45: 397-407.

Tsuda M, Mizokoshi A, Shigemoto-Mogami Y, Koizumi S, Inoue K. 2004. Activation of p38 mitogen-activated protein kinase in spinal hyperactive microglia contributes to pain hypersensitivity following peripheral nerve injury. *Glia*, 45: 89-95.

Tsuda M, Shigemoto-Mogami Y, Koizumi S, Mizokoshi A, Kohsaka S, Salter MW, Inoue K. 2003. P2X$_4$ receptors induced in spinal microglia gate tactile allodynia after nerve injury. *Nature*, 424: 778-783.

Twining CM, Sloane EM, Schoeniger DK, Milligan ED, Martin D, Marsh H, Maier SF, Watkins LR. 2005. Activation of the spinal cord complement cascade might contribute to mechanical allodynia induced by three animal models of spinal sensitization. *J Pain*, 6: 174-183.

Zhang J, Hoffert C, Vu HK, Groblewski T, Ahmad S, O'Donnell D. 2003. Induction of CB2 receptor expression in the rat spinal cord of neuropathic but not inflammatory chronic pain models. *Eur J Neurosci*, 17: 2 750-2 754.

Zhuang ZY, Gerner P, Woolf CJ, Ji RR. 2005. ERK is sequentially activated in neurons, microglia, and astrocytes by spinal nerve ligation and contributes to mechanical allodynia in this neuropathic pain model. *Pain*, 114: 149-159.

Part VIII Cortical Plasticity, Reorganization and Amputation

ACC Plasticity

CHAPTER 25

Min Zhuo*

MAJOR CONTRIBUTIONS

1. Wei F, Wang G-D, Kerchner GA, Kim SJ, Xu H-M, Chen Z-F and Zhuo M. 2001. Genetic enhancement of persistent pain by forebrain NR2B overexpression. *Nature Neuroscience*, 4: 164-169 (Comment in: *The Lancet*, 357:367, 2001; Nature Press Release).

2. Wei F and Zhuo M. 2001. Potentiation of synaptic responses in the anterior cingulate cortex following digital amputation in rat. *Journal of Physiology* (*Lond*), 532: 823-833.

3. Wei F, Qiu CS, Liauw J, Robinson DA, Ho N, Chatila T, Zhuo M. 2002. Calcium calmodulin-dependent protein kinase IV is required for fear memory. *Nature Neuroscience*, 5: 573- 579 (Comment in: *The Lancet* 360: 426, 2002).

4. Wei F, Qiu CS, Kim SJ, Muglia L, Maas JW, Pineda VV, Xu HM, Chen ZF, Storm DR, Muglia LJ, Zhuo M. 2002. Genetic elimination of behavioral sensitization in mice lacking calmodulin-stimulated adenylyl cyclases. *Neuron*, 36: 713-726.

5. Zhao MG, Toyoda H, Lee Y-S, We LJ, Ko SW, Zhang XH, Jia YH, Shum F, Xu H, Li B-M, Kaang B-K and Zhuo M. 2005. Roles of NMDA NR2B subtype receptor in prefrontal long-term potentiation and contexual fear memory. *Neuron*, 47: 1-14.

MAIN TOPICS

Synaptic transmission in the ACC undergo long-term potentiation

Long-term depression in the ACC

Long-term enhancement of synaptic responses in the ACC after injury

Loss of long-term depression after injury

Genetic enhancement of chronic pain by NR2B over-expression

Enhanced NR2B expression by injury

Genetic deletion of calcium-stimulated adenylyl cyclases

Activation of neuronal plasticity-related immediate early genes in the ACC after injury

Model for molecular mechanism of injury-related potentiation in the ACC

Activation of ACC triggered fear and aversive behaviors

Lesion or chemical blockade of ACC affects chronic pain in animals and humans

SUMMARY

Neurons and synapses in the central nervous systems are plastic, and can undergo longterm changes throughout life. Studies of molecular and cellular mechanisms of such changes not only provide important insight into how we learn and store new knowledge in our brains, but also reveal the mechanisms of pathological changes occurring following an injury. While neuronal mechanisms underlying physiological functions such as learning and memory may share some common signaling molecules with abnormal or injury-related changes in the brain during the induction, distinct synaptic and neuronal network mechanisms are involved in pathological pain as compared with that of cognitive learning and memory. Nociceptive information is transmitted and regulated at

---

* The introduction of Dr. Zhuo, please refer to Chapter 8.

different levels of the brain, from the spinal cord to forebrains. Furthermore, N-methyl-D-aspartate (NMDA) receptor-dependent, calcium-calmodulin (CaM) activated adenylyl cyclases (AC1 and AC8) in the anterior cingulate cortex (ACC) play important roles in the induction and expression of persistent inflammatory and neuropathic pain. Neuronal activity in the ACC can also influence nociceptive transmission in the spinal cord dorsal horn through activation of endogenous facilitatory system. Our results provide important synaptic and molecular insights into physiological responses to the injury, including behavioral, emotional and memory.

INTRODUCTION

In this chapter, we shall focus on forebrain areas. Among many different regions activated by injury, ACC and insular cortex are two major forebrain areas thought to be important for pain perception and persistent pain. Most of recent studies, in particular, those at molecular and cellular levels, are carried out in the ACC. We will discuss and explore the role of ACC. Future studies of molecular mechanism for insular cortex are clearly needed.

Animal and human studies consistently suggest that forebrain neurons play important roles in nociception and pain perception. In animal studies, lesions of the medial frontal cortex, including the ACC, significantly reduced acute nociceptive responses, and inhibited formalin injection induced aversive memory behaviors. In patients with frontal lobotomies or cingulotomies, the unpleasantness of pain is abolished. Electrophysiological recordings from the ACC neurons found that neurons within the ACC respond to noxious stimuli, including nociceptive specific neurons. Neuroimaging studies further confirm these observations and show that the ACC, together with other cortical structures, are activated by acute noxious stimuli (Fig.25.1). Thus, understanding of synaptic mechanism within the ACC will greatly help us to gain insights into plastic changes in the brain related to central pain.

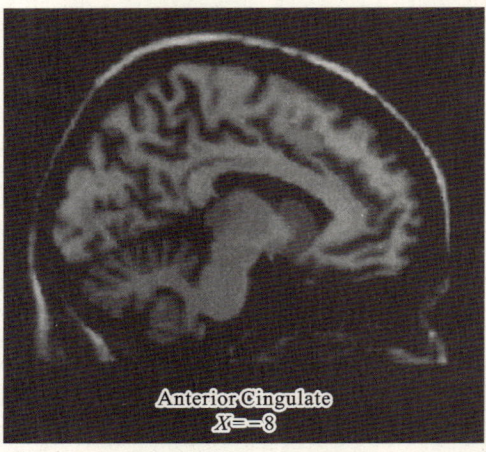

Fig.25.1 Activation of the ACC is related to pain unpleasantness (see also the color plate).

It is important to point out here that in addition to pain, the ACC has been proposed as the neurobiological substrate for executive control of cognitive and motor processes. Human imaging studies demonstrate that the ACC region is activated by different factors including motivational drive, reward, gain or loss, conflict-monitoring or error prediction, and attention or anticipation. The neuronal mechanisms for these different functions within the ACC remain mostly unknown due to the limitation of human studies. These "side-effect" or non-selective roles of the ACC further support the critical role of ACC in chronic pain-related mental disorders. The contribution of ACC in humans is unlikely to be limited for pain, but also include pain-related depression, drug addiction, suicide, and loss of interests.

SYNAPTIC TRANSMISSION IN THE ACC UNDERGO LONG-TERM POTENTIATION

Glutamate is the major fast excitatory transmitter in the ACC. Different types of glutamate receptors, including AMPA, KA, NMDA and metabotropic receptors (mGluRs) are found in the ACC. Fast synaptic responses induced by local stimulation or stimulation of thalamocortical projection pathways are mediated by AMPA/KA receptors, since bath application of CNQX completely blocks fast synaptic responses. Studies using selective AMPA receptor antagonist GYKI 53655 or KA GluR5 or GluR6 knockout mice found that postsynaptic KA receptor also contribute to synaptic transmission in adult neurons. Furthermore, genetic deletion of both GluR5 and GluR6 subtype receptors completely abolished KA mediated currents. It is still unclear if postsynaptic AMPA and KA receptor may mediate different ACC-related brain functions.

In addition to fast synaptic responses, in adult ACC slices at physiological temperatures, NMDA receptor mediated slow synaptic responses were also recorded from the ACC, suggesting that NMDA receptors are tonically active in this region. NMDA receptor mediated synaptic responses were further confirmed *in vivo* by electrophysiological recordings from freely moving animals. These findings indicate that synaptic responses recorded from *in vitro* brain slice preparations do not necessary completely represent those in physiological conditions.

Glutamatergic synapses in the ACC can undergo LTP in response to theta burst stimulation, a paradigm which more closely resembles the activity of ACC neurons. The potentiation lasted for at least 40 to 120 min. Interestingly, LTP can be also induced by different LTP inducing protocols using the whole-cell patch-clamp recording technique. Activation of NMDA receptors is critical for the induction of LTP in the ACC, including both NMDA NR2A and NR2B subtype receptors. Postsynaptic increases of calcium subsequent to the NMDA receptor activation are important for ACC LTP(Fig.25.2). Studies using gene knockout of calcium-CaM stimulated AC1 showed that postsynaptic cAMP is the key second messenger for ACC LTP. Unlike other central synapses, the expression of ACC LTP is likely to be postsynaptic. Future studies are needed to reveal detailed signaling pathways for ACC LTP.

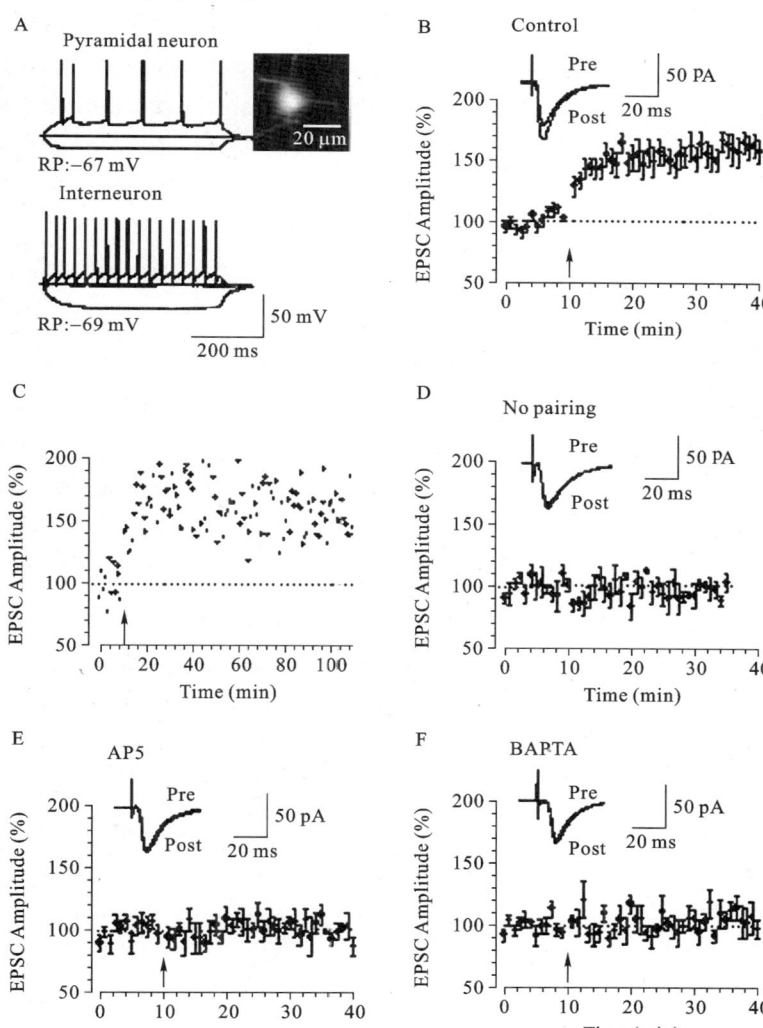

Fig.25.2 LTP is induced by postsynaptic NMDA receptor activation in the ACC. A. Current-clamp recordings to identify pyramidal neurons (upper) and interneurons (bottom) by current injections of −100, 0, and 100 pA. A labeled pyramid-like neuron was shown on the top right. RP, resting membrane potential. B. LTP was induced in pyramidal neurons ($n=15$) in adult ACC by the pairing training protocol (indicated by an arrow). The insets show averages of 6 EPSCs 5 min before and 25 min after the pairing training (arrow). The dashed line indicates the mean basal synaptic responses. C. An example showing long-lasting synaptic potentiation. Pairing training is indicated by an arrow. D. Basic synaptic transmission showing no change during recording without applying pairing training. The insets show averages of 6 EPSCs at the time points of 5 (pre) and 35 (post) min during the recording. E. and F. LTP was completely blocked by bath application of AP-5 ($n=7$) or addition of BAPTA ($n=7$) in the intracellular solution. The insets show averages of 6 EPSCs 5 min before and 25 min after the pairing training (arrow). The dashed line indicates the mean basal synaptic responses.

LONG-TERM DEPRESSION IN THE ACC

LTD has been thought to be reversed form of plasticity for LTP. In ACC slices of adult rats and mice, LTD can be induced by repetitive stimulation for a long period of time (15 min). Prolonged, low frequency stimulation (1 Hz for 15 min) produced long-lasting depression of synaptic responses. Depression is input-specific, and unstimulated pathways remain unchanged. As compared with LTD in the hippocampus, there are several properties of LTD in the ACC that differ from the hippocampus. First, repetitive stimulation at 5 Hz (3 min) induced LTD in the ACC but not in hippocampal slices. Second, unlike hippocampal LTD, which required activation of NMDA receptors, LTD induction required activation of mGluRs and L-type voltage-gated calcium channels (L-VDCCs). Finally, LTD in adult ACC slices is easily to be detected, while LTD in adult hippocampal slices are more difficult to be detected.

Recent studies using whole-cell patch recording technique further characterized ACC LTD. Unlike the hippocampus, both NMDA NR2A and NR2B subtype receptors are found to be important for the induction of LTD. Therefore, it is likely to be the case that different form of LTD may be induced in the brain ACC slices using different induction protocols and recording techniques.

LONG-TERM ENHANCEMENT OF SYNAPTIC RESPONSES IN THE ACC AFTER INJURY

One important question related to AC plasticity is whether injury causes prolonged or long-term changes in synaptic transmission in the ACC in whole animals. To test this question, we first measured synaptic responses to peripheral electrical shocks. We placed a recording electrode in the ACC of anesthetized rats. At high intensities of stimulation, sufficient to activate Aδ and C fibers, evoked field EPSPs were found in the ACC. The field EPSPs recorded from the ACC was obviously polysynaptic in nature, likely involving at least primary afferent fibers and spinothalamic and thalamocortical tracts (the estimated latency for the onset of field EPSPs was 12.0 ± 0.1 ms)(Fig.25.3). To detect central plastic changes, we performed amputation at the hindpaw contralateral to the one to which stimulation was delivered. Interestingly, after amputation of a central digit of the hindpaw, we observed a rapid enhancement of sensory responses to peripheral electrical shocks delivered to the normal hindpaw. The potentiation was long-lasting; evoked responses remained enhanced for at least 120 min(Fig.25.4). In order to address whether synaptic changes may occur locally within the ACC, we measured field EPSPs to focal ACC electrical stimulation. Consistently, we observed a long-lasting potentiation of field EPSPs after amputation that lasted for at least 90 min. The amount of potentiation is not significantly different from that in field recordings evoked by hindpaw stimulation. We hypothesize LTP within the ACC is likely due to abnormal activity during and after amputation. One important question is whether potentiated sensory responses required persistent activity from the injured hindpaw. To test this, we locally injected a local anesthetic, QX-314, into the hindpaw (5%, 50 μL) at 120 min after amputation. We found that QX-314 injection did not significantly affect the synaptic potentiation induced by amputation.

Intracellular recordings performed in anesthetized rats found that amputation caused prolonged depolarization in the ACC pyramidal cells, providing a key cellular mechanism for activation of postsynaptic NMDA receptors as well as voltage-gated ion channels. Although it is too early to speculate if the exact cellular changes in the ACC after amputation, it is hypothesized that excitatory synaptic transmission within the ACC is likely to undergo LTP.

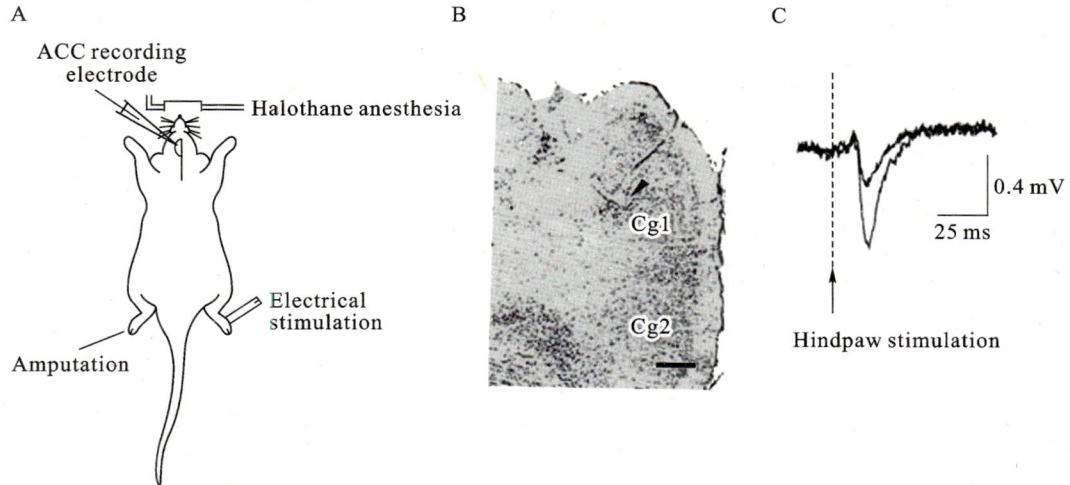

Fig.25.3   Sensory response of the anterior cingulate cortex to peripheral stimulation in adult rats.A. Diagram of *in vivo* recording from the ACC in an anaesthetised rat; animals were maintained at a lightly anaesthetised state by halothane. The recording electrode was placed into the ACC contralateral to the peripheral stimulation electrode. Amputation (the removal of the third digit of the hindpaw) was performed at the other hindpaw. During amputation, a higher concentration of halothane was used. B. An example of a histological section showing the recording site (arrowhead) labelled with neurobiotin and the track of recording electrode. C. Traces of synaptic responses to electrical stimulation applied to the hindpaw at a low intensity (5.0 V) and a higher intensity (25.0 V). An arrow indicates the time for hindpaw electrical stimulation. Cg1, Cingulate cortex, area 1; Cg2, Cingulate cortex, area 2.

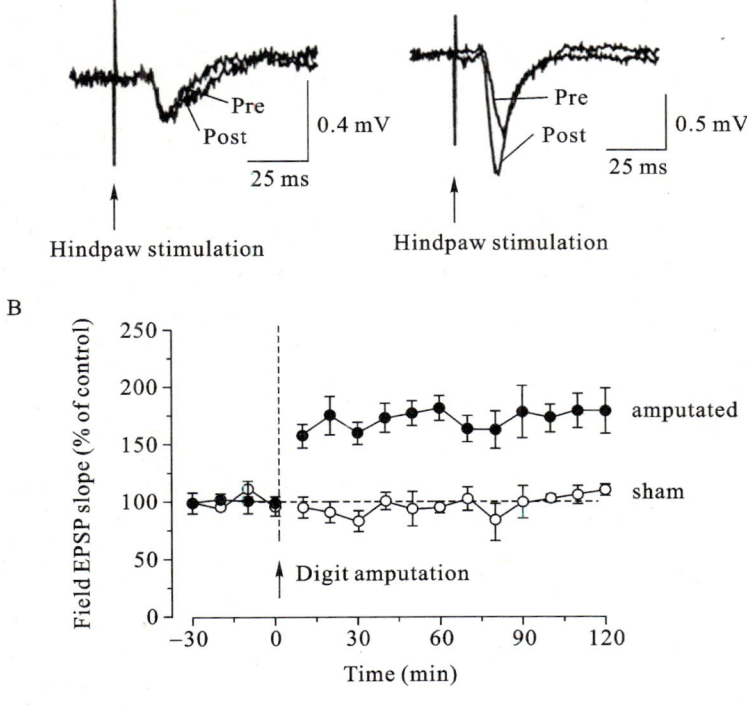

Fig.25.4   Long-lasting enhancement following amputation of a single hindpaw digit. A. Representative traces of EPSPs 5 min before amputation and 115–120 min after sham treatment (a) or amputation (b). In (b), the latency of sensory responses was not changed after the amputation, while the EPSP slope was increased. B. Amputation of a single digit of the contralateral hindpaw (see Fig.25. 1, indicated by an arrow) caused long-lasting enhancement of sensory responses (filled circles). Sensory responses were not significantly changed in sham-treated animals (open circles). The testing frequency was 0.01 Hz.

LOSS OF LONG-TERM DEPRESSION AFTER INJURY

In support of plastic changes in the ACC after injury, activity-dependent immediate early genes, such as c-fos, Egr1, adenosine 3′, 5′-monophosphate response element binding protein (CREB) are activated in the ACC neurons after tissue inflammation or amputation. Furthermore, these plastic changes persist for a long period of time, from hours to days. Studies using AC1&AC8 double knockout or NR2B overexpression mice show that NMDA receptors, AC1 and AC8 contribute to activation of immediate early genes by injury. In parallel with these dramatic changes in gene expression, synaptic plasticity recorded from *in vitro* ACC slices is also altered. In ACC slices of animals with amputation, the same repetitive stimulation produced less or no LTD. The loss of LTD is regionally selective, and no change was found in other cortical areas. One possible physiological mechanism for LTD in the ACC is to serve as an autoregulatory mechanism. LTD induced during low-frequency repetitive stimulation may help to maintain appropriate neuronal activity within the ACC by reducing synaptic transmission. In amputated or injured animals, the loss of autoregulation of synaptic tone may lead to overexcitation in the ACC neurons and contribute to enhancement of pain or unpleasantness related to the injury.

GENETIC ENHANCEMENT OF CHRONIC PAIN BY NR2B OVEREXPRESSION

In order to investigate molecular and cellular mechanisms for pain-related plasticity in the ACC, we decided to use genetic approaches together with integrative neuroscience techniques to investigate synaptic mechanisms in the ACC. First, we wanted to test if persistent pain may be increased by genetically enhanced NMDA receptor functions, a key mechanism for triggering central plasticity in the brain. Functional NMDA receptors contain heteromeric combinations of the NR1 subunit plus one or more of NR2A-D. While NR1 shows a widespread distribution in the brain, NR2 subunits exhibit regional distribution. In humans and rodents, NR2A and NR2B subunits predominate in forebrain structures. NR2A and NR2B subunits confer distinct properties to NMDA receptors; heteromers containing NR1 plus NR2B mediate a current that decays three to four times more slowly than receptors composed of NR1 plus NR2A. Unlike other ionotropic channels, NMDA receptors are 5–10 times more permeable to calcium, a critical intracellular signaling molecule, than to Na^+ or K^+. NMDA receptor mediated currents are long-lasting compared with the rapidly desensitizing kinetics of AMPA and KA receptor channels. In transgenic mice with forebrain-targeted NR2B overexpression, the normal developmental change in NMDA receptor kinetics was reversed. NR2B subunit expression was observed extensively throughout the cerebral cortex, striatum, amygdala, and hippocampus, but not in the thalamus, brainstem, or cerebellum. In both ACC and insular cortex, NR2B expression was significantly increased, and NMDA receptor mediated responses were enhanced. NMDA receptor mediated responses in the spinal cord, however, were not affected. NR2B transgenic and wild-type mice were indistinguishable in tests of acute nociception, NR2B transgenic mice exhibited enhanced behavioral responses after peripheral injection of formalin. Late phase nociceptive responses but not early responses were enhanced. Furthermore, mechanical allodynia measured in the complete Freund's adjuvant (CFA) model were significantly enhanced in NR2B transgenic mice. These findings provide the first genetic evidence that forebrain NMDA receptors play a critical role in chronic pain.

ENHANCED NR2B EXPRESSION BY INJURY

One critical question related to our hypothesis is whether NMDA NR2B receptors indeed undergo long-term upregulation in the ACC under physiological or pathological conditions. Our recent study provides the direct evidence that the upregulation of

NMDA NR2B receptors in the ACC contributing to inflammation-related persistent pain. After persistent inflammation, the expression of NMDA NR2B receptors in the ACC was upregulated; thereby increasing the NR2B component in NMDA mediated responses(BOX 25.1). Consistently, microinjection into the ACC and systemic administration of NR2B receptor selective antagonists inhibited behavioral responses to peripheral inflammation. These results are in good accordance with genetic studies showing that NR2B forebrain overexpression selectively enhanced inflammation-related persistent pain in transgenic mice.

BOX 25.1   Proposed model for the activity-dependent increases in NMDA receptor function in the ACC neurons.

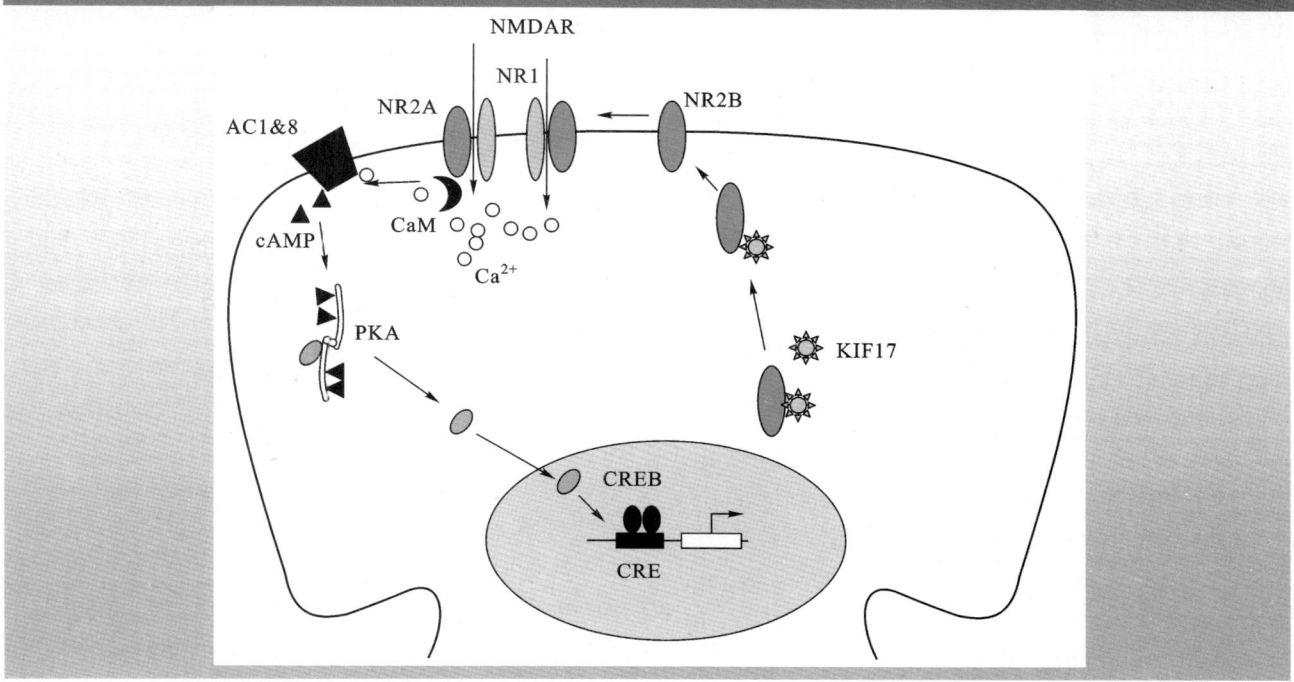

GENETIC DELETION OF CALCIUM-STIMULATED ADENYLYL CYCLASES

To determine downstream signaling pathways, we want to know if inhibition of NMDA receptor dependent, calcium-stimulated signaling pathways in the ACC may help to reduce chronic pain while keeping acute pain sensation intact (that is critical for animal or human self-protection). AC1 and AC8, the two major CaM-stimulated ACs in the brain, couple NMDA receptor activation to cAMP signaling pathways. In the ACC, strong and homogeneous patterns of AC1 and AC8 expression were observed in all cell layers. Behavioral studies found that wild-type, AC1, AC8 or AC1&AC8 double knockout mice were indistinguishable in tests of acute pain including the tail-flick test, hot-plate test, the mechanical withdrawal responses. However, behavioral responses to peripheral injection of two inflammatory stimuli, formalin and CFA, were reduced in AC1 or AC8 single knockout mice. Deletion of both AC1 and AC8 in AC1&AC8 double knockout mice produced greater reduction in persistent pain. More importantly, microinjection of an AC activator, forskolin, can rescue defects in chronic pain in AC1 and AC8 double knockout mice. Consistently, pharmacological intervenes of NMDA receptors as well as cAMP signaling pathways within the ACC also produced inhibitory effects on persistent pain in normal or wild-type animals, supporting the roles of ACC in persistent pain. Microinjection of NMDA receptor antagonists or cAMP-dependent protein kinase (PKA) inhibitors reduced or blocked mechanical allodynia related to inflammation. A recent study showed that persistent pain induced by tissue inflammation or nerve injury were significantly reduced in PDZ-93 knockout mice, in part due to the lower level of NR2B expression at the spinal and cortical levels of knockout mice.

ACTIVATION OF NEURONAL PLASTICITY-RELATED IMMEDIATE EARLY GENES IN THE ACC AFTER INJURY

As a marker for synaptic activity in the ACC, the expression of two major IEGs, c-Fos and Egr1/ NGFI-A, were examined at different time points after the injury. c-Fos and NGFI-A are transcription factors that are members of the leucine zipper and zinc finger families, respectively. In animals receiving sham treatment, there was little expression of c-Fos and a basal level of Egr1/NGFI-A. However, we found that single digit amputation in rats induced significant bilateral increases in the numbers of ACC cells expressing c-Fos or NGFI-A from 15 min to 2 days, with maximum expression at 45 min). c-fos has CRE (calcium/cAMP response element)-like sequences in its promoter regions, and its transcription is regulated by phosphorylated CRE-binding protein (pCREB). Significant increases in the expression of pCREB were also found bilaterally in ACC after amputation, compared to a basal level in sham-operated rats. Unlike c-Fos and NGFI-A, the level of pCREB two weeks later was lower than that in normal rats.

MODEL FOR MOLECULAR MECHANISM OF INJURY-RELATED POTENTIATION IN THE ACC

From pharmacological and genetic studies, we believe that molecular and cellular mechanisms for central plasticity in the ACC are starting to be revealed. Fig.25.5 is a model proposed based on current studies. Neural activity triggered by injuries release excitatory neurotransmitter glutamate in the ACC synapses. Activation of glutamate NMDA receptors leads to an increase in postsynaptic Ca^{2+} in dendritic spines. Ca^{2+} serves as an important intracellular signal for triggering a series of biochemical events that contribute to the expression of LTP. Ca^{2+} binds to CaM and leads to activation of calcium-stimulated signaling pathway.

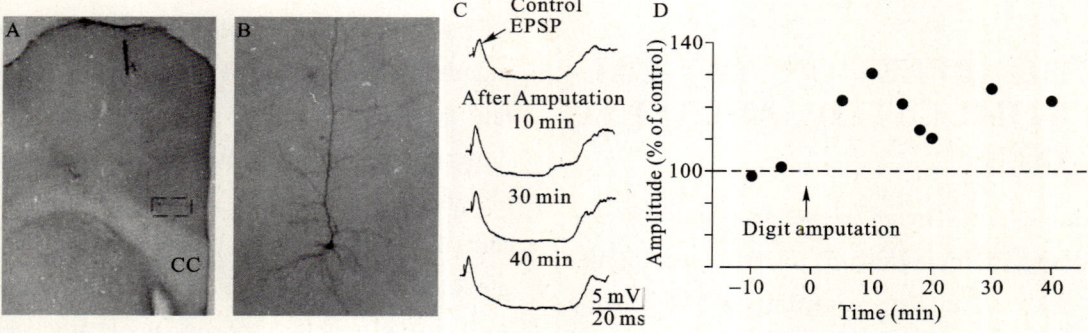

Fig.25.5 Prolonged membrane potential change of ACC neurons after digit amputation. A.   Light photomicrograph of a pyramidal neuron (square) in the ACC intracellularly stained with neurobiotin after recording. B. High magnification of the labeled pyramidal neuron in Fig. A. C. Representative recordings showing the response of ACC neuron to the contralateral third digit amputation. The upper panel is the membrane potential intracellularly recorded from a pyramidal neuron, the middle panel is the intracellularly applied hyperpolarizing current pulses (1 Hz, −0.5 nA, 200 ms), the lower panel is the simultaneous extracellular recording of DC potential in the ACC region. The arrows indicate the time of digit amputation. Approximately 2min after amputation, the baseline membrane potentials from both recording quickly depolarize for approximately 50 mV and gradually returned to the control level in about 55 min.

Among them, calcium-CaM stimulated ACs, including AC1 and AC8 and Ca^{2+}/CaM dependent protein kinases (PKC and CaMKII). The Ca/CaM dependent protein kinases phorsphorylate glutamate AMPA receptors, increase their sensitivity to glutamate. Activation of CaMKIV, a kinase predominantly expressed

in the nuclei, will trigger CaMKIV-dependent CREB. In addition, activation of AC1 and AC8 lead to activation of PKA, and subsequently CREB as well. CREB as well as other immediate early genes in turn activates targets that are thought to lead to structural changes (BOX25.2).

BOX 25.2   Signaling pathways from the postsynaptic membrane to the nuclei that lead to LTP in the ACC.

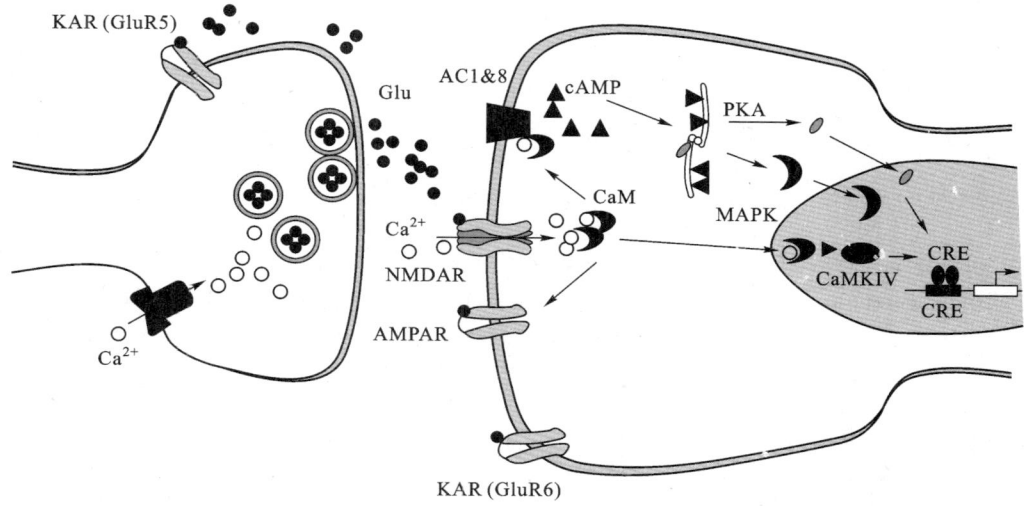

Neural activity triggered by injury releases glutamate in the ACC synapses. Subsequent to activation of glutamate NMDA receptors, Ca^{2+} binds to CaM and leads to activation of calcium-stimulated ACs, including AC1 and AC8 and Ca^{2+}/CaM dependent protein kinases (PKC, CaMKII and CaMKIV). Activation of CaMKIV, a kinase predominantly expressed in the

nuclei, will trigger CaMKIV-dependent CREB. In addition, activation of AC1 and AC8 lead to activation of PKA, and subsequently CREB. CREB and other immediate early genes (e.g., *Egr1*) in turn activate targets that are thought to lead to more permanent structural changes.

ACTIVATION OF ACC TRIGGERED FEAR AND AVERSIVE BEHAVIORS

What are behavioral effects of stimulating ACC in the freely moving mice? Using formalin induced aversive operative test, Howard Fields and his colleges show that chemical activation of glutamate receptors within the ACC form aversive behavioral responses. Furthermore, lesions or inhibition of excitatory synapses by K opioid receptors within the ACC blocked the formation of aversive operative responses induced by formation in freely moving rats. The major contribution of ACC to aversive behaviors is likely to cause pain-related unpleasantness. To test this possibility,

microelectrodes are implanted in the ACC of freely moving mice (Fig.25.6, 25.7). Consistent with chemical activation in the adult rats, electrical stimulation of the ACC paired with a non-noxious auditory tone cause long-term fear memory. Similar to classically conditioned fear memory induced by pairing foot-shock and tone, the activation of NMDA receptors in the amygdala is critical for the formation of auditory fear memory. Considering the high interconnection between the AC and hippocampus and amygdala, it is quite possible that cortical inputs from the ACC are important for the formation of pain-related fear memory. Recently, it has been also shown that inhibition of neuronal activity within the ACC also affect or reduce fear memory induced by foot-shock.

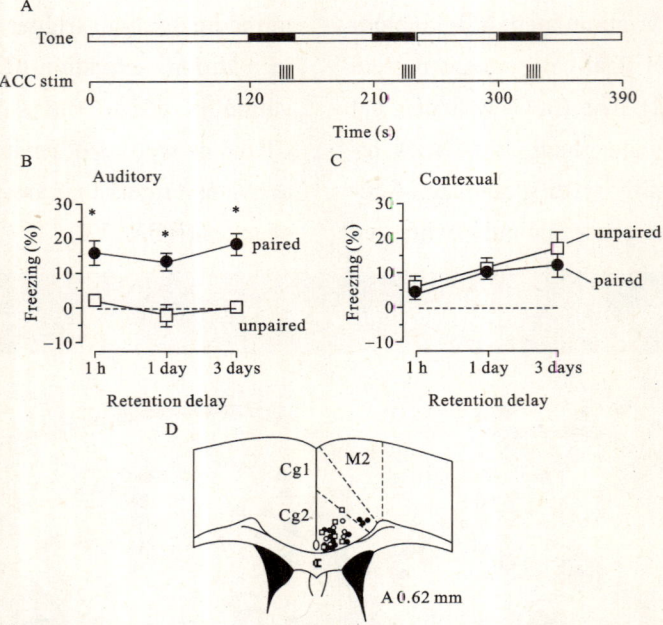

Fig.25.6 ACC stimulation induces long-term fear memory. A. Three pairings of 30 s tone and 10 s electrical train stimulation were delivered in the paired group on the conditioning day. B, C. Percentage freezing to the tone (B) and the conditioning context (C) measured at 1 hour, 1 day and 3 days after paired training. After paired training, long-lasting fear memory was detected in most of the mice (n=16 mice, filled circles), while some other mice showed no freezing across the test periods (n=5, data not shown). After unpaired training of tone and ACC stimulation, mice showed no freezing to the tone (n=6, open squares) but clear memory to the training environment; * $P<0.05$ compared with the unpaired group. D. Stimulating sites in ACC on the schematic representation of coronal section 0.62 mm anterior to the Bregma. Filled circles, effect sites of ACC paired group; open circles, no effect sites of ACC paired group; open squares, ACC unpaired group.

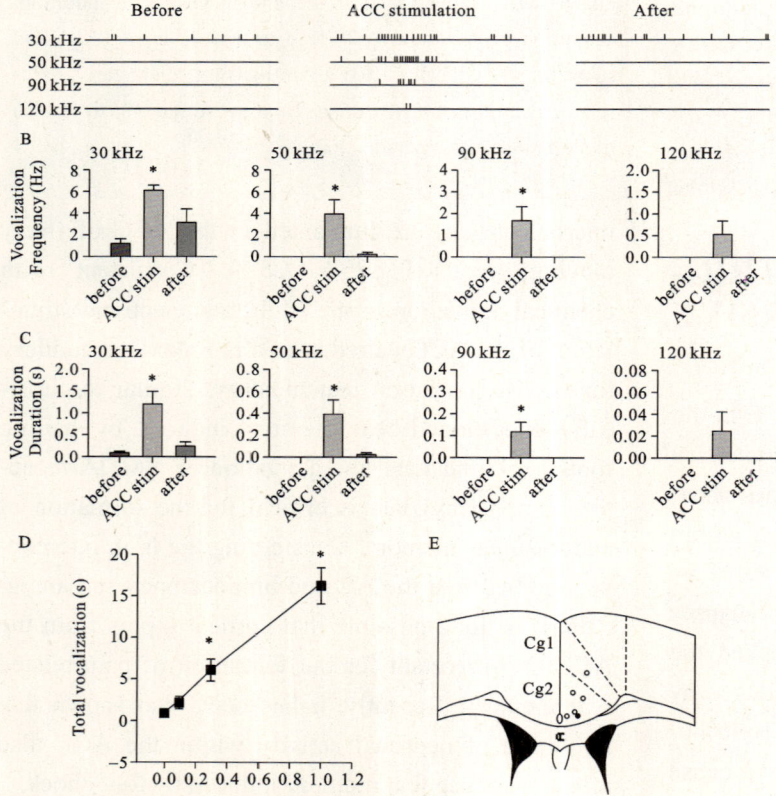

Fig.25.7 ACC stimulation induces ultrasonic vocalization in freely moving mice. A. An example of ultrasonic responses from a single mouse at four different frequencies before, during and after ACC stimulation (at 0.3 mA). 1 min duration; see filled circle for the stimulation site within the ACC in (E). B. ACC stimulation (0.3 mA; n=6) increased the frequency of individual ultrasonic responses; * $P<0.05$, comparing the frequency during ACC stimulation with baseline response before the stimulation. C. ACC stimulation (0.3 mA; n=6) also increased the duration of single ultrasonic response; * $P<0.05$, comparing the duration during ACC stimulation with baseline duration before the stimulation. D. Summarized data of ACC stimulation (n=6) produced ultrasonic responses at different intensities. Total vocalization responses (second) within 2 min ACC stimulation were plotted against the intensity of stimulation, E. Stimulating sites in ACC on the schematic representation of coronal section 0.62 mm anterior to the Bregma. Filled circle, for data shown in (A); open circles, other sites for data shown in B–D.

LESION OR CHEMICAL BLOCKADE OF ACC AFFECTED CHRONIC PAIN IN ANIMALS AND HUMANS

Studies from animals and humans demonstrate that local lesion of the ACC or pharmacological inhibition of neuronal activity in the ACC reduced chronic pain in patients and inhibited behavioral nociceptive responses in animals. In animal models of acute pain and persistent pain, lesions of the ACC produce antinociceptive effects. In freely moving animals, local administration of various opioid receptor agonists in the ACC produces powerful antinociceptive effects. Therefore, it is likely that the ACC is a novel target for treating chronic pain, in addition to traditional targets such as peripheral receptors and spinal cord dorsal horn.

BOX 25.3	A model explaining the neuronal pathways, which contribute to ACC activation, produced fear memory and descending facilitatory modulation of spinal nociception.

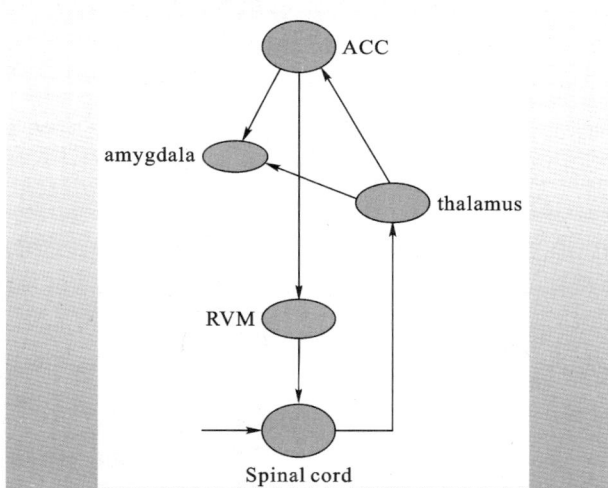

CONCLUSION AND FUTURE DIRECTIONS

Unlike neurons in the DRGs and spinal cord, it is proposed that neuronal activity in the ACC codes pain-related unpleasantness and pain perception. Similar to the other sensory synapses, glutamate is the major excitatory transmitter in the cingulate cortex.

Both AMPA and KA receptors contribute to normal synaptic transmission in the cingulate cortex, in some cases, postsynaptic NMDA receptor also contributes to synaptic transmission under physiological conditions. Synapses in the ACC can undergo biphasic long-term modulation. Theta burst stimulation or the pairing training of presynaptic activity and postsynaptic depolarization lead to long-term potentiation of AMPA receptor mediated EPSCs. NMDA receptor and/or L-type voltage-gated calcium channels trigger postsynaptic increases of calcium level, activating calcium-CaM dependent signaling pathways and lead to LTP. By contrast, repetitive stimulation for a prolonged period of time (15 min) or pairing the synaptic activity with slight postsynaptic depolarization lead to long-term depression of AMPA receptor mediated EPSCs. Prolonged changes in synaptic transmission observed in brain slice preparations are likely mimicking the pathological changes within the ACC after tissue and nerve injury. In addition, activation of several important activity-dependent immediate early genes may initiate the new synthesis of signaling molecules and proteins that may contribute to late, structural changes with in the ACC. Animal and human data suggest that inhibiting neuronal activity and/or plasticity may help reduce or block chronic or persistent pain. Understanding molecular and cellular mechanisms that lead to long-term plastic changes in the ACC not only help us to understand how noxious peripheral information is processed and stored in the brain, but also real new drug targets from treating various mental disorders.

GENERAL CITATIONS

Bush G, Luu P and Posner M I. 2000. Cognitive and emotional influences in anterior cingulate cortex. *Trends Cogn Sci*, 4: 215-222.

Devinsky O, Morrell MJ and Vogt BA. 1995. Contributions of anterior cingulate cortex to behaviour. *Brain*, 118 (Pt 1): 279-306.

Frankland PW and Teixeira CM. 2005.A pain in the ACC. *Mol Pain*, 1: 14.

Kaas JH, Florence SL and Jain N. 1999. Subcortical contributions to massive cortical reorganizations. *Neuron*, 22: 657-660.

Price DD. 2000. Psychological and neural mechanisms of the affective dimension of pain. *Science*, 288: 1769-1772 .

Rainville P. 2002. Brain mechanisms of pain affect and pain modulation. *Curr Opin Neurobiol*, 12: 195-204.

Sanders GS, Gallup GG, Heinsen H, Hof PR and Schmitz C. 2002. Cognitive deficits, schizophrenia, and the anterior cingulate cortex. *Trends Cogn Sci*, 6: 190-192.

Zhuo M. 2002. Glutamate receptors and persistent pain: targeting forebrain NR2B subunits. *Drug Discov Today*, 7: 259-267.

Zhuo M. 2005. Central inhibition and placebo analgesia. *Mol Pain*, 1: 21.

Zhuo M. 2005. Canadian Association of Neuroscience review: Cellular and synaptic insights into physiological and pathological pain. EJLB-CIHR Michael Smith Chair in Neurosciences and Mental Health lecture. *Can J Neurol Sci*, 32: 27-36.

DISCOVERY CITATIONS

Calejesan AA, Kim SJ and Zhuo M. 2000. Descending facilitatory modulation of a behavioral nociceptive response by stimulation in the adult rat anterior cingulate cortex. *Eur J Pain*, 4: 83-96.

Cooper SJ 1975. Anaesthetisation of prefrontal cortex and response to noxious stimulation. *Nature*, 254: 439-440.

Eisenberger NI, Lieberman MD and Williams KD. 2003. Does rejection hurt? An FMRI study of social exclusion. *Science*, 302: 290-292.

Florence SL, Taub HB and Kaas JH. 1998. Large-scale sprouting of cortical connections after peripheral injury in adult macaque monkeys. *Science*, 282: 1117-1121.

Follett KA and Gebhart GF. 1992. Modulation of cortical evoked potentials by stimulation of nucleus raphe magnus in rats. *J Neurophysiol*, 67: 820-828.

Hutchison WD, Davis KD, Lozano AM, Tasker RR and Dostrovsky JO. 1999. Pain-related neurons in the human cingulate cortex. *Nat Neurosci*, 2: 403-405.

Johansen JP, Fields HL and Manning BH. 2001. The affective component of pain in rodents: direct evidence for a contribution of the anterior cingulate cortex. *Proc Natl Acad Sci USA*, 98: 8077-8082.

Ko SW, et al. 2005. Selective contribution of Egr1 (*zif/268*) to persistent inflammatory pain. *J Pain*, 6: 12-20.

Ko S, Zhao MG, Toyoda H, Qiu CS and Zhuo M. 2005. Altered behavioral responses to noxious stimuli and fear in glutamate receptor 5 (GluR5)- or GluR6-deficient mice. *J Neurosci*, 25: 977-984.

Lee D E, Kim S J and Zhuo M. 1999. Comparison of behavioral responses to noxious cold and heat in mice. *Brain Res*, 845: 117-121.

Liauw J, Wu LJ and Zhuo M. 2005. Calcium-stimulated adenylyl cyclases required for long-term potentiation in the anterior cingulate cortex. *J Neurophysiol*, 94: 878-882.

Ploghaus A, et al. 1999. Dissociating pain from its anticipation in the human brain. *Science*, 284: 1979-1981.

Sah P and Nicoll RA. 1991. Mechanisms underlying potentiation of synaptic transmission in rat anterior cingulate cortex *in vitro*. *J Physiol*, 433: 615-630.

Sawamoto N, et al. 2000. Expectation of pain enhances responses to nonpainful somatosensory stimulation in the anterior cingulate cortex and parietal operculum/posterior insula: an event-related functional magnetic resonance imaging study. *J Neurosci*, 20: 7438-7445.

Singer T, et al. 2004. Empathy for pain involves the affective but not sensory components of pain. *Science*, 303: 1157-1162.

Tanaka E and North RA. 1994. Opioid actions on rat anterior cingulate cortex neurons *in vitro*. *J Neurosci*, 14: 1106-1113.

Tang J, et al. 2005. Pavlovian fear memory induced by activation in the anterior cingulate cortex. *Mol Pain*, 1: 6.

Tao YX, et al. 2003. Impaired NMDA receptor-mediated postsynaptic function and blunted NMDA receptor dependent persistent pain in mice lacking postsynaptic density-93 protein. *J Neurosci*, 23: 6703-6712.

Toyoda H, Zhao MG and Zhuo M. 2005. Roles of NMDA receptor NR2A and NR2B subtypes for long-term depression in the anterior cingulate cortex. *Eur J Neurosci*, 22: 485-494.

Wang CC and Shyu BC. 2004. Differential projections from the mediodorsal and centrolateral thalamic nuclei to the frontal cortex in rats. *Brain Res*, 995: 226-235.

Wei F, Li P and Zhuo M. 1999. Loss of synaptic depression in mammalian anterior cingulate cortex after amputation. *J Neurosci*, 19: 9346-9354.

Wei F, *et al*. 2001. Genetic enhancement of inflammatory pain by forebrain NR2B overexpression. *Nat Neurosci*, 4: 164-169.

Wei F, and Zhuo M. 2001. Potentiation of sensory responses in the anterior cingulate cortex following digit amputation in the anaesthetised rat. *J Physiol*, 532: 823-833.

Wei F, *et al*. 2002. Calcium calmodulin-dependent protein kinase IV is required for fear memory. *Nat Neurosci*, 5: 573-579.

Wei F, *et al*. 2002. Genetic elimination of behavioral sensitization in mice lacking calmodulin - stimulated adenylyl cyclases. *Neuron*, 36: 713-726.

Wei F, *et al*. 2003. Calmodulin regulates synaptic plasticity in the anterior cingulate cortex and behavioral responses: a microelectroporation study in adult rodents. *J Neurosci*, 23: 8402-8409.

Wu LJ, Zhao MG, Toyoda H, Ko SW and Zhuo M. 2005. Kainate receptor-mediated synaptic transmission in the adult anterior cingulate cortex. *J Neurophysiol*, 94: 1805-1813.

Wu MF, Pang ZP, Zhuo M and Xu ZC. 2005. Prolonged membrane potential depolarization in cingulate pyramidal cells after digit amputation in adult rats. *Mol Pain*, 1: 23.

Zhao M G, *et al*. 2005. Roles of NMDA NR2B subtype receptor in prefrontal long-term potentiation and contextual fear memory. *Neuron*, 47: 859-872.

Reorganization of the Sensorimotor System after Injury

CHAPTER 26

Huixin Qi, Jon H. Kaas

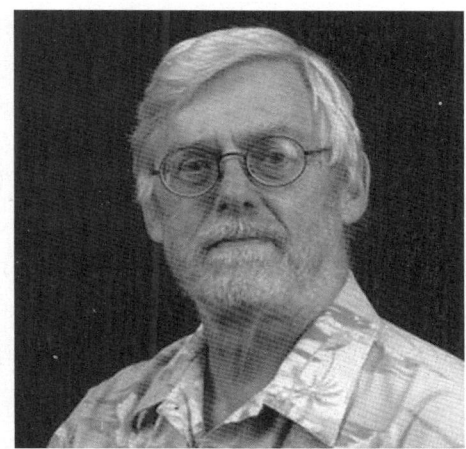

Dr. Kaas is a Distinguished, Centennial Professor and Senior Investigator in the Department of Psychology, Vanderbilt University. He obtained his PhD in Physiological Psychology from Duke University and pursued postdoctoral work at the Laboratory of Neurophysiology, University of Wisconsin.

MAJOR CONTRIBUTIONS

1. Kaas JH, Hackett TA. 1999. "What" and "where" processing in auditory cortex. *Nat Neurosci*, 2(12): 1045-1047.

2. Kaas JH, Collins CE. 2001. Evolving ideas of brain evolution. Nature, 411(6834): 141-142.

3. Collins CE, Lyon DC, Kaas JH. 2003. Responses of neurons in the middle temporal visual area after long-standing lesions of the primary visual cortex in adult new world monkeys. *J Neurosci*, 23(6): 2251-2264.

4. Lyon DC, Kaas JH. 2002. Evidence for a modified V3 with dorsal and ventral halves in macaque monkeys. *Neuron*, 33(3): 453-461.

5. Chino Y, Smith EL 3rd, Zhang B, Matsuura K, Mori T, Kaas JH. 2001. Recovery of binocular responses by cortical neu-

rons after early monocular lesions. *Nat Neurosci*, 4(7): 689-690.

6. Jain N, Diener PS, Coq JO, Kaas JH. 2003. Patterned activity via spinal dorsal quadrant inputs is necessary for the formation of organized somatosensory maps. *J Neurosci*, 23(32): 10321-10330.

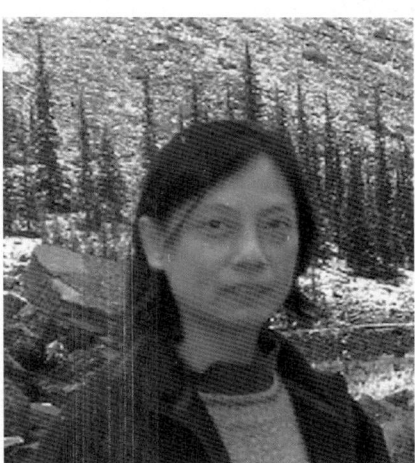

Dr. Qi is a Research Assistant Professor, Department of Psychology, Vanderbilt University. She obtained her PhD in Neurophysiology from Zurich University, Switzerland. She pursued her postdoctoral work at the Laboratory of Neuroscience led by Dr. Kaas, Vanderbilt University.

MAJOR CONTRIBUTIONS

1. Qi HX, Jain N, Preuss TM, Kass JH. 1999. Inverted pyramidal neurons in chimpanzee sensorimotor cortex are revealed by immunostaining with monoclonal antibody SMI-32. *Somatosens Mot Res*. 16(1): 49-56.

2. Qi HX, Stepniewska I, Kaas JH. 2000. Reorganization of primary motor cortex in adult macaque monkeys with

long-standing amputations. *J Neurophysiol*, 2133-2147.

3. Qi HX, Lyon DC, Kaas JH. 2002. Cortical and thalamic connections of the parietal ventral somatosensory area in marmoset monkeys (*Callithrix jacchus*). *J Comp Neurol*, 443(2): 168-182.

4. Qi HX, Stewart Phillips W, Kaas JH. 2004. Connections of neurons in the lumbar ventral horn of spinal cord are altered after long-standing limb loss in a macaque monkey. *Somatosens Mot Res*. 21(3-4): 229-239

5. Kaas JH, Qi HX. 2004. The reorganization of the motor system in primates after the loss of a limb. *Restor Neurol Neurosci*, 22(3-5): 145-152. (Review).

MAIN TOPICS

SUMMARY

The loss of sensory inputs or motor outputs to muscles can result from peripheral injury or the loss of a limb. Parts of the sensorimotor system may also be damaged by direct injuries, such as in stroke. After several decades of experiments and clinical observation, we know now that the damaged system is not static even in adults, but it adjusts and reorganizes following damage. Some of the reorganization may be beneficial and promote the recovery of lost functions. However, some reorganization may be detrimental and result in greater impairments, and misperceptions such as phantom pain. Research has increased our understanding of brain mechanisms that lead to recovery of lost functions in the sensorimotor system after injury, and an appreciation of therapeutic procedures that can maximize the desirable changes and minimize those changes that are damaging.

The loss of sensory inputs after nerve damage or the loss of a limb in the mature somatosensory system is followed by a gradual reactivation of parts of the system, such as primary somatosensory cortex, that had been devoted to the missing sensory input. This recovery appears to be the result of a number of neural mechanisms, including the growth of new connections at several levels of the somatosensory system. Some of this new growth and recovery occurs at the levels of the brainstem and thalamus, and the changes are relayed to cortex. This kind of reorganization can lead to misperceptions (touch on one skin surface is often perceived as on another) and phantom pain. This detrimental reorganization can be altered in several ways. Most importantly, the transplantation of a hand to replace an amputated hand can lead to reinnervation of the hand and the recovery of a more normal somatosensory and motor system. Other types of cortical reorganization after peripheral injury may lead to improvements in sensory and motor abilities based on the greater representation of remaining inputs.

Another type of injury, a lesion of motor cortex, results in an inactivated area of cortex. The size of the non-functional area of motor cortex increases during the period immediately following the lesion. This can be prevented or even reversed by treatments that involve training and increased use of the impaired limb. With training, the reduced representation of the impaired limb increases in extent in damaged motor cortex, partially compensating for the damage that removed part of the limb representation.

Finally, motor cortex reorganizes after the loss of a limb to increase the representation of preserved muscles in the limb stump and adjoining body parts. This reorganization may have some useful consequences for improved use of the preserved muscles, and it is based in part on changes in peripheral nerve connections, as well as adjustments in central nervous system connection strengths.

INTRODUCTION

When an individual suffers the loss of an arm or leg, they not only suffer mentally and physically from the difficulties of daily life, but 60%–80% of them also suffer phantom limb pain or residual limb pain. Phantom limb pain is defined as any painful sensation in the absent limb. A small percentage of patients have phantom limb sensations in the absent limbs that are not painful; others feel pain in the residual limb (stump pain). The majority of patients report that phantom limb pain and sensations begin immediately after surgery. It is common for phantom limb pain to occur in short episodes (lasting only seconds–minutes), and for the pain to recur several times a day. What changes happen to the peripheral nervous system (PNS) and central nervous system (CNS) that could cause phantom limb pain? What mechanisms could explain these phenomena, and therefore could suggest a strategy for treatment? Although useful data have been collected from humans with amputations, the types of experiments that can be done with humans are limited. Therefore, animal experiments are necessary to address some issues. Here we summarize the results of animal and human studies, especially new findings over the last two decades.

In mammals, in contrast to the peripheral nervous system (PNS) and the developing central nervous system (CNS), the adult CNS has been long considered to be incapable of modification and regrowth after damage. However, over the last two decades, it

gradually has become clear that the adult CNS is dynamic and mutable. It is capable of reorganizing in response to PNS and CNS injury and it is continuously modified by experience. Here we focus on the plasticity in the somatosensory and motor systems of primates including humans.

The somatosensory cortex is characterized by orderly representations of the body. In anterior parietal cortex of anthropoid primates (monkeys, apes, and humans), four histologically distinct strips of cortex, areas 3a, 3b, 1 and 2, individually represent the contralateral body surface and muscles. Body surface representations all proceed from medial representations of the foot to successively more lateral representations of the trunk, forelimb, face, and tongue. The representation of cutaneous receptors in area 3b is the most precise. Studies show that if part of the skin of the hand is denervated by cutting the median nerve at the wrist, the deactivated neurons in primary somatosensory (S1) cortex that represent the skin supplied by the median nerve recover responsiveness to touch on the skin of other parts of the hand over the course of a month. If the hand is amputated, the deactivated somatosensory areas in turn respond to the remaining part of the arm. When the dorsal columns of ascending afferents in the spinal cord are cut at a high cervical level, the forelimb, trunk and hindlimb portions of primary somatosensory cortex become unresponsive to tactile stimulation, while the preserved inputs from the face remain capable of activating the face portion of S1. However, after 6–8 months of recovery, the hand and upper limb portions of S1 become responsive to touch on the face.

The ability of the somatosensory system to reorganize after injury in adult anthropoid primates naturally raises the question of what happens to the motor system after loss of a limb? Modern neuroanatomical, electrophysiological and imaging techniques allow scientists get one step closer in revealing the insights of motor system reorganization after peripheral injury. For instance, we used intracortical microstimulation technique to "map" the motor cortex of normal primates or primates with an amputation. We found that many of the sites in the amputated animals that normally evoked movements in the missing muscles, evoked instead a movement of the muscles of the stump and shoulder or hip. Thus, cortical locations once devoted to moving digits of the hand became capable of moving the shoulder, or in the case of a leg amputation, cortical locations that normally represented foot and toes movements became capable of moving the hip. Such observations raised a further question: what changes in the sensorimotor system mediate the alterations in the representation in the cortex? Does the reactivation of areas affected by peripheral damage involve or depend on subcortical changes? As the loss of afferents from skin locations deprives parts of the representations in the brainstem and thalamus, as well as cortex, do similar reorganizations occur at these other levels? Furthermore, does the extent of the peripheral loss matter so that reactivations occur more fully or rapidly for a restricted lesion compared to more extensive losses of afferents and/or efferents? In addition, what are the functional consequences of cortical reorganization? Finally, can treatments alter the outcome so that they can be used to improve patients' quality of life after injury? These issues are addressed below.

PROGRESS IN CLINICAL STUDIES

Limb Amputation

After limb amputation, a patient may develop pain that is felt in the missing limb. The first medical description of phantom limb pain in a patient with an amputation was in the 16th century by Ambroise Pare. Over the centuries, there have been several theories attempting to explain the syndrome; the earliest of those are theories that postulate a peripheral nerve mechanism. In brief, this type of theory holds that the neuromas formed in the stump after amputation generate impulses that travel up to the spinal cord, thalamus and cerebral cortex and are perceived as pain. It was not until the last two decades that cortical reorganization was seen as one possible cause of phantom limb pain. During that time, our view of the mutability of the adult CNS has greatly changed.

By using modern electrophysiological and imaging techniques such as, magnetoencephalography, somatosensory evoked potentials, movement-related cortical potentials, focal transcranial magnetic stimulation and functional magnetic resonance imaging (fMRI), Flor and colleges found a strong direct relationship between the amount of cortical reorganization and phantom limb pain (but not phantom limb sensation). This correlation was not only with reorganization in primary somatosensory cortex, but also with primary motor cortex and secondary motor areas. They found a high correlation between the magnitude of the shift of the cortical representation of the face into the hand area in sensorimotor cortex and the degree of phantom limb pain. In addition, they found that a greater amount of motor cortex reorganization was associated with less daily use of a prosthesis, which tended to be related to more severe phantom limb pain. These data suggest a potential positive effect of prosthesis use on phantom limb pain and cortical reorganization. The spreading of representations of adjacent body parts to deafferented cortical areas in patients with an amputation was also reported by other studies, such as, those by Ramachandran.

Recently, the therapeutic transplantation of another hand to replace an amputated hand has been carried out in some patients. As in other studies of brain reorganization after hand amputation, Farne et al. (2002) found that following hand amputations, the hand territory in somatosensory cortex became responsive to facial cutaneous stimulation. However, this amputation-induced reorganization reversed 5 months after the missing hand was replaced by transplantation, as the grafted hand regained sensorimotor cortical representations. Interestingly enough, the newly acquired somatosensory awareness of stimuli on the grafted hand was strikingly hampered when the ipsilateral face was touched simultaneously, i.e., right face perception extinguished the right hand perception. Ipsilateral face-hand extinction was present in the formerly dominant right hand 5 months after transplant and eventually disappeared 6 months afterwards. The data suggest that ipsilateral face-hand extinction is a perceptual consequence of the reorganization that occurs after hand transplantation, and it demonstrates the inherently competitive nature of superimposed sensory representations. Apparently, the inputs from the grafted hand won the competition after 6 months.

In a double hand transplantation case, Sirigu and colleagues also found that amputation-induced cortical reorganization was reversed following hand transplantation. Before the transplants, the representations of unaffected muscles expanded such that the stump region representation expanded to parts of motor cortex previously devoted to the amputated hands. Parallel changes were also recorded in somatosensory cortex. After transplantation, a separate region of motor cortex for hand movements gradually emerged as the new hand became innervated and cortical organization became more normal. These results show that as motor control and sensation returns to the grafted hands, the somatotopic maps in motor and somatosensory cortex become more normal as reorganizational changes are reversed. Thus, the new peripheral inputs and hand use allowed a global remodeling of the limb cortical maps and reversed the functional reorganization induced by the amputation. The cortical rearrangement occurred in an orderly manner, and the hand and arm representations tended to return to their original cortical locus.

What are the mechanisms underlying this cortical reversibility? In monkeys with amputated limbs, remaining efferent motoneurons preserve their functional efficacy by targeting new muscles. As efferent and afferent central pathway neurons survive after the amputation, normal sensorimotor circuits may be preserved and can be reactivated after the graft. This could explain why cortical activity shifts are observed as early as two months after surgery. The intrinsic changes within M1 may result from a shift in the strengths of existing connections. If we assume that

cortical hand and elbow representations had preexisting connections, the elbow activation in the phase before surgery may emerge as a change in the weight of these connections. That is, the elbow connection may be enhanced at the expense of the deprived hand region. The hand transplant may have restored the efficacy of the original connections at the expense, this time, of the elbow representation, thus allowing typical features of cortical organization to reappear in the motor map. The use of hand transplants has proven a useful treatment option in selected cases. Up to 2004, only 18 patients had undergone 24 hand transplant operations. However, initial results have been extremely promising, and the functional results are highly superior to those obtained with prostheses artificial hand. Most notably, a patient that received two transplanted hands regained considerable sensorimotor function.

As a more common approach towards compensating for the loss of a hand, an artificial hand may be used. There are several kinds of technical aids that have been developed over recent decades to improve a patient's quality of life after injury. Commonly available motorized hands offer two degrees of freedom: the opening or closing of the grip by electromyographic signals from extensor and flexor muscles in the amputated stump, which are recorded by two surface electrodes. More complex models with several degrees of freedom, unfortunately, have proved too fragile and complicated and are not commonly in clinical use. Clearly, such hand prostheses are far from an ideal hand substitute. They lack dexterity, and they do not provide sensory feedback and conscious sensibility. Recently, a thought-controlled artificial hand was developed by Dhillon and colleagues. By using a longitudinal intrafascicular electrode implanted primarily in median and ulnar nerves, they recorded motor nerve impulses which allow patients to control the position of a cursor on a computer monitor. Patients could easily generate motor commands associated with the movements of the missing limb. This advance could lead to a greatly improved artificial hand. As another possibility, the use of transplants of body parts from one location to another (for example, a toe to replace a thumb) has gained increasing interest over the past few years.

Spinal Cord Injury

Sensorimotor cortical reorganizations and partial recoveries also occur after spinal cord injuries. Corbetta *et al.* (2002) used fMRI to investigate an individual with a high cervical spinal cord injury after a 5-year absence of nearly all sensorimotor function at and below the shoulders, and a rare recovery of some function in years 6–8 after intense and sustained rehabilitation therapies. There was no fMRI response to vibratory stimulation of the hand in the primary somatosensory cortex (S1) hand area. Instead, hand cortex responded to tongue movements that normally evoke responses only in the more lateral face area. In contrast, vibratory stimulation of the foot evoked topographically appropriate responses in S1 and in the second somatosensory cortex (S2). Motor cortex responses, tied to a visuomotor tracking task, displayed a near typical topography, although they were more widespread in premotor regions than in normal individuals. These findings suggest that some somatosensory cortical representation can return even after long-standing spinal cord injury.

Over the past decade, considerable effort has been directed toward promoting the recovery of walking after spinal cord injury. Advances in our knowledge of the neuronal control of walking have led to the development of a promising rehabilitative strategy in patients with partial spinal cord injury, e.g., treadmill training with partial weight support. Another strategy for improving walking in spinal cord injured patients is the use of electrical stimulation of nerves and muscles to assist stepping movements. This field has advanced significantly over the past decade as a result of developments in computer technology and the miniaturization of electronics. However, the most severe spinal cord injuries are still largely inaccessible to efficient therapy. Re-establishing functional activity in especially the lower limbs by reinnervating muscles below the spinal cord lesion represents an attractive therapeutic strategy. Liu *et al.* (1999, 2001) used peripheral nerve grafts to bridge a spinal cord lesion to avoid the glial barrier blocking the axonal regeneration and guide regenerating axons toward precisely defined targets (for example, lower limb muscles). In both primate and rats, they found considerable functional recovery with strong evidence of centrifugal axonal regeneration from the spinal cord above the lesion to the periphery. Furthermore, they developed a surgical procedure through which nerve autografts were implanted between the rostral spinal ventral horn and the caudal ventral roots, so that the rostral motor neuron axons could thus reach peripheral targets, leading to some return of motor function. In addition, Tadie *et al.* (2002) used a similar approach in a paraplegic patient with a stabilized clinical state three years after spinal cord traumatic damage at the thoracic 9 level. Three segments from autologous sacral nerves were implanted into the right and left antero-lateral quadrant of the cord at thoracic 7–8 levels, then connected to ipsilateral lumbar 2–4 ventral roots, respectively. Eight months after surgery, voluntary contractions of bilateral adductors and of the left quadriceps were observed. Muscular activity was confirmed by motor unit potentials in response to attempted muscle contraction and by recording muscle potentials evoked by transcranial magnetic stimulation. These data support the hypothesis that muscles can be reinnervated by motor neurons located rostral to the damaged spinal cord segments. They suggest that even a delayed surgical reconstruction of motor pathways may contribute to partial functional recovery.

Cortical Lesions

The most common cortical lesions seen in patients are those from stroke or trauma. Stroke is often characterized by incomplete recovery and chronic motor impairments. It is well known that immediate and intensive physiotherapy and pharmacotherapy are critically important for improving recovery from stroke. Recovery after damage to the cerebral cortex may depend on neuronal aggregates adjacent to the lesion progressively taking over the functions previously played by the damaged neurons. Recoveries from hemiplegic strokes are associated with a marked reorganization of the activation patterns in cortex.

Animal studies indicate that manipulations of brain activity in cortex adjacent to the damaged region can influence cortical reorganization and consequently promote functional recovery. Cohen and co-workers found that patients with hemiplegic stroke involving sensorimotor cortex usually experience dysfunction on the contralateral side of the body. Behavioral training for the immobilized limb, while restraining the intact limb, (which forces use but also may reduce somatosensory activation from the intact limb and reduce intrahemispheric inhibition), leads to improvement. Magnetically or electrically stimulating the affected hemisphere can enhance the ability of peri-infarct and nonprimary motor cortical regions to respond to motor training or other neuro-rehabilitative interventions. Stimulating the intact hemisphere can help down-regulate motor cortical excitability in the homonymous motor representation in the opposite hemisphere to balance the reciprocal inhibition through callosal connections. Recent studies have shown that this balance is disturbed in patients with cortical lesions. Specifically, some of these patients show an abnormally high interhemispheric inhibitory drive from M1 in the intact hemisphere to M1 in the affected hemisphere. Among the stimulating techniques, the repetitive transcranial magnetic stimulation (rTMS) is safe and noninvasive, with a high temporal resolution. Therefore rTMS is widely used in chronic stroke patients. This type of noninvasive cortical stimulation can enhance motor function in patients with chronic stroke.

In summary, the results from neuroanatomical and neurophysiological studies have demonstrated that undamaged cortical tissue near a cortical injury can remodel during the recovery period from weeks to months after injury. This remodeling likely contributes to recovery.

PROGRESS IN ANIMAL STUDIES

Studies of neural plasticity have greatly increased over the past two decades. The results of these studies clearly demonstrate the remarkable ability of the adult brain to be shaped by environmental inputs after lesions. An understanding of the mechanisms underlying functional recovery will promote better strategies of rehabilitation in patients. Some of the results from animal studies are discussed in the following section.

Somatosensory System

Much of the research on cortical plasticity has involved New World owl and squirrel monkeys, which have most of the primary somatosensory cortex (area 3b) exposed on the cortical surface (Fig.26.1). This allows for placement of electrode under visual guidance. This technical advantage allows for reliability, accuracy, and thoroughness in the multiunit mapping experiments. Old World macaque monkeys have also been studied in great detail, since they have a closer evolutionary relationship with humans. In addition, if similar results are obtained from more than one species, it can be reasonably concluded that the results reflect fundamental properties of the primate nervous system, not just peculiar features of a particular species. The results can then be more confidently generalized to humans.

Functional Reorganization of Somatosensory Cortex after Peripheral Injury

The somatosensory cortex is characterized by orderly representations of the body. In anterior parietal cortex of primates, four histologically distinct strips of cortex, area 3a, 3b, 1 and 2, individually represent the contralateral body surface and muscles. The representations all proceed from medial representations of the foot to successively more lateral representations of the trunk, forelimb, face, and tongue. The representation of cutaneous receptors in area 3b is the most precise. Once the detailed topographical organization was revealed, it became possible to determine the consequences of sensory loss on the somatotopy of these maps.

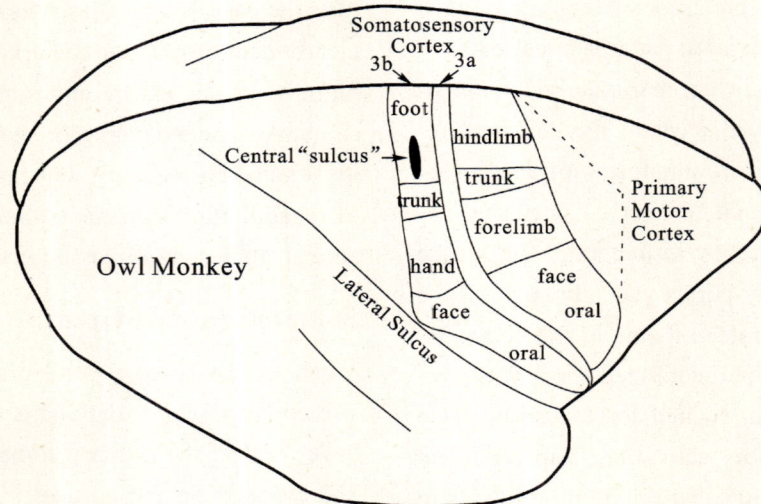

Fig.26.1 The basic organization of anterior parietal cortex (areas 3a, 3b, 1 and 2) and motor cortex (M1) in monkeys. M1 is located just rostral to somatosensory areas 3b and 3a, which contain orderly representations of cutaneous (3b) and muscle spindle (3a) receptors. These areas are shown on a dorsolateral view of the left cerebral hemisphere of a New World owl monkey, which provides the technical advantage in microelectrode mapping studies of having most of M1, 3a, and 3b exposed on the surface of the brain, as the central "sulcus" is only a shallow dimple. The somatotopic organization of the movement representation in M1 proceeds from tail, to hindlimb, to forelimb, to face, and then to tongue in a mediolateral sequence across cortex. M1 is organized in a similar manner in all of these primates. The somatotopic organization of area 3b (S1 proper) is shown for comparison with M1.

In the early 1980's, Merzenich and members of our laboratory studied the progression of changes in area 3b following median nerve section in adult squirrel and owl monkeys. We found that a fraction of novel receptive fields became apparent shortly after median nerve transection but most of the cortex failed to respond to tactile stimulation following nerve injury. However, after a recovery period of days or months, the deprived parts of the hand representation were no longer unresponsive to tactile stimuli. Instead, neurons responded vigorously to light touch on parts of the hand that adjoin the denervated region.

During that period, researchers did not know that the somatosensory system is capable of even more extensive reorganization. The first report of reorganization after the loss of a limb was from Rasmusson (1985) who had mapped somatosensory cortex in a single raccoon that had lost a forearm at some unknown time prior to its capture. The large representation of the forepaw in primary somatosensory cortex of this animal had been completely reactivated by an expanded representation of the stump. However, this finding from a single animal received little attention.

Several years later, a report of extensive cortical change after a major sensory loss convinced the research community that the adult brain is capable of enormous change. Pons and colleagues (1991) studied the impact of long-standing sensory deafferentation of the arm on somatosensory cortex of macaque monkeys. The sensory deafferentations eliminated the normal sources of activation from the large hand, wrist, and arm representations of four somatotopic fields (area 3a, 3b, 1 and 2 of anterior parietal cortex). Quite surprisingly, microelectrode recordings from the monkeys revealed that the deprived cortex was largely or completely reactivated by inputs from the face. Neurons throughout the explored zone of reactivated cortex responded vigorously to light touch and brushing of hairs on the face, much as in the normal cortical representations of the face. The reactivated cortex extended some 10–14 mm mediolaterally and 9–11 mm rostrocaudally, a much greater extent than found previously after more limited nerve damage. Moreover, similar reactivations undoubtedly took place in higher-level somatosensory representations such as the second somatosensory area, S2, and the parietal ventral area, PV, since these areas depended on inputs from anterior parietal cortex.

Functional Reorganization of Subcortical Structures after Peripheral Injury

To date, most studies of injury-induced reorganization have focused on the changes in cortical areas, and not many investigations have studied the organization of subcortical structures after injury. However, Garraghty (2001), Florence (1995, 2001), Rasmusson and coworkers used multi-unit electrophysiological recording techniques to assess the somatotopic organization of brainstem and thalamic areas following peripheral nerve cut and limb amputation in adult monkeys. They found that the denervation of the glabrous surface of the hand dramatically increased the size of the representation of the dorsal skin of the hand in both the cuneate nucleus of brainstem and the ventroposterior nucleus of the thalamus. The extent of cutaneously-driven reorganization in both somatosensory relay stations is comparable to that previously documented for area 3b of cortex. Similar results were found after long-standing limb loss. Neurons throughout the completely deprived portions of the ventroposterior nucleus of thalamus were responsive to light touch on the face or stump of the amputated arm (Fig.26.2, see also the color plate). Thus, subcortical centers contribute to the changes seen in cortex after injury as changes that occur in the ventroposterior nucleus are relayed to cortex.

Anatomical Substrates Underlying Functional Reorganization after Peripheral Injury

To investigate if peripheral nerve regeneration patterns are abnormal in damaged and regenerated peripheral nerves, Florence and colleagues studied the effects of median nerve cuts and regeneration on cortical organization. In three adult macaque monkeys, the median nerve was cut, sutured, and allowed to regenerate for 7-13 months. After regeneration, distributions of afferents to the dorsal horn of the spinal cord and the cuneate nucleus of the brainstem were determined by making injections of horseradish per-

oxidase conjugates into the distal phalanges of digit 1 or 2. While label from a single digit on the hand was normally confined to an appropriate, restricted location in the median nerve territories of the dorsal horn and cuneate nucleus of brainstem, label from the re-innervated digits spread out to cover most of the median nerve territories in those structures. These results are consistent with the interpretation that some proportion of primary sensory fibers normally innervating other digits and pads of median nerve skin erroneously reinnervated the skin of the injected digits. In the same monkeys, microelectrodes were used to record from an array of closely spaced sites across the representation of the hand in area 3b of somatosensory cortex. The reactivation pattern was abnormal, with neurons at many recording sites having more than one receptive field, larger than normal receptive fields, or receptive fields at abnormal skin locations. Thus, there is somatotopic disorder both in the regenerated median nerve and in reactivated cortex, indicating that primary somatosensory cortex does not reorganize to compensate fully for peripheral reinnervation errors in these adult primates. Nevertheless, some features of the organization of receptive fields in area 3b in these monkeys suggest the existence of some central selection of synapses.

While the reorganization of somatosensory cortex after peripheral nerve damage typically has been attributed to cortical plasticity, much of the large-scale cortical reorganization that occurs after a major loss of peripheral inputs reflects the sprouting or expansion of afferents from the remaining forelimb into deprived territories of the spinal cord and brainstem. To investigate if deafferentation resulting from limb amputation would have similar effects on cortical reorganization, Florence and colleagues studied the sensory afferent terminations in the spinal cord and brainstem, and the somatotopic organization of cortical area 3b in three adult monkeys with previous hand or forearm amputations, as a veterinary treatment of forelimb injuries. In each monkey, the distribution of labeled sensory afferent terminations from the remaining parts of the forelimb was much more exten-

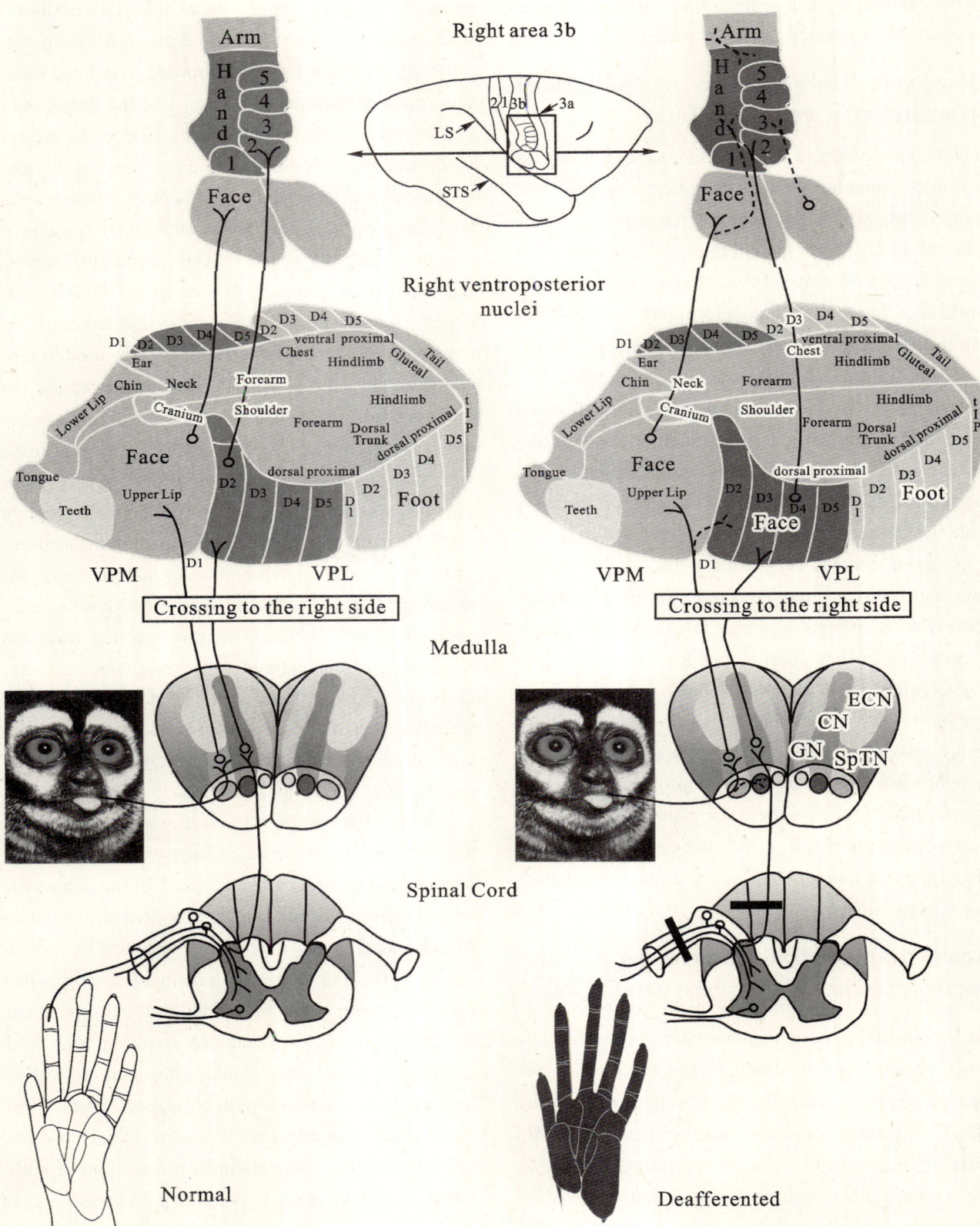

Fig.26.2 The relay of sensory information from the skin to somatosensory cortex in a normal monkey (left) and a monkey (right) with the loss of inputs from the hand by peripheral nerve injury (bar on dorsal root of nerve) or dorsal column pathway section (bar

sive than the normal distribution of inputs from the forelimb, and extended into portions of the dorsal horn of the spinal cord and the cuneate nucleus of the brainstem related to the amputated hand. In the same animals, tactile stimulation of the forelimb activated much of the deprived hand representation in area 3b of cortex; the lateral portion of the deprived region in area 3b appeared to be reactivated by inputs from the face. These data provide important new evidence that one of the mechanisms subserving large-scale reorganization in cortex is the growth of new subcortical connections and the relay of subcortical topographic changes to cortex. Presumably, the expanded primary sensory inputs from the forearm activate post synaptic neurons that are normally driven by inputs from the hand so that the neurons now have receptive fields on the forearm. Since the topographic representation of the body is greatly magnified in the relay to cortex, a limited amount of subcortical change can result in dramatic cortical map changes.

Reorganization after Complete or Partial Injury to the Dorsal Column Sensory Afferents in the Spinal Cord

An earlier study in owl and macaque monkeys showed that when the dorsal column of the spinal cord was completely sectioned at the cervical C3–C4

level, neurons in area 3b become immediately and perhaps permanently unresponsive to hand stimulation in spite of the remaining spinothalamic pathway. However, when the section of dorsal column afferents was not complete, and a few afferents from the hand remained to reach the cuneate nucleus in the brainstem, these fibers remained capable of activating their normal territory in the cortical hand representation. In addition, over weeks of recovery, this activated territory greatly expanded to encompass most of the deprived hand representation. Even in complete dorsal column sections, after prolonged recovery periods of six months or more, the deprived hand territory becomes responsive to inputs from the face (which are unaffected by spinal cord section). To further investigate the anatomical substrate for reactivating somatosensory cortex after dorsal column section, Jain and colleagues injected neuroanatomical tracers into subcutaneous skin on the chin of adult monkeys long after dorsal column sections. The results indicate that the afferents from the face to the trigeminal nucleus of the brainstem sprout and grow into the cuneate nucleus of the brainstem. This growth may underlie the large-scale expansion of the face representation into the hand region of somatosensory cortex that follows such deafferentations.

on spinal cord). Left. In the normal monkey (in the photograph, an owl monkey), inputs from the hand enter the cervical spinal cord while inputs from the face enter the lower brainstem. The hand inputs terminate in the cuneate nucleus of the lower brainstem (middle column), while the inputs from the face terminate in the trigeminal nucleus (outer column). Neurons receiving these inputs on the left side of the nervous system project to the ventroposterior nucleus (VP) on the right side of the brain (this crossing is not illustrated). The face inputs from the trigeminal nucleus terminate in the medial part of the ventroposterior nucleus (VPM), while the hand inputs from the cuneate nucleus terminate in the hand portion of the lateral portion of the ventroposterior nucleus (VPL). The locations of the representation of different body parts in the VP nucleus are indicated. Neurons in VP project to primary somatosensory cortex (area 3b) to create a somatotopic representation of the contralateral body surface. Only the face, hand and arm portions are shown here. The representational territories of digits 1–5 are outlined. The representation is not to scale, and it is bigger than the VP nucleus. The box on a small lateral view of the brain indicates where the hand and face portions of area 3b are located on the brain. Somatosensory areas 1, 2 and 3a are also shown. Arrows point to the lateral sulcus (LS) and the superior temporal sulcus (STS).Right. In a monkey with a long-standing loss of afferents from the hand (the black hand is the deafferented hand), neurons in the cuneate nucleus no longer respond to inputs from the hand. Instead, a few afferents from the face sprout and grow branches (dashed line) over months of recovery from the trigeminal nucleus to the cuneate nucleus where they activate neurons, which relay to the VPL hand region of the thalamus, where even more neurons are activated by touch on the face as a result of the altered significance of the inputs from the cuneate nucleus. It is also possible that some of the afferents from the trigeminal nucleus sprout into VPL to provide additional activation from the face, but there is no evidence for this possibility. Neurons in VPL that have become responsive to the face project to the hand portion of area 3b where neurons that are normally responsive to the hand become responsive to the face. It is also possible that neurons from the face representation in VPM branch from face cortex to hand cortex (dashed line) or neurons in face cortex or arm cortex grow branches into hand cortex to provide sources of activation, but anatomical studies suggest that this does not occur. As a result of the growth of new connections, and the amplification of the weak brainstem signal, area 3b becomes reorganized so that the hand region becomes responsive to touch on the face.

In a similar type of experiment, Darian-Smith and colleagues (2000, 2004) examined the role of primary afferent neurons in the somatosensory cortical "reactivation" that occurs after a localized cervical dorsal root lesion. After section of the dorsal rootlets that innervate the macaque's thumb and index finger (segments C6–C8), the cortical representation of these digits was initially silenced but then re-emerged for these same digits over 2–4 post lesion months. Cortical reactivation was accompanied by the emergence of physiologically detectable inputs from these same digits within dorsal rootlets bordering the lesion site. To investigate whether central axonal sprouting of primary afferents spared by the rhizotomy could mediate this cortical reactivation, neuroanatomical tracers were then injected into the thumb and index finger pads bilaterally to label the central terminals of any neurons that innervated these digits. The results indicated that labeled terminal bouton distributions were significantly larger on the side of the lesion in the dorsal horn and cuneate nucleus at 15–25 weeks after the dorsal rootlet section, than those mapped only 7 days post lesion. These results provide direct evidence for localized sprouting of spared (uninjured) primary afferent terminals in the dorsal horn and cuneate nucleus after a restricted dorsal root injury.

Reorganization after Behavioral Training in Developing Monkeys

Sensory perception can be severely degraded after peripheral injuries that disrupt the functional organization of the sensory maps in somatosensory cortex, even after nerve regeneration has occurred. Rehabilitation involving sensory retraining can improve perceptual function, presumably through plasticity mechanisms in the somatosensory processing network. However, until recently, little was known about the effects of rehabilitation strategies on brain organization, or where the effects are mediated. In one recent study, five macaque monkeys received months of enriched sensory experience after median nerve cut and repair early in life. Subsequently, the sensory representation of the hand in primary somatosensory cortex was mapped using multiunit microelectrodes. Additionally, the primary somatosensory relay in the thalamus, the ventroposterior nucleus, was studied to determine whether the effects of the enrichment were initiated subcortically or cortically. Age-matched controls included six monkeys with no sensory manipulation after median nerve cut and regeneration, and one monkey that had restricted sensory experience after the injury. The most substantial effect of the sensory environment was on receptive field sizes in cortical area 3b. Significantly greater proportions of the receptive fields for cortical neurons in the enriched monkeys were small and well localized compared to the controls, which showed higher proportions of abnormally large or disorganized fields. The refinements in receptive field size in somatosensory cortex likely provide better resolution in the sensory map and may relate to the improved functional outcomes after rehabilitation in humans.

MOTOR SYSTEM

The ability of the somatosensory system to reorganize after injury in adult primates naturally raises the question of what happens to the motor system after the loss of some of the targets of the spinal motor neurons. Research on this fundamental issue is an essential prerequisite to the development of improved, scientifically sound therapeutic and rehabilitation procedures for brain-injured humans. The following section provides an update on what is known about the functional recovery that takes place after peripheral injury or lesions in the primary motor cortex of nonhuman primates.

Based upon neurophysiologic, neuroanatomic, and neuroimaging studies conducted over the past two decades, the motor cortex can now be viewed as functionally and structurally dynamic. More specifically, the functional topography of the motor cortex (commonly called the motor homunculus or motor map), can be modified by a variety of experimental manipulations, including peripheral or central injury, electrical stimulation, pharmacologic treatment, and behavioral experience. Here we describe the functional changes that occur in M1 after the amputation of a limb, and the evidence that those changes depend in part on the formation of new connections in the motor system.

Reorganization of Motor Cortex after Long-Standing Limb Loss in Monkeys

Electrical stimulation of motor cortex was used to investigate the organization of primate primary motor cortex (M1) in macaque monkeys, squirrel monkeys and prosimian galagos years after the therapeutic amputation of an injured forelimb or hindlimb. Stimulation in the deprived part of M1 contralateral to the missing limb elicited movements of the remaining proximal muscles as well as movements from adjacent body representations in all cases. Stimulation in the deprived forelimb cortex evoked movements of the remaining arm stump and shoulder, whereas stimulation in the deprived hindlimb cortex evoked hip stump and trunk movements. Movements were evoked from all sites in the deprived cortex, so that there were no unresponsive zones. The minimal levels of current necessary to evoke these movements varied from those in the normal range to those at much higher levels. These results indicated that the functional organization of motor cortex had changed after amputations, and that the deprived cortex had become effective in activating new muscle groups.

These observations did not indicate what changes in the motor system mediate the alterations in the representation in motor cortex. Searching for changes in the connections of motor cortex and motor neurons of the spinal cord in these primates with amputations could provide an understanding of the mechanisms of cortical reorganization and functional recovery after peripheral injuries. Cortical reorganization might depend on changes in connections and connection strengths at several levels of the motor system.

To date, little is known about how connections of motor cortex and their subcortical targets are altered by the loss of a limb. Changes in the intrinsic connections of cortical areas are difficult to demonstrate unless they are relatively large, especially if only a few altered animals can be studied. Nevertheless, we had the opportunity to inject tracers in the arm region of M1 of four macaque monkeys with an arm amputation. The results revealed dramatically more widespread intrinsic connections in M1 in two of the monkeys compared to normal monkeys. The labeled intrinsic connections of the other two amputated monkeys were in the normal range. This result suggests that long standing limb loss may sometimes lead to a large-scale growth of new connections, and that these connections might contribute to cortical reorganization by spreading excitation from deactivated digit movement sites to preserved shoulder movement sites. Smaller, less detectable changes in growth of connections in M1 may also occur. Thus, persistent changes in the intrinsic horizontal connections of M1 may contribute to functional reorganization after limb amputations.

Another possibility is that some corticospinal neurons, those with axons that terminate on motor neurons previously projecting to the missing limb, are induced to grow and contact motor neurons projecting to preserved muscles in the stump and shoulder. The terminal arbors of corticospinal neurons are normally widespread, contacting motor pools related to several muscle groups. Thus, a limited increase in the number of relevant synaptic contacts at functionally intact locations in the motor neuron pool is all that would be needed for the cortical map to change. Unfortunately, there is no direct information on the stability or transformation of such terminal arbors after amputation. However, injections of tracers into the cervical spinal cord at C7–C8 levels in two squirrel monkeys with a forelimb amputation allowed the distributions of labeled corticospinal neurons in M1 of the "normal" and reorganized hemispheres to be compared in both the number of labeled cells and the extent of M1 with labeled cells, and there was no notable difference in the two sides. This result suggests that corticospinal neurons in the forelimb region of reorganized M1 neither gained nor lost overall synaptic contacts in the cervical spinal cord, but it does not address the issue of whether synaptic strengths were reweighted across motor pools. The motor neuron pools for the distal forelimb and the shoulder both occur at lower cervical levels of the spinal cord and local changes in connections at this level would not be distinguished by C7–C8 injections. Changes in the arrangements of terminal arbors of corticospinal neurons remain a possible contributor to the observed cortical plasticity, but there is no direct evidence.

To investigate whether motoneurons in the spinal cord could undergo sprouting therefore mediating the reactivation of the deprived motor cortex, we examined the integrity and connectivity of the spinal cord motoneurons in a macaque monkey (*Macaca mulatta*) that lost a hindlimb as a result of accidental injury more than 3.5 years earlier. To label motoneurons, multiple small injections of a neuroanatomical tracer were placed in the muscles of the hip just adjacent to the stump of the amputated leg, and in matched locations on the opposite side for control purposes. Injections of a second tracer were made in the intact foot. In the ventral horn that related to the intact hindlimb, motoneurons labeled by the hip injections were concentrated rostral and ventromedial to those labeled by the foot injections. Hip injections on the side of the amputation labeled neurons that were located well beyond the normal territory for motoneurons related to the hip and into the zone normally occupied by neurons projecting to the foot. Labeled motoneurons innervating the intact limb were significantly larger than neurons on the side of the amputation. Similar results were also obtained from squirrel monkeys. The data show that injections of anatomical tracers into the muscles proximal to the amputated stump labeled a larger extent of motoneurons than matched injections on the intact side or in normal animals, including motoneurons that would normally supply only the missing limb muscles. Although the total numbers of distal limb motoneurons remained normal, some distal limb motoneurons on the amputated side were smaller in size and simpler in form. These findings suggest that many motoneurons survived the long-standing amputations and made new connections with remaining intact muscles. These new patterns of connectivity likely contribute to the reorganization of motor cortex in amputees, and perhaps, to abnormal behaviors like those reported by human amputees.

Reorganization after Cortical Lesions

In humans, most cortical lesions are due to stroke or head trauma. Many people that suffer from stroke or head injury can have dramatic functional recovery. Recently, substantial progress has been made due to the use of noninvasive imaging and stimulation techniques. Some findings show that after a lesion on one side of the human brain, a dramatic reorganization of the hand representation occurs within either the ipsilateral primary motor cortex, nonprimary motor areas or both. The mechanisms underlying the functional recovery are largely unknown. Experiments conducted in monkeys by Nudo and coworkers have lead to great progress in understanding the nature of the functional recovery.

Nudo and collegues used a non-human primate model of cortical ischemia to evaluate the feasibility of using cortical stimulation combined with rehabilitative training to enhance behavioral recovery and cortical plasticity. Following pre-infarct training on a motor task, maps of movement representations in primary motor cortex were derived. Then, an ischemic infarct was produced which destroyed the hand representation in motor cortex. Several weeks later, a second cortical map was derived to guide implantation of a surface electrode over the peri-infarct motor cortex. After several months of spontaneous recovery, monkeys underwent subthreshold electrical stimulation combined with rehabilitative training for several weeks. Post-therapy behavioral performance was tracked for several additional months. A third cortical map was derived several weeks post-therapy to examine changes in motor representations. Monkeys showed significant improvements in motor performance (success, speed, and efficiency) following therapy, which persisted for several months. Cortical mapping revealed the emergence of new hand representations in peri-infarct motor cortex, primarily in cortical tissue underlying the electrode. Results support the feasibility of a therapy approach that combines peri-infarct electrical stimulation with rehabilitative training to reduce chronic motor deficits and promote recovery from cortical ischemic injury. Further, intensive task-specific practice with the impaired limb has a modulatory effect on the inevitable cortical plasticity. Taken together with parallel studies of forced use in human stroke patients, it is likely that use of the impaired limb can influence adaptive reorganizational mechanisms in the intact cerebral cortex, and thus, promote functional recovery.

Reorganization Induced by Motor Learning and Rehabilitation Training

Previous studies have shown that after incomplete injury to the hand representation in primary motor cortex (M1), the size of the spared portion of the hand representation decreased dramatically unless the unimpaired hand was restrained and the monkeys received daily rehabilitative training using the impaired fingers. Nudo and his colleagues investigated if restriction of the unimpaired hand was sufficient to retrain the spared hand area after injury or if the retention of the spared area required repetitive use of the impaired limb. After infarct to the hand area of M1 in adult squirrel monkeys, the unimpaired hand was restrained by a mesh sleeve over the unimpaired arm. Monkeys did not receive rehabilitative training. Electrophysiological maps of M1 were derived in anesthetized monkeys before infarct and 1 month after infarct by using intracortical microstimulation. One month after the lesion, the size of the hand representation had decreased. Areal changes were significantly smaller than those in animals in a previous study that had received daily repetitive training after infarct, and these areal changes were not different from those in a group of animals that received neither rehabilitative intervention nor hand restraint after injury. These results suggest that retention of the preserved portion of the hand area in M1 after a lesion requires repetitive

use of the impaired hand. In another set of experiments, retraining of skilled hand use after similar infarcts resulted in prevention of the loss of hand territory adjacent to the infarct of M1. In some instances, the hand representations expanded into regions formerly occupied by representations of the elbow and shoulder. Functional reorganization in the undamaged motor cortex next to the lesion was accompanied by behavioral recovery of skilled hand function. These results suggest that, after local damage to the motor cortex, rehabilitative training can shape subsequent reorganization in the adjacent intact cortex, and that reorganization of the undamaged motor cortex may play an important role in motor recovery.

In summary, the dynamic nature of sensorimotor representations in the adult brain gives us the lifelong potential to adapt to changes in our environment and to compensate for injury. Reorganizations in sensory systems typically involve relatively limited shifts in the topography of the functional representations, and in most reorganizations of the somatosensory cortex only neurons within 1–2 mm of the borders of the affected zone in cortex acquire new or altered receptive fields. In fact, for many years, it was assumed that this was the maximal distance for plasticity in the adult central nervous system. Evidence from human patients and from animal studies confirms that the adult brain is capable of much more extensive changes, involving much larger extents of the nervous system. Large-scale peripheral deafferentations, such as limb amputation or spinal cord damage, lead to extensive reactivations of large regions of somatosensory cortex deprived by the injury. These unusually large changes in cortical organization are not easily explained by cellular mechanisms involving the potentiation of previously existing connections. However, there is now evidence that new connections grow into regions deprived of primary afferent inputs as a result of injury. Subcortical sensory representations are smaller than their cortical counterparts; therefore, even limited new growth subcortically can lead to massive cortical reactivation.

OTHER MECHANISMS FOR RAPID REORGANIZATION: UNMASKED INHIBITION OF PRE-EXISTING CONNECTIONS AND INCREASED SYNAPTIC EFFICACY

One of the important questions in plasticity study is: "How do reactivations occur after injury?" A common explanation for most types of adult plasticity, both in cortex as well as subcortically, is that previously existing but hidden inputs in the normal anatomical framework of the somatosensory system become expressed. Connections with only subthreshold effects become potentiated through local modifications of synaptic weights and come to activate neurons that were previously unresponsive to the inputs.

The normal spread of the afferent terminals is larger than what is reflected in the physiologically determined excitatory receptive fields. The expression of latent inputs is inhibited at least partly by the inhibitory neurotransmitter—aminobutyric acid (GABA) ergic-or glycinergic interneurons. Deafferentation leads to the immediate expression of subthreshold inputs due to release of inhibition resulting from lack of excitatory inputs to the inhibitory cells. Over longer time periods, reduced activity levels could lead to a reduced expression of inhibitory transmitters. Experimental data appear to support this hypothesis. A decrease in immunostaining for GABA is observed two months after median and ulnar nerve transection and ligation in squirrel monkeys. Similarly, decreases in GABA receptor levels in the cortex and glutamic acid decarboxylase levels of ventroposterior nucleus of the thalamus have been observed in rats after peripheral deprivation. Thus the decrease in inhibition is not restricted to cortex, and disinhibition could operate at multiple levels.

AXON REGENERATION AND COLLATERAL SPROUTING

The potentiation of pre-existing connections, unmasked inhibition, and changes in synaptic strength cannot be the only mechanisms for the extensive reactivations seen after amputation and spinal cord lesion when the forearm representation comes to be largely reactivated by inputs from the face. The existing connectional framework allows for some overlap of the hand and face representations in cortex, but none that could account for the full extent of the injury-induced changes. The alternative explanation for the extensive reactivation is the new growth of connections. This would seem improbable, because there has been a long-held view that new growth, often called sprouting, is limited in the mature brain. Indeed, after injury to the adult CNS, axon outgrowth has two major obstacles to overcome: first, the inhibitors that are expressed, and second the blocking of a glial scar. There has been a recent explosion in the identification of specific myelin-associated inhibitors and receptors that prevent axon growth. An understanding of these mechanisms will greatly aid the development of therapeutic approaches toward functional recovery after injury. On the other hand, it is becoming increasingly clear that the adult CNS has more regenerative capacity than previously believed. As reviewed in previous sections, evidence has been accumulating in primates that sprouting does occur in the adult central nervous system. Injections of anatomical tracers into the stump of monkeys with long-standing arm amputations labeled sensory afferents from the arm that had sprouted beyond the original termination zones in the cuneate nucleus of the brain stem, into the hand and digit portions of the nucleus. More recently, similar injections were made into the skin of the face of two monkeys with an arm amputation and two monkeys with dorsal column section at a high cervical level. In these monkeys, sparse but obvious connections were observed from the trigeminal (face) nucleus to the cuneate (hand) nucleus. Thus, it appears that afferents from the face that normally terminate in the trigeminal nucleus had sprouted into the cuneate nucleus. This growth may underlie the large-scale expansion of the face representation into the hand region of somatosensory cortex that follows such deafferentations. We conclude that the adult primate CNS is capable of extensive new growth, and that the growth of even a few new connections can have a major impact on the functional organization of the brain. In cortex, there is evidence from monkeys with long-standing forelimb injuries that horizontal connections in cortex are more extensive than usual, so that neurons in the deprived cortical zones extend outside their normal territory and project to nearby non-deprived cortex; conversely, neurons in non-deprived cortical zones sprout into the deprived region of cortex. The new cortical growth no doubt contributes to the final pattern of reorganization that is expressed in cortex and perhaps participates in additional dynamic processes that reflect the experiential history of the individual.

In rats, Schwab and colleagues recently reported that after dorsal hemisection at mid-thoracic level of spinal cord, transected hindlimb corticospinal tract axons spontaneously sprout into the cervical gray matter to contact short and long propriospinal neurons. Over 12 weeks, contacts with long propriospinal neurons that bridged the lesion were maintained, and their axons arborized on lumbar motor neurons, creating a new intraspinal circuit relaying cortical input to the original spinal targets. Schwab and colleagues confirmed that these new anatomical contacts formed a novel circuit by retrograde transsynaptic tracing with Bartha-pseudorabies virus. Finally, electrophysiology and behavioral testing confirmed that recovery is mediated, at least in part, through sprouting of the corticospinal tract and thus most likely involved the newly formed spinal detour circuit.

New growth of axons also may accompany the plastic changes that have been reported in other systems. Sprouting of horizontal connections has been reported in the deprived portion of visual cortex after retinal lesions in cats. The new connections are proposed to provide new sources of activation for neurons in deprived cortex. In the auditory system, the possibility of new growth has not been addressed; however, much as in other sensory systems, primary auditory cortex that is deprived by peripheral lesions comes to be reactivated by other intact inputs. In the

motor system, the basis for much of the cortical reorganization that has been described in human amputees is proposed to be a reduction of GABAergic inhibition. However, as reviewed above, changes in the innervation of muscles by spinal cord motoneurons do occur, and it seems likely that changes in central nervous system structures also occur.

In summary, the new growth and sprouting of axons can take place at a minimum of four levels in the sensorimotor system. In the somatosensory system (Fig.26.2), the new growth can occur at the levels of corticocortical, thalamocortical, brainstem and dorsal column connections. In the motor system, the new growth can occur at the levels of corticocortical, cortical and subcortical nuclei, corticospinal, and between spinal cord and peripheral nerves.

CONCLUSIONS AND FUTURE DIRECTIONS

The mature brain is capable of reorganization in response to peripheral nerve cut, amputations, or spinal cord injury. Mechanisms underlying these changes may range from altered tonic inhibition and synaptic efficacy to neuronal sprouting. An understanding of these mechanisms could facilitate the development of strategies for improving functional recovery after such injuries.

GENERAL CITATIONS

Kaas JH. 2001. *Mutable Brain: Dynamic and Plastic Features of the Developing and Mature Brain (Brain Plasticity and Reorganization)*. Amsterdam, The Netherlands: Harwood Academic Publishers.

DISCOVERY CITATIONS

Bareyre FM, Kerschensteiner M, Raineteau O, Mettenleiter TC , Weinmann O, and Schwab ME. 2004. The injured spinal cord spontaneously forms a new intraspinal circuit in adult rats. *Nat Neurosci*, 7: 269-277.

Churchill JD, Arnold LL, and Garraghty PE. 2001. Somatotopic reorganization in the brainstem and thalamus following peripheral nerve injury in adult primates. *Brain Res*, 910: 142-152.

Corbetta M, Burton H,   Sinclair RJ, Conturo TE, Akbudak E, and McDonald JW. 2002. Functional reorganization and stability of somatosensory-motor cortical topography in a tetraplegic subject with late recovery. *Proc Natl Acad Sci USA*, 99: 17066-17071.

Darian-Smith C and Gilbert CD. 1994. Axonal sprouting accompanies functional reorganization in adult cat striate cortex. *Nature*, 368: 737-740.

Darian-Smith C and Brown S. 2000. Functional changes at periphery and cortex following dorsal root lesions in adult monkeys. *Nat Neurosci*, 3: 476-481.

Darian-Smith C. 2004. Primary afferent terminal sprouting after a cervical dorsal rootlet section in the macaque monkey. *J Comp Neurol*, 470: 134-150.

Dhillon GS, Lawrence SM, Hutchinson DT, and Horch KW. 2004. Residual function in peripheral nerve stumps of amputees: implications for neural control of artificial limbs. *J Hand Surg [Am]*, 29: 605-615; discussion 616-618.

Farne A, Roy AC, Giraux P, Dubernard JM, and Sirigu A. 2002. Face or hand, not both: perceptual correlates of reafferentation in a former amputee. *Curr Biol*, 12: 1342-1346.

Flor H, Elbert T, Knecht S, Wienbruch C, Pantev C, Birbaumer N, Larbig W, and Taub E. 1995. Phantom-limb pain as a perceptual correlate of cortical reorganization following arm amputation. *Nature*, 375: 482-484.

Florence SL, Garraghty PE, Wall JT, and Kaas JH. 1994. Sensory afferent projections and area 3b somatotopy following median nerve cut and repair in macaque monkeys. *Cereb Cortex*, 4: 391-407.

Florence SL and Kaas JH. 1995. Large-scale reorganization at multiple levels of the somatosensory pathway follows therapeutic amputation of the hand in monkeys. *Journal of Neuroscience*, 15: 8083-8095.

Florence SL, Taub HB, and Kaas JH. 1998. Large-scale sprouting of cortical connections after peripheral injury in adult macaque monkeys. *Science*, 282: 1117-1121.

Florence SL, Boydston LA, Hackett TA, Lachoff HT, Strata F, and Niblock MM. 2001. Sensory enrichment after peripheral nerve injury restores cortical, not thalamic, receptive field organization. *Eur J Neurosci*, 13: 1755-1766.

Friel KM, Heddings AA, and Nudo RJ. 2000. Effects of postlesion experience on behavioral recovery and neurophysiologic reorganization after cortical injury in primates. *Neurorehabil Neural Repair*, 14: 187-198.

Giraux P, Sirigu A, Schneider F, and Dubernard JM. 2001. Cortical reorganization in motor cortex after graft of both hands. *Nat Neurosci*, 4: 691-692.

Jain N, Florence SL, Qi H-X, and Kaas JH. 2000. Growth of new brain stem connections in adult monkeys with massive sensory loss. *Proceedings of the National Academy of Sciences USA*, 97: 5546-5550.

Karl A, Birbaumer N, Lutzenberger W, Cohen LG, and Flor H. 2001. Reorganization of motor and somatosensory cortex in upper extremity amputees with phantom limb pain. *J Neurosci*, 21: 3609- 3618.

Liu S, Kadi K, Boisset N, Lacroix C, Said G, and Tadie M. 1999. Reinnervation of denervated lumbar ventral roots and their target muscle by thoracic spinal motoneurons via an implanted nerve autograft in adult rats after spinal cord injury. *J Neurosci Res*, 56: 506-517.

Liu S, Aghakhani N, Boisset N, Said G, and Tadie M. 2001. Innervation of the caudal denervated ventral roots and their target muscles by the rostral spinal motoneurons after implanting a nerve autograft in spinal cord-injured adult marmosets. *J Neurosurg*, 94: 82-90.

Lotze M, Grodd W, Birbaumer N, Erb M, Huse E and Flor H. 1999. Does use of a myoelectric prosthesis prevent cortical reorganization and phantom limb pain? *Nat Neurosci*, 2: 501-502.

Nudo RJ, Wise BM, SiFuentes F, and Milliken GW. 1996. Neural substrates for the effects of rehabilitative training on motor recovery after ischemic infarct. *Science*, 272: 1791-1974.

Plautz EJ, Barbay S, Frost SB, Friel KM, Dancause N, Zoubina EV, Stowe AM, Quaney BM, and Nudo RJ. 2003. Post-infarct cortical plasticity and behavioral recovery using concurrent cortical stimulation and rehabilitative training: a feasibility study in primates. *Neurol Res*, 25: 801-810.

Pons TP, Garraghty PE, Ommaya AK, Kaas JH, Taub E, and Mishkin M. 1991. Massive cortical reorganization after sensory deafferentation in adult macaques [see comments], *Science*, 252: 1857- 1860.

Ramachandran VS and Rogers-Ramachandran D. 2000. Phantom limbs and neural plasticity. *Arch Neurol*, 57: 317-320.

Rasmusson DD, Turnbull BG, and Leech CK. 1985. Unexpected reorganization of somatosensory cortex in a raccoon with extensive forelimb loss. *Neurosci Lett*, 55: 167-172.

Tadie M, Liu S, Robert R, Guiheneuc P, Pereon Y, Perrouin-Verbe B, and Mathe JF. 2002. Partial return of motor function in paralyzed legs after surgical bypass of the lesion site by nerve autografts three years after spinal cord injury. *J Neurotrauma*, 19: 909-916.

Yang TT, Gallen C, Schwartz B, Bloom FE, Ramachandran VS, and Cobb S. 1994. Sensory maps in the human brain. *Nature*, 368: 592-593.

Part IX   Endogenous Analgesia and Other Form of Analgesia

Endogenous Biphasic Modulation

CHAPTER 27

Min Zhuo*, Gerald F. Gebhart

Dr. Zhuo MAJOR CONTRIBUTIONS

1. Zhuo M, Gebhart GF. 1990. Characterization of descending inhibition and facilitation from the nuclei reticularis gigantocellularis and gigantocellularis pars alpha in the rat. *Pain*, 42:337-350.
2. Zhuo M, Gebhart GF. 1992. Characterization of descending facilitation and inhibition of spinal nociceptive transmission from the nuclei reticularis gigantocellularis and gigantocellularis pars alpha in the rat. *Journal of Neurophysiology*, 67: 1599-1614.
3. Li P, Zhuo M. 1998. Silent glutamatergic synapses and nociception in mammalian spinal cord. *Nature*, 393: 695-698.
4. Calejesan A A , Kim S J, Zhuo M. 2000. Descending facilitatory modulation of a behavioral nociceptive response by stimulation in the adult rat anterior cingulate cortex. *Eur J Pain*, 4:83-96.
5. Zhuo M, Sengupta J N and Gebhart GF. 2002. Biphasic modulation of spinal visceral nociceptive transmission from the rostroventral medial medulla in the rat. *J Neurophysiology*, 87: 2225-2236.

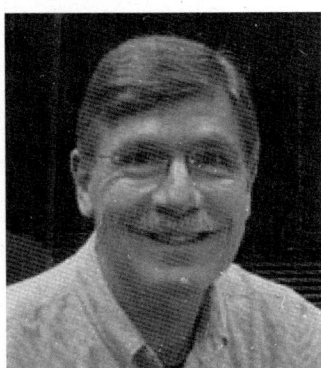

Dr. Gebhart is Director of the Center for Pain Research at the University of Pittsburgh. He completed his Ph.D. at the

* The introduction of Dr. Zhuo, please refer to Chapter 8.

University of Iowa and continued post-doctoral research at the Center for Research in Neurologic Sciences,University of Montreal, Canada (H. H. Jasper, Sponsor).

MAJOR CONTRIBUTIONS

1. Zhuo M, Gebhart GF. 1990. Characterization of descending inhibition and facilitation from the nucleireticularis gigantocell- ularis and gigantocellularis pars alpha in the rat. *Pain*, 42:337-350.
2. Porreca F, Ossipov MH, Gebhart GF. 2002. Chronic pain and medullary descending facilitation. *Trends Neurosci.* 25(6):319- 325. (Review).
3. Zhuo M, Gebhart GF. 2002. Modulation of noxious and non-noxious spinal mechanical transmission from the rostral medial medulla in the rat. *J Neurophysiol*, 88(6): 2928-2941.
4. Zhuo M, Sengupta, JN, Gebhart GF. 2002. Biphasic modulation of spinal visceral nociceptivetransmission from the rostro- ventral medial medulla in the rat. *J Neurophysiology*, 87:2225- 2236.
5. Gebhart GF. 2004. Descending modulation of pain. *Neurosci Biobehav Rev.*, 27(8):729-737. (Review)

MAIN TOPICS

Endogenous facilitatory systems

Biphasic modulation

Stimulus-response function and latency

Unmasking effects of descending facilitation

Neuronal vs cardiovascular effects of Stimulation

Supraspinal inputs to the RVM

Different approaches for studying spinal molecular mechanisms

Stimulation-produced facilitation and drug pretrea-

SUMMARY

It is well documented that sensory transmission, including pain, is subject to endogenous inhibitory influences at the dorsal horn of the spinal cord. Recent results, from behavioral to molecular studies, demonstrate that endogenous modulatory systems are bi-phasic, including inhibitory and new facilitatory systems. In this review, we propose the existence of endogenous facilitatory systems in the brain, and review evidence supporting the hypothesis. We believe that understanding the molecular and cellular basis of endogenous facilitatory systems hold the hope for better future treatment of patients with chronic pain.

INTRODUCTION

Brain activity is able to affect sensory transmission through descending modulatory systems. For many years, it has been believed that endogenous modulatory systems are mainly inhibitory, or "analgesic". Cumulative studies, however, reveal that descending modulation of spinal sensory transmission is biphasic, including inhibitory and facilitatory influences. Descending influences from supraspinal, central nuclei directly or indirectly modulate spinal sensory transmission and include the anterior cingulate cortex (ACC), amygdala, periaqueductal gray (PAG), and rostroventral medial medulla (RVM), which may function as the last relay between brain centers and the spinal cord. Biphasic modulation of spinal nociceptive transmission from the RVM, perhaps reflecting the different types of neurons identified in this area, offer fine regulation of spinal sensory thresholds and responses. Integrative approaches have been used to investigate the mechanisms for descending facilitation, including electrophysiological, pharmacological, behavioral, and biochemical studies. In this review, we will summarize data using whole animal preparation, *in vitro* spinal and brain slices, and genetically manipulated mice to support the hypothesis that the positive feedback mechanism within the synapses or between different brain regions is a key mechanism for persistent pain caused by injury.

ENDOGENOUS FACILITATORY/ SYSTEMS

The investigation of descending facilitatory systems has been carried out systematically in the brainstem RVM. At the whole animal level, electrophysiological, pharmacological, and behavioral experiments have been performed to characterize facilitation of responses of spinal sensory neurons to peripheral noxious stimuli as well as behavioral responses to noxious stimuli. Facilitation affects spinal nociceptive transmission from somatocutaneous areas as well as from visceral organs. Furthermore, facilitation is a common form of modulation of sensory transmission, affecting both noxious and non-noxious inputs. These unique features indeed raise the possibility that descending facilitation may serve as a key central mechanism to contribute to injury-related central pain or allodynia.

BIPHASIC MODULATION

A key feature of descending facilitation is that it is intensity-dependent. Whether facilitation or inhibition is observed, in part, depends on the intensity of stimulation applied. According to effects on spinal sensory

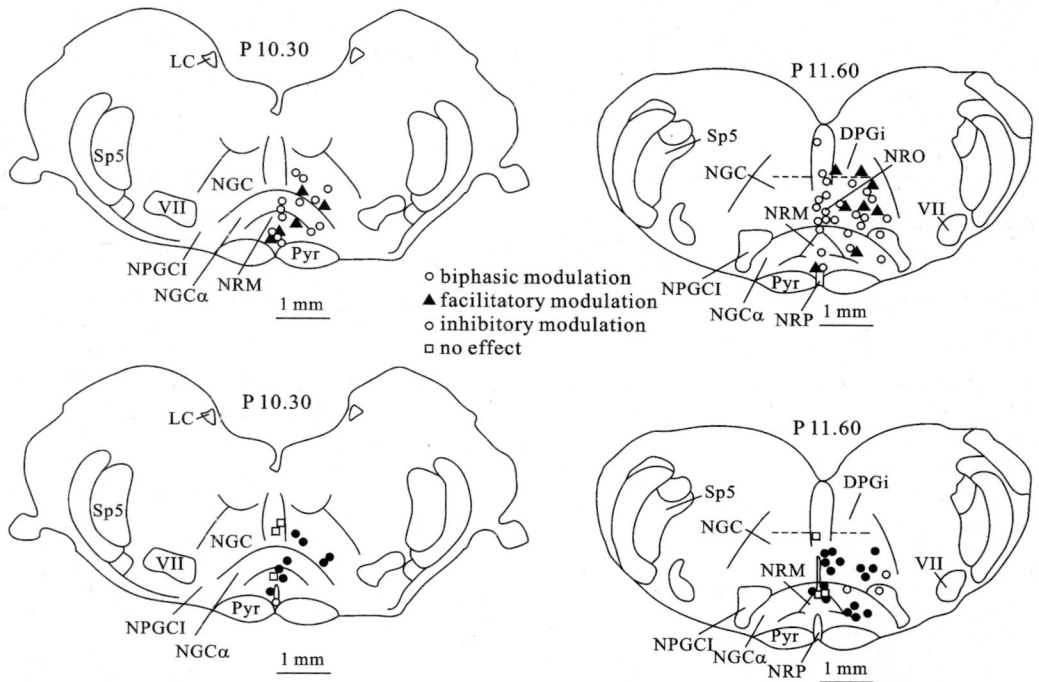

Fig.27.1   Brainstem sites for micro-electrical stimulation to produce biaphsic, inhibitory or facilitatory modulation of spinal visceral pain transmission.

neuronal responses, we characterize sites within the brainstem into three different groups: biphasic, inhibitory and facilitatory sites. At biphasic sites of stimulation, it is typical that electrical stimulation facilitates spinal nociceptive transmission at lesser intensities (5–25 µA) and inhibits responses of the same neurons at greater intensities (50–100 µA). At inhibitory sites, electrical stimulation only reduces and inhibits responses of spinal sensory neurons. At facilitatory sites, we found that electrical stimulation only caused increases in responses of spinal sensory neurons. To determine if facilitatory or inhibitory effects were simply due to different groups of spinal dorsal horn neurons recorded, we also investigated the effects of electrical stimulation at one intensity, but different sites in the RVM on the same spinal neuron. We found that the responses of the same spinal sensory neurons can be either inhibited or facilitated by electrical stimulation applied to different sites in the brainstem. Thus, spinal units receive both facilitatory and inhibitory influences descending from the brainstem.

There is no clear anatomical separation between these different effects produced by stimulation in the brainstem. Biphasic effects are often produced at sites of stimulation adjacent to those from which only inhibition is produced by similar intensities of stimulation. Further, inhibitory effects are produced at biphasic sites of stimulation adjacent to other biphasic sites from which facilitatory effects are produced (Fig.27.1). It is unlikely that effects are simply due to activation of fibers passing through the RVM because microinjection of glutamate or selective receptor agonists into the RVM also produces similar biphasic effects (Fig.27.3).

STIMULUS-RESPONSE FUNCTION AND LATENCY

For studying the effects of facilitation on stimulation-response functions (SRFs), responses of spinal neurons to graded, noxious cutaneous or visceral stimuli were studied. In most cases, in particular within the range of noxious intensities of cutaneous or visceral stimulation, descending inhibition significantly reduced the slopes of SRFs. In contrast, descending facilitation enables responses and causes a parallel shift of the

SRF to the left without changing its slope. These different outcomes on the encoding properties of spinal neurons suggest that descending facilitation is likely to be mechanistically different from descending inhibition. The latency to stimulation-produced facilitation and inhibition is determined by employing a cumulative sum technique and bin-by-bin analysis of unit responses and further supports that the mechanisms and pathways leading to inhibition and facilitation are different. Brainstem stimulation is given during a relatively stable rate of neuronal response to noxious stimulation. The first 500 ms period of recording is averaged to generate a reference baseline, and the cumulative sum of unit activity 500 ms before and 1500 ms after the onset of stimulation is plotted. The latency to effect is defined as the time from the onset of stimulation to the point when the cumulative sum of the histogram departs steadily from the reference baseline. The mean latency of stimulation-produced inhibition from the RVM is about 90 ms whereas the apparent mean latency to facilitation by electrical stimulation is greater than 200 ms. This suggests that descending facilitatory influences likely involve sites rostral to the RVM (e.g. ACC, see below).

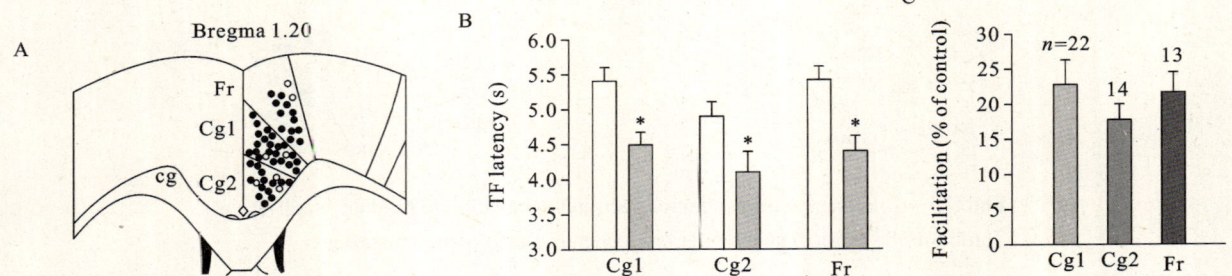

Fig.27.2 Facilitation of the spinal noiceptive tail-flick reflex produced by electrical stimulation in the ACC. A. Stimulation sites in the ACC, illustrated on representative coronal brain sections. Filled circles are sites where electrical stimulation produced facilitation. Open circles are sites where stimulation did not produce any significant effect. Differing from the brainstem, stimulation at intensities tested did not produce significant inhibition of the tail-flick reflex. B. Summarized data for the reduction in response latencies induced by micro-electrical stimulation in three sub-regions of the cortex. C. Percentage facilitation induced by electrical stimulation.

Table 27.1	Comparison of endogenous facilitation and analgesia systems.	
	Endogenous facilitation	Endogenous analgesia
Central origins	ACC; RVM	PAG; RVM
Central transmitters	Glutamate; neurotension	Opioids, glutamate
Stimulation intensity	5–25 μA	50–100 μA
Stimulation-response functions	Reducing threshold	Reducing peak response without changing threshold
Response latency	200 ms	90 ms
Laterality	Bilateral	Bilateral
Spinal pathways	Ventrolaterla funiculi (VLF)/ventral funiculi (VF)	Dorsolateral funiculi (DLF)
Spinal transmitters	5-HT	Ach, Ne, 5-HT
Synaptic mechanism	Postsynaptic AMPAR trafficking	Inhibition of presynaptiic elease
	Enhanced AMPAR mediated EPSCs	Reduced AMPAR mediated EPSCs
Sensory modality	Non-nociceptive responses	Non-nociceptive responses
	Nociceptive responses	Nociceptive responses
Origin of sensory inputs	Somatosensory	Somatosensory
	Visceral	Visceral

UNMASKING EFFECTS OF DESCE-NDING FACILITATION

Facilitatory influences are observed only at lesser intensities of stimulation (or lesser concentrations of glutamate). In early studies, the presence of descending facilitation from the brainstem may have been missed because brain stimulation intensity-dependent functions were not performed. Descending inhibitory and facilitatory influences are likely to be simultaneously activated, and prepotent inhibitory effects masked facilitatory effects. This notion has been confirmed in experiments investigating spinal pathways for descending modulation. Bilateral transections of the dorsolateral funiculi (DLFs) in the thoracic spinal cord not only abolished descending inhibition produced by electrical or chemical stimulation in the RVM, but also unmasked descending facilitatory influences on spinal sensory neurons at the same high intensities of stimulation that only produced inhibition before the DLF transactions. These findings suggest that descending inhibitory and facilitatory influences can be simultaneously engaged by activation of sites in the RVM and that removal of the route conveying the inhibitory influences uncovers descending facilitatory effects on spinal sensory neurons.

NEURONAL VS CARDIOVASCULAR EFFECTS OF STIMULATION

It is well documented that brainstem sites are important for regulation of cardiovascular functions. In biphasic sites of stimulation in the RVM, electrical stimulation (10 μA) that facilitated responses of spinal neurons to noxious stimuli did not affect mean arterial blood pressure. At intensities of electrical stimulation that significantly inhibited responses of spinal neurons, mean arterial pressure was decreased, increased, or unaffected. The latency for electrical stimulation-produced increases or decreases in blood pressure was estimated by employing the cumulative sum technique described above. The mean apparent latency to increase blood pressure was about 4.0 s. The estimated latency to decrease arterial blood pressure was about 3.0 s. The latency for cardiovascular changes is about 100 times slower than changes in spinal neuronal responses, indicating that modulation of sensory transmission in the spinal cord precedes effects on the cardiovascular system, suggesting independence of these descending systems, at least from the RVM.

SUPRASPINAL INPUTS TO THE RVM

Recent studies from both humans and non-human animals consistently suggest that the ACC and its related areas are important for processing pain perception. Lesions of the medial frontal cortex, including the ACC, significantly increased acute nociceptive responses as well as injury-related aversive memory behaviors. In patients with frontal lobotomies or cingulotomies, the unpleasantness of pain is abolished. Electrophysiological recordings from both non-human animals and humans demonstrate that neurons within the ACC respond to noxious stimuli and include neurons that respond only to noxious input. Neuroimaging studies further confirm these observations and show that the ACC, together with other cortical structures, is activated by acute noxious stimuli. It has been proposed that the ACC may activate the endogenous pain modulatory system due to its projecting connections to the PAG in the midbrain. To investigate the roles of the ACC in descending modulation, we applied electrical stimulation or chemical microinjection into the ACC and found that activation of ACC neurons only produces facilitation of spinal nociceptive reflexes (Fig.27.2). Furthermore, activation of glutamate mGluRs in the ACC also produced similar facilitatory effects. The descending facilitatory modulation from the ACC is likely conveyed through the RVM because blockade of activity in the RVM or AMPA receptor antagonists given into the RVM attenuated or abolished the facilitation (Fig.27.4).

DIFFERENT APPROACHES FOR STUDYING SPINAL MOLECULAR MECHANISMS

Molecular mechanisms for descending facilitation in the spinal cord are carried out using different approaches, including *in vivo* and *in vitro* experiments. For *in vivo* experiments, intrathecal (i.th.) application of neurotransmitter receptor antagonists is used to identify spinal transmitters/receptors that mediate the facilitatory effects. For *in vitro* experiments, the effects of a prominent spinal neurotransmitter, serotonin (5-HT), on AMPA receptor-mediated excitatory postsynaptic currents in spinal neurons have been investigated. Genetic studies have also been performed to examine roles of two major calcium-stimulated adenylyl cyclases subtype 1 (AC1) and subtype 8 (AC8) in spinal facilitation.

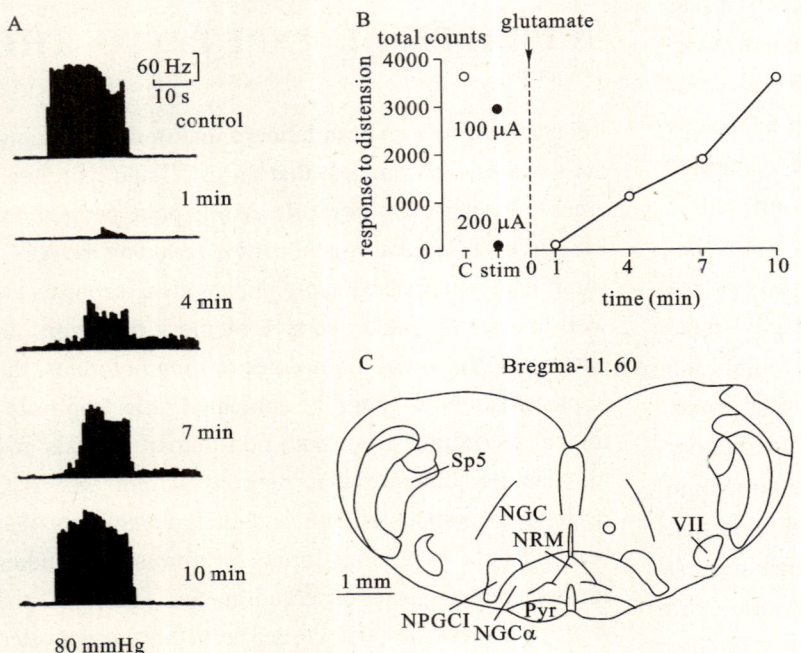

Fig.27.3 Microinjection of glutamate into the brainstem (shown by the open circle in C) inhibits behavioral responses (shown in A) to visceral pain induced by colorectal distension (at 80 mmHg). The total responses at each time points are given in the plot shown in B. Electrical stimulation at high intensities (100 and 200 μA) delivered to the same brainstem sites produced inhibitory effects (indicated by filled circles).

STIMULATION-PRODUCED FACILITATION AND DRUG PRETREATMENT

5-HT-containing neurons in the RVM send descending projection fibers to targets in the spinal cord, including the superficial dorsal horn. Activation of these descending pathways can facilitate or inhibit spinal nociceptive transmission. Behavioral and pharmacological experiments have been performed to determine the spinal receptors that mediate descending modulation from the RVM. The advantage of intrathecal administration of drugs is that it allows rapid, reversible and localized blockade of neurotransmitter receptors (e.g., in the lumbosacral spinal cord). Intrathecal pretreatment with the non-selective 5-HT receptor antagonist methysergide completely reversed the facilitatory effect of electrical stimulation in the RVM. Interestingly, the baseline nociceptive reflex response latency as well as the mean arterial blood pressure was not affected by i.th. pretreatment with the same dose of methysergide. Neither the opioid receptor antagonist naloxone nor the cholinergic nicotinic receptor antagonist mecamylamine affected the facilitatory effect of electrical stimulation in the RVM. Intrathecal pretreatment with the cholinergic muscarinic receptor antagonist atropine or the adrenergic α receptor antagonist phentolamine also failed to influence the facilitation of nociceptive reflexes produced by stimulation in the RVM.

FACILITATION OF SPINAL SYNAPTIC TRANSMISSION BY 5-HT

It is important to show that these modulatory effects are due to changes in spinal sensory synaptic transmission, and not due to modulation of pre-motor spinal interneurons or spinal local inhibitory synapses. Consistent with the biphasic modulatory effects of 5-HT on spinal nociceptive transmission and behavioral reflexes, we found that 5-HT produced biphasic modulation of excitatory synaptic responses in spinal cord slices. 5-HT at high doses produces inhibition of AMPA/kainate receptor mediated excitatory postsynaptic currents (EPSCs), while a low dose of 5-HT or a selective 5-HT$_2$ receptor agonist induces facilitation of fast EPSCs in the lumbar spinal cord. 5-HT at low doses could facilitate fast EPSCs in the presence of a NMDA receptor antagonist, AP-5 (50 μM), indicating that the facilitatory effect is NMDA receptor independent. Furthermore, the facilitatory effect induced by 5-HT at low doses persisted during washout of 5-HT. While activation of 5-HT receptors is important for the induction of the facilitation, continuous activation of these receptors is not necessary for the expression of the facilitation. Application of methysergide after administration of a serotonergic receptor agonist, DOI, failed to reverse the facilitatory effect of 5-HT. These results indicate that 5-HT triggers long-term plastic changes in spinal dorsal horn synapses and continuous activation of 5-HT receptors are not required for the expression of the facilitation.

5-HT may affect spinal sensory transmission by acting on presynaptic or postsynaptic receptors. Postsynaptic application of G protein inhibitors, introduced through the recording pipette, abolish the effect of 5-HT to facilitate synaptic transmission, suggesting that postsynaptic 5-HT receptors are critical for the effect In support of this notion, we found postsynaptic Ca^{2+}-dependent processes to be required for 5-HT-induced facilitation. In experiments with chelating postsynaptic Ca^{2+} with BAPTA in the pipette solution, the facilitatory effect of 5-HT was abolished, indicating that an increase in postsynaptic Ca^{2+} is required. Additional evidence against a mechanism of 5-HT-induced synaptic facilitation involving modulation of presynaptic glutamate release comes from the observation that while 5-HT application clearly caused AMPA receptor mediated EPSCs, NMDA receptor mediated EPSCs were significantly decreased by 5-HT in the same neurons. This result suggests that postsynaptic enhancement of AMPA receptor mediated currents by 5-HT are selective.

COACTIVATION OF CALCIUMSTIMULATED ADENYLYL CYCLASES IN ADULT SENSORY NEURONS

Possible developmental factors have been raised as concerns in the study of silent synapses because most such experiments are performed in spinal cord slices from young animals (e.g., postnatal days 2⁻4 old). Recordings from adult neurons have been reported, and less or no silent synapses have been found. To study synaptic regulation by 5-HT, we performed intracellular recordings in adult mouse spinal cord slices. We found that in sensory synapses of the adult mouse, some synaptic responses (26.3 % of a total of 38 experiments) between primary afferent fibers and dorsal horn neurons were almost completely mediated by NMDA receptors. Dorsal root stimulation did not elicit any detectable AMPA/kainate receptor-mediated responses in these synapses. Unlike young spinal cord, 5-HT alone does not produce any long-lasting synaptic enhancement in adult spinal dorsal horn neurons.

cAMP signaling pathways have been implicated in the function of spinal dorsal horn neurons. Activation of several receptors for sensory transmitters such as glutamate and calcitonin gene related peptide (CGRP) has been reported to raise cAMP levels. In slices or isolated cells from young animals, a cAMP analogue enhanced glutamate receptor mediated synaptic responses or had no effect on AMPA/kainate receptor mediated synaptic responses. In a recent study, application of forskolin did not significantly affect synaptic responses induced by dorsal root stimulation in slices of adult mice. However, co-application of 5-HT and forskolin produced long-lasting facilitation of synaptic responses. Possible contributors to the increase in the cAMP levels are calcium-sensitive adenylyl cyclases (AC). We found that the facilitatory effect induced by 5-HT and forskolin was completely blocked in mice lacking AC1 or AC8, indicating that calcium-sensitive adenylyl cyclases are important. Our results demonstrate that in adult sensory synapses, cAMP signaling pathways determine whether activation of 5-HT receptors causes facilitatory or inhibitory effects on synaptic responses. Unlike synapses from young animals, 5-HT alone did not induce reliable and long-lasting facilitation of synaptic responses. Instead, 5-HT at the same low dose induced no effects, short-lasting increases or inhibition in neurons from adult animals. However, co-application of the same dose of 5-HT with forskolin produced significant long-lasting enhancement of synaptic responses. This finding provides a possible explanation for regulation of two different signaling pathways under physiological or pathological conditions. Postsynaptic increases in cAMP levels by sensory transmitters may favor 5-HT-induced facilitation. The interaction between cAMP and 5-HT may provide an associative heterosynaptic form of central plasticity in the spinal dorsal horn to allow sensory inputs from the periphery to act synergistically with central modulatory influences descending from the brainstem RVM. We think it is unlikely that cAMP acts in addition to 5-HT signal pathways. First, 5-HT at a higher dose produces opposite effects—that is, inhibition of synaptic responses—and forskolin alone did not produce facilitation. Second, in neurons from young animals, it has been reported that PKC is required for the effects of 5-HT.

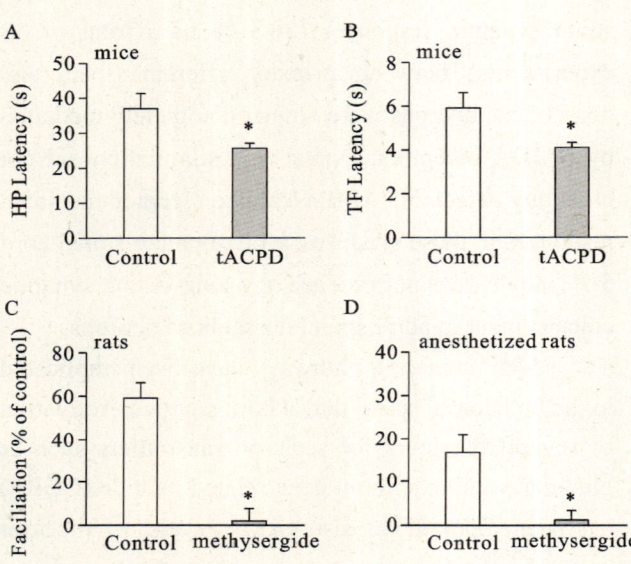

Fig.27.4 Spinal serotonin receptors contribute to descending modulation from the ACC. A, B. Microinjection of tACPD (0.25 μg in 0.5 μL) in the ACC facilitated the hot-plate responses (A, i.e., reduced response latency) and spinal nociceptive tail-flick reflex (B) in freely moving mice. C,D. In freely moving (C) or anesthetized rats (D), tACPD microinjection in the ACC also facilitated the tail-flick reflex. Intrathecal injection of a serotonergic receptor antagonist methysergide (32.0 nmoles/10 μL) at a dose that blocked descending facilitation also blocked the facilitation of the tail-flick reflex.

DESCENDING PROJECTIONS AND CHRONIC PAIN

Neurons in the brain that contribute to descending modulatory systems are clearly important to the normal processing of nociceptive input. Peripheral noxious stimuli activate not only neurons in the spinal cord, but also neurons in the RVM and ACC. Such activation is brief, but when peripheral tissues are injured, long-lasting changes in neuronal activity can occur in these brain areas. Here, we propose a positive feedback model, then provide evidence to support its contribution to chronic pain.

Positive Feedback Model

A positive feedback control is proposed to serve as the key pathophysiological mechanism for chronic pain (Fig.27.5). Such positive enhancement occurs not only at single synapses, but also between multiple neuronal synapses in different parts of the brain. Several mechanisms may contribute to synaptic enhancement: (i) postsynaptic regulation of glutamate receptors, including phosphorylation and dephosphorylation of the receptor; (ii) recruitment of functional glutamate receptors (for example, in spinal dorsal horn neurons, recruitment of postsynaptic functional AMPA receptors); (iii) presynaptic enhancement of glutamate release; and (iv) structural changes in synapses. At the level of neuronal networks, heterosynaptic facilitation or dis-inhibition can lead to enhancement as well. It is well documented that dorsal horn neurons receive descending facilitatory modulation from brainstem neurons. The consequence of this *positive feedback control* will lead central neurons to an enhanced and overexcited status. Accordingly, a weak input can lead to significantly greater consequences than would normally obtain from that intensity input (e.g., significantly more neuron action potentials). The enhanced excitability of central nervous system neurons has been termed "central sensitization" and most likely contributes to chronic pain states characterized by allodynia and including central pain. Studies on the mechanisms of central sensitization have primarily focused on the spinal cord and have generally excluded consideration of brain contributions such as positive feedback from supraspinal sites.

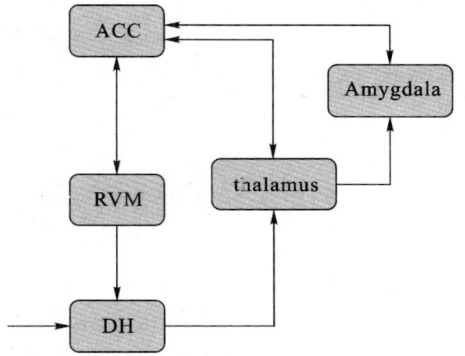

Fig.27.5   Endogenous facilitatory systems.

RVM

RVM neurons have been classified by Fields and colleagues into three physiological classes. Among them, the lack of response of cells termed "neutral" to acute noxious stimulation and to morphine suggested that this cell class might not play an important role in acute nociception or opioid-dependent antinociception. Our recent results, however, suggest that NEUTRAL cells may participate in the response to prolonged nociceptive stimulation or inflammation.

Considerable evidence reveals a significant contribution of supraspinal influences to development and maintenance of hyperalgesia. For example, spinal cord transection, which removes descending modulatory influences on the spinal cord, prevents development of secondary, but not primary mechanical and/or thermal hyperalgesia after topical mustard oil application,

carrageenan inflammation or nerve-root ligation. In all of these models, hypersensitivity to stimuli applied to uninjured tissue adjacent to or at some distance from the site of tissue injury either does not develop or is not maintained. Similarly, inactivation of the RVM attenuates hyperalgesia and central sensitization in several models of persistent pain. As in the spinal cord, inhibition of medullary NMDA receptors or generation of one of its downstream mediators, NO, attenuates both somatic and visceral hyperalgesia. In support, topical mustard oil application or colonic inflammation increases expression of NO synthase in the RVM. These data suggest a significant role for the RVM in mediating the sensitization of spinal neurons and development of secondary hyperalgesia. Results to date suggest that peripheral injury and persistent input engage spinobulbospinal mechanisms that may be important contributors to some chronic pain states. Thus, like the ACC, the RVM is an important contributor, and may be the final common pathway, in positive feedback control of spinal nociceptive processing.

ENDOGENOUS ANALGESIA SYSTEMS

Stimulation-morphine-induced Analgesia

Spinal nociceptive transmission is modulated by an endogenous antinociceptive or analgesic system, consisting of the midbrain periaqueductal gray (PAG) and the rostral ventral medulla (RVM). The RVM serves as an important relay for descending influences from the PAG to the spinal cord, since not all neurons in the PAG send their descending projecting fibers to the spinal cord dorsal horn. In animals under light anesthesia, activation of neurons in the RVM inhibits spinal nociceptive transmission and behavioral nociceptive reflexes.

Descending Pathways

The inhibitory effect is mediated directly by descending pathways projecting bilaterally in the dorsolateral funiculi, and indirectly by descending activation of local spinal inhibitory neurons. In the spinal cord, muscarinic, noradrenergic and serotonergic receptors are important for descending inhibition of behavioral nociceptive reflexes.

In Vivo Intracellular Recordings

Electrophysiological studies using intracellular or whole-cell patch-clamp recordings of dorsal horn neurons allow for the investigation of the cellular mechanisms underlying antinociceptive or analgesic effects induced by these transmitters. In anesthetized whole animals, electrical stimulation applied to sites within the nucleus raphe magnus or PAG produced inhibitory postsynaptic potentials (IPSPs) in dorsal horn neurons including ascending projection spinothalamic tract cells. More detailed pharmacological analyses came from studies using an *in vitro* brain/spinal cord slice preparation. In trigeminal nuclei, all three major transmitters, acetylcholine, serotonin and norepinephrine are reported to inhibit glutamatergic transmission. In the lumbar spinal cord, less is known about the synaptic mechanisms underlying sensory inhibition by carbachol, clonidine and serotonin.

Cholinergic

Animal studies consistently demonstrate that activation of spinal cholinergic muscarinic systems is antinociceptive in various acute behavioral tests. Intrathecal injection of carbachol, the same agonist used in the current study, inhibits different behavioral responses to acute noxious stimuli. Recent studies showed that muscarinic receptor agonists, injected systemically or intrathecally, inhibited behavioral responses in animals with inflammatory pain or neuropathic pain. Analgesic effects of cholinergic drugs were also reported in patients in experimental, acute postoperative and chronic pain.

Two different types of synaptic regulation in the dorsal horn could potentially contribute to cholinergic inhibition of sensory transmission: inhibition of excitatory transmission and enhancement of inhibitory transmission. In the present study, we showed that in the lumbar spinal cord, carbachol inhibited glutamatergic

transmission through postsynaptic muscarinic receptors. Using intracellular recordings, we reported that the amplitude of excitatory postsynaptic potentials (EPSPs) were inhibited by carbachol, although postsynaptic inhibition of G-proteins had not been performed. Secondly, inhibitory transmission in the dorsal horn may be affected as well. Because the inhibitory influences were removed in our experiments, it is unlikely that the observed effect was due to indirect changes in inhibitory tone. Both Travagli (1996) and Baba *et al.* (1998) reported that inhibitory postsynaptic potentials (IPSPs) or currents (IPSCs) were enhanced in the trigeminal nuclei and dorsal horn neurons, respectively. Therefore, postsynaptic inhibition of glutamate-mediated responses and enhancement of inhibitory responses likely contribute to behavioral antinociception and clinical analgesia caused by cholinergic drugs. Carbachol may also affect spinal sensory transmission and central plasticity mediated by neuropeptides, including substance P and CGRP, although our study does not address this possibility.

Although the central source of acetylcholine is mainly within local spinal neurons, these spinal cholinergic systems can be activated by descending modulatory pathways from supraspinal structures. In addition, systemic morphine administration or visceral nociceptive stimuli such as corolectal distension also activated spinal cholinergic inhibitory systems. Descending inhibition from different regions of the brain is reported to be mediated by spinal muscarinic receptors, although the transmitters that activate spinal cholinergic neurons remain obscure. Thus, spinal cholinergic systems play an inhibitory role in spinal sensory transmission and provide an important target for the management of pain in patients. Although previous pharmacological studies exclude the involvement of spinal nicotinic receptors in descending inhibition from the RVM, we cannot rule out a possible role for nicotinic compounds in modulating spinal sensory transmission.

Noradrenergic

It is well known that intrathecal administration of

noradrenergic receptor agonists, including clonidine, is antinociceptive/analgesic. Intrathecal administration of the nonselective α-adrenergic antagonist phentolamine or the selective α_2-adrenergic antagonist yohimbine was found to attenuate descending inhibition of nociceptive reflexes produced by electrical and/or chemical stimulation in the PAG, nucleus raphe magnus, nucleus reticularis paragigantocellularis and locus coerleus. Unlike cholinergic terminals, norepinephrine-containing fibers mainly originate from supraspinal structures. PAG stimulation-induced inhibition of nociceptive dorsal horn neurons in rats was associated with the release of norepinephrine, serotonin, and amino acids.

Both presynaptic and postsynaptic receptors are indicated in spinal inhibition produced by noradrenergic compounds. Clonidine produced significant inhibition of fast excitatory sensory responses in the spinal cord, and the inhibition was significantly but incompletely reduced by postsynaptic inhibition of G-protein signaling, indicating a role for postsynaptic G-protein-coupled receptors. Incomplete blockade may be due to partial inhibition of postsynaptic G-proteins and/or the involvement of presynaptic receptors. In animal studies, it has been reported that spinal noradrenergic systems are tonically active, and blockade of spinal noradrenergic receptors significantly decreases mechanical and thermal withdrawal thresholds. In spinal slice experiments, application of phentolamine did not lead to significant enhancement of synaptic responses, indicating that any tonic inhibition depends upon other inputs which may be removed in slice preparations.

Serotonergic

Intrathecal administration of serotonin has been reported to be antinociceptive or facilitatory. Different types of serotonin receptors in the spinal cord are believed to be involved in inhibitory and facilitatory effects. Spinal serotonin-containing fibers orginate mainly from supraspinal structures, including a variety of brainstem nuclei such as the nuclei raphe magnus, obscurus, pallidus, reticularis gigantocellularis, and gigantocellularis pars alpha. It has been consistently shown that both descending inhibition and facilitation of a behavioral spinal nociceptive reflex from various supraspinal structures are mediated in part by serotonergic receptors. The facilitatory effect of serotonin has been recently examined in the dorsal horn and found to be related to the regulation of postsynaptic AMPA receptor function. Inhibitory mechanisms, however, may contain both presynaptic actions on primary afferent terminals and a postsynaptic action on spinal dorsal horn neurons. Our results provide direct evidence of a postsynaptic mechanism but do not rule out a possible additional contribution of presynaptic receptors, as postsynaptic inhibition of G-proteins did not completely block the effects of serotonin. More studies are needed to investigate the molecular mechanisms for pre- and post-synaptic inhibition as well as possible regulatory effects of serotonin on spinal inhibitory synaptic transmission.

CONCLUSIONS AND FUTURE RESEARCH DIRECTIONS

Understanding the molecular and cellular mechanisms underlying central changes in various pain-related states holds hope for improved treatment of chronic pain. From the basic science point of view, it is important to understand molecular and cellular mechanisms for long-term plastic changes in the ACC, RVM and spinal dorsal horn after peripheral tissue insult. At the level of neuronal circuits or networks, it is necessary to understand how ascending and descending projection fibers affect local neuronal activity and contribute to neuronal plasticity. Such information will provide clues for testing new drug targets—for example, blocking descending facilitatory influences at different levels of the central nervous system (e.g., the ACC and RVM). Two simplified neuronal circuit models for descending facilitation (Fig.27.5) and inhibition (Fig.27.6) are proposed. It is critical for future studies to address the mechanisms at molecular, cellular, and circuit levels for these endogenous modulatory systems.

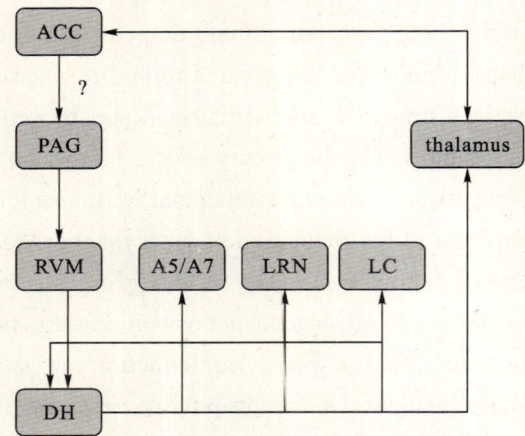

Fig.27.6 Endogenous inhibitory/analgesia systems.

It is clear that improved understanding of endogenous facilitatory systems provides not only knowledge about the basic physiological mechanisms related to sensory transmission, modulation and neuron plasticity, but also knowledge that can lead to improved management of persistent and chronic pain states in patients.

GENERAL CITATIONS

Fields H. 2004. State-dependent opioid control of pain. *Nat Rev Neurosci*, 5:565-575.

Fields HL, Heinricher MM and Mason P. 1991. Neurotransmitters in nociceptive modulatory circuits. *Annu Rev Neurosci*, 7:309-338.

Gebhart GF. 2004. Descending modulation of pain. *Neurosci Biobehav Rev*, 27:729-737.

Mason P. 2005. Deconstructing endogenous pain modulation. *J Neurophysiol*, 94: 1659-1663.

Mason P 1999. Central mechanisms of pain modulation. *Curt Opin Neurobiol*, 9: 436-441.

Millan MJ. 1999. The induction of pain: an integrative review. *Progress in Neurobiology*, 57:1-164.

Porreca F, Ossipov MH, Gebhart GF. 2002. Chronic pain and medullary descending facilitation. *Trends Neurosci,* 25: 319-325.

Robinson DA, Calejesan AA, Wei F, Gebhart GF, Zhuo M. 2004. Endogenous facilitation: from molecular mechanisms to persistent pain. *Curr Neurovasc Res*, 1: 11-20.

Sandkuhler J. 1996. The organization and function of endogenous antinociceptive systems. *Prog Neurobiol*, 50:49-81.

Urban MO, Gebhart GF. 1999. Supraspinal contributions to hyperalgesia. *PNAS*, 96:7687-7692.

Zhuo M. 2000. Silent glutamatergic synapses and long- term facilitation in spinal dorsal horn neurons. *Progress in Brain Research*, 129:101-113.

Zhuo M. 2002. Glutamate receptors and persistent pain: targeting forebrain NR2B subunits. *Drug Discov Today*, 7:259-267.

DISCOVERY FINDINGS

Almeida A, Storkson R, Lima D, Hole K, Tjolsen A. 1999. The medullary dorsal reticular nucleus facilitates pain behaviour induced by formalin in the rat. *Eur J Neurosci*, 11:110-122.

Calejesan AA, Kim SJ, Zhuo M. 2000. Descending facilitatory modulation of a behavioral nociceptive response by stimulation in the adult rat anterior cingulate cortex. *Eur J Pain*, 4:83-96.

Donovan-Rodriguez T, Urch CE, Dickenson AH. 2005. Evidence of a role for descending serotonergic facilitation in a rat model of cancer-induced bone pain. *Neurosci Lett*, 393:237-242.

Gardell LR, Vanderah TW, Gardell SE, Wang R, Ossipov MH, Lai J, Porreca F. 2003. Enhanced evoked excitatory transmitter release in experimental neuropathy requires descending facilitation. *J Neurosci*, 23:8370-8379.

Hori Y, Endo K and Takahashi T. 1996. Long-lasting synaptic facilitation induced by serotonin in superficial dorsal horn neurones of the rat spinal cord. *J Physiol (Lond)*, 492:867-876.

Johansen JP, Fields HL, Manning BH. 2001. The affective component of pain in rodents: direct evidence for a contribution of the anterior cingulate cortex. *PNAS*, 98:8077-8082.

Kaplan H, Fields HL. 1991. Hyperalgesia during acute opioid abstinence: evidence for a nociceptive facilitating function of the rostral ventromedial medulla. *J Neurosci*, 11:1433-1439.

Lima D, Almeida A. 2002. The medullary dorsal reticular nucleus as a pronociceptive centre of the pain control system. *Prog Neurobiol*, 66:81-108.

Lopez-Garcia JA and King AE. 1996. Pre-and post-synaptic actions of 5-hydroxytryptamine in the rat lumbar dorsal horn *in vitro*: implications for somatosensory transmission. *Eur J Neurosci*, 8:2188-2197.

Meng ID, Manning BH, Martin WJ, Fields HL. 1998. An analgesia circuit activated by cannabinoids. *Nature*, 395:381-383.

Morgan MM, Fields HL. 1994. Pronounced changes in the activity of nociceptive modulatory neurons in the rostral ventromedial medulla in response to prolonged thermal noxious stimuli. *J Neurophysiol*, 72:1161-1170.

Neugebauer V, Schaible HG. 1990. Evidence for a central component in the sensitization of spinal neurons with joint input during development of acute arthritis in cat's knee. *J Neurophysiol*, 64:299-311.

Pan ZZ, Tershner SA, Fields HL. 1997. Cellular mechanism for anti-analgesic action of agonists of the kappa-opioid receptor. *Nature*, 389:382-385.

Robinson DA, Calejesan AA and Zhuo M. 2002. Long-lasting changes in rostral ventral medulla neuronal activity following inflammation in the adult rat. *Journal of Pain*, 3:292-300.

Sikes RW and Vogt BA. 1992. Nociceptive neurons in area 24 of rabbit cingulate cortex. *Journal of Neurophysiology*, 68:1720-1732.

Suzuki R, Rahman W, Hunt SP, Dickenson AH. 2004. Descending facilitatory control of mechanically evoked responses is enhanced in deep dorsal horn neurones following peripheral nerve injury. *Brain Res*, 1019:68-76.

Talbot JD, Marrett S, Evans AC, Meyer E, Bushnell MC and Duncan GH. 1991. Multiple representations of pain in human cerebral cortex. *Science*, 251:1355-1358.

Tang YP, Xhimizu E, Dube GR, Rampon C, Kerchner GA, Zhuo M, Liu G and Tsien JZ. 1999. Genetic enhancement of learning and memory in mice. *Nature*, 401:63–69.

Thomas DA, McGowan MK, Hammond DL. 1995. Microinjection of baclofen in the ventromedial medulla of rats: antinociception at low doses and hyperalgesia at high doses. *J Pharmacol Exp Ther*, 275: 274-284.

Urban MO, Gebhart GF. 1999. Supraspinal contributions to hyperalgesia. *Proc Natl Acad Sci USA*, 96:7687-7692.

Urban MO, Jiang MC, Gebhart GF. 1996. Participation of central descending nociceptive facilitatory systems in secondary hyperalgesia produced by mustard oil. *Brain Res*, 737:83-91.

Vanegas H, Schaible HG. 2004. Descending control of persistent pain: inhibitory or facilitatory? *Brain Res Brain Res Rev*, 46:295-309.

Wang GD and Zhuo M. 2002. Synergistic enhancement of glutamate-mediated responses by serotonin and forskolin in adult mouse spinal dorsal horn neurons. *J Neurophysiology*, 87:732-739.

Wei F and Zhuo M. 2001. Potentiation of synaptic responses in the anterior cingulate cortex following digital amputation in rat. *J Physiology (Lond)*, 532:823-833.

Wei F, Li P and Zhuo M. 1999. Loss of synaptic depression in mammalian anterior cingulate cortex after amputation. *J of Neuroscience*, 19:9346-9354.

Wei F, Wang GD, Kerchner GA, Kim SJ, Xu HM, Chen ZF. and Zhuo M. 2001. Genetic enhancement of inflammatory pain by forebrain NR2B overexpression. *Nature Neuroscience*, 4:164-169.

Wei F, Qiu CS, Kim SJ, Muglia L, Maas JW, Pineda VV, Xu HM, Chen ZF, Storm DR, Muglia LJ and Zhuo M. 2002. Genetic elimination of behavioral sensitization in mice lacking calmodulin-stimulated adenylyl cyclases. *Neuron*, 36:713-726.

Wei F, Dubner R, Ren K. 1999. Nucleus reticularis gigantocellularis and nucleus raphe magnus in the brain stem exert opposite effects on behavioral hyperalgesia and spinal Fos protein expression after peripheral inflammation. *Pain*, 80:127-141.

Xie JY, Herman DS, Stiller CO, Gardell LR, Ossipov MH, Lai J, Porreca F, Vanderah TW. 2005. Cholecystokinin in the rostral ventromedial medulla mediates opioid-induced hyperalgesia and antinociceptive tolerance. *J Neurosci*, 25:409-416.

Zhang L, Zhang Y, Zhao ZQ. 2005. Anterior cingulate cortex contributes to the descending facilitatory modulation of pain via dorsal reticular nucleus. *Eur J Neurosci*, 22: 1141-1148.

Zhuo M and Gebhart GF. 1990a. Characterization of descending inhibition and facilitation from the nuclei reticularis gigantocellularis and gigantocellularis pars alpha in the rat. *Pain*, 42:337-350.

Zhuo M and Gebhart GF. 1990b. Spinal cholinergic and monoaminergic receptors mediate descending inhibition from the nuclei reticularis gigantocellularis pars alpha in the rat. *Brain Research*, 535: 67-78.

Zhuo M and Gebhart GF. 1991. Spinal serotonin receptors mediate descending facilitation pfs nociceptive reflex from the nuclei reticularis goigantocellularis and gigantocellularis pars alpha in the rat. *Brain Research*, 550:35-48.

Zhuo M and Gebhart GF. 1992. Characterization of descending facilitation and inhibition of spinal nociceptive transmission from the nuclei reticularis gigantocellularis and gigantocellularis pars alpha in the rat. *J Neurophysiol*, 67:1599-1614.

Zhuo M and Gebhart GF. 1997. Biphasic modulation of spinal nociceptive transmission from the medullary raphe nuclei in the rat. *J Neurophysiol*, 78: 746-758.

Zhuo M and Gebhart GF. 2002a. Biphasic modulation of a visceral nociceptive reflex from the rostroventral medial medulla in the rat. *Gastroenterology*, 122:1007-1019.

Zhuo M and Gebhart GF. 2002b. Modulation of noxious and non-noxious spinal mechanical transmission from the rostral medial medulla in the rat. *J Neurophysiology*, 88:2928-2941.

Zhuo M, Sengupta JN and Gebhart GF. 2002. Biphasic modulation of spinal visceral nociceptive transmission from the rostroventral medial medulla in the rat. *J Neurophysiology*, 87:2225-2236.

Paradoxical Analgesic and Hyperalgesic Effects of Stress

CHAPTER 28

Meredith Turnbach Robbins, Timothy J. Ness

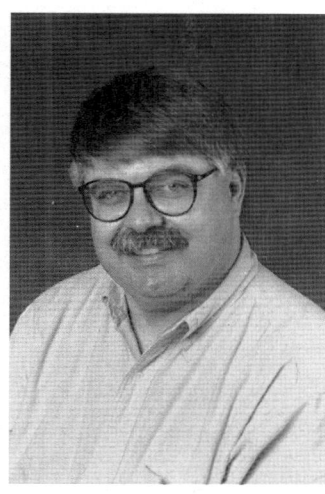

Dr. Ness is a Professor and Co-Director, Fellowship in Pain Management, Department of Anesthesiology, University of Alabama at Birmingham. After graduating from Luther in the College, Decorah Iowa, he went on to complete MD and PhD degrees at the University of Iowa, College of Medicine. He continued postdoctoral work in Anesthesia Residency and trained as Fellow in Pain Management at the University of Iowa Hospitals and Clinics, Iowa City, IA.

MAJOR CONTRIBUTIONS

1. Ness TJ, Gebhart GF. 1988. Colorectal distension as a noxious visceral stimulus: physiologic and pharmacologic characterization of pseudaffective reflexes in the rat. *Brain Res*, 450:153-169.
2. Ness TJ, Gebhart GF. 1990. Visceral pain: a review of experimental studies. *Pain*, 41:167-234.
3. Ness TJ, Metcalf AM, Gebhart GF. 1990. A psychophysiological study in humans using phasic colonic distension as a noxious visceral stimulus. *Pain*, 43:377-386.
4. Ness TJ, Gebhart GF. 2001. Inflammation enhances reflex and spinal neuron responses to noxious visceral stimulation in rats. *Am J Physiol Gastrointest Liver Physiol*, 280:G649-G657.
5. Ness TJ, Lewis-Sides A, Castroman P. 2001. Characterization of pressor and visceromotor reflex responses to bladder distension in rats: sources of variability and effect of analgesics. *J Urol*, 165:968-974.

MAIN TOPICS

Animal models of stress
Stress-induced effects on nociception
Early-in-life stress inducers
Mechanisms of stress-induced analgesia (SIA)
  General considerations
  Oxytocin
  Neurotensin
  Endothelin-1
  Nociceptin/Orphanin FQ
Mechanisms of stress-induced hyperalgesia (SIH)
  General considerations
  Amygdala
  Neurotensin
  Mitogen-activated protein kinase
  Corticotropin releasing factor
  Ovarian steroids
  Neurokinins

SUMMARY

Stress is a mentally or emotionally disruptive condition produced by adverse external influences which affects physical health. It is one of the most common human experiences, and the stress response which involves activation of the hypothalamic-pituitary-adrenocortical (HPA) axis and subsequent behavioral, neurochemical and immunological changes, is key to adapting to a constantly changing environment. The heightened anxiety and arousal accompanying the stress response is generally considered to be motivating rather than debilitating. However, when stress is sustained or perceived as uncontrollable, the biological changes that, short-term, are usually adaptive, can have long-term pathophysiological consequences.

Stressors may be physiological and/or psychological, and both types have been utilized to study stress effects on various experiences, including pain. The use of animal models of stress led to the observation of two pain-related phenomena. Following exposure to stressful situations, animals may exhibit antinociception to noxious cutaneous stimuli, a phenomenon known as stress-induced analgesia. It is easy to understand how there would be survival value in suppressing pain so that an animal could react ("fight or flight") to a dangerous situation. Interestingly, stress-induced hyperalgesia, which involves enhanced nociceptive responses, often occurs simultaneously. Although it has been less extensively studied in the laboratory than SIA, SIH has been well-documented in the clinic, especially in functional gastrointestinal disorders such as irritable bowel syndrome (IBS), which are characterized by visceral hypersensitivity. Stressful life events, particularly early in life, may predispose individuals to or exacerbate symptoms of functional GI disorders.

How these two, seemingly paradoxical, phenomena can co-exist is of great interest. SIA and SIH do share some common neurotransmitters (opioids, neurotensin) and supraspinal sites (rostral ventromedial medulla (RVM), amygdala). fMRI studies reveal that visceral and cutaneous pain activate a common neural network including somatosensory and parietal cortices, cerebellum, thalamus and basal ganglia. However, these different stimuli also evoke differential activation patterns in various brain regions. Thus,

it is likely that there is not one single pain pathway, but rather separate pathways subserving the phenomena of SIA and SIH. Determining the components of these pathways would enable scientists and clinicians to develop better pain treatments.

INTRODUCTION

Exposure to "stress" is one of the most common human experiences and which modifies many other experiences including pain. Defined as a mentally or emotionally disruptive condition produced by adverse external influences which affects physical health, its etiology may be physical or psychological. What an individual considers stressful is subjective and so a universally accepted scientific definition remains to be found. Physiological stress occurs when tissue is injured and in this context the "stress response" is a combination of neural and humoral responses to cytokine release and primary afferent nerve activation. One component of this stress response is enhanced activation of the hypothalamic-pituitary-adrenocortical (HPA) axis, a feedback loop by which signals from the brain trigger the release of hormones necessary to respond to stress. Stress results in the release of corticotropin-releasing hormone (CRH) from the paraventricular nucleus (PVN) of the hypothalamus. CRH then causes the pituitary gland to release adrenocorticotrophic hormone (ACTH), which stimulates the synthesis and release of cortisol, epinephrine, norephinephrine and endorphins from the adrenal cortex. The HPA axis exerts effects on the autonomic nervous system and glandular systems and communicates with a number of different brain regions, including the limbic system, amygdala, hippocampus, and areas that control body temperature, appetite and pain perception. Once activated, the stress response turns off hormonal systems regulating growth, immunity, metabolism, and reproduction, essentially redirecting biochemical resources to dealing with the threat. Once the threat has passed, cortisol exerts a negative feedback effect on the hypothalamus, inhibiting the production of CRH. It is notable that psychological stress, or anxiety, also activates the same HPA axis-related mechanisms, but to varying degrees. When one evaluates models of stress-related phenomena, it is therefore prudent to assess whether a physiological stimulus is evoking the stress response, or whether a behavioral situation is the source of stress. Although similar in many ways, the two types of stress are not exactly the same.

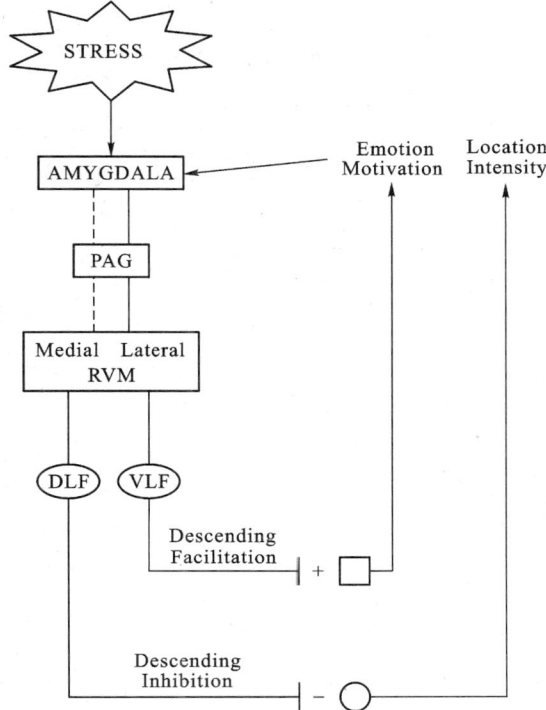

Fig. 28.1   Schematic diagram of proposed mechanisms of stress-induced changes.

ANIMAL MODELS OF STRESS

A number of different animal models of stress are used in research (Table 28.1). While some clearly fall into a physiological versus psychological category,

others have components that are from both categories. Water avoidance and forced swimming are psychological stressors, while cold-water swim might be considered physiologic as well. Other common psychological stressors include the elevated "plus" maze, open-field exposure, immobilization and neonatal maternal separation. Another, less commonly employed psychological stressor is the communication box. Its use involves placing animals in separate, adjacent compartments through which they can hear and see each other. Some of the animals receive footshock, while others do not. However, the unshocked animals hear the vocalizations and see the reactions of the shocked animals. Operant conditioning paradigms, where an unconditioned stimulus (i.e., footshock) is either paired or unpaired with a conditioned stimulus (i.e., tone), may fall into both categories since the unconditioned stimulus is usually a physical stimulus. Footshock alone and hypertonic saline injection are examples of stressors that are purely neurogenic.

The constant flux of the demands of daily life requires continuous adjustments to changing surroundings, and the stress response is critical in making those adjustments. For example, recognizing that a situation is dangerous requires appraisal of the situation, behavioral changes, coping, and body responses, all characteristics of a stress response. In most situations, heightened anxiety and arousal are motivating (i.e., fight or flight) rather than debilitating, and stress may generally be considered an adaptive process with clear survival value.

Table 28.1 Animal models used to assess effects of stress.		
Category of Stimulus	Psychological	Physiological
Post-surgical	X	X
Forced swim	X	X
Water avoidance	X	
Open field exposure	X	
Predator exposure	X	
Communication box	X	
Elevated "plus" maze	X	
Immobilization	X	X
Inescapable footshock	X	X
Hypertonic saline injection	X	X
Maternal fetal separation	X	X
Amygdala steroid injections	(X)*	X

STRESS-INDUCED EFFECTS ON NOCICEPTION

A variety of stressful stimuli, such as those described above, have been shown to produce analgesia or antinociception, a phenomenon referred to as stress-induced analgesia (SIA). After exposure to these stressors, animals exhibited antinociception to noxious cutaneous stimuli. It is easy to understand why, when faced with a stressor such as a predator, an animal would need to be able to react, fight or flee, without experiencing the pain of an injury. However, one hallmark of stress is the inability to carry out an appropriate coping response. Stress that is perceived as uncontrollable, chronic or unpredictable may result in abnormal behavior, higher than normal activity of the autonomic nervous system, enhanced secretion of hormones, and an increased tendency toward disease. Thus, what is usually considered a short-term adaptive response may, over time, induce long-term pathophysiological changes. In these cases, instead of being inhibited, as in SIA, nociceptive responses become augmented, a phenomenon known as stress-induced hyperalgesia (SIH).

SIH has been demonstrated in the lab as hypersensitivity to stimulation of viscera, such as the colon or urinary bladder and as increased operant behavioral responses to noxious somatic stimuli. Wistar-Kyoto rats, a strain that is predisposed to enhanced levels of anxiety, exhibit exaggerated responses to colorectal distension compared to other strains of rats. Visceral hyperalgesia has also been observed following exposure to restraint-induced stress, water avoidance-related stress and thermal stimuli-related behavioral paradigms.

EARLY-IN-LIFE STRESS INDUCERS

It is well-known that adverse early life experiences are epidemiologically associated with gastrointestinal diseases such as the irritable bowel syndrome (IBS) and with urinary tract disorders such as interstitial cystitis (IC). Consequently, one particular stressor, neonatal maternal deprivation, has been extensively used as an animal model believed relevant to clinical disease. The neonatal period is often referred to as a stress hyporesponsive period characterized by diminished adrenocorticotropin and corticosterone responses to most stressors. However, this diminished response can be overcome by a severe stressor, such as prolonged maternal deprivation, resulting in permanent alterations in the HPA axis.

Major stresses occurring in early childhood cause the HPA feedback loop to become stronger and stronger with each new stressful experience, producing an adult with an extremely sensitive stress circuit. The quality of the early life environment helps shape an organism's response to psychological stressors, increasing the risk of maladaptive responses to stressors throughout life. Adult rats exposed to repeated neonatal stress in the form of maternal separation demonstrate increases in plasma cortiosterone levels and an enhanced synthesis and release of CRH in response to acute stressors. Maternal deprivation increases colonic paracellular permeability, which favors bacterial translocation into the liver, spleen and mesenteric lymph nodes and stimulates the mucosal immune system. Dysregulation of the mucosal immune system and excessive production of inflammatory cytokines are key factors in the pathogenesis of inflammatory bowel disease. More importantly, early maternal separation induces long-term (into adulthood) hypersensitivity to rectal distension, the main pathophysiological characteristic of IBS in humans. It is likely that most of the time stress is an adaptive process involving behavioral, neurochemical, and immunological changes which help an organism cope with an ever-changing environment. However, if these short-term changes are sustained, what is normally considered an adaptive process can have long-term, pathophysiological consequences.

MECHANISMS OF STRESS-INDUCED ANALGESIA (SIA)

General Considerations

SIA has generally been divided into two types:

low-intensity stress-induced analgesia is naloxone-sensitive and is mediated by an antinociceptive circuit that includes the amygdala, PAG and RVM; high-intensity stressors induce analgesia via a μ-opioid receptor independent pathway that involves the hypothalamus and PAG. The latter appears to be linked to N-methyl-D-aspartate (NMDA) ligand-gated glutamate receptor/cation channel complexes since the NMDA antagonist MK-801 antagonized that form of SIA. Gender and strain differences are robust in both rats and mice and selective inbreeding for stress-related effects suggests a strong link to genetic influences. Sex-specific quantitative trait loci have been identified on chromosome 8 in relation to non-opioid SIA in female mice. Opioid SIA has been abolished by site-directed mutagenesis of the pro-opiomelanocorticotin gene in mice. Notably, these transgenic mice had normal HPA axis function and exhibited robust non-opioid SIA which was accentuated by naloxone treatment suggesting a compensatory upregulation of alternative pain inhibitory mechanisms. Other neurotransmitters have been implicated in SIA and are discussed individually.

Oxytocin

Oxytocin is a neuropeptide synthesized in the paraventricular nucleus (PVN) and supraoptic nucleus (SON) of the hypothalamus. It not only plays a prominent neuroendocrine role, but has also been implicated in the modulation of pain and nociception. Immunostaining studies revealed that oxytocin-containing neurons in the PVN project to the superficial dorsal horn and are activated in response to stressful conditions. Oxytocin knockout mice respond similarly to wild-type mice in tail-flick, tail mechanical withdrawal threshold and hot-plate tests. Cold water swim stress and restraint stress induce significant antinociception in wild-type mice, an effect that was drastically reduced in knockout mice. Electrophysiological recordings from lumbar dorsal horn neurons demonstrate that oxytocin also inhibit EPSPs evoked by dorsal root stimulation. This suggests that oxytocin modulates stress-induced antinociception by inhibiting glu-

tamate-mediated synaptic transmission between primary afferent fibers and dorsal horn neurons.

Neurotensin

As noted before, there are two distinct pathways involved in SIA. Evidence suggests that neurotensin (NT) signaling is plays a role in both pathways. Administration of a NT antagonist into the PAG attenuates analgesia produced by administration of a μ-opioid receptor agonist into the amygdala. Cold-water swim, a high-intensity stressor, increases NT expression in the lateral hypothalamus (LH) and medial preoptic nucleus of the hypothalamus (MPO), two areas implicated in SIA. Furthermore, chemical stimulation of the MPO activates PAG neurons, an effect that is blocked by microinjection of a NT antagonist into the PAG.

Endothelin-1

The endothelins are potent vasoconstrictive peptides expressed in a variety of tissues and cell types. Endothelin-1 (ET-1) is widely distributed in the central nervous system, including the hypothalamus, PAG, and LC, areas involved in endogenous pain modulation, and a number of behavioral studies have implicated ET-1 in nociceptive processing. Central administration of ET-1 has antinociceptive effects. In ET-1 knockout mice, acute, inflammatory, and neuropathic pain responses are decreased relative to wild-type controls. Furthermore, the degree of analgesia following swim-stress was less in the knockout mice. These reports suggest that there is basal release of neuronal ET-1 that is augmented in persistent pain states and acts to suppress pain. The observation that peripheral inflammation increases ET-1 release in the hypothalamus, which is closely linked with other structures involved in pain modulation, provides further support for a role of ET-1 in endogenous pain inhibitory systems.

Nociceptin/Orphanin FQ

The opioid receptor-like 1 (ORL1) receptor is a novel member of the opioid receptor family, and its endogenous ligand is nociception/orphanin FQ (N/OFQ). The peptide and its receptor are expressed in the spinal cord, DRG and various brain regions. N/OFQ was initially found to produce hyperalgesia when injected supraspinally but more recent studies support a role for N/OFQ in stress-induced analgesia. N/OFQ knockout mice exhibit elevated levels of basal nociception and impaired adaptation to stress. In models of neuropathic pain, N/OFQ significantly impairs thermal hyperalgesia and cold allodynia. Intracerebroventricular injections of N/OFQ decrease anxiety-related behaviors as evidenced by an increase in the time spent in the open arms of an elevated plus maze and the time spent in the light compartment of a light-dark box. Central administration also enhances circulating concentrations of ACTH and corticosterones in unstressed rats and augments those hormonal responses in mildly stressed rats. Thus, N/OFQ can activate the HPA axis.

Electrophysiological experiments in substantia gelatinosa neurons demonstrate that N/OFQ decreases the amplitude of glutamatergic EPSCs evoked by stimulation of Aδ-or C-fibers. In contrast, mIPSCs mediated by GABA$_A$ or glycine receptors were unaffected by N/OFQ. N/OFQ also inhibits Ca^{2+} currents in DRG neurons. These data suggest that N/OFQ suppresses excitatory but not inhibitory synaptic transmission to spinal neurons, accounting for its inhibitory action on pain transmission.

MECHANISMS OF STRESS-INDUCED HYPERALGESIA (SIH)

General Considerations

SIH is a phenomenon noted only recently in basic science studies related to stress and nociception, but has long been observed in clinical pain states. Stressful life events, unless coupled with other major physiological events such as pregnancy, almost universally lead to an exacerbation of underlying pain disorders. Recent investigation using visceral pain stimuli have demonstrated that stress can accentuate pain responses in a fashion similar to clinical observa-

tions. A notable study by researchers at UCLA (Coutinho et al, 2002) demonstrated seemly paradoxical simultaneous SIA in relation to somatic stimuli (tail heating) and SIH in relation to visceral stimuli (gut distension). These investigators noted that this paradox also manifests clinically in IBS patients who experience increased sensitivity to rectal distension (visceral hypersensitivity) that is frequently associated with diminished cutaneous pain sensitivity. One might propose that SIH was only due to a difference between visceral (diffuse) and cutaneous (discrete) sensation, but other studies have demonstrated that acute restraint stress will inhibit licking and guarding responses to thermal stimuli (SIA), but will magnify learned operant escape responses to the same stimuli. An enhanced motivational response to the thermal stimulus would be a form of SIH. The neurotransmitters and pathways associated with the SIH phenomenon have not been as extensively investigated as those of SIA, but some patterns of organization have been identified and are listed according to their main topic.

Amygdala

The amygdala, particularly the central amygdaloid nucleus (CeA) is a key limbic structure involved in fear and anxiety. The amygdala has a high density of glucocorticoid and mineralocorticoid receptors, both of which are involved in anxiety and fear responses. This, together with the observation that patients with functional bowel or urinary disorders exhibit symptoms following anxiety or stress, suggests a role for the amygdala in visceral responses to stressful situations. Stereotaxic delivery of adrenal steroids into the amygdala produces increased behavioral indices of anxiety. At the same time it also produces visceral hyperalgesia as measured using reflex responses to gut distension and enhanced responsiveness of lumbosacral spinal neurons to noxious visceral stimulation (gut or bladder distension.) The number of CRF-containing neurons in the amygdala, as well as the level of CRF mRNA in those neurons is increased after corticosterone into the amygdala. Thus, the amygdala exerts descending modulatory effects on lumbosacral spinal neurons receiving inputs from visceral structures to produce central sensitization to noxious visceral stimuli. This likely occurs via the release of CRF and suggests how anxiety and the generation of the stress response may be linked to altered gastrointestinal function in individuals with functional bowel and urinary disorders.

Neurotensin

Just as there is evidence for the involvement of NT in SIA, there is also suggestion of the importance of this neurotransmitter to SIH as well as evidence that endogenous NT signaling is required for normal visceral nociceptive processing. In NT knockout mice, visceromotor responses to noxious colorectal distension are significantly less robust than those observed in wild-type counterparts. Similarly, rats pretreated with an NT antagonist exhibited reduced abdominal muscle contractions in response to colorectal distension. However, under conditions of intense stress, NT signaling appears to contribute to analgesia. For example, water avoidance stress enhanced visceral nociceptive responses in NT knockout mice. Rats pretreated with an NT receptor antagonist do not exhibit SIA. The precise role of NT in both SIA and SIH may be complex since NT has been shown to facilitate and inhibit visceral and somatic nociception depending on the site and dose of administration. Low doses microinjected into the RVM facilitate pain responses, while high doses are analgesic. Thus, endogenous NT signaling may affect nociception via a descending facilitatory pathway. Intense stress increases NT signaling and likely activates a descending inhibitory pathway to produce analgesia. These differential effects of NT may be due to activation of subtypes of NT receptors with different binding affinities.

Mitogen-activated Protein Kinase

One pathway that appears to be involved in chronic SIH is the mitogen-activated protein kinase (MAPK) pathway. MAPK is important in numerous cellular and physiological processes such as cell proliferation, differentiation and survival, synaptic plasticity, learning and memory. Chronic restraint stress induces hyperalgesia to thermal stimulation and central changes in phosphorylated MAPK/extracellular signal-regulated kinase (ERK) levels. Specifically, phosphorylated ERK was significantly increased in the RVM and significantly decreased in the locus coeruleus (LC), two areas involved in descending modulation of nociceptive processing. Phosphorylation of MAPK activates transcription of TPH, the ratelimiting enzyme in serotonin biosynthesis. Chronic restraint stress also increased TPH levels in the RVM. Taken together, these observations suggest that as a result of chronic stress, prolonged ERK activation increases the transcription of TPH, which subsequently enhances serotonin biosynthesis, producing central sensitization of dorsal horn neurons via descending serotonergic projections from the RVM. The stress-induced decrease in activated ERK in LC neurons may blunt the inhibitory noradrenergic projections from this area to the dorsal horn, resulting in hyperalgesia to thermal stimuli.

Corticotropin Releasing Factor

Corticotropin releasing factor (CRF) is critical to the regulation of the HPA axis in response to a stressful event and has recently been implicated in stress-related visceral hypersensitivity. Colonic motility is enhanced by a variety of stressors in humans and laboratory animals, and altered bowel function is a characteristic symptom of IBS. This effect is mimicked by central or peripheral administration of CRF or its agonists. Studies using receptor specific antagonists and knockout mice implicate the CRF1 receptor in the colonic motor response to various stressors. Intracerebroventricular administration of CRF elicits visceral hyperalgesia to colorectal distension in rats. Central or peripheral administration of CRF1 receptor antagonists prevented the restraint-or water avoidance-induced hyperalgesia to colorectal distension in rats exposed to neonatal stress and the visceral hypersensitivity observed in a high anxiety strain of rats. In humans, peripheral injection of CRF1 receptor agonists increased colonic sensation to distension in a manner similar to that observed after stress. Other clinical studies revealed that intravenous administration of CRF lowered the threshold for pain sensation to colorectal distension in healthy individuals and stimulated colonic motility in both healthy subjects and those with IBS. Studies in primates and rodents demonstrate that adverse events early in life are associated with CRF neuronal hyperactivity in adulthood. As mentioned previously, early-in-life events may also increase vulnerability to developing visceral hypersensitivity as an adult. Taken with the findings described above, it is clear that hyperactivity of the CRF1-dependent signaling pathways contributes to stress-induced colonic motility and hypersensitivity to colorectal distension.

Ovarian Steroids

A number of studies have demonstrated that responses to noxious stimuli and analgesic substances are differentially affected by gonadal hormones as evidenced by changes during differing stages of the menstrual or estrous cycles. Following maternal separation and exposure to a stressor, female rats exhibit an enhanced response to rectal distension but males do not. This partial restraint stress-induced visceral hyperalgesia does not occur in ovariectomized rats unless receiving 17β-estradiol or 17β-estradiol and progesterone. Thus, there is evidence for a major role of estrogens in stress-induced visceral hypersensitivity. One way by which ovarian steroids may exert their effects is via various stress mediators. Regulating the synthesis of CRH or ACTH could alter the HPA response to stress in female rats. Indeed, the CRF gene contains the estrogen response element, enabling estrogens to directly affect CRF expression.

Neurokinins

A neurokinin-1 (NK1) receptor antagonist blocks stress-induced increases in abdominal muscle responses to rectal distension, suggesting that visceral sensitivity may be enhanced by stress via NK1 receptor activation, presumably by the neurotransmitter Substance P (SP). Sex steroids differentially regulate the expression of uterine tachykinin receptors, and intestinal NK1 receptors have been implicated in stress-induced bowel dysfunction, suggesting yet another mechanism by which estrogens influence visceral hypersensitivity. NK1 receptors are expressed on mast cells, visceral afferent nerves, and endothelial cells. SP may directly activate mast cells, amplifying a feedback loop involving SP, histamine and nerve growth factor. Alternatively, SP may bind to visceral afferents and release neurotransmitters that stimulate mast cells to release inflammatory mediators. Subsequent sensitization of afferents would increase responses to painful stimuli.

CONCLUSIONS

In this Chapter we have discussed the concept of stress, animal models of stress used in the laboratory, and the phenomena of SIA and SIH. What is probably most interesting about these two phenomena is that they often co-exist which does beg the question of how these two phenomena could occur simultaneously? The answer to the reverse question perhaps sheds light on a possible answer: the only way that they could not occur simultaneously was if there was a single pain pathway through the central nervous system.

There has been ample evidence given through the years that multiple sites in the spinal cord, subcortical structures and cortex of the brain appear to have importance to differing aspects of nociception. One of the oldest concepts that relate to spinal cord processing proposes an "old" pathway (e.g., the *paleospinothalamic* tract that encodes for affective and motivational aspects of pain sensation and which project to those sites of the brain associated with emotion and motivation) and the "new" pathway (e.g., the *neospinothalamic* tract that encodes for intensity and location of pain sensation). Logic would suggest that there might be survival value in the suppression of "distracting" information such as pain intensity or location and in the suppression of reflexes that might slow the "fight or flight" response of a stressed or injured organism. Similarly, magnification of the emotional and motivational aspects of pain-related responses would likewise appear to be of survival value. Hence, a stress-induced system which differentially suppressed one pathway while enhancing the other could produce an evolutionary advantage. The site of pathway splitting and/or site of inhibitory/excitatory actions could be at the spinal, subcortical or cortical level, but a suppression of spinal reflexes by SIA mechanisms suggests action at that early step in sensory processing. It is possible that differential effects could even be "prespinal" due to differential effects on A β-versus C-fiber activation.

To date, with the exception of one study demonstrating differential effects of stress on nociceptive reflexes versus operant responses to thermal stimuli, the studies demonstrating SIH have been in visceral pain systems and so may demonstrate a visceral versus cutaneous pain difference. fMRI studies have demonstrated that visceral and cutaneous stimuli equated for perceived pain intensity activate a common neural network including S2, posterior parietal cortex, cerebellum, thalamus and basal ganglia but also have differential effects with cutaneous stimulation producing greater activation in the insular cortex and ventrolateral prefrontal cortex, and visceral stimulation activating a more anterior area in the anterior cingulate cortex, bilateral inferior primary somatosensory cortex, and bilateral primary motor cortex. These activation patterns may explain differential motor, autonomic and emotional responses associated with each stimulus and therefore differential sensitivity to SIA versus SIH mechanisms.

Another explanation for differential SIA versus SIH effects could include temporal characteristics of the stimulus being administered and duration of the stress-induced effects. Most stimuli in which SIA has been demonstrated were brief stimuli evoking escape responses whereas the operant behavioral studies and visceral pain studies used stimuli of longer duration. A differential effect on brief stimuli versus long stimuli could therefore explain some of the findings. In studies of pain and stress effects, SIA is short-lived, but SIH may persist for up to one month. Hence, time of stress-related effect measurement also contributes to the possible differential effects.

Many explanations for presumably paradoxical phenomena can be put forth in the absence of data that addresses these phenomena in a simultaneous fashion.

Although it is possible that SIA and SIH may prove to be epiphenomena specific to particular experimental paradigms, it is our opinion that a determination of the differences between SIA and SIH will help to dissect out the many components of pain sensation and allow future scientists and clinicians to better treat the more global phenomenon of pain.

GENERAL CITATIONS

Barreau F, Ferrier L, Fioramonti J, Bueno L. 2004. Neonatal maternal deprivation triggers long term alterations in colonic epithelial barrier and mucosal immunity in rats. *Gut*, 53:501-506.

Mayer EA, Naliboff BD, Chang L, Coutinho SV. 2001. Stress and irritable bowel syndrome. *Am J Physiol Gastrointest Liver Physiol*, 280:G519-524.

Schafer M, Mousa SA, Stein C. 1997. Corticotropin- releasing factor in antinociception and inflammation. *Eur J Pharmacol*, 323:1-10.

DISCOVERY CITATIONS

Barreau F, Ferrier L, Fioramonti J, Bueno L. 2004. Neonatal maternal deprivation triggers long term alterations in colonic epithelial barrier and mucosal immunity in rats. *Gut*, 53:501-506.

Bradesi S, Eutamene H, Garcia-Villar R, Fioramonti J, Bueno L. 2003. Stress-induced visceral hypersensitivity in female rats is estrogen-dependent and involves tachykinin NK1 receptors. *Pain*, 102:227-234.

Bradesi S, Schwetz I, Ennes HS, Lamy CM, Ohning G, Fanselow M, *et al.* 2005. Repeated exposure to water avoidance stress in rats: a new model for sustained visceral hyperalgesia. *Am J Physiol Gastrointest Liver Physiol*, 289:G42-53.

Clarke S, Chen Z, Hsu MS, Hill RG, Pintar JE, Kitchen I. 2003. Nociceptin/orphanin FQ knockout mice display up-regulation of the opioid receptor-like 1 receptor and alterations in opioid receptor expression in the brain. *Neuroscience*, 117:157-168.

Coutinho SV, Plotsky PM, Sablad M, Miller JC, Zhou H, Bayati AI, *et al*. 2002. Neonatal maternal separation alters stress-induced responses to viscerosomatic nociceptive stimuli in rat. *Am J Physiol Gastrointest Liver Physiol*, 282:G307-316.

Fernandez F, Misilmeri MA, Felger JC, Devine DP. 2004. Nociceptin/orphanin FQ increases anxietyrelated behavior and circulating levels of corticosterone during neophobic tests of anxiety. *Neuropsychopharmacology*, 29:59-71.

Greenwood-van Meerveld B, Gibson M, Gunter W, Shepard J, Foreman R, Myers D. 2001. Stereotaxic delivery of corticosterone to the amygdala modulates colonic sensitivity in rats. *Brain Res*, 893: 135-142.

Gui X, Carraway RE, Dobner PR. 2004. Endogenous neurotensin facilitates visceral nociception and is required for stress-induced antinociception in mice and rats. *Neuroscience*, 126:1023-1032.

Gunter WD, Shepard JD, Foreman RD, Myers DA, Greenwood-van Meerveld B. 2000. Evidence for visceral hypersensitivity in high-anxiety rats. *Physiol Behav*, 69:379-382.

Hasue F, Kuwaki T, Kisanuki YY, Yanagisawa M, Moriya H, Fukuda Y, *et al*. 2005. Increased sensitivity to acute and persistent pain in neuron-specific endothelin-1 knockout mice. *Neuroscience*, 130:349-358.

Imbe H, Murakami S, Okamoto K, Iwai-Liao Y, Senba E. 2004. The effects of acute and chronic restraint stress on activation of ERK in the rostral ventromedial medulla and locus coeruleus. *Pain*, 112:361-371.

Kalinichev M, Easterling KW, Holtzman SG. 2001. Repeated neonatal maternal separation alters morphine- induced antinociception in male rats. *Brain Res Bull*, 54:649-654.

King CD, Devine DP, Vierck CJ, Rodgers J, Yezierski RP. 2003. Differential effects of stress on escape and reflex responses to nociceptive thermal stimuli in the rat. *Brain Res*, 987:214-222.

Qin C, Greenwood-van Meerveld B, Foreman RD. 2003. Visceromotor and spinal neuronal responses to colorectal distension in rats with aldosterone onto the amygdala. *J Neurophysiol*, 90:2-11.

Qin C, Greenwood-van Meerveld B, Foreman RD. 2003. Spinal neuronal responses to urinary bladder stimulation in rats with corticosterone or aldosterone onto the amygdala. *J Neurophysiol*, 90:2180-2189.

Robinson DA, Wei F, Wang GD, Li P, Kim SJ, Vogt SK, *et al*. 2002. Oxytocin mediates stress-induced analgesia in adult mice. *J Physiol*, 540:593-606.

Soderholm JD, Yates DA, Gareau MG, Yang PC, MacQueen G, Perdue MH. 2002. Neonatal maternal separation predisposes adult rats to colonic barrier dysfunction in response to mild stress. *Am J Physiol Gastrointest Liver Physiol*, 283:G1257-1263.

Strigo IA, Duncan GH, Boivin M, Bushnell MC. 2003. Differentiation of visceral and cutaneous pain in the human brain. *J Neurophysiol*, 89:3294-3303.

Acupuncture Analgesia

CHAPTER 29

Zhi-Qi Zhao

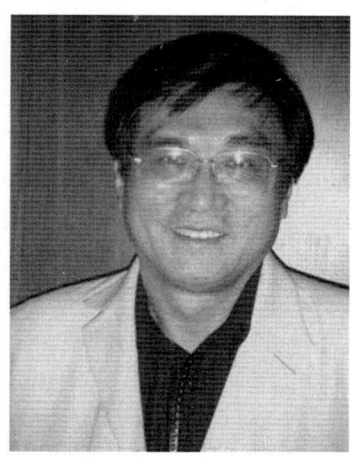

Dr. Zhao is a Professor and Head of Pain Research Unit in the Institute of Neurobiology, Fudan University in Shanghai. He graduated from Department of Biology, Peking University and completed PhD degree at John Curtin School of Medical Research, Australian National University. He worked at Shanghai Institute of Physiology and Shanghai Brian Research Institute, Chinese Academy of Sciences until 1999. He is interested in peripheral and spinal transmission of nociceptive information, neuroplasticity of pain and neural mechanisms underlying acupuncture analgesia.

MAJOR CONTRIBUTIONS

1. Xu G-Y, Huang L-Y M, Zhao Z-Q. 2000. Activation of silent mechanoreceptive cat C and Aδ sensory neurons and their SP expression following peripheral inflammation. *J Physiol*, 528: 339-348.
2. Hu J-Y and Zhao Z-Q. 2001. Differential contributions of NMDA and non-NMDA receptor to spinal c-Fos expression evoked by superficial tissue and muscle inflammation in the rat. *Neuroscience*,106:823-831.
3. Song P and Zhao Z-Q. 2001. Involvement of glia in the development of morphine tolerance. *Neurosci Res*, 39:281-286.
4. Zhang Y-Q, Ji G-C, Wu G-C, Zhao Z-Q. 2002. Excitatory Amino Acid Receptor Antagonists and Electroacupuncture Synergetically Inhibit Carrageenan-induced Behavioral Hyperalgesia and Spinal Fos Expression in Rats. *Pain*, 99: 523-535.
5. Gao Y-J, Ren W-H, Zhang Y-Q, Zhao Z-Q. 2004. Contributions of the anterior cingulate cortex and amygdala to pain- and fear-conditioned place avoidance in rats. *Pain*, 110:343-353.

MAIN TOPICS

Meridians and acupuncture points (acupionts)

Acupuncture feeling closely related to muscle contraction between acupoints

Activation of receptors and afferent nerve fibers by acupuncture

Segmental mechanism underlying the functional specificity of acupoints

Neural pathway and central mechanisms of acupuncture analgesia

Neurochemical basis of acupuncture analgesia
　Opioid peptides
　Cholecytokinin octapeptide
　5-hydroxytryptamine and Noradrenalin
　Glutamate

Molecular mechanisms of acupuncture analgesia

Neuroimage in acupuncture analgesia

SUMMARY

Acupuncture is an age-old healing art in traditional

Chinese medicine in which diverse pains, particularly chronic pain, can effectively be alleviated by impaling thin needle into certain specific "acupuncture point" (acupoint) on the patient's body. Increasing great attention was paid to neural mechanisms underlying acupuncture analgesia. (i) "Acupoint" is an anatomical small locus rather than a tiny point on the skin, which may be excitable muscle/skin-nerve complexes with high density of nerve endings expressing multireceptors. (ii) Acupuncture analgesia is manifest only when the intricate feeling of acupuncture (soreness, numbness, heaviness and distension) in human occurs. Such feeling mainly originates from acupuncture-induced impulses from muscle. (iii) The types of activated afferent nerve fibers by acupuncture are diversity, depending upon the different manipulation methods of acupuncture and the individual difference of acupuncture sensitization. The manual acupuncture (MA): all types (Aβ, Aδ and C) of afferent fibers are activated and mediate analgesia. The electroacupuncture (EA): electrical current via acupuncture needles at intensity enough to excite Aβ- (group II) and partial Aδ-type afferent fibers (group III) can produce analgesic effect. The electrical acupuncture-like stimulation (EALS): current via surface electrodes activates Aβ- and partial Aδ-afferent fibers induce analgesia. (iv) Segmental mechanism in the spinal cord contributes to the functionally relative-specificity of acupoints. (v) Neural pathway and central mechanisms of acupuncture analgesia: impulses from acupoints are ascended mainly through the ventrolateral funiculus, which is the spinal pathway of pain and temperature sensation. Many brain structures are involved in modulation of acupuncture in pain, including the nucleus raphe magnus (NRM), periaqueductal gray (PAG), locus cerules (LC), arcuate nucleus, preoptic area, centromedian nucleus, habenular nucleus, nucleus accumbens, caudate nucleus septal nucleus and amygdala etc. (vi) Neurochemical basis of acupuncture analgesia: many signal molecules play an important role in acupuncture analgesia, such as opioid peptides (μ-, δ- and κ-receptors), glutamate (NMDA and AMPA/KA receptors), 5-hydroxytryptamine, noradrenalin and cholecytokinin octapeptide (CCK-8).

INTRODUCTION

It is well known acupuncture is an age-old healing art in traditional Chinese medicine in which diverse pains, particularly chronic pain, can effectively be alleviated by impaling thin needle into certain specific "acupuncture point" (acupoint) on the patient's body. Such acupuncture-induced analgesic effect is commonly termed acupuncture analgesia. However, acupuncture therapy is not limited only to pain. The 42 diseases listed by WHO are recommended to use acupuncture treatment. In 1997, NIH reported that: "Promising results have emerged, for example, showing efficacy of acupuncture in adult postoperative and chemotherapy nausea and vomiting and in postoperative dental pain. There are other situations such as addiction, stroke rehabilitation, headache, menstrual cramps, tennis elbow, fibromyalgia, myofacial pain, osteoarthritis, low back pain, carpal tunnel syndrome, and asthma where acupuncture may be useful as an adjunct treatment or acceptable alternative or be included in a comprehensive management program". However, this chapter is limited in the field of acupuncture analgesia.

Generally, it is inevitable that psychological factors are involved in acupuncture treatment. One may wonder whether acupuncture analgesia is simply attributed to hyponosis or some other psychological effects. Consequently, increasing great attention was paid to neural mechanisms underlying acupuncture analgesia. In the past decades, our understanding of how the brain processes signals induced by acupuncture has developed rapidly. To apperceive peripheral and central mechanisms of acupuncture analgesia, some basics should be highlighted firstly. (i) The so-called "acupoint" is an anatomical small locus rather than a tiny point on the skin, in which electrical resistance is ordinarily lower than that on the surrounding skin. (ii) A large amount of clinical observations reveal that acupuncture analgesia is manifest only when the intricate feeling of acupuncture in patients occurs. This special feeling of human is described as soreness, numbness, heaviness and disten-sion in the deep tissue beneath the acupuncture point. In parallel there is the local feeling of acupuncturist's fingers, the so-called "De-Qi", which is similar with the finger's feeling of fisher when a fish is gnawing the bait. In the paraplegic patients, the acupuncture needles delivered to the lower limbs fail to produce such feeling. Consequently, there is no any analgesic effect on the upper part of the body. (iii) Acupuncture analgesia is persistent when acupuncture stimulation is terminated (Fig.29.1). (iv) Many manipulations of acupuncture are clinically used, including three main manipulations: the manual manipulation, electrical acupuncture and electrical acupuncture-like stimula-tion. That the acupuncture needle is penetrated into the acupoint of the body by hand without electrical stimulation is titled the manual acupuncture (MA),

which is commonly used by traditional acupuncturists. That the stimulating current via acupuncture needles connected with an electrical stimulator is delivered to acupoints of the body is titled electrical acupuncture (EA). The surface electrode delivered on the skin over acupoint instead of insertion of acupuncture needles is titled electrical acupuncture-like stimulation (EALS). The mechanism underlying acupuncture analgesia produced by three kinds of manipulation is homolo-gous, but exhibits difference. (v) The analgesic effect of acupuncture is characterized by obvious individual difference. (vi) The efficacy of acupuncture in the pathological pain is much potent than that in the physiological pain.

The following discussion will mainly focus on neurophysiological and neurochemical foundation of acupuncture analgesia.

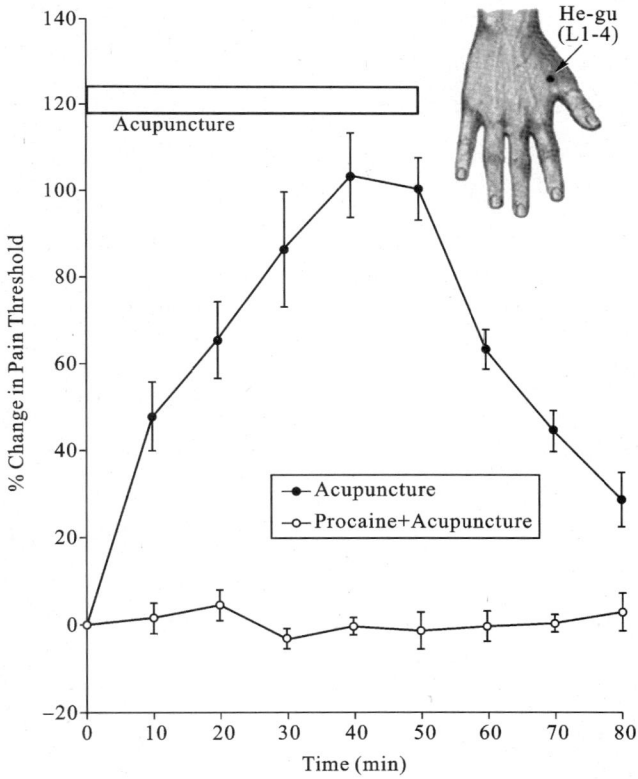

The Analgesic Effect of Acupuncture in Human Volunteers

Fig.29.1   Acupuncture analgesia in human. Manual acupuncture at He-Gu point (LI-4) gradually produced an increase in pain threshold with a peak increase occur-ring 20–40 min after the needle insertion in volunteers. The analgesic effect was completely prevented by the injection of procaine into the Ho-Gu point prior to ne-edling (modified with permission from Ulett *et al.*, 1998).

MERIDIANS AND ACUPUNCTURE POINTS (ACUPIONTS)

The acupoints used by acupuncturists are based on the ancient meridian theory. As shown in Fig.29.2, the

meridians are referred to as channels (jing) and their branches (luo), where acupoints locate. Traditional acupuncturists are convinced of meridians being a network system to link acupoints. However, a huge of studies suggests that the meridians might be a functio-nal, but not anatomical, conception. It might resemble the conception of the constellation, in which the fic-tive lines (channels) link various stars (acupoints).

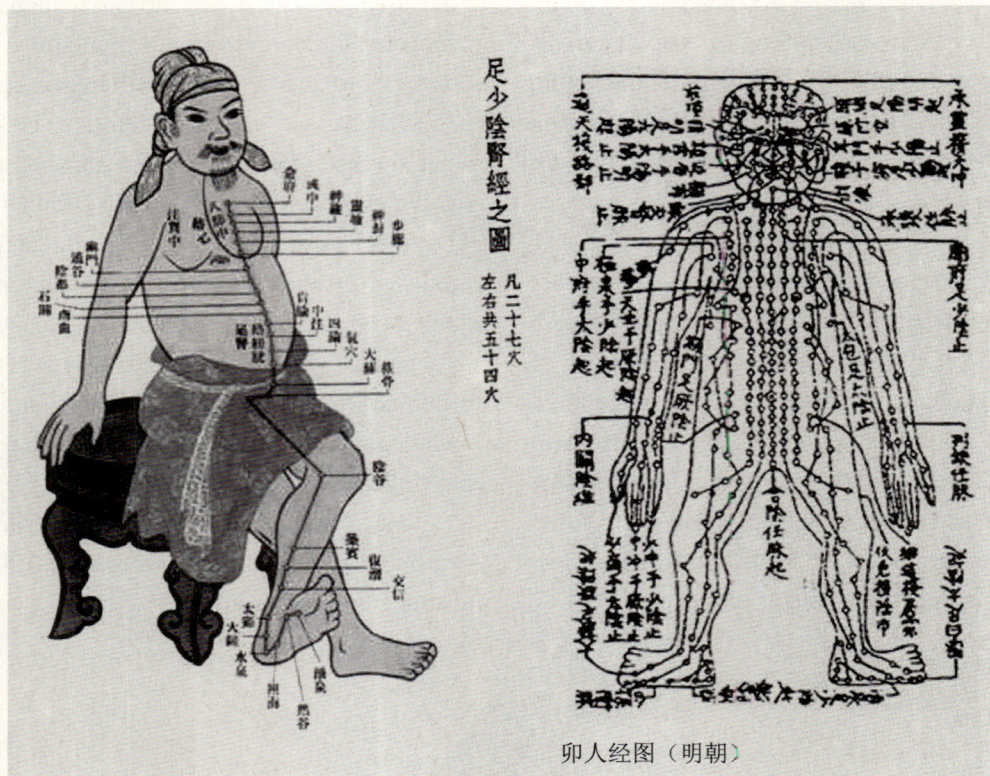

卯人经图（明朝）

Fig.29.2 Meridians and acupuncture points. Twenty-seven acupoints locate on one, Zushaoyin medredian (left picture made in Ming Dynasty), of ventral meridians (right).

In the early 1960's, the topographical relation-ship between 325 acupoints of 12 meridians as well as Ren meridian and the distributions of the peripheral nerves was examined in 8 adult cadavers, 49 detached extremities and 24 lower extremities. All of the me-ridians were traced to certain peripheral nerves. Out of 325 acupoints located on the meridians, 324 exhib-ited the rich innervation. Based on the fact that rat hind limbs are anatomically identical to those of hu-mans, a recent study explored the distribution of af-ferent nerve endings with acupoints in the rat hind limbs by means of combining single fiber recordings with the Evans blue extravasation. The location of the receptive fields (RFs) for each identified unit was marked on scaled diagrams of the hind limb. Noxious antidromic stimulation-induced Evans blue extravasa-tion was used to map the RFs of C-fibers in the skin or muscles. Results indicate that, for both A-and C-fibers, the distribution of RFs was closely associ-ated with acupoints. In the skin, the RFs concentrate either at the sites of acupoints or along the orbit of meridian channels. Similarly, the majority of sarcous sensory receptors are located at acupoints in the mus-cle. It strongly suggests that A-and C-type afferent fiber terminals in the skin and muscles of rats are dis-tributed in close association with the loci of acupoints in humans. The authors assume that acupoints in hu-mans may be excitable muscle/skin-nerve complexes with high density of nerve endings. Needle feeling may result from the activation of multireceptors within an acupoint or from the communication be-tween nonsarcous acupoints and sarcous acupoints.

ACUPUNCTURE FEELING CLOS-ELY RELATED TO MUSCLE CON-TRACTION BENEATH ACUPOINTS

As mentioned above, so-called acupuncture feeling described as soreness, numbness, heaviness and distension in the deep tissue beneath the acupoints plays a key role in acupuncture analgesia. Electromyographic studies in volunteers showed that the magnitude of EMG recording from the insulated acupuncture needles in the muscle beneath acupoint is intimately related to the intensity of the subjective sensation derived from acupuncture manipulation and also with the local "De-Qi" feeling of acupuncturist's fingers. Both the subjective acupuncture feeling and acupuncturist's finger sensation are blocked after injection of procaine into the muscle beneath acupoints. It is conceivable that the acupuncture feeling mainly originates from acupuncture-induced impulses from muscle, although the other deep tissues are not ruled out.

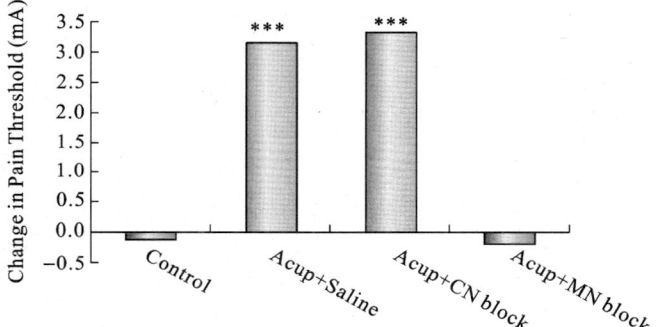

To obtain the strong efficacy of acupuncture, commonly, acupuncture needles are repetitively penetrated up and down in the different directions by acupuncturists. Therefore, the deep tissues, particularly muscle, are locally injured by such manipulation, where proinflammatory mediators, such as histamine, bradykinin, PGE2, 5-HT and ATP etc., release and excite nociceptors directly or indirectly. Clinically, the acupuncture feeling retains several hours even a few days after withdrawal of acupuncture needles, suggesting involvement of C-type afferent fibers mainly in acupuncture analgesia. The early experimental studies provided compelling supports for this view. By means of single-fiber recording from the cat deep peroneal nerve innervating the anterior tibial muscle at where "Zu-San-Li" acupoint locates in the cat, following the needle was twisted to penetrate into the anterior tibial

ACTIVATION OF RECEPTORS AND AFFERENT NERVE FIBERS BY ACUPUNCTURE

The types of activated afferent nerve fibers by acupuncture are diversity, depending upon the different manipulation methods of acupuncture and the individual difference of acupuncture sensitization.

Manual acupuncture: the fact that manual acupuncture-induced analgesia in volunteers is abolished by blockade of conduction of the muscle nerve, but not the cutaneous nerve innervating the impaled acupoint, indicates activation of afferent fibers predominately from muscle.

Fig.29.3 The muscle nerve innervating the impaled acupoint mediated acupuncture analgesia. Blockade of cutaneous branches of the radial nerve (CN) innervating the skin at He-Gu point by procaine failed to alter acupuncture-induced increase in pain threshold in volunteers. Blockade of the muscular nerves (MN), deep branches of the ulnar nerve and the median nerve innervating muscles at He-Gu point, completely abolished acupuncture analgesia.

muscle by hand, firing of a C-type afferent fiber persisted for a prolong period. Using selective blockade of conduction in Aδ-type and C-type afferent fibers by applied capsaicin to the bilateral sciatic nerves, manual acupuncture-induced analgesia was completely abolished in the rat. C-type fibers-mediating analgesia by the manual acupuncture seems to be similar to that provoked by so-called the diffuse noxious inhibitory control (DNIC), which is mediated by Aδ-type and C-type afferent fibers.

Electroacupuncture (EA): The stimulating current at diverse parameters applied to acupoints through acupuncture needles can produce analgesic effect in human subjects and experimental animals. From last 1970's up to now, it has being argued which kinds of afferent fibers mediate EA analgesia. The bone of contention is whether C-type afferent fibers are involved in EA analgesia. In the electrophysiological, animal behavioral and human experimental studies, lines of evidence demonstrated that electrical current via acupuncture needles at intensity enough to excite Aβ-type afferent fibers (group II) and partial Aδ-type afferent fibers (group III) can produce analgesic effect. At this degree of stimulating current, evoked feeling unusually is acceptable, even comfortable for some one. However, some results showed that C afferent fibers play key role in EA analgesia. EA analgesia still retained in the rat, when conduction of Aβ- and Aδ-type fibers was blocked, which suggests importance of C-type afferent fibers. Additionally, the clinical observations seem to be propitious to the latter. In patients with Syringomyelia, when the anterior commissure of the spinal cord is damaged, pain and temperature sensation deficits, and along with it, their acupuncture effect and acupuncture feeling are reduced or abolished. But then, it must be pointed out that excitation of C afferent fibers by synchronously strong electrical impulses will inevitably elicit insufferable pain in clinical practice, despite involvement of C afferent fibers in EA analgesia in the animal experiment.

Electrical acupuncture-like stimulation (EALS): The surface electrode is delivered on the skin over acupoint instead of insertion of acupuncture needles. EALS is similar to transcutaneous electrical nerve stimulation (TENS), but the difference between EALS and TENS is location of surface electrodes delivered as well as stimulation intensity and frequency. The former is delivered on the skin over acupoints with low-frequency and high-intensity and the latter on the site of pain with high-frequency and low-intensity. The kinds of afferent fibers activated by EALS are corresponding to that by EA. Excitation of Aβ-type afferent fibers (group II) and partial Aδ-type afferent fibers (group III) is involved in EALS-induced analgesia. Han's group develops a HANS stimulator, which is widely used to as an EALS for acupuncture analgesia and other treatments. It will be discussed in details in the following part.

SEGMENTAL MECHANISM UNDERLYING THE FUNCTIONAL SPECIFICITY OF ACUPOINTS

Clinically, acupuncturists are based on the ancient meridian theory to select acupoints and emphasize the functional specificity of acupoints. A general principle has been found when the sites of pain locate in the upper part of the body such as the head, neck and arm, acupoints on the arms are usually used for treatment, whereas acupoints on the legs are used to relieving pain in the lower part of the body such as sciatica, abdominalgia etc. Consequently, it is comparable with a spinal segmental innervating principle in the modern neurophysiology. The finding of animal experiments provides a strong support for this view. Inhibition of nociceptive thermal responses in the spinal dorsal horn neurons was more powerful when acupoints used located in the same segmental innervating regions than that those in the remote spinal segments. The most efficacious inhibition occurred when acupoints were selected in the same nerve innervating the receptive field of pain. Therefore, spinal segmental relationship between pain site and acupoints partially underlies the functional specificity of acupoints.

Despite importance of the spinal segmental principle, many distant acupoints from the pain sties are efficient for relieving pains.

NEURAL PATHWAY AND CENTRAL MECHANISMS OF ACUPUNCTURE ANALGESIA

The analgesic effect of acupuncture is considered essentially to be attributable to an interaction of afferent impulses from the region of pain and those from acupoints. It is well documented the main ascending and descending pathways of pain. There are two leading ascending pain pathways: the spinoparabrachial tract and spinothalamic tract. The former originates from the superficial dorsal horn in the spinal cord and projects to the parabrachial nucleus connecting to the brain areas involved in processing pain emotion, whereas the latter originates the superficial and deep dorsal horn and projects to thalamus connecting to the cortex areas involved in the sensory discrimination and emotion of pain. The descending pathways have described in other chapters in details. The clinical observations and experimental studies suggest that pathways of acupuncture signals are interwoven with pain pathways.

Spinal pathway: Patients with a deficit of deep sensation or diseases of spinal motor neuron, such as Tabes Dosalis involving posterior column, sequelae infantile paralysis and Amyotrophic Lateral Selerosis, still remained acupuncture feeling at all affected acupoints, but quickly disappeared after ceasing acupuncture stimulation, compared with a long-lasting in normal subjects. However, in patients with Syringgomyclia involved in anterior commisssure and posterior horn in the spinal cord, the acupuncture feeling was markedly weakened or completely abolished in the related acupoints with pain and temperature deficits. These observations were supported by the animal experiments. Section of the spinal dorsal column failed to affect acupuncture stimulation-induced the inhibitory effect of nociceptive responses of the thalamic neurons. The acupuncture-induced increase in pain threshold to noxious heating was similar in the chronically dorsal chordotomized animals and intact animals. However, unilateral section of the ventral of two-thirds of the spinal lateral funiculus at spinal segmental T_{12}-L_1 analgesia produced by stimulation of acupoints located in the contralateral, but not ipsilateral, leg was almost abolished. Taken together, it is suggested that impulses from acupoints are ascended mainly through the ventrolateral funiculus, which is the spinal pathway of pain and temperature sensation.

Relevant Brain areas: On the basis of clinical and experimental evidence, a fascinating postulation has been made that under certain conditions any innocuous sensory input may have some inhibitory effects of pain, but the characteristic sensory impulses produced by acupuncture are the most effective. It is

well known that many areas in the CNS, particularly the reticular formation, receive a convergence of heterosensory impulses from various sources. Marked potential changes by acupiont stimulation could be recorded in many brain areas. A large of studies have showed involvement of many brain structures in modulation of pain by acupuncture, including the nucleus raphe magnus (NRM), periaqueductal gray (PAG), locus cerules (LC), arcuate nucleus, preoptic area, centromedian nucleus, habenular nucleus, nucleus accumbens, caudate nucleus, septal area and amygdala etc., by means of stimulation or lesion techniques. Some of these structures such as the NRM and PAG play a predominant role in the descending inhibitory system. Electroacupuncture could facilitate spontaneous firing in some NRM neurons in responsive to noxious stimuli, but inhibited their nociceptive responses. Stimulation of the NRM potentiated acupuncture-induced inhibitory effect, whereas lesion of this nucleus or the dorsolateral funiculi (DLF) containing descending fibers from the NRM significantly reduced acupuncture effect. Also, the similar results were observed in the PAG, arcuate nucleus, centromedian nucleus, caudate nucleus, nucleus accumbens and amygdale. Contrarily, activity of the LC and habenular nucleus deceases acupuncture analgesia. These nuclei make up of intricate neural circuits implicating in acupuncture analgesia (Fig.29.4).

Acupuncture analgesia as a result of sensory interaction: The clinical and experimental evidence indicates that pain can be alleviated by various procedures such as acupuncture, forceful pressure, mechanical vibration and heating on the body as well as white noise and flicker etc., suggesting that one kind of sensation may be suppressed by other kind of sensation. The afferent impulses produced by acupuncture are probably the most effective. It is, therefore, conceivable that acupuncture analgesia is essentially a manifestation of integrative processes in different levels of the CNS between the afferent impulses from the pain regions and impulses from acupoints. As shown in Fig.29.4, convergence of impulses originating from pain sites and acupoints occur in the spinal dorsal horn and many brain nuclei, where integration of two kinds of impulses take place resulting in analgesic effect.

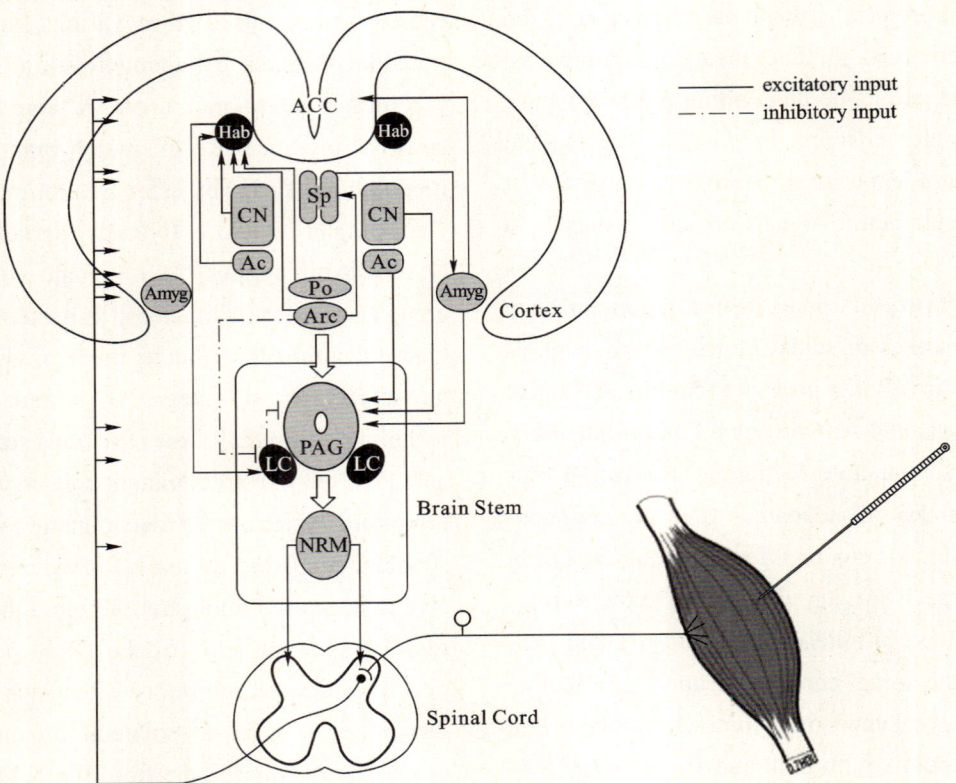

Fig.29.4 Putative central circuit underlying acupuncture analgesia. Many brain region and nuclei are involved in processing signals from acupoints. Activity and lesion of nuclei (green) produce potentiation and reduction of acupuncture analgesia, respectively, except two nuclei (Hab and LC) which exert an inverse action. ACC, anterior cingulated cortex; Hab, habenular n.; Sp, septal area; CN, caudate n.; Ac, accumbens n.; Amyg, amygdala n.; Po, peoptic area; Arc, arcuate n.; PAG, periqueductal grey; LC, locus cerulers; NRM, n. raphe magnus.

NEUROCHEMICAL BASIS OF ACUPUNCTURE ANALGESIA

In the early 1970's, it was found when the cerebrospinal fluid of donor rabbits given acupuncture was infused into the cerebral ventricles of recipient rabbits; the pain threshold of the recipients was increased, strongly suggesting involvement of central chemical mediators in acupuncture analgesia. From then on, a great deal of findings in human and animal studies demonstrated that acupuncture analgesia is a complicated physiological process mediated by various transmitters and modulators.

Opioid Peptides

The discovery of endogenous opioid peptides intensely magnetized to explore the role of opioid peptides in acupuncture analgesia. The first stimulating finding in 1977 showed that naloxone, a specific opioid receptor antagonist, partially reversed the analgesic effect of acupuncture on electrical stimulation-induced tooth pulp pain in human subjects. This result was swiftly evaluated by sensory detection theory in healthy subjects and confirmed in patients with chronic pain. Also, it was found that electroacupuncture (EA)-induced inhibition of nociceptive responses in the dorsal horn neurons was blocked by naloxone in the cat. Further, acupuncture analgesia could be potentiated by protection of endogenous opioid peptides using peptidase inhibitors, such as D-amine acids, D-phenylalanine and bacitracin. Subsequently, on the basis of these finding, the effects of opioid peptides on acupuncture analgesia have being studied widely and our understanding of opioid mechanisms underlying acupuncture analgesia has made profound progress in the past three decades.

The three main groups of opioid peptides, β-endorphin, enkephalins and dynorphins, and their μ-, δ- and κ-receptors are widely distributed in the areas of the CNS related to nociception and pain, which play a pivotal role in antinociceptive process. As shown in Fig.29.4, many brain nuclei and regions are involved in processing acupuncture signals, in which the most of them contain opioid peptides and μ-, δ- and κ-receptors.

Immunohistochemical studies have showed enkephalins and μ-receptors are densely distributed in laminae I–II of the spinal cord. Intrathecal administration of various specific antagonists of the opioid receptor subtypes produced differential effects on different frequencies of EA-induced analgesia. Low-and high-frequency EA are mediated by μ-/δ-receptors and κ-receptors, respectively, in physiological pain, whereas low- and high-frequency EA are mediated by μ-/δ-receptors, but not κ-receptors, in inflammatory hyperalgesia. In the supraspinal structures, decrease in acupuncture analgesia was observed when activity of opioid receptors of the given brain areas were blocked by opioid receptor antagonist. The PAG contains high density of opioid receptors, which is a critical region in the descending pain inhibitory system for morphine- and brain stimulation-induced analgesia. In addition to lesion, blockade of opioid receptors in the PAG by naloxone or antibody against μ-or δ-receptors also attenuated EA analgesia. Similar blockade of EA analgesia was observed when microinjection of naloxone into the preoptic area, nucleus habenula, septal area, nucleus accumbens, amygdala and caudate nucleus. The arcuate nucleus is an important structure in endogenous opioid peptide system, in which β-endophin-containing neurons are densely located. Their axons project to the lateral septal area, nucleus accumbens, PAG and LC. Arcuate-PAG projection is implicated in mediating acupuncture analgesia. Arcuate stimulation-induced excitation of NRM neurons was blocked by section of β-endophinergic tract or micro-

injection of naloxone into the PAG. In addition to lesion of the arcuate instead of stimulation, the same procedure almost completely blocked EA analgesia, indicating importance of Arcuate-PAG-NRM-Dorsal horn pathway in acupuncture analgesia.

As mentions above, an important finding is frequency-dependent EA analgesia mediated by the different opioid receptor subtypes. By means of detecting release of opioid peptides in the spinal cord, 2 Hz electrical acupuncture-like stimulation elicited a significant increase in the content of enkephalin-ir, but not dynorphin-ir, whereas 100 Hz stimulation increased dynorphin-ir, but not enkephalin-ir in rats and human subjects. When lesion of the arcuate nuclei abolished low-frequency EA-induced analgesia but not high-frequency EA, selective lesion of the parabrachial nuclei attenuated high-frequency EA-induced analgesia but not low-frequency EA. The PAG as a common stage mediates both of descending modulation. Box 29.1 shows a putative mechanism underlying frequency-dependent EA analgesia.

Recent studies indicate involvement of the novel opioid peptide orphanin FQ (OFQ) in modulation of nociception. Administration of OFQ (i.c.v.) produced a dose-dependent antagonism of the analgesia induced by electroacupuncture (EA, 100 Hz) in the rat, whereas antisense oligonucleotides (i.c.v) to OFQ mRNA potentiated EA-indcued analgesia, suggesting that endogenous OFQ in the brain exerts a tonic antagonistic effect on EA-induced analgesia. However, intrathecal administration of OFQ enhanced EA-induced analgesia rather than antagonism in the spinal cord. These findings are consistent with the experimental results obtained in rats where morphine induced analgesia is antagonized by i.c.v. OFQ and potentiated by i.t. OFQ.

OFQ is an endogenous ligand for opioid receptor-like-1 (ORL1) receptor. Besides, in the sciatic nerve chronic constriction injury model, EA decreased in expression of preproorphanin FQ mRNA and increased in OFQ immunoreactivity in the NRM of rats, suggesting that EA modulated OFQ synthesis and OFQ peptide level in NRM of the neuropathic pain.

BOX 29. 1   Frequency-dependent EA analgesia mediated by the different opioid receptor subtypes.

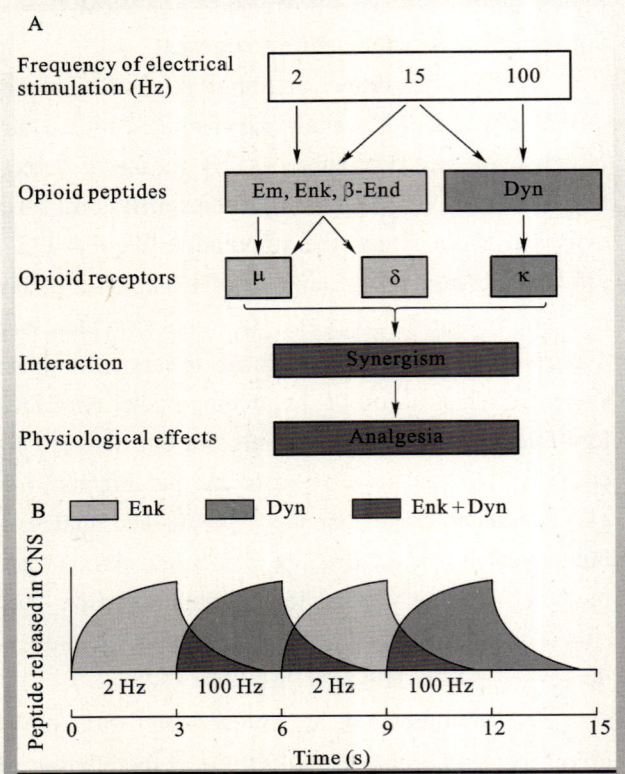

A

Frequency of electrical stimulation (Hz)

Opioid peptides

Opioid receptors

Interaction   Synergism

Physiological effects   Analgesia

B   Enk   Dyn   Enk + Dyn

Peptide released in CNS

2 Hz   100 Hz   2 Hz   100 Hz

Time (s)

Opioid peptides and opioid receptors involved in analgesia elicited by electroacupuncture of different frequencies (A). Opioids and receptors involved at 2 Hz are in light shadow, those involved at 100 Hz, in shadow. At 15 Hz, there is a partial involvement of components involved at both of the other two frequencies (dark shadow). Dyn, dynorphin A; b-End, b-endorphin; Em, endomorphin; Enk, enkephalins. Simultaneous activation of all three types of opioid receptor elicits a synergistic analgesic effect. Note that simultaneous receptor activation does not necessarily mean that the opioids are released simultaneously—it could be that the residual presence of one opioid overlaps with newly induced release of another. B. Model for the synergistic analgesic effect produced by alternating low and high frequency stimulation (referred to as model A in the text). Stimulation at 2 Hz facilitates the release of enkephalin; that at 100 Hz stimulates the release of dynorphin. The overlapping areas indicate the synergistic interaction between the two peptides (with permission from Han, 2003).

Cholecytokinin Octapeptide (CCK-8)

CCK-8 is widely distributed in various brain areas and the spinal cord and exerts many physiological functions, in which CCK-8 as the most potent neuropeptide involves in processing an anti-opioid activity. In the behavioral test, intrathecal administration of CCK-8 and CCK_B receptor antagonists significantly depressed and potentiated electroacupunture (EA)-induced antinociception, respectively. Radioimmunoassay revealed when EA-like stimulation was delivered to the acupoints in the rat hind-leg, high-frequency EA was found to be more effective than low-frequency EA in raising CCK release. Further observation showed that rats with weak EA-induced analgesia, low responders, had a remarkable increase in CCK release by high-frequency EA, wheareas rats with strong EA-induced analgesia, high responders, had little increase in CCK release. Particularly, following i.c.v. microinjection of antisense oligonucleotides to CCK

mRNA, a responder rat could be changed into a non-responder by inducing over-expression of CCK in the brain.

Monoamines: 5-hydroxytryptamine (5-HT) and Noradrenalin (NA)

The NRM is a crucial site in descending pain modulation system and contains an abundance of 5-HT. Compelling evidence has testified that both serotonergic descending and ascending pathways originated from the NRM are implicated in mediating acupuncture analgesia. Following the selective chemical lesion of 5-HT-ergic fibers with 5, 6-DHT, blockade of 5-HT biosynthesis by pCPA or antagonism of 5-HT receptors by cyproheptadine or methysergide, acupuncture analgesia was obviously weakened in the different species tested. Contrarily, following delivering 5-HT precursor such as 5-HTP or tryptophan, blockade of 5-HT degradation by monoamine oxidase inhibitor pargyline or reduction of 5-HT uptake by clomipramine, acupuncture analgesia was potentiated. The finding that acupuncture stimulation increased in the central content of 5-HT and its metabolic products particularly in the NRM and the spinal cord provides an explanation for involvement of 5-HT in acupuncture analgesia. A electrophysiological study using specific receptor antagonists suggested that serotonin receptor subtypes play different roles in acupuncture analgesia. $5-HT_1$, $5-HT_2$ and $5-HT_3$, may mediate electroacupuncture analgesia, whereas $5-HT_{1A}$ and $5-HT_{2A}$ antagonize EA analgesia.

Large number of studies showed that the role of noradrenalin (NA) in acupuncture analgesia is complicated and paradoxical. NA seems to exert the different action in the spinal and supraspinal level. By means of increase or decrease of activity of NA system with lesion of the LC, degeneration of NA, extragenous administration of NA receptor agonist or antagonist in the brain and spinal cord, it is inclined to refer that NA may produce inhibition of acupuncture analgesia in the brain nuclei, but potentiation in the spinal cord. Acupuncture analgesia is closely related to activation of $\alpha 2$ adrenergic receptors in the spinal dorsal horn.

Glutamate and Its Receptor

Excitatory amino acids, such as glutamate and aspartate, are richly contained in nociceptive primary afferent fiber terminals and NMDA, AMPA/KA and metabotropic receptors are distributed densely in the superficial dorsal horn of the spinal cord where primary nociceptive afferents terminate. It is well-documented that glutamate and its receptor play a pivotal role in spinal transmission of nociceptive information and central sensitization.

Increasing evidence suggests involvement of NMDA and AMPA/KA receptors in acupuncture analgesia. In the spinal nerve ligation model, immunochemical study revealed that neuropathic pain-induced increase of NMDA receptor subtype NR1 immunoreactivity in the spinal superficial laminae could be reduced by low-frequency electroacupunctur (EA) in the rat. Moreover, EA decreased in spinal nerve

ligation-induced mechanical allodynia. A combination of ketamine, a NMDA receptor antagonist, with EA produced more potent anti-allodynic effect than that induced by EA alone. A similar phenomenon was observed in the carrageenan-induced inflammation model. Although neither i.t. injection of NMDA receptor antagonist AP5 (0.1 nmol) nor AMPA/KA receptor antagonist DNQX (1 nmol) alone had an effect on inflammation-induced thermal hyperalgesia, both significantly potentiated EA-induced analgesia in carrageenan-injected rats, especially AP5. In the Fos expression study, when a combination of electroacupuncture with AP5 or DNQX was used, the level of Fos expression in the spinal cord induced by carrageenan was significantly lower than electroacupuncture or i.t. injection of AP5 or DNQX alone. These results demonstrate that electroacupuncture and NMDA or AMPA/KA receptor antagonists have a synergetic anti-nociceptive action against inflammatory pain.

MOLECULAR MECHANISMS OF ACUPUNCTURE ANALGESIA

As mentioned above, opioid peptides, monoamines and excitatory amino acids in the CNS contribute to central mechanism of acupuncture analgesia. Among them, opioid peptides may be primarily responsible to processing acupuncture signals. The genes are regulated primarily at the transcriptional level. Moreover, transcription factors serve as a power of target genes. A line of evidence has demonstrated that EA obviously induce a rapid expression of c-fos gene in various brain regions, especially in the PAG, suggesting transcription factors are also related in processing acupuncture signals. Using antisense oligodeoxynucleotides ODNs of c-fos and/or c-jun, the role of Fos and Jun proteins in EA-induced transcription of the opioid genes preproenkephalin (PPE), preprodynorphin (PPD) and proopiomelanocortin (POMC) was addressed. EA-induced Fos and Jun expression was blocked efficiently and specifically by c-fos and c-jun antisense ODNs, respectively. The antisense ODNs markedly deceased in EA-induced PPD, but not PPE, mRNA expression. These results suggest that Fos and Jun proteins are involved in PPD rather than PPE gene transcription activated by EA stimulation.

Nuclear factor-kappa B (NF-kB) is another crucial regulator of the inducible genes, which, as a transcriptional activator, is implicated in multiple functional processes including inflammation-induced hyperalgesia. The NF-kB family consists of NF-kB1 (p50/p105) and NF-kB2. In the NF-kB1 knockout mice, deletion of the NF-kB1 gene induced a significant decrease of the analgesic effect after EA, comparing with that in the wild-type mice, suggesting that NF-kB1 plays a crucial role in EA analgesia.

A revelatory study analyzed the effect of genotype on sensitivity to EA analgesia in 10 common inbred mouse strains. B10 strain was the most sensitive, and the SM strain was the least sensitive to both 2 and 100 Hz EA. However, the relative sensitivities of other strains to these two EA frequencies suggested some genetic dissociation between them as well. An intriguing finding was the significant difference in 2 Hz EA-induced analgesia between the B6 and B10 strains. It has known that there is allelic variation in microsatellite of delta gene between sublines B10 and B6. This raises the possibility that B10 and B6 may have different allelic forms of the delta gene and hence show variation in their analgesic responses to electroacupuncture. These findings provide a role of inherited genetic factors for a possible explanation of individual differences in acupuncture analgesia.

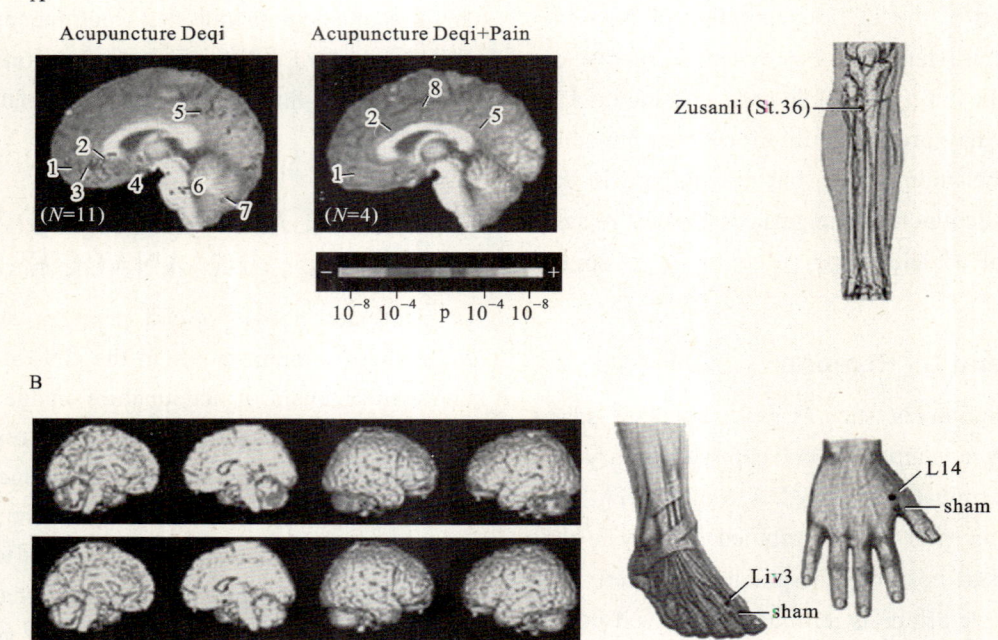

Fig.29.5 Acupucture-induced change in brain neuroimage (see also the color plate)

A. Relationship of changes in "De-Qi" sensations and fMRI signal changes of the brain during acupuncture performed at Zusanli (St.36). Brain area: 1, frontal pole; 2, subgenual anterior cingulated, Brodmann area 24; 3, ventromedial prefrontal (VMPF) cortex; 4, hypothalamus; 5, posterior cingulate; 6. reticular formation; 7, cerebellar vermis; 8, middle cingulate, Brodmann area 32. Left image: Acupuncture with De-Qi sensations but without sharp pain resulted in widespread signal decreases, including the frontal pole, VMPF cortex, cingulated cortex, hypothalamus, reticular formation and the cerebellar vermis. Right image: Acupuncture with De-Qi and sharp pain sensations resulted in signal increases in several areas, including the frontal pole and the anterior, middle and posterior cingulated (modified with permission from Hui *et al.*, 2005).
B. The difference of acupuncture-induced changes in fMRI image between acupoints Liv3 (Taichong)/LI4 (Hegu) and sham points. In the up image, Acupuncture at Liv3 evoked specific activation at the postcentral gyrus, posterior cingulate, parahippocampal gyrus, BA 7, 19 and 41, but deactivation at the inferior frontal gyrus, anterior cingulate, BA 17 and 18, compared with acupuncture at its sham point. In the down image, Acupuncture at LI4 evoked specific activation at the temporal pole, but deactivation at the precentral gyrus, superior temporal gyrus, pulvinar and BA 8, 9 and 45, compared with acupuncture at its sham point (modified with permission from. Yan *et al.*, 2005).

NEUROIMAGE IN ACUPUNCTURE ANALGESIA

The understanding of central mechanism of acupuncture analgesia is predominately depended on the data from animal experiments. Recently, the studies on correlation between functional neuroimage and acupuncture in the human brain are increasing by means of functional magnetic resonance imaging (fMRI) and positron emission tomography (PET)

Several fMRI studies have revealed that stimulation of acupoints (Hegu, Zusanli, or Yanlinquan) modulates human central nervous system including cerebral limbic/paralimbic and subcortical structures. When stimulation evoked acupuncture feeling (so-called De-Qi) in subjects, the activated brain regions included the PAG and NRM from midbrain, insular, dorsomedial nucleus of thalamus, anterior cingulate cortex, hypothalamus, nucleus accumbens, and primary somatosensory–motor cortex, while some regions exhibited deactivation such as the rostral part of the anterior cingulate cortex, amygdala formation and hippocampal complex. The similar data were acquired by scanning in 3-D mode of PET. Clinically, De-Qi sensation is closely associated with the efficiency of acupuncture analgesia, therefore, De-Qi-induced changes in brain images are very important for understanding central mechanism of acupuncture. Intriguingly, stimulation of classical acupoints elicited significantly higher activation than stimulation of non-acupoints over the hypothalamus and primary somatosensory–motor cortex and deactivation over the rostral segment of anterior cingulate cortex. When the so-called vision-related acupoints located in the lateral aspect of the foot was stimulated, activation of occipital lobes was observed by fMRI. Stimulation of the eye by directly using light results in similar activation in the occipital lobes by fMRI. But there was no activation in the occipital lobes following stimulation of non-acupoints.

These findings greatly deepen our insight of central mechanism underlying acupuncture analgesia and impel to explore puzzle of acupuncture.

GENERAL CITATIONS

Cao XD. 2002. Scientific bases of acupuncture analgesia. *Acup Electro-Therap Res, INT J*, 27:1-14.

Chang HT. 1980. Neurophysiological interpretation of acupuncture analgesia. *Endeavour*, 3:92-96.

Han J-S. 2003. Acupuncture: neuropeptide release produced by electrical stimulation of different frequencies. *Trends in Neurosci*, 26:17-22.

He LF. 1987. Involvement of endogenous opioid peptides in acupuncture analgesia. *Pain*, 31:99-121.

Pomeranz B. 2001. Scientific basis of acupuncture. In: Stux G, Hammerschlag R, (eds), *Clinical Acupuncture: Scientific Basis*. Hedelberg, Germany: Springer.

DISCOVERY CITATIONS

Chang HT. 1973. Intergrative action of thalamus in the process of acupuncture for analgesia. *Sci Sin*, 16:25-60.

Chiang CY, Chang CT, Chu HC, *et al.* 1973. Peripheral afferent pathway for acupuncture analgesia. *Sci Sin*, 16:210-217.

Cho ZH, Chung SC, Jones JP, *et al.* 1998. New findings of the correlation between acupoints and corresponding brain cortices using functional MRI. *Proc Natl Acad Sci USA*, 95: 2670-2673.

Cui KM, Li WM, Gao X, *et al.* 2005. Electro-acupuncture relieves chronic visceral hyperalgesia in rats. *Neurosci Lett*, 376:20-23.

de Medeiros MA, Canteras NS, Suchecki D, *et al*, 2003. Analgesia and c-Fos expression in the periaqueductal gray induced by electroacupuncture at the Zusanli point in rats. *Brain Res*, 973: 196-204.

Dong Z-Q, Ma F, Xie H, *et al.* 2005. Changes of expression of glial cell line-derived neurotrophic factor and its receptor in dorsal root ganglions and spinal dorsal horn during electroacupuncture treatment in neuropathic pain rats. *Neurosci Lett*, 376:143-148.

Du HJ, Zhao YF. 1975. Central Localization of descending inhibition of visceral-somatic reflex produced by acupuncture. *Sci Sin*, 18:631-639.

Guo HF, Tian JH, Wang XM, *et al.* 1996. Brain substrates activated by electroacupuncture EA of different frequencies II: role of Fos/Jun proteins in EA-induced transcription of preproenkephalin and preprodynorphin genes. *Molecular Brain Res*, 43: 67-173.

Guo ZL, Moazzamia AR, Longhursta JC. 2004. Electroacupuncture induces c-Fos expression in the rostral ventrolateral medulla and periaqueductal gray in cats: relation to opioid containing neurons. *Brain Res*, 1030: 103-115.

Han J-S, Terenius L. 1982. Neurochemical basis of acupuncture analgesia. *Ann Rev Pharmacol Toxicol*, 22:193-220.

He LF, Lu RL, Zhuang SY, *et al.* 1985. Possible involvement of opioid peptides of caudate nucleus in acupuncture analgesia. *Pain*, 23:83-93.

Hu ZL. 1979. A study on the histological structure of acupuncture points and types of fibers conveying needling sensation. *Chin Med J*, 92:233.

Huang C, Long H, Shi Y-S, *et al.* 2003. Nocistatin potentiates electroacupuncture antinociceptive effects and reverses chronic tolerance to electroacupuncture in mice. *Neurosci Lett*, 350:93-96.

Hsieh J-C, Tu C-H, Chen F-P, *et al.* 2001. Activation of the hypothalamus characterizes the acupuncture stimulation at the analgesic point in human: a positron emission tomography study. *Neurosci Lett*, 307: 105-108.

Hui KKS, Liu J, Marina O, *et al.* 2005. The integrated response of the human cerebro-cerebellar and limbic systems to acupuncture stimulation at ST 36 as evidenced by fMRI. NeuroImage, 27: 479-496.

Kima HW, Kwon YB, Han HJ, *et al.* 2005. Antinociceptive mechanisms associated with diluted bee venom acupuncture (apipuncture) in the rat formalin test: involvement of descending adrenergic and serotonergic pathways. *Pharmacol Res*, 51: 183-188.

Koo ST, Parka YI, Lim KS, *et al.* 2002. Acupuncture analgesia in a new rat model of ankle sprain pain. *Pain*, 99: 423-431.

Lao LX, Zhang RX, Zhang G, *et al.* 2004. A parametric study of electroacupuncture on persistent hyperalgesia and Fos protein expression in rats. *Brain Res*, 1020: 18-29.

Le Bars D, Willer J-C. 2002. Pain modulation triggered by high-intensity stimulation: implication for acupuncture analgesia? *International Congress Series*, 1238:11-29.

Lee G, Rho S, Shin MK, *et al.* 2002. The association of cholecystokinin-A receptor expression with the responsiveness of electroacupuncture analgesic effects in rat. *Neurosci Lett*, 325: 17-20.

Lee G-S, Han J-B, Shin M-K, *et al.* 2003. Enhancement of electroacupuncture-induced analgesic effect In cholecystokinin-A receptor deficient rats. *Brain Res Bull*, 62: 161-164.

Li A-H, Zhang JM, Xie Y-K. 2004. Human acupuncture points mapped in rats are associated with excitable muscle/skin-nerve complexes with enriched nerve endings. *Brain Res*, 1012: 154-159.

Mayer DJ, Price DD, Raffi A. 1977. Antagonism of acupuncture analgesia in man by narcotic antagonist naloxone. *Brain Res*, 121:368-372.

Parka HJ, Leeb HS, Leeb HJ, *et al.* 2002. Decrease of the electroacupuncture-induced analgesic effects in nuclear factor-kappa B1 knockout mice. *Neurosc Lett*, 319: 141-144.

Shen E, Wu WY, Du HJ, *et al.* 1973. Electromyographic activity produced locally by acupuncture manipulation. *Chin Med J*, 9:532- 535.

Shen E, Cai TD, Lan Q. 1974. Effects of supraspinal sturcures on acupuncture-induced inhibition of visceral-somatic reflex. *Chin J Med*, 10:628-633.

Takagi J, Yonehara N. 1998. Serotonin receptor subtypes involved in modulation of electrical acupuncture. *Jpn J Pharmacol*, 78:511-514.

Toda K. 2002. Afferent nerve characteristics during acupuncture stimulation. *International Congress Series*, 1238: 49-61.

Ulett GA, Han SP, Han JS. 1998. Electroacupuncture: mechanisms and clinical application. *Biol Psychiatry*, 44: 129-138.

Wan Y, Wilson SG, Han J-S, *et al.* 2001. The effect of genotype on sensitivity to electroacupuncture analgesia. *Pain*, 91: 5-13.

Wang K, Yao S, Xian Y, *et al.* 1985. A study on the receptive field of acupoints and the relationship between characteristics of needling sensation and groups of afferent fibers. *Sci Sin(Ser B)*, 28:963-971.

Wei JY, Feng CC, Chu TH, *et al.* 1973. Observation on activity of deep tissue receptors in cat hindlimb during acupuncture. *Kexue Tongbao (Science Bulletin)*, 18:184-186.

Wu C-P, Chao C-C(Zhao Z-Q), Wei J-Y. 1974. Inhibitory effect produced by stimualtion of afferent nerves on responses of cat dorsolateral fasciculus fibers to nocuous stimulus. *Sci Sin*, XVII:688-697.

Yan B, Li K, Xu JX, *et al*. 2005. Acupoint-specific fMRI patterns in human brain. *Neurosci Lett*, 383: 236-240.

Zhang R-X, Lao L, Wang LB, *et al*. 2004. Involvement of opioid receptors in electroacupuncture-produced anti-hyperalgesia in rats with peripheral inflammation. *Brain Res*, 1020:12-17.

Zhang YQ, Ji GC, Wu GC, *et al*. 2002. Excitatory amino acid receptor antagonists and electroacupuncture synergetically inhibit carrageenan-induced behavioral hyperalgesia and spinal Fos expression in rats. *Pain*, 99:523-535.

Zhang Y-Q, Ji G-C, Wu G-C, *et al*. 2003. Kynurenic acid enhances electroacupuncture analgesia in normal and carrageenan-injected rats. *Brain Res*, 966:300-307.

Zhou PH, Qian PD, Huang DK, *et al*. 1979. A study of the relationships between the points of the channels and peripheral nerves. *National Symposia of Acupucture-Moxibustion & Acupuncture Anesthesia*. Beijing. 302.

Zhu B, Xu W-D, Rong PJ, *et al*. 2004. A C-fiber reflex inhibition induced by electroacupuncture with different intensities applied at homotopic and heterotopic acupoints in rats selectively destructive effects on myelinated and unmyelinated afferent fibers. *Brain Res*, 1011: 228-237.

Mechanisms of Opioid Tolerance

CHAPTER 30

Zhizhong Z. Pan[*]

MAIN TOPICS

Desensitization

Internalization

Glutamate Receptors

Chronic Opioid-Induced Pain and Hyperalgesia

Cyclic AMP-PKA

SUMMARY

Opioid tolerance, defined by decreased analgesic efficacy of opioid analgesics after repeated and prolonged use, is a significant clinical problem limiting adequate treatment of pain with opioids, the most effective analgesics available today. After decades of research, multiple mechanisms at molecular, cellular and network levels have been proposed to account for the behavioral observation of opioid analgesic tolerance. Major mechanisms include those mediated by opioid receptor desensitization and internalization, glutamate receptors, chronic opioid-induced hyperalgesia and the cAMP-protein kinase A (PKA) pathway. Phosphorylation-dependent opioid receptor desensitization decreases opioid receptor function and agonist efficacy by uncoupling of opioid receptors from downstream effectors, but its rapid time course and recovery of surface receptor functions may limit its contribution to only the early stage of opioid tolerance.

Opioid receptor internalization and subsequent downregulation, on one hand, decrease receptor density on surface membrane and reduce number of receptors available for agonist activation. On the other hand, differential ability of various opioid agonists to induce internalization appears to reflect their potency to induce analgesic tolerance, indicating receptor internalization as a key signal for downstream adaptive responses that lead to tolerance. Glutamate receptors, both NMDA and AMPA receptors, have long proved a key component in the synaptic networks responsible for behavioral tolerance, but their detailed role in the network has just begun to emerge. A mechanism of opioid tolerance from a system point of view states that chronic opioids induce sensitized pain, which counteracts the analgesic effect of sustained opioids. Our understanding of the underlying synaptic mechanisms for this counteraction has significantly improved. Finally, although superactivation of the cAMP signaling cascade has long been recognized as a typical molecular adaptation to chronic opioids, its physiological consequences on cell functions and its mechanistic significance for opioid tolerance have been characterized lately.

INTRODUCTION

Poppy-derived opium has been used to treat pain for thousands of years. Nowadays, morphine, the main

---

[*] For the introduction of Dr. Pan, please refer to Chapter 11.

ingredient of opium, and other opioid-based drugs are still the most widely used analgesics for the treatment of moderate to severe pain, particularly, cancer pain. This is because opioid analgesics remain the most effective among different analgesics available for many types of pain in current clinical practice. Many pain conditions, such as cancer pain and neuropathic pain, are chronic and require repeated use of opioid analgesics to maintain a desired analgesic level during the period when pain persists. However, it is well known that the analgesic efficacy of opioids gradually decreases after repeated and prolonged use of opioids, a phenomenon termed *opioid tolerance*. The analgesic tolerance to chronically used opioids significantly diminishes their analgesic effectiveness such that increased doses are constantly necessary to maintain the desired analgesic level and sufficiently control pain. Unfortunately, opioids at high doses cause several severe side effects and are fatal at extreme doses. Opioid tolerance, combined with the side effects at high opioid doses, significantly limits the clinical use of opioid analgesics to efficiently and sufficiently control pain, resulting in a possible forced termination of opioid treatment and replacement by other less effective alternatives, leaving millions of chronic pain patients under-treated. Because the mechanisms for opioid tolerance are only partially understood, current opioid therapies for chronic pain are largely empirical. Since opioid analgesics are envisioned to remain the major choice for pain control with no other better replacement drugs available in the foreseeable future, improving the current opioid therapies by circumventing the problem of opioid tolerance is both practical and in great need. The key to such a goal is our understanding of the neurobiological mechanisms underlying opioid tolerance. Tremendous research efforts have been made in the last several decades to study the mechanisms of opioid tolerance at multi-disciplinary levels, and remarkable progress has been achieved in terms of chronic opioid-induced adaptive changes in the brain and spinal cord related to opioid analgesia, and the behavioral contributions of these changes to analgesic tolerance to chronic opioids. Chronic opioid-induced adaptations have been characterized at the molecular, receptor, cellular, network and system levels with various mechanisms proposed for analgesic tolerance. This chapter will focus on several typical, well-studied mechanisms at each representative levels, as we currently understand. Their behavioral significance in mediating opioid tolerance is also discussed.

DESENSITIZATION

Receptor desensitization is a process in which a receptor, after binding to an agonist, uncouples to its downstream effectors, mostly G proteins. Desensitization is a common feature for the G protein-coupled receptor super family, including opioid receptors. Receptor desensitization, which occurs rapidly within minutes, diminishes agonist efficacy. Most studies on the mechanisms of desensitization used *in vitro* cultured cell lines expressing a single type of opioid receptors, taking advantage of the simple receptor-signaling system to determine the extent of desensitization. While detailed mechanisms may differ among specific receptor types, a consensus of desensitization mechanism involves receptor phosphorylation by various protein kinases. The targeted phosphorylation sites in both the μ-opioid receptor (MOR) and the δ-opioid receptor locate within the third intracellular loop and the carboxyl tail (Capeyrou *et al.*, 1997; Trapaidze *et al.*, 1996).

A common mechanism for MOR desensitization involves MOR phosphorylation by the G protein-coupled receptor kinase (GRK) (see review by Law and Loh in General Citations). Agonist binding-induced GRK phosphorylation uncouples MOR from the G proteins and promotes MOR binding to β-arrestin for receptor internalization through endocytosis (Fig.30.1). For example, desensitization of MOR expressed in *Xenopus oocytes* requires GRK2 (Kovoor *et al.*, 1997). However, in locus coeruleus neurons, acute desensitization of MOR, measured by its coupling to the inwardly rectifying potassium channels, appears independent from the GRK (Harris and Williams, 1991). Mice lacking β-arrestin-2 do not show MOR desensitization by chronic morphine and fail to develop morphine tolerance (Bohn *et al.*, 2000). Protein kinase C (PKC) may induce MOR desensitization through an indirect mechanism rather than direct phosphorylation of MOR (Zhang *et al.*, 1997; Ueda *et al.*, 1995). PKA generally lacks a significant role in opioid receptor desensitization (Harris and Williams, 1991; Hasbi *et al.*, 1998). Other protein kinases that may play a role in opioid receptor desensitization include calmodulin kinase II and tyrosine kinase.

The extent of contribution of MOR desensitization to chronic opioid-induced analgesic tolerance is a contentious issue and remains unclear at present. Although MOR desensitization reduces agonist efficacy and could potentially contribute to tolerance with reduced MOR effects, there is a general lack of link between MOR desensitization and behavioral tolerance. There are several issues that may limit the demonstration of MOR desensitization for its role in tolerance. First, most desensitization studies are carried out in cultured cell lines *in vitro* and limited studies in native neurons. It is technically difficult to link results from these studies to behavioral measurement of tolerance in an *in vivo* system. Second, desensitization occurs rapidly within minutes and readily reversible while behavioral tolerance develops over a much longer period (hours to days). This limits the possible contribution of MOR desensitization largely to the initiation or early stage of tolerance development. Finally, receptor desensitization often leads to β-arrestin-mediated receptor internalization and a series of downstream events that regulate the function of opioid receptors on surface membrane. Identifying the specific role of receptor desensitization in tolerance development in an *in vivo* system would be a significant technical challenge.

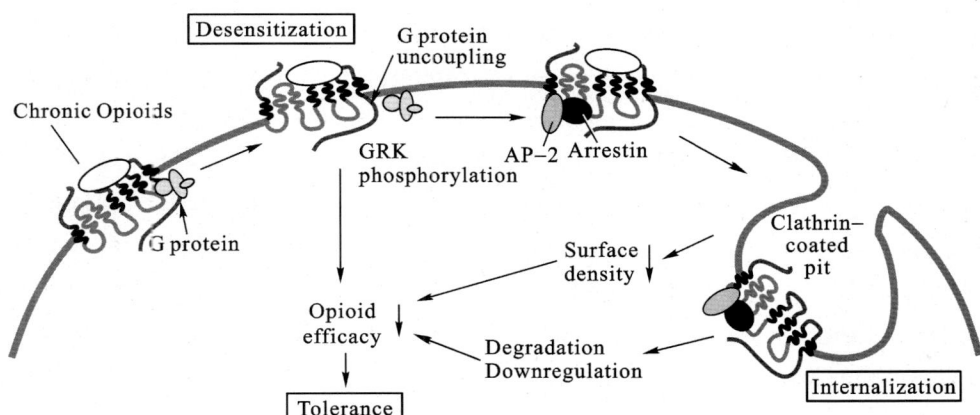

Fig.30.1   Mechanisms of opioid tolerance through receptor desensitization and internalization. In the presence of chronic opioids, agonist-bound μ-opioid receptor (MOR) is phosphorylated by G protein-coupled receptor kinase (GRK), which induces an increased uncoupling of MOR from G proteins and downstream effectors, such as potassium channels. This increased uncoupling reduces the efficacy of opioid agonists and their cellular effects, contributing to tolerance. Phosphorylated MOR may undergo a conformational change with increased affinity for binding to β-arrestin and the regulatory proteins AP-2. This process promotes MOR internalization in a clathrin-coated pit through classic endocytosis. The internalized MOR is then degraded, resulting in a MOR downregulation and a net decrease in surface MOR density, diminishing agonist effects and contributing to tolerance.

INTERNALIZATION

The mechanism for the internalization of opioid receptors has been described in another chapter (Chapter 11). There are two internalization-related mechanisms that may contribute to opioid tolerance: receptor internalization-induced receptor downregulation and differential properties of opioid agonists in inducing receptor internalization.

Receptor downregulation can be induced by receptor internalization. After prolonged agonist exposure, opioid receptors undergo β-arrestin-dependent internalization through the typical endocytosis process. Internalized opioid receptors may be subject to degradation, resulting in a decreased receptor density on surface membrane for agonist activation and contributing to tolerance (Fig.30.1). However, a direct connection between receptor downregulation and opioid tolerance has yet to be demonstrated. Importantly, controversial results have been reported in terms of effects of chronic opioids on surface density of opioid receptors. Chronic morphine has been shown to downregulate MOR density in some brain regions, but induce no change in other brain areas (Bhargava and Gulati, 1990; Tao et al., 1998), or even upregulate MOR (Rothman et al., 1998). In general, although chronic opioid-induced receptor desensitization, internalization and downregulation have been shown to mediate cellular tolerance measured by cellular effects of agonists in vitro, its magnitude is much smaller than that of the behavioral tolerance observed in vivo, and therefore cannot account for a large part of the mechanisms mediating in vivo tolerance. This suggests that additional critical mechanisms exist at the cellular network and system levels.

The other internalization-related mechanism for opioid tolerance may result, at least partly, from the ability of opioid agonists to induced MOR internalization. An important finding that contradicts the mechanisms of desensitization and internalization-induced downregulation for opioid tolerance is that morphine, a strong tolerance inducer, causes only weak MOR desensitization (Yu et al., 1997) and does not induce significant MOR internalization (Arden et al., 1995). Comparison of different MOR agonists reveals that agonist ability to induce MOR internalization is inversely related to its potency for induction of tolerance (Whistler et al., 1999). Recent studies have considerably advanced our understanding of the downstream regulating processes for the internalized receptors (see review by Tan et al.). In addition to degradation, internalized receptors also can be dephosphorylated and resensitized through the receptor-recycling pathway and be trafficked back to surface membrane. Representing a new hypothesis for tolerance, He et al. shows that sub-threshold DAMGO that does not induce internalization by itself, causes MOR internalization in the presence of morphine, inhibits chronic morphine-induced supersensitivity of adenylyl cyclase and enhances analgesia induced by chronic morphine (He et al., 2002). From these findings, they propose that receptor internalization is a critical signal for preventing sustained MOR signaling and consequent tolerance. For example, because morphine does not induce MOR internalization, its activation of MOR persists and sustained MOR signaling promotes other compensatory mechanisms to counteract MOR signaling, resulting in tolerance. In contrast, DAMGO induces MOR internalization, which rapidly desensitizes MOR signaling and also triggers receptor resensitization, causing less tolerance (Fig.30.2). Further studies are necessary to clarify the detailed mechanisms for DAMGO-morphine interaction in opioid analgesia and tolerance development, and to determine the role of MOR trafficking pathways in MOR signaling and opioid tolerance.

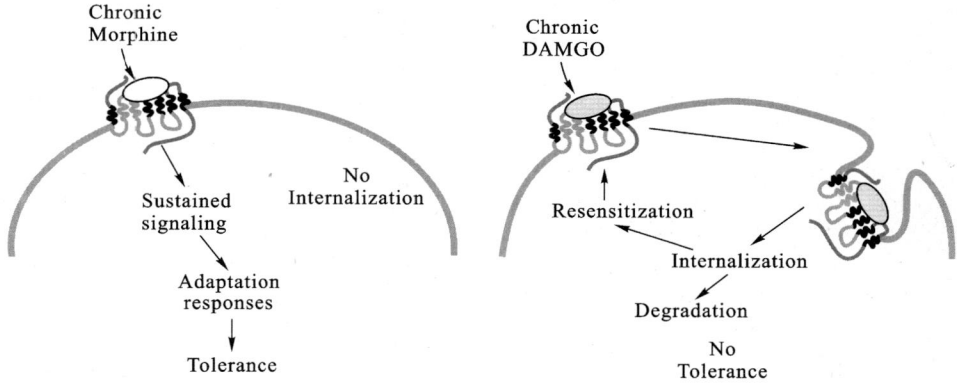

Fig.30.2   Mechanisms of opioid tolerance through agonist-regulated internalization. Persistent stimulation of MOR by chronic morphine does not induce significant internalization, which maintains MOR signaling and its activation of downstream effectors, causing various adaptive responses to counteract the sustained MOR stimulation. These adaptations oppose the morphine action, contributing to tolerance. In contrast, persistent activation of MOR by DAMGO induces considerable MOR internalization. Most of the internalized MOR can be resensitized and trafficked back for insertion on surface membrane through yet unidentified recycling pathways and regulatory proteins. Thus, the internalization signal triggers the recycling of MOR traffic, which maintains surface MOR for agonist activation, resulting in less tolerance.

GLUTAMATE RECEPTORS

Glutamate receptors mediate many forms of synaptic plasticity in the CNS. It has been well established that glutamate receptors play a crucial role in the development of opioid tolerance. The first strong evidence came from a study by Trujillo and Akil in which they showed that systemic application of a non-competitive NMDA receptor antagonist MK-801 significantly attenuated morphine tolerance (Trujillo *et al.*, 1991). Subsequent studies demonstrated that blockade of AMPA receptors also reduced morphine tolerance (Mao *et al.*, 1994; Kest *et al.*, 1997). Recent studies using mice deficient in a specific subunit of both NMDA and AMPA receptors further confirm the critical role of both types of glutamate receptors in the development of opioid tolerance (Inoue *et al.*, 2003; Vekovischeva *et al.*, 2001).

Despite the clear demonstration of a crucial involvement of glutamate receptors in opioid tolerance, the mechanism by which glutamate receptors mediate behavioral tolerance remains largely unclear. In spinal trigeminal neurons *in vitro*, MOR agonists activate PKC and enhance NMDA current through PKC-mediated removal of Mg^{2+} blockade (Chen

and Huang, 1992). However, how such an opioid-mediated enhancement in NMDA receptor function contributes to analgesic tolerance to chronic morphine in the spinal cord has yet to be illustrated. In rats *in vivo*, chronic morphine significantly increases GABA synaptic current, but induces no change in glutamate synaptic transmission in several brain areas examined, including the ventral tegmental area and the periaqueductal gray (Ingram *et al.*, 1998; Bonci and Williams, 1997). In recent studies, we have found that *in vivo* administration of chronic morphine significantly increases presynaptic release of glutamate in neurons of the nucleus raphe magnus (NRM), a critical brainstem site for opioid analgesia (Bie *et al.*, 2005; Bie and Pan, 2005). These NRM neurons contain MOR and are thought to have a facilitating action on pain transmission in the spinal cord through their descending projections (Pan *et al.*, 1997). Opioids produce analgesia at least partly by hyperpolarizing these neurons and removing their pain-facilitating action. Thus, we have proposed that chronic morphine enhances the activity of glutamate synaptic inputs onto these neurons, which increases their excitability and thereby counteracts the inhibitory effect of analgesic opioids, contributing to opioid tolerance (Fig.30.3).

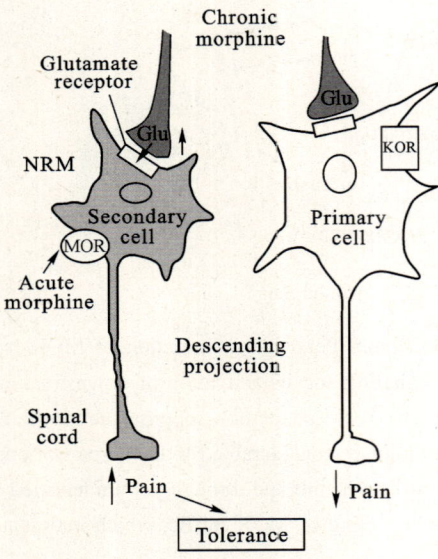

Fig.30.3 Mechanisms of opioid tolerance through glutamate synaptic transmission in NRM neurons and increased pain. Chronic morphine stimulates glutamate synaptic inputs only in secondary cells of the NRM, increasing their excitability and descending pain-facilitating actions on spinal pain transmission. As acute morphine produces analgesia partly by hyperpolarizing these cells, this chronic morphine action and resultant pain counteract morphine analgesia, contributing to tolerance.

CHRONIC OPIOID-INDUCED PAIN AND HYPERALGESIA

There is accumulating evidence showing that chronic exposure to opioids induces abnormal pain and an increase in pain sensitivity in both clinical reports and animal studies (see review by Ossipov *et al.*). It has been demonstrated that repeated administration of opioids in the spinal cord causes tactical allodynia (nociceptive responses to non-noxious stimulation) and thermal hyperalgesia (increased sensitivity to noxious stimulation) in rats (Mao *et al.*, 1994; Vanderah *et al.*, 2000). The same abnormal pain state also can be induced by systemic application of chronic opioids (Vanderah *et al.*, 2001). Interestingly, recent studies clearly show that chronic opioid-induced pain hypersensitivity is largely mediated by neurons in the rostral ventromedial medulla (RVM) of which NRM is a major component. In fact, RVM has been implicated in the sensitized pain states induced by many different pathologic conditions, including nerve injury, inflammation, sickness response as well as chronic opioids (see review by Pan). In the case of chronic opioids, inactivation of RVM with lidocaine or bilateral lesion of the dorsolateral faniculus, where the descending projections from RVM to spinal dorsal horn travel, blocks tactical allodynia and thermal hyperalgesia induced by spinal or systemic administration of chronic opioids (Vanderah *et al.*, 2001).

The mechanism underlying chronic opioid-induced pain hypersensitivity has been largely unknown. Numerous studies implicate the NMDA receptor as an important player in the mechanism. Actually, it has been well recognized that the hyperalgesia induced by chronic opioids or neuropathy and opioid tolerance may share important mechanisms. The most apparent feature common to the hyperalgesia and tolerance is the sensitivity to NMDA antagonists, as both can be effectively antagonized by blocking the NMDA receptors. Based on these observations, a hypothesis has emerged that chronic opioids induce hyperalgesia somehow through activation of NMDA receptors and the enhanced pain counteracts the analgesic effect of opioids, contributing to opioid tolerance. How the NMDA receptor operates in the mechanism for the hyperalgesia and tolerance development remains to be investigated. Apparently, that requires studies in a well-characterized local circuit that contains NMDA receptors and is involved in opioid analgesia and tolerance. As mentioned above, we have shown recently that in opioid-tolerant rats, glutamate synaptic transmission is enhanced in NRM neurons whose activity facilitates spinal pain (Bie and Pan, 2005). The hyperalgesia induced by opioid withdrawal after chronic morphine treatment is blocked by local NRM application of glutamate receptor antagonists (Bie *et al.*, 2005). These findings are consistent with the hypothesis that chronic opioid-induced pain contributes to opioid tolerance. Thus, in the NRM, chronic opioids increase the activity of pain-facilitating neurons by enhancing their glutamatergic inputs, which produces an increase in pain sensitivity through their descending actions in the spinal dorsal horn, counteracting the analgesic effect of sustained opioids and contributing to opioid tolerance (Fig.30.3).

CYCLIC AMP-PKA

A hallmark molecular adaptation to chronic opioids is the supersensitization of the cAMP-PKA pathway. It has been well documented that acute opioids inhibit the activity of adenylyl cyclase (AC) and cAMP production whereas chronic opioids induce a compensatory increase in AC activity, causing an increase in intracellular cAMP concentration to pre-opioid level. Originally identified in cultured cell lines with *in vitro* application of opioids, this AC supersensitization has now been confirmed with *in vivo* administration of chronic opioids in many brain regions involved in major opioid effects, including analgesia and drug addiction (see review by Nestler). We have also demonstrated such an AC supersensitization in the NRM (Bie *et al.*, 2005). The neurobiochemical mechanisms underlying chronic opioid-induced superactivation of the cAMP cascade are still unclear and remain an intensively pursued issue. Supporting an important role of the sensitized cAMP cascade in chronic opioid actions, AC and PKA inhibitors significantly attenuate opioid withdrawal in opioid-dependent rats after chronic morphine treatment (Punch *et al.*, 1997).

The critical question next is, what are the cellular and behavioral actions of the sensitized AC and elevated cAMP level, and how those actions are related to opioid tolerance. In various cell preparations *in vitro*, AC activators and cAMP analogs have been found to have two major modulating effects on cell functions, enhancing neurotransmitter release and augmenting the hyperpolarization-activated cation

current (I_h). However, the physiological effects of a superactivated cAMP cascade by chronic opioids administered *in vivo* have just begun to emerge. Until recently, the only effect of a sensitized cAMP system induced by chronic opioids administered *in vivo* is an increase in GABA synaptic transmission. The behavioral significance of this enhanced GABA synaptic activity has yet to be illustrated. Further advancing the field, our recent study shows that *in vivo* administered chronic morphine induces AC supersensitization, which increases glutamate synaptic transmission and enhances the I_h in the same NRM neurons (Bie *et al.*, 2005). Both an increased glutamate synaptic input and an enhanced membrane-depolarizing I_h are expected to increase the excitability of these NRM neurons and consequently their descending pain-facilitating actions, promoting pain in a morphine-tolerant state (Fig.30.4). Upon opioid withdrawal, when inhibition of these neurons by sustained morphine is removed, their activity is further increased, producing withdrawal-induced pain. This notion of cAMP mediated mechanisms is validated by behavioral observations that NRM microinjection of cAMP/PKA inhibitors, glutamate receptor antagonists and I_h blockers all diminishes morphine withdrawal-induced hyperalgesia (Bie *et al.*, 2005).

CONCLUSION AND FUTURE DIRECTIONS

Decades of intensive research have remarkably improved our understanding of the mechanisms for opioid tolerance. While early studies mostly focus on receptor desensitization and regulation using simple receptor-expression systems, later studies increasingly emphasize the dynamic regulation of opioid receptor functions though agonist-receptor interactions, functional interactions between different opioid receptor types and between opioid receptors and other receptor systems. An increasing recognition and need in current tolerance research is the mechanisms at the network level with a link to behavioral analysis, where

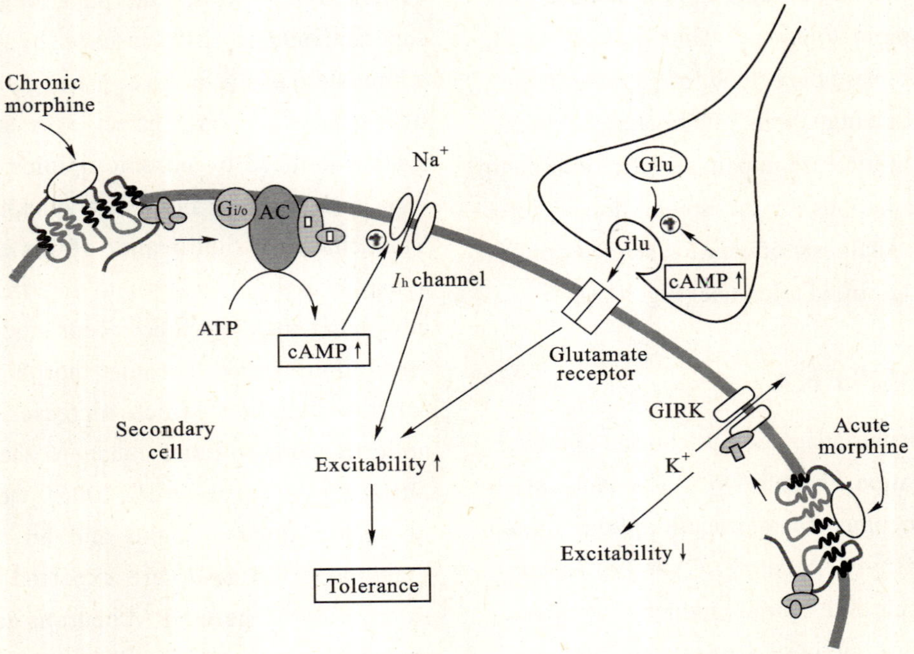

Fig.30.4 Mechanisms of opioid tolerance through cAMP-mediated actions in NRM neurons. Chronic morphine upregulates adenylyl cyclase (AC) activity and increases cAMP concentration in both cell bodies of secondary cells and glutamatergic terminals innervating these cells. Elevated cAMP level enhances the membrane-depolarizing current of the hyperpolarization-activated channel (I_h) on postsynaptic membrane, and increases glutamate release from the glutamatergic terminals. Both of the cAMP-mediated actions increase the excitability of secondary cells, counteracting the inhibitory action of acute morphine on these cells and contributing to tolerance (see Fig.30.3).

our knowledge lacks the most. An emerging notion is that opioid receptor trafficking may play a crucial role in the development of opioid tolerance. Studies using opioid receptor knockout mice have provided valuable information regarding the role of each opioid receptor types in tolerance development. Particularly, MOR has been demonstrated as a key triggering component that leads to all behavioral effects of chronic opioids, including analgesic tolerance. Presently, what is more important is to understand a series of adaptive responses downstream from MOR. One of such adaptations is receptor trafficking, which receives increasing research interests in current opioid studies. For example, chronic morphine has recently been found to upregulate the function of δ-opioid receptors in both the brain and the spinal cord. Multiple other receptor-transmission systems, such as δ-opioid receptors, glutamate receptors and the anti-opioid peptide cholecystokinin system, also likely undergo plastic changes through receptor trafficking after chronic MOR stimulation. The pathways and proteins

that regulate receptor trafficking, particularly receptor resensitization and insertion back to surface membrane, are poorly understood at present. In summary, opioid tolerance is a complex behavioral manifestation of chronic opioid-induced adaptations involving multiple mechanisms at all levels. Understanding of these mechanisms and identifying key components that lead to behavioral tolerance will be critical for the development of new pharmacological strategies and the improvement of current opioid therapies to overcome the problem of opioid tolerance.

GENERAL CITATIONS

Kieffer BL and Evans CJ. 2002. Opioid tolerance-in search of the holy grail. *Cell*, 108: 587-590.

Law PY and Loh HH. 1999. Regulation of opioid receptor activities. *J Pharmacol Exp Ther*, 289: 607-624.

Nestler EJ. 2001. Molecular basis of long-term plasticity underlying addiction. *Nat Rev Neurosci*, 2: 119-128.

Ossipov MH, Lai J, Vanderah TW, Porreca F. 2003. Induction

of pain facilitation by sustained opioid exposure: relationship to opioid antinociceptive tolerance., *Life Sci* 73: 783-800.

Pan ZZ. 2003.An intensified descending pain-facilitating pathway. *Drug Discovery Today: Disease Models*, 1: 121-125.

Tan CM, Brady AE, Nickols HH, Wang Q, and Limbird LE. 2004 .Membrane trafficking of G protein-coupled receptors. *Annu Rev Pharmacol Toxicol*, 44: 559-609.

DISCOVERY CITATIONS

Arden JR, Segredo V, Wang Z, Lameh J, Sadee W. 1995. Phosphorylation and agonist-specific intracellular trafficking of an epitope-tagged mu-opioid receptor expressed in HEK 293 cells. *J Neurochem*, 65: 1636-1645.

Bhargava HN and Gulati A. 1990. Down-regulation of brain and spinal cord mu-opiate receptors in morphine tolerant-dependent rats. *Eur J Pharmacol*, 190: 305-311.

Bie B and Pan ZZ. 2005. Increased glutamate synaptic transmission in the nucleus raphe magnus neurons from morphine-tolerant rats. *Mol Pain*, 1: 7.

Bie B, Peng Y, Zhang Y, Pan ZZ. 2005. cAMP-mediated mechanisms for pain sensitization during opioid withdrawal. *J Neurosci*, 25: 3824-3832.

Bohn LM, Gainetdinov RR, Lin FT, Lefkowitz RJ，Caron MG. 2000. Mu-opioid receptor desensitization by beta-arrestin-2 determines morphine tolerance but not dependence. *Nature*, 408: 720-723.

Bonci A and Williams JT. 1997. Increased probability of GABA release during withdrawal from morphine. *J Neurosci*, 17: 796-803.

Capeyrou R, *et al.* 1997. Agonist-induced signaling and trafficking of the mu-opioid receptor: role of serine and threonine residues in the third cytoplasmic loop and C-terminal domain. *FEBS Lett*, 415: 200-205 .

Chen L and Huang LY. 1992. Protein kinase C reduces Mg^{2+} block of NMDA-receptor channels as a mechanism of modulation. *Nature*, 356: 521-523.

Harris GC and Williams JT. 1991. Transient homologous mu-opioid receptor desensitization in rat locus coeruleus neurons. *J Neurosci*, 11: 2574-2581.

Hasbi A, *et al.* 1998. Desensitization of the delta-opioid receptor correlates with its phosphorylation in SK-N-BE cells:

involvement of a G protein-coupled receptor kinase. *J Neurochem*, 70: 2129-2138.

He L, Fong J, von Zastrow M, Whistler JL. 2002. Regulation of opioid receptor trafficking and morphine tolerance by receptor oligomerization. *Cell*, 108: 271-282.

Ingram SL, Vaughan CW, Bagley EE, Connor M, Christie MJ.1998. Enhanced opioid efficacy in opioid dependence is caused by an altered signal transduction pathway. *J Neurosci*, 18: 10269-10276 .

Inoue M, Mishina M, Ueda H. 2003. Locus-specific rescue of GluRepsilon1 NMDA receptors in mutant mice identifies the brain regions important for morphine tolerance and dependence. *J Neurosci*, 23: 6529-6536.

Kest B, McLemore G, Kao B, Inturrisi CE. 1997. The competitive alpha-amino-3-hydroxy-5-methyliso-xazole-4-propionate receptor antagonist LY293558 attenuates and reverses analgesic tolerance to morphine but not to delta or kappa opioids. *J Pharmacol Exp Ther*, 283: 1249-1255.

Kovoor A, Nappey V, Kieffer BL, Chavkin C. 1997. Mu and delta opioid receptors are differentially   desensitized by the coexpression of beta-adrenergic receptor kinase 2 and beta-arrestin 2 in *Xenopus oocytes*. *J Biol Chem*, 272: 27605-27611.

Mao J, Price DD, Mayer DJ. 1994. Thermal hyperalgesia in association with the development of morphine tolerance in rats: roles of excitatory amino acid receptors and protein kinase C. *J Neurosci*, 14: 2301-2312.

Pan ZZ, Tershner SA, Fields HL. 1997. Cellular mechanism for anti-analgesic action of agonists of the kappa-opioid receptor. *Nature*, 389: 382-385.

Punch LJ, Self DW, Nestler EJ, Taylor JR. 1997. Opposite modulation of opiate withdrawal behaviors on microinfusion of a protein kinase A inhibitor versus activator into the locus coeruleus or periaqueductal gray. *J Neurosci*, 17: 8520-8527.

Rothman RB, *et al.* 1989. Chronic administration of morphine and naltrexone up-regulate mu-opioid binding sites labeled by [3H][D-Ala2, MePhe4,Gly-ol5] enkephalin: further evidence for two mu-binding sites. *Eur J Pharmacol*, 160: 71-82.

Tao PL, *et al.* 1998. Immunohistochemical evidence of down-regulation of mu-opioid receptor after chronic PL-017 in rats. *Eur J Pharmacol*, 344: 137-142.

Trapaidze N, Keith DE, Cvejic S, Evans CJ, Devi LA. 1996. Sequestration of the delta opioid receptor. Role of the C terminus in agonist-mediated internalization. *J Biol Chem*, 271: 29279-29285.

Trujillo K A and Akil H. 1991. Inhibition of morphine tolerance and dependence by the NMDA receptor antagonist MK-801. *Science*, 251: 85-87.

Ueda H, *et al.* 1995. Protein kinase C involvement in homologous desensitization of delta-opioid receptor coupled to Gi1-phospholipase C activation in *Xenopus oocytes*. *J Neurosci*, 15: 7485-7499.

Vanderah TW, *et al.* 2000. Dynorphin promotes abnormal pain and spinal opioid antinociceptive tolerance. *J Neurosci*, 20: 7074-7079.

Vanderah TW, *et al.* 2001. Tonic descending facilitation from the rostral ventromedial medulla mediates opioid-induced abnormal pain and antinociceptive tolerance. *J Neurosci*, 21: 279-286.

Vekovischeva OY, *et al.* 2001. Morphine-induced dependence and sensitization are altered in mice deficient in AMPA-type glutamate receptor-A subunits. *J Neurosci*, 21: 4451-4459.

Whistler JL, Chuang HH, Chu P, Jan LY, von Zastrow M. 1999. Functional dissociation of mu opioid receptor signaling and endocytosis: implications for the biology of opiate tolerance and addiction. *Neuron*, 23: 737-746.

Yu Y, *et al.* 1997. Mu opioid receptor phosphorylation, desensitization, and ligand efficacy. *J Biol Chem*, 272: 28869-28874.

Zhang J, Barak LS, Winkler KE, Caron MG, Ferguson SS. 1997. A central role for beta-arrestins and clathrin-coated vesicle-mediated endocytosis in beta2-adrenergic receptor resensitization. Differential regulation of receptor resensitization in two distinct cell types. *J Biol Chem*, 272: 27005-27014.

Part X Models for Studying Pain and Searching for Pain Killers

Models in Pain Research

Timothy J. Ness[*]

MAIN TOPICS

SUMMARY

Pathological conditions producing pain in humans lead to the perception of damaged tissue (nociception) from multiple sites within the body, are evoked by multiple different types of stimuli and produce behavioral, reflex and neurophysiological responses. Models of pain in nonhuman animals have allowed for an improved understanding of the mechanisms of pain and serve as predictors of the potential clinical efficacy of analgesic manipulations. Nonhumans are not able to report pain in the sophisticated way of humans and so experimental paradigms need to be assessed regarding their validity as models of pain. Ideal models use an easily controlled, reproducible stimulus which is pain-producing in humans to produce aversive behaviors in the species being tested. Ideally, responses to this stimulus are quantifiable, reliable, reproducible and are altered by modifiers known to affect a particular clinical pain such as known analgesics or conditions producing hypersensitivity (i.e., inflammation). Using a site-stimulus-response-modifier descriptive nomenclature, the present chapter will describe currently employed models of pain.

INTRODUCTION

Our understanding of pain has increased markedly in the recent past with an expansion of model systems from the use of brief cutaneous stimuli to clinically relevant stimuli and models of specific disease processes. With the characterization of such models it is possible to move beyond general statements related to "pain" and "pain mechanisms" and instead investigate the sensory consequences of specific pathophysiologies. Clinically, pain is not a single entity and so there is value in developing models of the various types of pain. In order to maintain scientific integrity related to such pain models, certain criteria should be met that

---

[*] For the introduction of Dr. Ness, please refer to Chapter 28.

establish the validity of the particular model in relation to a particular pathophysiology.

ADEQUATE NOXIOUS STIMULI

Key considerations in the development of models for the study of pain relates to understanding what constitutes an "adequate" stimulus and what constitutes a "noxious" stimulus. The Nobel laureate, Sherrington, considered by many to be the father of modern neurophysiology, provided a definition of an adequate stimulus as that which optimally and selectively activated a particular neural structure or produced a particular response. He also defined noxious stimuli to be those stimuli which produce or predict tissue damage. These definitions have remained in place with only minor modification to this day. There are special conditions of pain in which these definitions do not wholly apply. One of these is pain arising from the internal organs of the body where frank tissue damage does not reliably produce pain and in which non-tissue damaging stimuli such as filling of the gall bladder may produce pain. Hence, it is more correct to describe nociceptive stimuli as "pain-producing" (which requires it to have been tested in humans) or "algogenic" rather than as noxious.

Use of non-human animal subjects which cannot report a sensation as painful has prompted a need for additional "evidence" that stimuli are likely algogenic within a given species. Such evidence is that the same stimulus which produces pain in humans also produces aversive behaviors in the studied species and produces responses which are modified by analgesic manipulations known to reduce that type of pain in humans (e.g., morphine). What constitutes aversive behaviors is a matter of debate but the best evidence of the aversiveness of a stimulus would be the use of learning models employing operant behavioral paradigms. The simple demonstration of reflex responses that appear related to pain (i.e., alterations in blood pressure), although supportive of the stimulus being algogenic, are too nonspecific to be definitive.

ALGOGENIC STIMULI

Stimuli which have been employed in studies related to pain can be generally categorized into four groups: electrical stimuli, mechanical stimuli, chemical stimuli and ischemia. Electrical stimuli have utilized implanted electrodes or probes which allow direct tissue contact. This stimulus is easily quantified, easily controlled and can produce pain, but also produces other sensations which are generally described as "unnatural." Thermal stimulation is provided by radiant heat (including pulsed laser), by immersion in solutions and using contact probes of constant or variable temperatures. Highly quantifiable and controllable, thermal stimuli can be relatively "modality specific" for thermal pain with minimal uncontrolled aspects of stimulation. Mechanical stimuli have included pinch, probing and stretch. Mechanical stimuli are also easily quantified, easily controlled, can be isolated and are related to a natural stimulus. Chemical stimuli have been applied topically or by injection to produce direct activation of neural structures or to induce alterations in tissue chemistry such as happens with inflammation. Quantification, control, isolation and modality-specificity of chemical stimuli are very preparation dependent. Ischemia has been produced by either internal or external occlusion of vasculature which also produces a mechanical stimulus. The effects of such occlusion are dependent upon collateral bloodflow and metabolic activity of the selected organ.

NOCICEPTIVE RESPONSES

Humans use tissue damage-related descriptors (e.g., burning) when describing their pain. Hence, the term *nociception,* defined as the perception of damaged tissue, is appropriate to use in relation to studies of pain. A perception of tissue damage is present even if none is occurring. It is presumed that non-human animals have similar perceptions. Reflex responses to algogenic stimuli were termed by Sherrington to be pseudaffective responses. In decerebrate animals these included growling, grimacing, muscle contractions (limb and abdominal), pupillary dilation, respiratory changes and alterations in heart rate and blood pressure. Pseudaffective responses have been proven to be reliable, but non-specific in that numerous alterations unrelated to pain can produce similar autonomic and motor reflexes. These responses appear to be profoundly affected by the presence of anesthesia. This effect of anesthesia on responses to algogenic stimuli has significant ethical ramifications since it would argue that all studies should perhaps be performed in unanesthetized animals. Many experimentally employed algogenic stimuli utilize invasive surgical procedures to place stimulation equipment and many use stimuli which are neither of short duration nor escapable. Hence, validity of specific preparations as models of pain is of paramount importance if one is to justify the use of such stimuli in the absence of anesthetics or analgesics.

Neurophysiological responses to visceral stimuli have proved to be reliable, but due to the invasive surgery necessary to perform neurophysiological experiments, animals are anesthetized or have undergone spinal transection and/or decerebration. Other responses include neuronal early-intermediate gene induction (e.g., *c-fos*), but this response lacks specificity since virtually all stimuli (e.g., hair brushing) produce the response.

Due to the non-specificity of many measured responses to algogenic stimuli, additional support for the validity of the particular response to a particular stimulus is necessary. To be of utility, responses should therefore be reliable (and ideally reproducible), should not be inhibited by known non-analgesics (excluding obvious interactions such as the effect of paralytics on motor responses) and should be inhibited by manipulations known to produce analgesia. These criteria establish that models of pain must correlate with known human conditions prior to their use in assessing novel hypotheses related to nociception.

MODEL OF TYPE OF PAIN VERSUS TYPE OF DISEASE

An important consideration when assessing an experimental paradigm related to pain is whether the proposed system is attempting to model a type of pain or a type of painful disease. Those whose professional life is dependent upon grant support know that the clinical significance of pain-related studies is enhanced when there is direct relevance to a particular disease entity. As a consequence, great verbal hyperbole is expended in attempts to promote specific models as representative of specific diseases.

The goal of a model is to be predictive of subsequent observations and this is clearly the case in relation to numerous pain models that are able to predict analgesic efficacy for various types of clinical pain. Pharmaceutical companies utilize "standard" models in the process of drug discovery to determine whether there is potential benefit in relation to the treatment of pain. A good example of such a screening test is the rat tail flick test of D'Amour and Smith. In this test a radiant light is focused on a portion of tail skin and the latency for the evocation of a withdrawal reflex is measured. Analgesics such as opioids produce a robust increase in this latency in a rank order fashion that is consistent with their clinical effects on post-operative pain. Hence, in this situation the tail flick reflex is predictive of effects on post-operative pain although it is clearly not a model of post-operative pain in humans. Simply, one must assess specifics of any paradigm to determine whether there is sufficient evidence to support predictability of a particular response in relation to a specific pain.

In recent years there has been a greater emphasis on the use of pain models that more closely mimic the actual pathophysiological processes of specific diseases. In most cases, a "modifier" has been added to an existent pain-related paradigm. For example, the administration of chemotherapy to cancer patients may often result in painful neuropathy. As a consequence, several different models of chemotherapy-induced pain have been presented which modify the organism by treating the animal with chemotherapy and then assessing responses to "standard" thermal and mechanical stimuli presented to cutaneous fields most affected by the chemotherapy. The precise relevance to a particular disease state requires a back-and-forth process of testing manipulations known or thought to modify clinical pain responses. Only after predictability of responses has been determined can a particular model system be identified as of value.

MODEL NOMENCLATURE

There is no universally accepted method of model description or comparison. One method is through use of the following organizational scheme: Site-Stimulus-Response-Modifier. The "Site" designation indicates the source of pain generation being tested. The "Stimulus" types are one of the following: thermal vs. mechanical vs. ischemic vs. electrical vs. chemical. The "Response" types can be many, some examples being flexion reflexes, vocalization, cardiovascular reflexes, spontaneous grooming, operant behavior and so forth. The most extensive designation category relates to the "Modifier" employed which may be analgesics, inflammation, nerve injuries and so forth. Using this organizational scheme it is possible to group together various model systems that relate to one another, while maintaining the unique differences between them.

SCOPE OF DISCUSSION

The present, limited discussion of the topic of pain models can not give an assessment of all possible model systems related to pain that have been described. As a consequence, a specific attempt was made to address model systems that have been utilized in publications in the past three years. Representative references, including primary references, will be cited. As noted above, use of reduced or deeply anesthetized experimental preparations limits the interpretations that can be formed in regards to neurophysiological

measures of neuronal activity since these very manipulations significantly alter the very sensations being studied. As a consequence, neurophysiological experimental paradigms will be viewed as correlates of model systems rather than model systems in their own right and so will have minimal discussion. This is due, in part, to basic difficulties associated with current technology and due to some of the ambiguity that is inherent to these types of studies. Neurophysiological studies in awake animals may resolve some of these issues, but may raise others due to behavioral and postsurgical variables that are added by this form of testing. Further, studies of neuronal components of nociception within the spinal cord and higher order sites of processing have demonstrated profound convergence of both nociceptive and non-nociceptive information which adds ambiguity related to the interpretation of neuronal activity as representative of pain. This in no way reduces the importance of such studies, but at present we must view neurophysiological information as representative of a complex organization of sensory processing that may or may not be predictive of effects in the whole organism.

MODEL SYSTEMS

Models using brief cutaneous stimuli

The most commonly employed stimuli utilized in studies related to pain are brief cutaneous stimuli such as pinching, poking or heating. Such stimuli can be easily and reproducibly administered, are readily quantified, are known to produce or predict tissue damage in humans and produce pain at known intensities of stimulation. Electrical stimuli are also brief, controllable and quantifiable but produce a global activation of all sensory structures. Thermal, mechanical and electrical stimuli evoke robust flexion reflexes and localized behavioral responses and so in most settings are "escapable" in that the evoked behavioral responses typically lead to the termination of the stimulus. This gives some element of control to test subjects and therefore minimizes ethical concerns in the performance of studies in both humans and non-human subjects. Chemical stimuli are also frequently used in cutaneous sites, but the responses are neither brief nor particularly escapable and so will be discussed in a separate sections.

Thermal stimuli are presented using either radiant heat focused onto a test site (e.g., the tail in the tail flick test), by immersion in hot water or by using a thermal contact probe. In the self-descriptive hot plate test, the entire test surface is a contact probe heated to and maintained at algogenic intensities (typically 48–52°C). Responses include flinching, foot licking, foot withdrawal and escape behaviors and are quantified as the latency from placement onto the plate and evocation of a response. The Hargreaves test determines the latencies of similar foot withdrawal or foot licking responses, but uses radiant light focused onto footpads through a glass chamber floor. A difference score comparing affected versus unaffected limbs is often employed in this test. Tail immersion in hot or cold water has been used to evoke escape responses and quantified as the latency to response.

Mechanical stimuli are presented in various ways using needles, forceps or clamps in a crude fashion, or more elegantly using calibrated forceps which produce a quantifiable force over a defined area. The Randall-Sellitto test provides a progressively increasing pressure to the footpad of a loosely restrained hindpaw and measures the force of pressure applied at the time of evocation of a withdrawal reflex. Von Frey hairs, named for the German psychophysisist who first devised their use from horsehairs, are calibrated filaments that provide a fixed force of punctate pressure before bending. Electronic versions have been constructed which provide a punctate stimulus of measurable force. Attachment of a disc of known area to the end of von Frey hairs has been utilized to allow for the quantification of nonpunctate mechanical stimuli.

Electrical stimuli have been frequently used to evoke behavioral responses such as operant behaviors, classical conditioning or avoidance behaviors. Sophisticated models, such as the shock titration paradigm in primates, teach the animal subjects to minimize algogenic electrical stimuli by an operant behavior. When animals allow higher or longer intensities of stimulation to occur, they are rewarded with food or drink. In this way animals titrate the stimulus to a "tolerable" level. Administration of analgesics has been demonstrated to allow the subject to tolerate higher levels of stimulation.

Using brief mechanical and thermal stimuli and withdrawal responses as endpoints, numerous model systems have examined the effects of various modifiers (Tables 31.1, 31.2). Analgesic manipulations have been used in virtually all model systems as part of the validation-of-method process and so are not listed separately as modifiers. The concepts of allodynia and hyperalgesia come into play in most clinically relevant models. Allodynia is defined as pain produced by normally nonpainful stimuli such as hair movement or light pressure. The nonhuman animal correlates to this are responses suggestive of nociception evoked by typically nonalgogenic stimuli. "Cool" stimuli or low intensities of mechanical stimulation such as those produced by very fine von Frey hairs are nonalgogenic in humans and so commonly employed in the nonhuman models. Hyperalgesia is defined as greater than normal intensities of pain evoked by normally painful stimuli or pain evoked by lower than normal intensities of stimuli which are algogenic at high intensities (a lowering of "threshold"). The nonhuman animal correlates of hyperalgesia are decreased intensities of stimuli needed to evoke nociceptive responses or increased vigor of responses to suprathreshold stimuli. Frequently, the lowering-of-threshold component of hyperalgesia is difficult to dissociate from allodynia. As a consequence, a common convention is to restrict discussions of hyperalgesia to the continuum of temperatures associated with cutaneous "hot" stimuli and to describe alterations in mechanical and "cool" thermal stimuli as representative of allodynia. Discussions of "beta" allodynia has been typically restricted to mechanical stimuli that optimally activate $A\beta$ sensory fibers (vibration, hair movement, very light pressure).

Cutaneous tissue modifiers such as incisions, burns and local inflammation as well as numerous deep tissue-related modifiers (e.g., bony injury, visceral stimulation, cancer) produce evidence of *secondary* cutaneous hyperalgesia or allodynia (Table31.1). Likewise, nerve injury at either peripheral or central locations also leads to similar phenomena (Table31.2). These model systems are therefore defined more by their sites of pain generation and the modifiers employed and not by their test stimuli and responses.

Table 31.1   Cutaneous site-thermal/mechanical stimuli-flexion/withdrawal responses—multiple modifiers.

Type of modifier	Description of model
Analgesic manipulations	Tail flick reflex evoked by radiant heat
(drugs, SIA, SPA)	Hot plate – foot lift/lick
Bony injury	Tibial fracture model of CRPS
	Osteotomy
Burn	Footpad – contact UV radiation
Cancer	Breast cancer cells in femur
	Hepatocarcinoma cells into thigh
	Melanoma cancer cells in femur
Incision	Plantar incision
	Thoracotomy
	Stab wound
Inflammation	Footpad subcutaneous injection
	(capsaicin, carageenan, CFA, zymosan)
Ischemic injury	Chronic post-ischemia model of CRPS
Muscle acidity	Repeated acid injection – Gastrocnemius
Pancreatitis	Dibutyl tin & alcohol-induced
Parotiditis	CFA to parotid – hyperalgesia
Visceral irritants	Turpentine, mustard oil
(secondary somatic hyperalgesia)	

SIA: stress-induced analgesia, SPA: stimulation-produced analgesia, CFA: Complete Freund's adjuvant, CRPS: complex regional pain syndrome.

MODELS USING CHEMICAL STIMULI

Numerous model systems have employed subcutaneous injections of algogenic substances. Their pain-producing qualities have typically been validated by responses to topical application, injection into blister bases or injection into other body sites. In recent years, a popular model using such stimuli is the formalin test of Duboisson and Dennis. In this model, formalin is injected subcutaneously into the foot of a rodent and "flicking," "licking" or "lifting" of the affected limb quantified. A two phase reaction is typically noted with initial activity for a few minutes (Phase 1 response) followed by a brief period of reduced activity, subsequently followed by renewed activity (Phase 2 response). The neurochemistry of responses related to Phase 1 appears to differ from those of Phase 2. Others have also injected formalin into numerous other body sites ranging from the face to the colon and observed correlative behaviors.

The injection of the natural substance, bradykinin, has also utilized in numerous models employing chemical stimuli. Generated by tissue injury, bradykinin, when injected into the subcutaneous tissues as well as muscle and other deep tissues leads to brief responses that appear nociceptive in nature. Other inflammatory compounds in addition to chemicals such as capsaicin produce robust motor responses that can be quantified (Table31.2). A "standard" pharmaceutical screening tool since its initial description in the 1950s, the "writhing test" consists of the intraperitoneal injection of a chemical irritant (most commonly phenylquinone or acetic acid) followed by the subsequent counting of "writhes" —a characteristic contraction of abdominal muscles accompanied by a hindlimb extensor motion. Methodology has been varied with the use of endothelin, bradykinin, ATP, acetylcholine, magnesium sulfate, hypertonic saline, and iodinated radio-contrast agents as intraperitoneal irritants. This model of pain has proven predictive value as a screening tool for analgesic actions but ethical concerns have presented significant constraints to use of the model. It has been described as a model of visceral pain due to the intraperitoneal delivery of algogenic agent, but is perhaps more correctly described as a peritoneal-viscero-inflammatory model with multiple sites of action and multiple actions.

Table 31.2 Chemical stimulus - motor responses—multiple sites—multiple modifiers.		
Site	**Chemical**	**Response**
Foot	Formalin	Posturing/licking/shaking
Intraperitoneal	Bradykinin Acetic Acid Phenylquinone	Writhing (characteristic postures and movements)
Intrapancreatic	Bradykinin	Posturing/ambulation
Intravesical	Xylene, capsaicin resiniferotoxin	Licking/biting
Orofacial	Formalin, capsaicin	Facial grooming, movements
Pericardial	Inflammatory soup	Posturing
Uterine Mustard oil		Posturing

NEUROPATHIC PAIN MODELS

Pain that occurs secondary to nervous tissue injury has proven to be difficult to treat clinically and difficult to understand neurophysiologically. As a consequence, a plethora of models exist with varying correlation to clinical conditions (Table31.3). Argument for the validity for some of the model systems has been made by the demonstration of a lack-of-effect of traditional analgesics with varying success. Sites of nervous tissue injury can be central or peripheral with a majority of the pain models employing peripheral nerve injury as their modifier. Most models have described the effects of nervous tissue injury on evocable responses invoking the concepts of cutaneous allodynia and hyperalgesia noted above. A hallmark feature of clinical neuropathic pain is the presence of a spontaneous component. Namely, pain occurs without cause. For this reason, models examining spontaneous behaviors such as autotomy, altered postures and "grooming" after nervous system injury (Table31.4) have special value in relation to neuropathic pain.

Although allodynia and hyperalgesia are frequently present in neuropathic pain, they are often not the problematic component of the pain that brings them to their physician for treatment.

CANCER-RELATED PAIN MODELS

Cancer pain is by definition pain due to the presence or treatment of cancer. This means that at least two different types of cancer pain models exist—those related to the presence of a cancer and those related to sequelae of treatment. The latter include neuropathic pains produced by surgery or by treatments such as chemotherapy. Models of vincristine-induced, cisplatin-induced and paclitaxel-induced peripheral neuropathies with associated alterations in cutaneous sensory processing have been described. Anti-ganglioside antibodies used in the treatment of certain types of neuroblastoma produce a generalized neuritis resulting in a neuropathic pain. The chemotherapeutic agent, cyclophosphamide, produces a cystitis which results in a type of visceral pain. The presence of cancer can be pain producing and models employing mammary cancer cells, hepatocarcinoma cells, melanoma cells and fibrosarcoma cells implanted into femurs with re-sultant bony destruction, somatic allodynia/hyperalgesia and altered gait/postures have all been described.

Table 31.3   Cutaneous site-thermal/mechanical stimuli- flexion/withdrawal response – nerve injury modifier.

Type of nerve injury	Type of change in measure
AIDS-related neuropathy	Allodynia/hyperalgesia
Autoimmune Encephalomyelitis	Hyperalgesia
Brachial plexus avulsion	Hyperalgesia
Cancer chemotherapy	
Cisplatin-peripheral neuropathy	Allodynia/Hyperalgesia
Vincristine-peripheral neuropathy	Allodynia/Hyperalgesia
Paclitaxel-peripheral neuropathy	Allodynia
Anti-ganglioside antibodies	Allodynia/Hyperalgesia
Diabetic neuropathy	Allodynia/Hyperalgesia
Infraorbital nerve lesion	Allodynia/Hyperalgesia
Nucleus pulposus application	Allodynia/Hyperalgesia
Sacral nerve transection	Allodynia/Hyperalgesia
Sciatic nerve partial injury	Allodynia/Hyperalgesia
Sciatic nerve constriction	Allodynia/Hyperalgesia
Sciatic nerve inflammation	Allodynia/Hyperalgesia
Spinal segmental nerve ligation	Allodynia/Hyperalgesia
Spinal Cord Inflammation	Allodynia
Spinal Cord Contusion	Allodynia
Spinal Cord Transection	Allodynia/Hyperalgesia
Spinal Cord Excitotoxic Injury	Allodynia
Spinal Cord ischemic injury	Allodynia
Varicella zoster virus infection	Allodynia

Note also spontaneous behaviors related to nervous system injury in Table.31.4.

Table 31.4   Spontaneous behaviors — multiple sites & modifiers.

Description of behavior	Modifier
Autotomy (self-mutilation)	Deafferentation
"Grooming", scratching	Excitotoxic spinal cord injury
Limb disuse	Femur inj fibrosarcoma
Posturing	Post-laparotomy
Decreased locomotion	Bladder inflammation
	Pancreatitis

ARTICULAR-MUSCULOSKELETAL PAIN MODELS

Painful arthritis comes in many forms ranging from focal, single-joint versions produced by local trauma to panarticular versions produced by rheumatological disease. Model systems have produced experimental modifiers that affect either single joints or which cre-ate a systemic immunological response in which many joints of the body come under attack (Table31.5). Complete Freund's adjuvant (CFA) has been used to create both systemic as well as localized responses with progressive joint destruction as a sequelae of the treatment. Altered positioning, altered gait, decreased toleration of joint compression and alterations in cu-taneous sensory responses (hyperaglesia and allodynia responses) are produced by the joint manipulations and allow quantification of the phenomenon. Ankle ligamentous trauma or intra-articular injections produce local tissue inflammatory responses and can be similarly quantified. Bony injury such as that produced by fracture or osteotomy leads to altered gaits as well as alterations in cutaneous sensation. Interestingly, Houghton *et al.* demonstrated that the cutaneous hypersensitivity that follows a tibial or calcaneal oste-

otomy requires the dorsal columns of the spinal cord to be intact. A model of muscular pain has been described by Sluka *et al.* in which repeated injections of acidic solution are injected into muscle and resultant effects on cutaneous sensation (e.g., hyperalgesia and allodynia).

Table 31.5   Joint site-mechanical stimuli-behavioral response—inflammation modifier.

Source of inflammation	Observed effect
Ankle ligament trauma	Reduced weightbearing
Cervical facet injury	Allodynia
Intra-articular CFA	Gait alterations
	"Freezing" and scratching
Intra-articular Iodoacetate	Reduced weightbearing
Intra-articular kaolin	Increased vocalization
Intra-articular urate	Decreased weightbearing
Partial meniscectomy	Allodynia/Hyperalgesia
Lumbar laminectomy	Allodynia and posturing

Note also spontaneous behaviors related to joints in Table31.4.CFA – Complete Freund's Adjuvant.

Table 31.6   Visceral sites-multiple stimuli/responses/modifiers.

Visceral site-stimulus	Responses
Artificial urolithiasis	Posturing behaviors
Bladder distension	Visceromotor, CV responses
Colorectal distensions	Visceromotor, CV responses
Cyclclophosphamide cystitis	Posturing behaviors
Duodenal distension	Posturing behaviors
Gall bladder distension	CV responses, behaviors
Ureter distension	CV responses
Uterine Cervix Distension	Abdominal Contractions
Vaginal Distension	Operant behavior modifications

Note also secondary somatic hyperalgesia produced by visceral stimulation in Table 31.1 and spontaneous behaviors evoked by visceral stimulation in Table31.4.

VISCERAL PAIN MODELS — GENERAL

When the site of pain origin is an internal organ of the body, the pain is referred to as visceral pain. The characteristics of visceral pain differ from cutaneous pain with the hallmark features of poor localization, referral of pain to other somatic sites and greater emotional/autonomic responses to a given intensity of pain. Current models of visceral pain utilize me-

chanical stimuli, generally of controllable duration, or chemical stimuli applied directly to relevant targets with time-limited periods of observation, thus permitting selectivity with respect to site of stimulation. Thermal sensitivity of viscera is low and so uncommonly applied. Electrical stimuli have been employed but with limitations similar to that noted in other systems (e.g., nonspecificity of responses). Occlusion of blood supply to most viscera is associated with pain. Accordingly, models of coronary artery occlusion and ischemia of abdominal visceral organs have been reported but found limited utility due to the profound secondary effects on physiology.

MECHANICAL VISCERAL STIMULI

Balloon distension of hollow organs, principally the gastrointestinal tract, is the most widely used experimental stimulus of the viscera. Experimental balloon distension of the gastrointestinal tract in humans has been established to reproduce pathologically experienced pain in terms of intensity, quality and the area to which the sensation is referred. Responses to distending stimuli in the small bowel, colon/rectum, biliary system and urinary bladder include quantifiable pseudaffective responses (e.g., changes in blood pressure, heart rate and in contractions of the abdominal wall musculature). Traditional analgesics (e.g., morphine) produce inhibition of most distension-related responses. A variety of irritants/inflammogens (trinitrobenzene sulfonic acid, turpentine, acetic acid, zymosan, mustard oil) have been shown to enhance responses to mechanical distending visceral stimuli. Typically, the stimulus-response function generated by visceral stimulation in the presence of inflammation is shifted leftward with response thresholds decreased and response vigor increased. A novel distending mechanical visceral stimulus is provided by an artificial ureteral calculosis in a model which has been characterized in rats. Kidney stones are undeniably painful in humans and produce a mechanical distension of the ureter. Characteristic postures are spontaneously generated in the presence of an artificial stone placed surgically into the upper third of the ureter by injecting 0.02 mL of dental resin cement (while still liquid) through a fine needle. Rats are allowed to recover from surgical anesthesia and then continuously observed for typically four days for "visceral episodes" demonstrating behaviors similar to those observed in the writhing test (e.g. abdominal contractions, hindlimb extensions).

A newly presented model of uterine pain has utilized the mechanical stimulus of uterine cervix dis-

tension to evoke robust abdominal contraction reflexes that are inhibited by analgesics. Berkley has used vaginal distension as a stimulus to modify operant behaviors demonstrating the aversiveness of the stimulus.

Distension of the gallbladder and associated biliary system produces pathological pain when the gallbladder is inflamed and/or associated ducts obstructed and has been experimentally reproduced in humans. Vigorous cardiovascular reflexes can also be evoked by biliary system distension and these responses have been used to discriminate nociceptive neuronal responses from non-nociceptive responses. "Escape" behaviors in cats and dogs to gallbladder distension have been noted.

INFLAMMATION OF VISCERA

Inflammation of internal organs commonly produces reports of pain. Experiments in non-human animals have artificially inflamed the urinary bladder, uterus, colon and esophagus with the intraluminal administration of irritants which include turpentine, mustard oil, croton oil, acetic acid, acetone, xylene and capsaicin and its analogues. McMaho and Abel performed an extensive characterization of visceromotor and micturition reflexes following inflammation of the bladder. Following the administration of irritants, increased responses to urinary bladder filling correlated with measures of inflammation such as tissue edema, plasma extravasation and leukocyte infiltration. Rats became hyper-responsive to noxious stimuli applied to the lower abdomen, perineum and tail and thereby secondary somatic hyperalgesia demonstrated. Modulatory effects of traditional and non-traditional analgesics have all been noted.

Another well-characterized model using visceral irritant administration is the injection of substances such as xylene or vanilloids (capsaicin, resiniferotoxin) through a surgically implanted intravesical catheter. Immediate behavioral responses include abdominal/perineal licking, headturns, hindlimb hyperextension, head grooming, biting, vocalization, defecation, scratching and salivation. Analgesics including peripherally administered opioids produced dose-dependent inhibition of these behavioral responses. Another method of irritant delivery to the bladder uses cyclophosphamide (CP; 100 mg/kg) administered intraperitoneally which is metabolized and excreted as urinary acrolein. Beginning approxi- mately one hour after systemic administration rats demonstrate alterations in postures and behaviors which are graded. Inhibition by analgesics has been reported.

CONCLUSION

There are many models which have been put forward attempting to describe pain of different origins. Clinical pains are often prolonged and "relatively" inescapable as are some of the models examined here. This article has examined models that are in current use with a focus on their validity as defined by proposed criteria. In this way it may assist decisions related to the value of the knowledge to be gained versus the cost of that knowledge. Distinct patterns of response are apparent when model systems are grouped according to the four basic criteria of SITE-STIMULUS-RESPONSE-MODIFIER.

CITATIONS

Abelli L, Conte B, Somme V, Maggi CA, Girliani S, Meli A. 1989. A method for studying pain arising from the urinary bladder in conscious, freely-moving rats. *J Urol*, 141:148-151.

Aicher SA, Silverman MB, Winkler CW, Bebo BF Jr. 2004. Hyperalgesia in an animal model of multiple sclerosis. *Pain*, 110: 560-570.

Allen JW and Yaksh TL. 2004. Tissue injury models of persistent nociception in rats. *Methods Mol Med*, 99: 25-34.

Ammons WS and Foreman RD. 1984. Cardiovascular and T2-T4 dorsal horn cell responses to gallbladder distension in the cat. *Brain Res*, 321:267-277.

Authier N, Gillet JP, Fialip J, Eschalier A, Coudore F. 2003. An animal model of nociceptive peripheral neuropathy following repeated cisplatin injections. *Exp Neurol*, 182: 12-20.

Back SK, Sung B, Hong SK, Na HS. 2002. A mouse model for peripheral neuropathy produced by a partial injury of the nerve supplying the tail. *Neurosci Letts*, 322:153-156.

Beitz AJ, Newman A, Shepard M, Ruggles T, Eikmeier L. 2004. A new rodent model of hind limb penetrating wound injury characterized by continuous primary and secondary hyperalgesia. *J Pain*, 5: 26-37.

Bennett GJ and Xie YK. 1998. A peripheral mononeuropathy in rat that produces disorders of pain sensation like those seen in man. *Pain*, 33: 87-107.

Berkley KJ, Wood E, Scofield SL, Little M. 1995. Behavioral responses to uterine or vaginal distension in the rat. *Pain*, 61:121-131.

Bon K, Lichtensteiger CA, Wilson SG, Mogil JS. 2003. Characterization of cyclophosphamide cystitis, a model of visceral and referred pain in the mouse: species and strain differences. *J Urol*, 170: 1008-1012.

Brennan TJ. 1999. Postoperative models of nociception. *ILAR J*, 40: 129-136.

Buvanendran A, Kroin JS, Kerns JM, Nagalla SN, Tuman KJ. 2004. Characterization of a new animal model for evaluation of persistent postthoracotomy pain. *Anesth Analg*, 99: 1453-1460.

Carroll MN Jr and Lim RKS. 1958. Mechanisms of phenylquinone writhing. *Fed Proc* 17:357.

Cervero F. 1982. Afferent activity evoked by natural stimulation of the biliary system in the ferret. *Pain,* 13: 137-151.

Chernov HI, Wilson DE, Fowler F, Plummer AJ. 1967. Non-specificity of the mouse writhing test. *Arch Int Pharmacodyn*, 167:171-178.

Chidiac JJ, Rifai K, Hawaa NN, Masaad CA, Jurjus AR, Jabbur SJ, Saade NE. 2002. Nociceptive behaviour induced by dental application of irritants to rat incisors: a new model for tooth inflammatory pain. *Eur J Pain*, 6: 55-67.

Coderre TJ and Wall PD. 1987. Ankle joint urate arthritis (AJUA) in rats: an alternative animal model of arthritis to that produced by Freund's adjuvant. *Pain*, 28: 379-393.

Coderre TJ, Xanthos DN, Francis L, Bennett GJ. 2004. Chronic post-ischemia pain (CPIP): a novel animal model of complex regional pain syndrome-type I (CRPS-I; reflex sympathetic dystrophy) produced by prolonged hind-paw ischemia and reperfusion in the rat. *Pain*, 112: 94-105.

Colburn RW, Coombs DW, Degnen CC, Rogers LL. 1989. Mechanical visceral pain model: chronic intermittent intestinal distension in the rat. *Physiol Behav*, 45:191-197.

Coulthard P, Pleuvry BJ, Brewster M, Wilson KL, Macfarlane TV. 2002. Gait analysis as an objective measure in a chronic pain model. *J Neurosci Methods*, 116: 197-213.

Courteix C, Eschalier A, Lavareen J. 1993. Streptozocin-induced diabetic rats: behavioral evidence for a model of chronic pain. *Pain*, 53: 81-88.

Craft RM, Carlisi VJ, Mattia A, Herman RM, Porreca F. 1993. Behavioral characterization of the excitatory and desensitizing effects of intravesical capsaicin and resiniferatoxin in the rat. *Pain*, 55: 205-215.

D'Amour FE and Smith DL. 1941. A method for determining loss of pain sensation. *J Pharmacol Exp Ther*, 72: 74-79.

Dalziel RG, Bingham S, Sutton D, Grant D, Champion JM, Dennis SA, Quinn JP, Bountra C, Mark MA. 2004. Allodynia in rats infected with varicella zoster virus — a small animal model for post-herpetic neuralgia. *Brain Res - Brain Res Rev*, 46: 234-242.

DeCastro Costa M, DeSutter P, Gybels J, van Hees J. 1981. Adjuvant-induced arthritis in rats: a possible animal model of chronic pain. *Pain*, 10: 173-186.

Dubuisson D and Dennis S. 1977. The formalin test: a quantitative study of the analgesic effects of morphine, meperidine and brainstem stimulation in rats and cats. *Pain*, 4: 161-174.

Euchner-Wamser I, Meller ST, Gebhart GF. 1994. A model of cardiac nociception in chronically instrumented rats: behavioral and electrophysiological effects of pericardial administration of algogenic substances. *Pain*, 58:117-

128.

Fernihough J, Gentry C, Malcangio M, Fox A, Rediske J, Pellas T, Kidd B, Bevan S, Winter J. 2004. Pain related behavior in two models of osteoarthritis in the rat knee. *Pain*, 112: 83-93.

Gazda LS, Milligan ED, Hansen MK, Twining CM, Poulos NM, Chacur M, O'Connor KA, Armstrong C, Maier SF, Watkins LR, Myers RR. 2001. Sciatic inflammatory neuritis (SIN): behavioral allodynia is paralleled by peri-sciatic proinflammatory cytokine and superoxide production. *J Periph Nerv Syst*, 6: 111-129.

Giamberardino MA, Valente R, de Bigontina P, Vecchiet L. 1995. Artificial ureteral calculosis in rats: behavioural characterization of visceral pain episodes and their relationship with referred lumbar muscle hyperalgesia. *Pain*, 61:459-469.

Gillardon F, Morano I, Zimmermann M. 1991. Ultraviolet irradiation of the skin attenuates calcitonin gen-related peptide mRNA expression in rat dorsal root ganglion cells. *Neurosci Lett*, 124: 144-147.

Guo TZ, Offley SC, Boyd EA, Jacobs CR, Kingery WS. 2004. Substance P signaling contributes to the vascular and nociceptive abnormalities observed in a tibial fracture rat model of complex regional pain syndrome type I. *Pain*, 108: 95-107.

Han JS, Bird GC, Li W, Jones J, Neugebauer V. 2005. Computerized analysis of audible and ultrasonic vocalizations of rats as a standardized measure of pain-related behavior. *J Neurosci Methods*, 141: 261-269.

Hargreaves K, Dubner R, Brown F, Flores C, Joris J. 1988. A new and sensitive method for measuring thermal nociception in cutaneous hyperalgesia. *Pain*, 32:77-88.

Hendershot LC, Forsaith J. 1959. Antagonism of the frequency of phenylquinone-induced writhing in the mouse by weak analgesics and nonanalgesics. *J Pharmacol Exp Ther*, 125:237-240.

Higuera ES and Luo ZD. 2004. A rat pain model of vincristine-induced neuropathy. *Methods Mol Med*, 99: 91-98.

Holguin A, O'Connor KA, Biedenkapp J, Campisi J, Wieseler-Frank J, Milligan ED, Hansen MK, Spataro L, Maksimova E, Bravmann C, Martin D, Fleshner M, Maier SF, Watkins LR. 2004. HIV-1 gp120 stimulates proinflammatory cytokine-mediated pain facilitation via activation of nitric oxide synthase-I (nNOS). *Pain*, 110: 517-530.

Houghton AK, Hewitt E, Westlund KN. 1999. Dorsal column lesion prevents mechanical hyperalgesia and allodynia in osteotomy model. *Pain*, 82: 73-80.

Houghton AK, Kadura S, Westlund KN. 1997. Dorsal column lesions reverse the reduction of homecage activity in rats with pancreatitis. *Neuroreport*, 8:3795-3800.

Joseph EK, Chen X, Khaser SG, Levine JD. 2004. Novel mechanism of enhanced nociception in a model of AIDS therapy-iinduced painful neuropathy in the rat. *Pain*, 107: 147-158.

Kim SH and Chung JM. 1992. An experimental model for peripheral neuropathy produced by segmental spinal nerve ligation in the rat. *Pain*, 50: 355-363.

Kobayashhi K, Imaizumi R, Sumichika H, Tanaka H, Goda M, Fukunari A, Komatsu H. 2003. Sodium iodoace-tate-induced experimental osteoarthritis and associated pain model in rats. *J Vet Med Sci*, 65: 1195-1199.

Koo ST, Park YI, Lim KS, Chung K, Chung JM. 2002. Acupuncture analgesia in a new rat model of ankle sprain pain. *Pain*, 99: 423-431.

Koster R, Anderson M, de Beer EJ. 1959. Acetic acid for analgesic screening. *Fed Proc,* 18:412.

Lanteri-Minet M, Bon K, de Pommery J, Michiels JF, Mene-trey D. 1995. Cyclophosphamide cystitis as a model of visceral pain in rats: model elaboration and spinal structures involved as revealed by the expression of c-fos and Krox-24 proteins. *Exp Brain Res*, 105:220-232.

Lee BH, Seong J, Kim UJ, Won R, Kim J. 2005. Behavioral characteristics of a mouse model of cancer pain. *Yonsei Med J*, 46: 252-259.

Lee BH, Won R, Baik DH, Lee CH, Moon CH. 2000. An animal model of neuropathic pain employing injury to the sciatic nerve branches. *NeuroReport*, 11: 657-661.

Lee KE, Thinnes JH, Gokhin DS, Winkelstein BA. 2004. A novel rodent neck pain model of facet-mediated behavioral hypersensitivity: implications for persistent pain and whiplash injury. *J Neurosci Methods*, 137: 151-159.

Martin TJ, Buechler NL, Kahn W, Crews JC, Eisenach JC. 2004. Effects of laparotomy on spontaneous exploratory activity and conditioned operant responding in the rat: a model for postoperative pain. *Anesthesiology*, 101: 191-203.

Massie JB, Huang B, Malkmus S, Yaksh TL, Kim CW, Garfin SR, Akeson WH. 2004. A preclinical post laminectomy rat model mimics the human post laminectomy pain syndrome. *J Neurosci Methods*, 137: 283-289.

McMahon SB and Abel C. 1987. A model for the study of visceral pain states: chronic inflammation of the chronic decerebrate rat urinary bladder by irritant chemicals. *Pain*, 28:109-127.

Medhurst SJ, Walker K, Bowes M, Kidd BL, Glatt M, Muller M, Hattenberger M, Vaxelaire J, O'Reilly T, Wotherspoon G, Winter J, Green J, Urban L. 2002. A rat model of bone cancer pain. *Pain*, 96: 129-140.

Meller ST and Gebhart GF. 1997. Intraplantar zymosan as a reliable, quantifiable model of thermal and mechanical hyperalgesia in the rat. *Eur J Pain*, 1: 43-52.

Mills CD, Grady JJ, Hulsebosch CE. 2001. Changes in exploratory behavior as a measure of chronic central pain following spinal cord injury. *J Neurotrauma*, 18: 1091-1105.

Ness TJ, Lewis-Sides A, Castroman P. 2001. Characterization of pressor and visceromotor reflex responses to bladder distension in rats: sources of variability and effect of analgesics. *J Urol*, 165: 968-974.

Ness TJ and Elhefni H. 2004. Reliable visceromotor responses are evoked by noxious bladder distension in mice. *J Urol*, 171: 1704-1708.

Ness TJ and Gebhart GF. 1988. Colorectal distension as a noxious visceral stimulus: physiologic and pharmacologic characterization of pseudaffective reflexes in the rat. *Brain Res*, 450:153- 169.

Ogawa A, Ren K, Tsuboi Y, Morimoto T, Sato T, Iwata K. 2003. A new model of experimental parotiditis in rats and its implications for trigeminal nociception. *Exp Brain Res*, 152: 307-316.

Ohtori S, Takahashi K, Aoki Y, Doya H, Ozawa T, Saito T, Moriya H. 2004. Spinal neural cyclooxygenase-2 mediates pain caused in a rat model of lumbar disk herniation. *J Pain*, 5: 385-391.

Pelissier T, Pajot J, Dallel R. 2002. The orofacial capcaicin test in rats: effects of different capsaicin concentrations and morphine. *Pain*, 96: 81-87.

Pioli EY, Gross CE, Meisser W, Bioulac BH, Bezard E. 2003. The deafferented nonhuman primate is not a reliable model of intractable pain. *Neurol Res*, 25: 127-129.

Randall LO, Selitto JJ. 1957. A method for measurement of analgesic activity on inflamed tissue. *Arch Int Pharmacodyn Ther*, 111: 409-419.

Ren K and Dubner R. 1999. Inflammatory models of pain and hyperalgesia. *ILAR J*, 40: 111-118.

Rodrigues-Filho R, Santos ARS, Bertelli JA, Calixto JB. 2003. Avulsion injury of the brachial plexus triggers hyperalgesia and allodynia in the hindpaws: a new model for the study of neuropathic pain. *Brain Res*, 982: 186-194.

Roughan JV and Flecknell PA. 2004. Behaviour-based assessment of the duration of laparotomy-induced abdominal pain and the analgesic effects of carprofen and buprenorphine in rats. *Behav Pharmacol*, 15: 461-472.

Roza C and Laird JM. 1995. Pressor responses to distension of the ureter in anaesthetised rats: characterisation of a model of acute visceral pain. *Neurosci Lett*, 198:9-12.

Sandner-Kiesling A, Pan HL, Chen SR, James RL, DeHaven-Hudkins DL, Dewan DM, Eisenach JC. 2002. Effect of kappa opioid agonists on visceral nociception induced by uterine cervical distension in rats. *Pain*, 96: 13-22.

Scheifer C, Hoheisel U, Trudrung P, Unger T, Mense S. 2002. Rats with chronic spinal cord transection as a possible model for the at-level pain of paraplegic patients. *Neurosci Letts*, 323: 117-120.

Seltzer Z, Dubner R, Shir Y. 1990. A novel behavioural model of neuropathic pain disorders produced in rats by partial sciatic nerve injury. *Pain*, 43: 205-218.

Sherrington CS. 1906. *The Integrative Action of the Nervous System*. New Haven: Yale University Press.

Siddall P J, Xu C L, Cousins M J. 1995. Allodynia following traumatic spinal cord injury in the rat. *NeuroReport*, 6: 1241-1244.

Slart R, Yu AL, Yaksh TL, Sorkin LS. 1997. An animal model of pain produced by systemic administration of an immunotherapeutic anti-ganglioside antibody. *Pain*, 69: 119-125.

Sluka KA, Kalra A, Moore SA. 2001. Unilateral intramuscular injections of acidic saline produce a bilateral, long-lasting hyperalgesia. *Muscle Nerve*, 24: 37-46.

Smiley MM, Lu Y, Vera-Portocarrero LP, Zidan A, Westlund KN. 2004. Intrathecal gabapentin enhances the analgesic effects of subtherapeutic dose morphine in a rat experimental pancreatitis model. *Anesthesiology*, 101: 759-765.

Smith SB, Crager SE, Mogil JS. 2004. Paclitaxel-induced neuropathic hypersensitivity in mice: responses in 10 inbred mouse strains. *Life Sci*, 74: 2593-2604.

Stulrajter V, Pavlasek J, Strauss P, Duda P, Gokin AP. 1978. Some neuronal, autonomic and behavioral correlates to visceral pain evoked by gall-bladder stimulation. *Activ Nerv Sup (Praha)*, 20:203-209.

Vera-Portocarrero LP, Lu Y, Westlund KN. 2003. Nociception in persistent pancreatitis in rats: effects of morphine and neuropeptide alterations. *Anesthesiology*, 98: 474-484.

Vermeirsch H, Nuydens RM, Salmon PL, Meert TF. 2004. Bone cancer pain model in mice: evaluation of pain behavior, bone destruction and morphine sensitivity. *Pharmacol Biochem Behav*, 79: 243-251.

Vos BP, Strassman AM, Maciewicz RJ. 1994. Behavioral evidence of trigeminal neuropathic pain following chronic constriction injury to the rat infraorbital nerve. *J Neurosci*, 14: 2708-2723.

Wesselmann U, Czakanski PP, Affaitati G, Giamberardino MA. 1998. Uterine inflammation as a noxious visceral stimulus: behavioral characterization in the rat. *Neurosci Lett*, 246: 73-76.

Wuarin-Bierman L, Zahnd GR, Kaufmann F, Burcklen L, Adler J. 1987. Hyperalgesia in spontaneous and experimental models of diabetic neuropathy. *Diabetologia*, 30:

653-658.

Xu X J, Hao J X, Aldskogius H, Seiger A, Wiesenfeld-Hallin Z. 1992. Chronic pain-related syndrome in rats after ischemic spinal cord lesion: a possible animal model for pain in patients with spinal cord injury. *Pain*, 48: 279-290.

Yaksh TL and Reddy SV. 1981. Studies in the primate on the analgetic effects associated with intrathecal actions of opiates, alpha-adrenergic agonists and baclofen. *Anesthesiology*, 54: 451-467.

Yezierski RP, Liu S, Ruenes GL, Kajander KJ, Brewer KL. 1998. Excitotoxic spinal cord injury: behavioral and morphological characteristics of a central pain model. *Pain*, 75: 141-155.

Models for Studying Pain and Searching for Pain Killers *in Vitro* Electrophysiological Studies of Pain

Chapter 32

Peter Goldstein, Jianguo Gu[*]

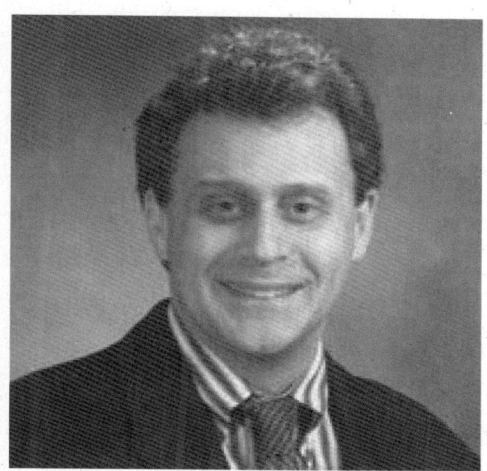

Dr. Goldstein is an Assistant Professor in the Weill Medical College, Cornell University, New York. Following graduation from Cornell University, he pursued a MD degree at the Mount Sinai School of Medicine, City University of New York. He completed residency and fellowship work at the Presbyterian Hospital, New York, and College of Physicians and Surgeons, Columbia University, New York.

MAJOR CONTRIBUTIONS

1. Goldstein PA, Lee CJ, MacDermott AB. 1995. Variable distributions of Ca(2+)-permeable and Ca(2+)-impermeable AMPA receptors on embryonic rat dorsal horn neurons. *J Neurophysiol*, 73(6):2522-2534.
2. Okamoto M, Baba H, Goldstein PA, Higashi H, Shimoji K, Yoshimura M. 2001. Functional reorganization of Sensory pathways in the rat spinal dorsal horn following peripheral nerve injury. *J Physiol*, 532(Pt 1): 241-250.
3. Goldstein PA, Elsen FP, Ying SW, Ferguson C, Homanics GE, Harrison NL. 2002 Prolongation of hippocampal miniature inhibitory postsynaptic currents in mice lacking the GABA(A) receptor alpha1 subunit. *J Neurophysiol*, 88(6):3208-3217.
4. Jia F, Pignataro L, Schofield CM, Yue M, Harrison NL, Goldstein PA. 2005. An extrasynaptic GABAA receptor mediates tonic inhibition in thalamic VB neurons. *J Neurophysiol*, 94(6):4491-4501.
5. Ying SW, Goldstein PA. 2005. Propofol-block of SK channels in reticular thalamic neurons enhances GABAergic inhibition in relay neurons. J Neurophysiol, 93(4):1935-1948.

MAIN TOPICS

Patch-clamp techniques

Acutely dissociated sensory neurons for pain research

Acutely dissociated DRG and TG neurons

Acutely dissociated DH neurons

Massive dRG and DH co-cultures

Microisland DRG-DH co-culture

Neonatal spinal cord transverse slice preparation

Whole-patch clamp recording from neonatal spinal cord slices

Adult spinal cord transverse slice preparation

Whole-patch clamp recording from adult spinal cord slices

Thalamocortical slice preparation

---

[*] For the introduction of Dr. Gu, please refer to Chapter 10.

SUMMARY

Studying pain and searching for pain killer have been involved at several different levels, including behavioral test on whole animals of pain models, studies on pain related neuronal pathways and circuits at tissue levels, research on nociceptive mechanisms and therapeutic targets at cellular, subcellular and molecular levels. Electrophysiological approaches have been applied at each of these levels for addressing fundamental questions including nociceptive signal initiation, encoding, transmission, modulation, and perception. Modern pain therapy and management rely on the understating of cellular, subcellular, and molecular mechanisms of pain under both physiological and pathological conditions. These mechanisms can be studied using electrophysiological approaches, particularly the patch-clamp recordings in *in vitro* tissue and cell model systems.   Combination of *in vitro* electrophysiological approaches with molecular biological and other neurobiological methods provides a powerful tool in pain research and in searching for pain killers.

INTRODUCTION

Sensory signals including pain are usually initiated at peripheral nerve endings and encoded as nerve membrane depolarization followed by action potential firings. These electrical events are propagated from peripheral sensory nervous system (somatosensory and trigeminal nerves) to the central sensory nervous system (e.g. spinal cord dorsal horn, thalamus, sensory cortex). Sensory signals are propagated by means of electrical conduction on nerve fibers and transmitted synaptically between sensory neurons. Pathological pain conditions, at the most basic neurological level, are due to the abnormality of electrical events encoding for sensory stimuli. Electrophysiology is the most important approach to study electrical events in sensory system. Electrophysiological studies have provided many understandings of basic functions and dysfunctions of sensory nervous systems, mechanisms of physiological and pathological pain, and therapeutic targets for pain management. Electrophysiological approaches can be applied to many model systems including both *in vivo* and *in vitro* preparations. This chapter is to introduce a number of *in vitro* preparations used in studies of sensory functions and pain mechanisms at circuitry, cellular, subcellular and molecular levels. Although conventional electrophysiology such as extracellular recording technique and intracellular recording technique are still often used in studies of sensory nervous systems and pain, we will only describe patch-clamp recording technique and its applications in *in vitro* preparations. A closely related approach is *in vivo* patch-clamp recording technique, which is covered in Chapter 33.

PATCH-CLAMP TECHNIQUES

It is worth of briefly describing the patch-clamp recoding technique before introducing *in vitro* models for studying sensory physiology and pain. Patch-clamp technique has been used extensively to study a wide range of electrophysiological properties of sensory neurons. Fundamentally, this is a technique measures cell membrane conductance. Membrane conductance of a cell is mainly determined by ion channels expressed on cell membranes. Membranes of sensory neurons express many ion channels and these channels can open upon membrane potential changes or ligand binding. Sensory neurons also express receptors or ion channels that open by natural stimuli including temperature changes and mechanical forces, producing thermal and touch sensations. The major charge carrying ions for cells are sodium (Na^+), potassium (K^+), chloride (Cl^-) and calcium (Ca^{2+}). In sensory neurons, ion channels open to become permeable to these ions when stimulated electrical, thermally, mechanically, or chemically. Patch-clamp technique, invented by Sakmann and Neher about twenty years ago (Pflugers Arch 375: 219-228, 1978), remains to be the most sensitive technique so far for characterizing and studying membrane ion channels. This technique allows for the direct electrical measurement of currents flowing through ion channels at very high resolution. There are four major configurations of patch-clamp recordings, including cell-attached configuration, whole-cell configuration, inside-out configuration and outside-out configuration. These patch-clamp configurations can be used to address a broad spectrum of biological questions including biophysical and pharmacological characteristics of ion channels, modulation of ion channels by second messengers and protein kinases, and specific neuronal functions associated with a type of ion channels. Among the four configurations, three of them (cell-attached patch, inside-out patch, and outside-out patch) allow to study single ion channels, which provide the most specific biophysical properties of ion channels and their modulation under different conditions. The whole-cell configuration is the most widely used patch-clamp technique. Whole-cell configuration allows recording of the "macroscopic" or total currents flowing through all channels in the entire cellular membrane. Therefore, it can be used to characterize functions and modulation of ion channels, pharmacology of ion channels, synaptic transmission and plasticity, and other applications.

In research on sensory physiology and pathology, patch-clamp techniques have been applied to *in vitro* preparations including acutely dissociated sensory neurons, sensory neuron cultures, spinal cord and brain tissue slices. These cell and tissue preparations, or *in vitro* models, provide a number of advantages over whole animals. First, these models are much simplified systems that allow good controls of experimental conditions, which avoid influence by multiple variables seen in whole animal experiments. Second, pharmacological manipulations are much easy and precise, which allow good characterizations of ion channels and their modulation, and thereby researchers can answer many physiological and pharmacological questions at the cellular and molecular levels. Another advantage of these *in vitro* models is that they are suitable for the use of molecular and genetic techniques. Indeed, the combination of electrophysiology and molecular biology is a very powerful tool, which has lead to the identification of a number of sensory molecules and their functions in pain.

ACUTELY DISSOCIATED SENSORY NEURONS FOR PAIN RESEARCH

One of the most often used *in vitro* cell preparations for pain research is acutely dissociated sensory neurons. Sensory neurons can be dissociated enzymatically and mechanically, and then used for patch clamp recordings shortly after the dissociation. Most dissociated sensory neurons are healthy, and they can be clearly visualized under microscope for application of patch-clamp recordings. Surrounding solutions and drugs can be applied in a precisely controlled manner, allowing reliable pharmacological and electrophysiological characterization of ion channels. Neuronal processes of dissociated neurons are truncated and because of this, there is less problem of space clamp on acutely dissociated neurons than other cell preparations. Therefore, this preparation is suitable for studying biophysical properties of ion channels including channel kinetics. Because neurons are acutely dissociated and used within a few hours, it is general believe that changes in receptor expression is minimum compared with cultured sensory neurons. Neurons at each level of sensory systems can be acutely dissociated for research on sensory physiology and pain. For peripheral sensory system, most studies use acutely dissociated neurons of dorsal root ganglions (DRG), the neurons of somatosensory system. One reason for the use of DRG neurons is because of their abundance; one can easily harvest over thirty DRGs from a rat. Trigeminal ganglion (TG) neurons are cranial sensory neurons functionally equivalent to DRG neurons. Acutely dissociated TG neurons have also been used for *in vitro* electrophysiological studies, but their uses are not as often as DRGs because each animal only has one pair of TGs. For sensory neurons in the CNS, cells acutely dissociated from spinal cord dorsal horn have been widely used. Application of patch clamp recordings is more difficulty on acutely dissociated neurons than culture cells because the former often have tissue debris attached to cell membranes, making it more difficult to form tight seal between patch-electrode and cells.

ACUTELY DISSOCIATED DRG AND TG NEURONS

DRG or TG neuron dissociation involves mild enzyme digestion followed by gentle mechanical dissociation. Both peripheral and central processes of these sensory neurons are usually completely lost during the tissue preparation procedures, making cells to be almost perfect round shape. Fig.32.1 shows acutely dissociated DRG neurons from adult rats and their responses to P2X receptor agonist α, β methylene-ATP (α, β mATP) with several different current types. The results suggested the expression of different subtypes of P2X receptors on DRG neurons.

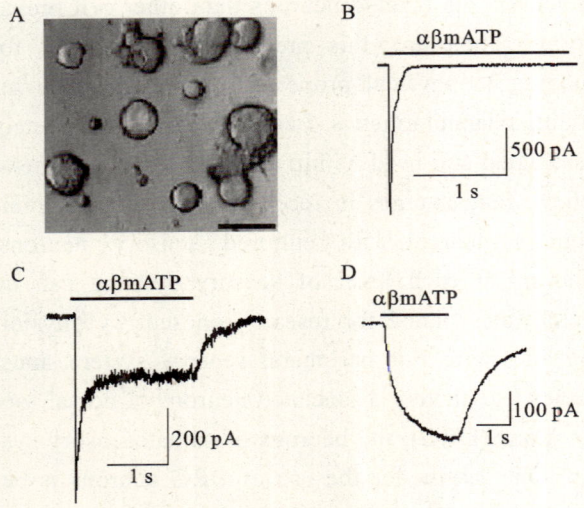

Fig.32.1 Acutely dissociated DRG neurons used for studying P2X receptors. A. Acutely dissociated DRG neurons from adult rats. For neuron dissociation, DRGs were dissected out from animals and incubated with dispase II at 5 mg/mL (Boehringer Mannheim, Germany) and type I collagenase at 2 mg/mL (Sigma, St. Louis, MO) for 45 min. After a rinse, DRGs were triturated to dissociate the neurons. Dissociated neurons were then plated on coverslips pre-coated with poly-D-lysine (Sigma, St. Louis, MO). B–D. Whole-cell patch-clamp recordings were made from three different DRG neurons. The P2X receptor agonist α, β mATP (α, β-methylene-ATP) evoked three different types of inward currents.

The rationale of using acutely dissociated DRG

or TG neurons for studies on sensory physiology and pathology is based on the assumption that sensory molecules expressed on peripheral terminals are also expressed on cell bodies. Based on this assumption, functional characteristics of a sensory molecule observed on cell bodies represent those on peripheral nerve endings. This assumption is applicable for most sensory molecules. For example, consistent with the recording of P2X receptor currents in acutely dissociated DRG neurons, subcutaneously injection of P2X receptor agonist ATP to human subjects produces painful sensation. Acutely dissociated DRG and TG neurons have been characterized morphologically, immunochemically, and electrophysiologically. One of the purposes of these characterizations is to try to make differentiation between nociceptive and non-nociceptive neurons. For example, it has been generally thought that nociceptive sensory neurons have small diameter. Many small-sized neurons (diameter<30 µm) acutely dissociated from rat DRGs showed rapidly desensitizing P2X currents. On the other hand, slowly desensitizing P2X currents were not usually seen in small-sized DRG neurons. Combination of electrophysiological recordings with immunostaining is often used to explore receptor functions. For example, patch-clamp recordings of P2X currents have been performed in conjunction with IB4 staining and P2X3 immunostaining (Fig.32.2). P2X3 receptors were found to be predominantly expressed on IB4-positive neurons. Furthermore, rapidly desensitizing P2X currents were mainly recorded from IB4-positive and P2X3 immunoreacitve DRG neurons and these neurons were also sensitive to capsaicin. Because IB4-positive and capsaicin-sensitive neurons are believed to be heat nociceptive neurons, the results provide strong evident for the involvement of P2X3 receptors in nociception.

Application of patch-clamp recordings on acutely dissociated DRG neurons from animals with inflammatory and neuropathic pain conditions can provide insights into the role of a receptor in pathological pain conditions. For example, it has been shown that $P2X_{2+3}$ subtype currents become significantly increased in DRG neurons after peripheral inflammation. Together with behavioral tests in whole animals of pathological pain models and with other approaches such as the use of P2X receptor knock mice, a role of P2X receptors in nociception under both physiological and pathological conditions have been established. There are many other examples of using *in vitro* electrophysiology on acutely dissociated sensory neurons for the studies of pain.

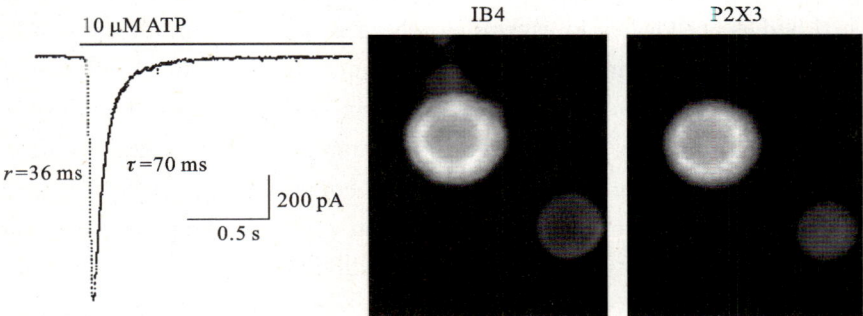

Fig.32.2 Combination of staining and electrophysiology on acutely dissociated DRG neurons from adult rats to study functions of P2X3 receptors. Acutely dissociate DRG neurons were first tested with ATP using whole cell patch-clamp recording technique. After recordings, IB4 stainging and P2X3 immunostaining were performed sequentially. In this figure, ATP evoked a rapidly desensitizing inward current in the cell which was both IB4-positive and P2X3-immunoreactive.

Patch-clamp recordings have been combined with Ca^{2+}-imaging technique and this combination has multiple applications. One of the applications is to use Ca^{2+} imaging technique to pre-identify neurons that response to a certain type of sensory stimuli. This is to take the advantage that Ca^{2+} imaging technique allows to observe responses of cells in a whole optical field rather than a single cell. This is particularly helpful for studies on sensory receptors that are expressed only on a small population of neurons. Many sensory molecules are only expressed on subpopulations of sensory neurons, making it difficult to sample these neurons when randomly select cells for electrophysiological recording without pre-identification. For example, TRPM8 receptors are only expressed on ~7% of DRG neurons or TG neurons. It becomes very labor intensive to perform electrophysiological study on TRPM8-expressing neurons without pre-identification. Fig.32.3 (see also the color plate)shows the use of Ca^{2+} imaging technique to pre-identify neurons that potentially express TRPM8 receptors. In this example, acutely dissociated DRG neurons were tested with 100 μM menthol, a TRPM8 receptor agonist. Menthol responsive neurons showed increased intracellular Ca^{2+} levels. Whole-cell patch-clamp recordings were then performed on those cells and menthol evoked inward currents from almost all the pre-identified sensory neurons.

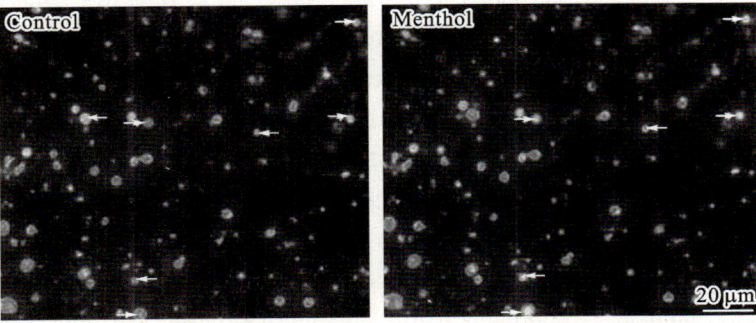

Fig.32.3 Identification of menthol-sensitive neurons. Acutely dissociated DRG neurons were tested with TRPM8 receptor agonist menthol (100 μM). Only subpopulation of neurons showed response (indicated by arrows).

Retrograde labeling has been used to pre-identify functional subgroups of sensory neurons for *in vitro* electrophysiological recordings. One such example is the retrograde labeling of trigeminal neurons that innervate tooth-pulp. The tooth-pulp is innervated extensively by unmyelinated and small myelinated nerve fibers whose cell bodies are located in trigeminal ganglions. These afferent fibers enter the pulp chamber by way of the root apex. Axons branch has extensive ramification and formation of a dense plexus near the odontoblast layer. The sensory afferent fibers that innervate tooth-pulp are believed to be mainly, if not exclusively, nociceptive. For this reason trigeminal neurons innervating tooth-pulp has been used as a model system to study sensory receptors associated with nociception. The use of these neurons for *in vitro* electrophysiological recordings requires a means of distinguishing these cells from other neurons in the trigeminal ganglions. A widely used approach to identify pulpal neurons in the trigeminal ganglion has been the introduction of retrograde nerve tracers into open pulp. For examine, us-ing retrograde labeled trigeminal neurons as *in vitro* nociceptive neuron model system, and in comparison with afferent fibers innervating muscles, Cook *et al.* have shown distinct ATP receptors on pain-sensing and stretch-sensing neurons and demonstrated different functions of P2X receptor subtypes. However, because the exposure of the tooth pulp for tracer application produces local inflammation and necrosis, a recent study has made modification by application of the tracer to shallow dentin cavities to retrograde label cell bodies of pulpal afferents in the trigeminal ganglion while avoiding exposure of the pulp (Fig.32.4). In addition to pulpal afferents, retrograde labeling has also been used to preidentify visceral afferent neurons for *in vitro* electrophysiological recordings. For example, retrograde labeling has been performed for identifying afferent neurons that innervate stomach, cardiac, and bladder. *In vitro* electrophysiological recordings showed that lactate acid activate acid-sensing ion channel (ASIC) on afferent neurons innervating cardiac tissues, providing an explanation for the pain sensation during cardiac ischemia.

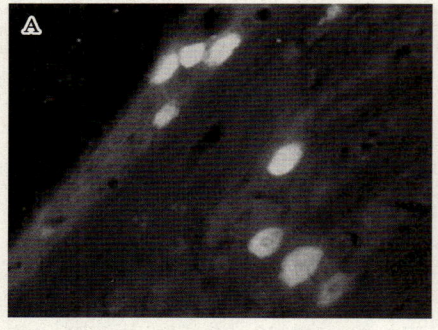 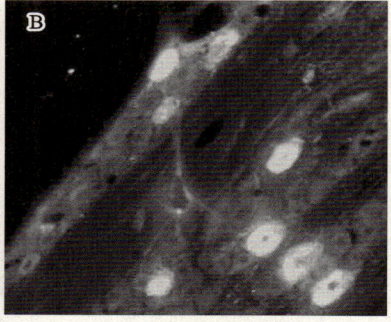

Fig.32.4 Retrograde labeling of trigeminal ganglion neurons that innervate tooth-pulp. Trigeminal ganglion cell bodies labeled by FG 3 weeks after application of the tracer to shallow dentin cavities in the first maxillary molar (A) were also immunostained for WGA (B) 2 days after subsequent application of WGA to open pulp of the same tooth (Pan *et al.* 2003, *J Neurosci Methods*, 126(1):99-109).

ACUTELY DISSOCIATED DH NEURONS

Similar to DRG and TG neurons, DH neurons can be acutely dissociated enzymatically followed by mechanical dissociation. Enzymatically dissociated DH neurons have been used in many patch-clamp studies on receptors expressed on DH neurons, and will not be described here. The observation that enzymes can alter the properties of some receptors and channels prompted Vorobjev to mechanically dissociate neu-rons from brain slices without enzyme digestion. Mechanical dissociation is achieved by applying a vertically vibrating glass "ball" pipette to the slice surface. This technique was then modified and adopted to be used to prepare acutely dissociated DH neurons in the spinal cord. Interestingly, many presynaptic boutons were found to be attached to the dissociated neurons. The attached synaptic boutons can be seen using the dye FM1-43. Patch-clamp recordings made from such preparations showed spontaneous inhibitory postsynaptic currents (sISPCs) and spontaneous excitatory postsynaptic currents (sEPSCs) in most, if not all dissociated neurons. As such this preparation is also called "nerve-boutton preparation". The nerve-bouton preparation is a simple approach to study neurotransmitter release from presynaptic nerve terminals. Using this preparation, it has been shown that P2X receptor activation facilitates the release of GABA and glycine on dorsal horn neurons. This highly simplified system may be useful for high throuput screening of pain drugs that modulate neurotransmitter release.

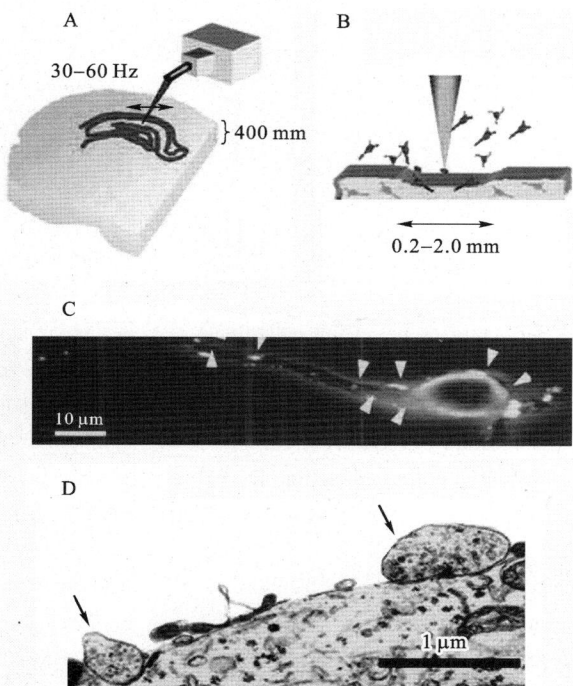

Fig.32.5 Mechanically dissociated neurons with presynaptic boutons. A, B. Schematic representation of the mechanical dissociation technique leading to the liberation of single neurons. Brain slices are first prepared using standard techniques and incubated at room temperature for >1 h before securing a single slice to a dish. A heavily fire-polished blunt pipette is horizontally vibrated across the surface of the neuronal area of interest at a frequency of 30–60 Hz and with an amplitude displacement of 0.2–2.0 mm. This amplitude, and the pipette tip size, can be adjusted according to the size of the neuronal region of interest. Successful liberation of viable neurons (and debris) results in a fine mist originating from the dissociation site. The procedure takes ~2–5 min. The treated slice is then removed and the liberated neurons are left to settle onto the base of the dish. C. An isolated hippocampal CA1 neuron with presynaptic terminals (boutons) stained with FM1–43. Arrowheads indicate patches of FM1–43 fluorescence. D. Electron micrograph showing presynaptic boutons (arrowheads) adherent to a dissociated CA1 hippocampal neuron from a 14-day-old rat. **** with permission.

Mono-culture of DRG, TG, or DH neurons

DRG, TG, and DH neurons can be cultured and then used for electrophysiological experiments to study, for example, sensory receptor functions and their modulations by different inflammatory mediators. For DH neuron cultures, neurons from animals at embryonic age of 16 days (E16) are often used, and DH neurons culture cannot be made using adult animals. Unlike DH neurons, DRG and TG neurons form animals at different ages, including adults, can be used for preparing cultures. The use of cultured sensory neurons has a technical advantage over acutely dissociated sensory neurons when performing patch-clamp recordings. This is because cell surface of a cultured sensory neuron is very smooth, which facilitates the formation of good seal between a patch-clamp electrode and cell membrane so that it becomes much easy to do patch-clamp recordings on cultured sensory neurons compared with acutely dissociated sensory neurons. NGF is usually added in culture medium because many DRG and TG neurons require NGF support for survival. On the other hand, DH neuron cultures don't need NGF. Cultured sensory neurons can change their phenotypes. For examine, in the presence of NGF, mot of cultured DRG neurons express SP and CGRP. Sensory receptors such as VR1 receptors and P2X receptors change their expression levels and patterns in cultured conditions, and these changes can be affected inflammatory mediators. For example, using cultured DRG, it has been shown that TNFα upregulate VR1 receptors. Thus, cultured sensory neurons provide useful *in vitro* models in studying sensory receptor regulation by inflammatory mediators and other factors.

MASSIVE DRG AND DH CO-CULTURES

DRG neurons, when plated in the dishes together with DH neurons (Fig.32.6), form synapses with DH neurons. In massive DRG and DH co-cultures, each DH neuron may receive synaptic contacts from DRG neurons. All synapses formed between DRG and DH neurons are glutamatergic, representing those formed between the central terminals of afferent fibers and DH neurons *in vivo*. This co-culture system can be used to study sensory transmission and modulation using double-patch recordings made from a DRG neuron and a DH neuron. As shown in Fig.32.6, double-patch recordings were made to study effects of menthol, a TRPM8 receptor agonist, on paired-pulse evoked EPSCs. Menthol produced synaptic potentia-

tion and changed paired-pulse ratio, implicating the activation of TRPM8 receptors can modulate sensory plasticity through a presynaptic mechanism. Presynaptic action of menthol at sensory synapses was also evidenced by testing the effects of menthol on mEPSC frequency in the DRG-DH coculture system. It was shown that menthol increased mEPSC frequency without affecting mEPSC amplitude.

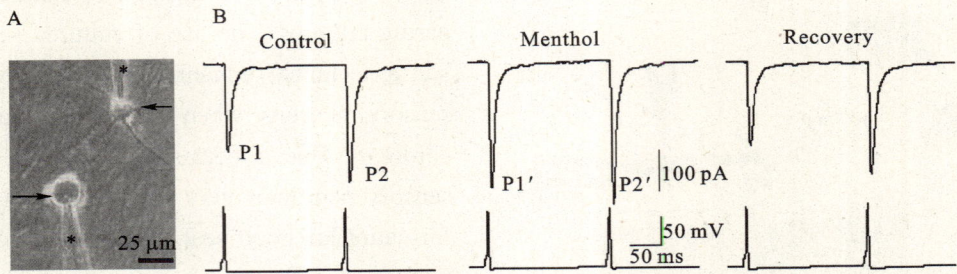

Fig.32.6   DRG-DH neuron pair in massive DRG-DH co-culture system and double patch-clamp recordings. A. Micrograph shows an example of double-patch recording from a DRG-DH neuron pair.   Asterisks indicate two patch-electrodes on a DRG neuron (arrow) and a DH neuron (arrowhead). B. Three sets of traces on the upper panel show paired-pulse eEPSCs recorded from the DH neuron in the absence (left), the presence of 1 μM menthol (middle), and washout of menthol (right). Three sets of traces on the lower panel show action potentials recorded from the DRG neuron after the paired-pulse stimulation. Paired-pulse interval was 200 ms. Each trace represents the average of 10 sweeps at time interval of 10 s. P_1 and P_2 represent the amplitudes of eEPSC-pair in control, and P_1' and P_2' represent those after menthol application.

For preparing massive DRG-DH co-cultures, DH neurons are dissociated from the spinal cord dorsal horn of rat embryos 16 days *in utero*. The embryos are removed, decapitated, and the dorsal half of the spinal cord is isolated. The tissue is then incubated for 20 min at 37℃ in MEM (minimum essential medium) modified for suspension culture (Gibco) plus 0.25% trypsin (from trypsin 2.5% Gibco). The cells are triturated in standard culture medium that consists of MEM containing 5% heat-inactivated horse serum (Gibco), 8 mg/mL glucose and MEM vitamin (Gibco). Similarly, DRGs are isolated separately from E16 embryos, exposed to trypsin and dissociated. DH and DRG neurons are plated on glass coverslips previously prepared with a monolayer of rat cortical astrocytes. 2.5S NGF (10 ng/mL) and 5-flouro-2'-deoxyuridine (10 mM) are added at the time of plating. 2.5S NGF is added once every week when cells are fed with fresh media. The neurons are maintained at 37℃ in a humidified atmosphere of 95% air and 5% CO_2 and fed weekly.

The above example shows that massive DRG-DH co-culture system is a useful *in vitro* cell model in studying sensory synaptic transmission and modulation. However, synaptically paired DRG and DH neurons are found to be less that 25% in massive co-culture system. Therefore, it is quite labor-intensive to search for synaptically coupled neuron pairs to perform experiments. Alternatively, microisland DRG-DH co-culture system may be used to overcome this technique difficulty.

MICROISLAND DRG-DH CO-CULTURE

Derived from agarose-collagen microisland cultures made by Segal and Furshpan for hippocampal neurons, a microisland DRG-DH co-culture system was developed for study of synaptic transmission and modulation at the first sensory synapses *in vitro*. In this culture system, sensory synapses are formed between

DRG and DH neurons. Microislands, about a few hundreds of micrometer in diameter, are made of agarose-collagen droplet and astrocytes bedding, and upon which DRG and DH neurons are plated to form a co-culture system in confined areas (Fig.32.7). A microisland confines the extension of axons and dendrites of neurons within the island, making a high probability of synaptic contacts between neurons. Indeed almost every DRG-DH neuron pairs on a microisland form synapses. All these synapses are glutamatergic, representing those formed between the central terminals of sensory afferent fibers and dorsal horn neurons *in vivo*. This co-culture system is more desirable that massive co-culture system in studying sensory synaptic transmission and modulation using double patch-clamp recordings. Stimulation of DRG neurons by injection of depolarizing currents can reliably evoke eEPSC recorded from dorsal horn neurons. Synaptic failures in normal bath solution are rare, probably because of multiple synapses formed between DRG and DH neurons in the microisland co-culture system. Stimulation of DH neurons, on the other hand, does not produce synaptic-like events on DRG neuron, indicating that glutamatergic synaptic transmission between DRG and DH neuron is unidirectional, i.e., from DRG to DH neuron. By using the DRG-DH microisland co-culture system, it has been demonstrated that P2X receptors are localized at presynaptic sites of sensory synapses and that activation of presynaptic P2X receptors modulate glutamate release at the sensory synapses.

In addition to the DRG-DH microisland co-culture system described above, several other forms of sensory neuron microisland culture system can be made for studies on sensory synaptic transmission and modulation. For example, if only a single dorsal horn neuron is plated on a microisland, the axon of the neuron will form synapses onto its own dendrites. This type of synapses is called autoptic synapses. Autoptic synapses of hippocampal neurons in microislands have been used for studying synaptic plasticity. Similarly, autoptic synapses of dorsal horn neurons may be used to study synaptic plasticity of sensory neurons and cellular mechanisms. A microisland may have a pair of DH neurons and they can be either glutamatergic or GABAergic, or one glutamatergic and one GABAergic. These will allow one to study excitatory and inhibitory synaptic transmission between these neuron pairs. A microisland may also have three more neurons for application of triple-patch or multiple-patch recordings to study synaptic circuitry and integration.

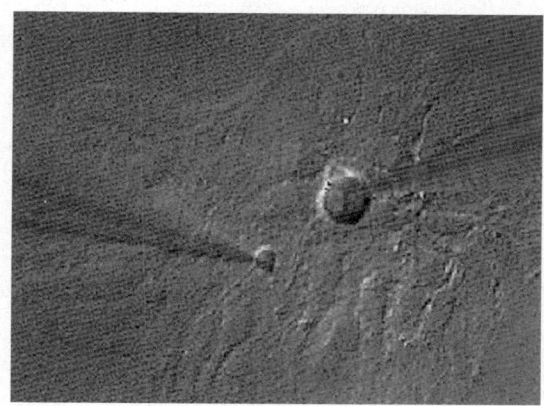

Fig.32.7   DRG-DH microisland co-culture system. Microisland co-culture is prepared as follow. Coverslips are pre-coated with PDL and then dipped in 0.5% agarose (type I - low EEO, from Sigma) and allowed to dry for 1 h. Once dry, the dishes are sprayed with rat tail collagen (2 mg/mL in a 0.2% acetic acid solution) using an atomizer. The collagen droplets can be examined under microscope to see if the sizes are desirable. If the sizes of most droplets are bigger than 1000 μm,   a finer atomizer is needed for spraying collagen. The dishes   are then plated with astrocytes, which will be only grown on collagen droplets. After 3 to 7 days, neurons are plated on top of the astrocytes. The plating density is usually 10,000 to 30,000 DH neurons per dish and 30,000–50,000 DRG neurons per dish. On the astrocyte microisland, DH neurons and DRG neurons are settled down randomly. Some microislands receive a single DH neuron and a single DRG neuron, producing a DRG and DH pair. A microisland may receive a few more neurons, which may be useful for *in vitro* neuronal circuitry study. Some microisland may only receive a single DH neuron, and autoptic synapses can be formed on such microisland.

Acutely prepared spinal cord slices present an excellent model for studying molecular and cellular mechanisms participating in synaptic transmission in the spinal cord dorsal horn (DH). The model readily permits investigations into basic functional physiology, developmental changes in synaptic circuitry, pharmacological modulation of synaptic transmission, and the pathophysiological changes observed in chronic and inflammatory pain models.

Both transverse and longitudinal slices can be prepared, but we will focus on transverse slices; readers interested in longitudinal slices should refer to work from de Koninck's group. The techniques for performing whole cell patch clamp recordings from neurons located in the spinal cord DH will be described for tissue obtained from both neonatal and adult rats, although in principle the same general techniques can be applied to tissue obtained from mice.

NEONATAL SPINAL CORD TRANSVERSE SLICE PREPARATION

Transverse sections can be prepared from any level of the spinal cord, although in young animals, it may be technically easier to prepare slices from the cervical spinal cord as it is larger in size than either the thoracic or lumbar spinal cord. The spinal cord from a neonatal rat (as young as P0) is obtained after sacrifice. Following the methods of Takahashi and others, a pup is briefly anesthetized (typically with a volatile anesthetic — either isoflurane or halothane administered in a closed chamber until loss-of-righting reflex is observed) and decapitated. The cervical spinal column is rapidly removed en bloc and submerged in ice-cold artificial cerebrospinal fluid (aCSF) saturated with 95% O_2/5% CO_2. In most cases, using aCSF (containing: 125 mM NaCl, 2.5 mM KCl, 2 mM $CaCl_2$, 1 mM $MgCl_2$, 25 mM $NaHCO_3$, 1 mM NaH_2PO_4, 25 mM D-glucose, mOsm adjusted to 320 with sucrose) will suffice, but if cell viability is a problem, one can try using a sucrose-substituted slicing solution (containing: 234 mM sucrose, 2.5 mM KCl, 10 mM $MgSO_4$, 0.5 mM $CaCl_2$, 24 mM $NaHCO_3$, 1.25 mM NaH_2PO_4, and 11 mM D-glucose).

With the spinal column fully submerged in, and continuously perfused by, the appropriate solution, ventral and dorsal laminectomies are performed with an angled spring-loaded scissor (such as Fine Science Tools [FST], Foster City, CA; No. 15006-09) and the spinal cord exposed (using a paraffin-coated petri dish and dissecting pins can help stabilize the preparation during the dissection); both ventral and dorsal spinal roots will be visible, and the ventral roots should be cut as close to the cord as possible (using for example, Vannas style spring scissors with fine small blades, FST No. 15000-08). One has the option of cutting the dorsal roots or trying to preserve them depending on the nature of the experiment; keep in mind, however, that in young animals, the dorsal roots are very fragile and the dorsal root entry zone is easily damaged. With the assistance of a dissecting stereomicroscope, the meninges are carefully removed using an angled-to-side Vannas style spring scissor (such as FST No. 15002-08); note, the pia is not nearly as well developed in neonatal animals as compared to adults, where it will appear as a highly reflective, closely applied, layer surrounding the white matter, much like a casing covering a sausage.

WHOLE-PATCH CLAMP RECORDING FROM NEONATAL SPINAL CORD SLICES

Neurons can be directly visualized in neonatal spinal cord slices on an upright microscope using video-enhanced infrared (IR) microscopy and differential-interference contrast (DIC) optics. A spinal cord slice is transferred to a recording chamber and the residual agar removed; the slice is secured in place by a platinum wire grid with nylon threads, and the chamber is placed on the stage of an upright microscope fit with a 10× dry lens, a 40× water immersion lens, and a 775 nm infrared bandpass filter. Slices are continuously superfused with aCSF at 5–10 mL/min; technically, it is easier to patch when the extracellular solution is at room temperature, but clearly, more physio-

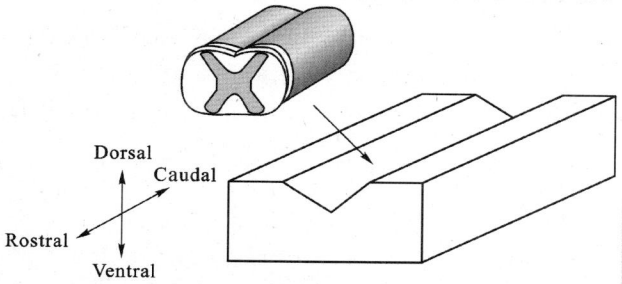

Dorsal

Caudal

Rostral

Ventral

The spinal cord is trimmed to 1-1.5 cm in length and supported against a previously prepared 3% (w/v) agar block in which a shallow V-shaped groove has been cut; the groove should be deep enough such that the dorsal surface of the cord is roughly at the same level as the horizontal surface of the block (Box 32.1). With neonatal tissue, a thin layer of cyanoacrylate glue is used to hold the tissue in place. The spinal cord is placed ventral side down in the groove and the spinal cord and agar block trimmed at the rostral end such that the coronal face of the spinal cord is flush with the agar and is perpendicular to the long axis of the block. The preparation is then glued rostral end down to a vibratome stage with the dorsal surface facing the cutting blade.

The stage is filled with ice-cold solution (either aCSF or sucrose-substituted slicing solution) saturated with O_2 / CO_2, and transverse slices of the desired thickness prepared. Typically, slow forward motion of the blade coupled with near maximal oscillation frequency will yield the best slices. If compression of the cord occurs while slicing, consider decreasing the advance rate of the blade, increasing the oscillation rate (or both), and double check to make sure that the meninges have been completely removed. Slices are transferred to a beaker filled with aCSF continuously bubbled with O_2 / CO_2 and allowed to recover for 1 h at 37 ℃. A fine nylon mesh platform should be used so that the slices are not resting on the bottom of the beaker; this will enable better circulation of saturated solution around the slices; an excellent description of the incubating chamber has been provided elsewhere.

logical responses are obtained if the perfusate is closer to animal body temperature. Using the 10×lens, lamina II (or substantia gelatinosa) is identified, and individual neurons visualized using the 40×lens. The recording electrode is advanced through the tissue towards an identified neuron while applying positive pressure through the back of the electrode, thereby clearing a path to the neuron and preventing the tip from becoming clogged (application of positive pressure through the recording electrode replaces the earlier method of "surface cleaning"). Once the electrode tip touches the cell membrane (as evidenced by dimpling and possibly a small displacement of the membrane), the positive pressure is released and gentle negative pressure rapidly applied so as to obtain a high-resistance seal ($>1G\Omega$). Whole-cell recordings in either voltage or current clamp are obtained in the usual manner following rupture of the membrane under the pipette tip. The electrode solution can contain markers such as biocytin or vital fluorescent dyes (such as Lucifer Yellow) to allow subsequent determination of cell morphology and anatomic location. The specific ionic composition of the intracellular solution, here and in the subsequent sections, will vary with the nature of the experiments being performed and the reader should refer to the literature for more specific information before choosing one solution or another.

Evoked postsynaptic responses can be obtained using focal stimulation. This approach, unfortunately, does not permit identification of the stimulated presynaptic element (fiber or interneurons). Evoked responses can also be obtained by stimulating the dorsal root or the root entry zone. Obtaining an undamaged dorsal root of sufficient length for use with a suction electrode, while technically demanding, is possible in immature (P21-23) rats; stimulating a small section of root near the root entry zone is technically much easier, but will not provide sufficient tissue for analysis to distinguish between Aβ-, Aδ-, and C-fiber mediated responses (BOX 32.2).

BOX 32.2   Schematic diagram for recording and dorsal root stimulation, and representative synaptic currents obtained from mature rats

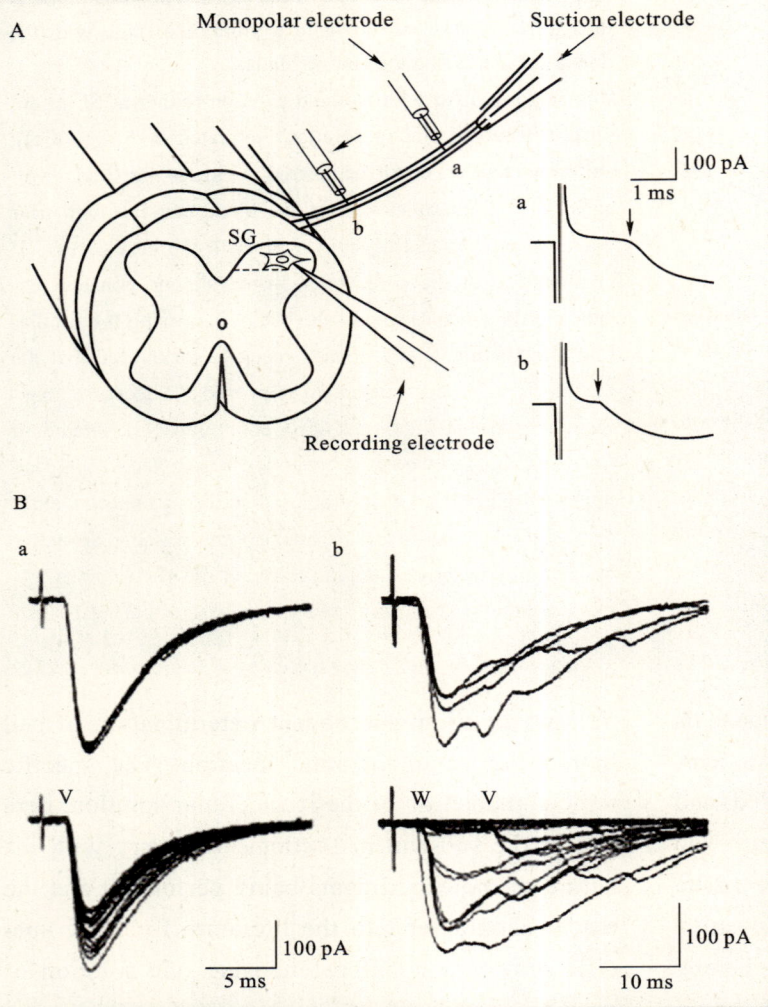

A. Whole-cell patch-clamp recordings were made from neurons in lamina II in a transverse slice that retained an attached dorsal root. The dorsal root was stimulated by a suction electrode that was used for intracellular recordings from dorsal root ganglion neurons or by monopolar stimulating electrodes positioned at a and b. Monosynaptic fast EPSCs were evoked by single low intensity stimuli applied at two different points (a and b). The difference in latency of the EPSCs permitted calculation of the conduction velocity of the fibers. Arrowheads indicate the onset of EPSCs. B. Mono/polysynaptic EPSCs in lamina II neurons in response to primary afferents stimulation. a, Monosynaptic EPSCs evoked by low frequency stimulation (0.1 Hz) of Aδ afferents (upper trace). The monosynaptic nature was clarified based on their constant latencies and absence of failures with high-frequency repetitive stimulation (20 Hz; lower trace). b, Polysynaptic EPSCs evoked by Aδ afferents (upper trace). The latency of EPSCs was constant when the dorsal root was stimulated at low frequency (0.1 Hz), but the latency became variable and failures were observed with high-frequency repetitive stimulation at 20 Hz (lower trace) (from Park *et al.*, 1999).

ADULT SPINAL CORD TRANSVERSE SLICE PREPARATION

The method for preparing and recording from transverse adult rat spinal cord slices is well described by Yoshimura and colleagues. An adult rat (100–250) is anesthetized with urethane (1.2 mg/kg, i.p), and 0.5% lidocaine with 1:10000 epinephrine (10 μg/mL) is injected into the subcutaneous tissue overlying the thoracolumbar vertebral column. Body temperature is maintained at 37–39℃ using a heating pad placed beneath the animal, and supplemental humidified oxygen is delivered via a plastic nose cone. The skin overlying the spinal column from the mid-thorax to the sacrum is removed and the paraspinous musculature exposed for a length of 4–5 cm, and lidocaine with epinephrine is injected bilaterally into the paraspinous muscles adjacent to the thoracolumbar vertebral column using a 25 g needle. The muscle should be cut along the spinous processes as closely as possible using a pair of sharp curved scissors (such as FST No. 14059-11); next, extend the cuts laterally to sever the connections to the transverse processes, thereby exposing the transverse processes. Do not cut deep to the processes, especially in the thoracic region as this can result in a pneumothorax. Irrigate as necessary with room temperature aCSF (117 mM NaCl, 3.6 mM KCl, 2.5 mM CaCl$_2$, 1.2 mM MgCl$_2$, 25 mM NaHCO$_3$, 1.2 mM NaH$_2$PO$_4$, 11 mM D-glucose, bubbled with O$_2$/CO$_2$).

The laminectomy is performed using a pair of curved blunt scissors (consider FST No. 14077-10) starting at the mid- to low thoracic spine and proceeding caudally. A transverse cut is made between the spinous processes (but not through the cord), and lifting the more caudal edge up with a pair of medium tooth forceps, the tip of the scissor is inserted into the canal with the tips facing up and away from the cord; the incisions are extended caudally proceeding from one side then to the other until the cauda equina is exposed. Thoroughly irrigate with aCSF, but do not aim the irrigation solution directly onto the cord. Cover the cord with warm mineral oil and allow the animal to rest for 30–60 min; administer supplemental urethane as needed.

After the rest period, cover the bottom of a large glass petri dish with a piece of filter paper and fill the dish with ice-cold aCSF solution bubbled with O$_2$ / CO$_2$. Transect the rostral spinal cord (FST No. 15024-10) and cut the dorsal and ventral roots lateral to the cord (FST No. 15023-10); the dorsal roots should be 1–2 cm in length. Transfer the cord to the petri dish and rinse with fresh ice-cold aCSF solution. Cut the ventral roots (which will be smaller than the dorsal roots) as close to the cord as possible. Depending on the experiments to be performed, cut all the remaining dorsal roots or leave one dorsal root at L$_5$ or L$_6$ for use with a stimulating electrode; if stimulating the nerve, select one that is not too large for the suction electrode and that is attached to the spinal cord by a single root rather than multiple rootlets.

It is critical that the arachnoid and pia are removed prior to sectioning. Make parallel dorsolateral slits through the meninges along the length of the cord, but do not cut into the white matter. Holding the cord gently but firmly, and proceeding in a rostral to caudal direction, remove the arachnoid/pia on the ventral surface to the level of the root; this can be accomplished using a pair of fine forceps and "peeling" the arachnoid/pia in strips from the white matter. Finally, remove the arachnoid/pia from the dorsal surface (except around the region of the root entry zone); be sure to carefully remove the pia from the region just caudal to root so as prevent tethering of the root. The spinal cord should be white without any visible blood vessels once the pia is removed. Remember, once the root enters the cord, the fibers ascend 1–2 levels before forming synaptic connections, so removing the meninges below the level of the root is not nearly as important. Trim the spinal cord using a fresh razor or scalpel blade to a length of ~1.5 cm.

As before, a prepared agar block is used to stabilize the spinal cord during sectioning. Here, the channel is more rectangular in shape than was the case for use with neonatal spinal cord; the channel should be approximately as wide the spinal cord and half as deep. Place the spinal cord ventral side down while keeping the dorsal root (if preserved) free; the root entry zone should be aligned with the vertical axis of the groove and should not be off-center. Trim the agar and the rostral spinal cord so that the cut surfaces are flush, and affix the agar and spinal cord to the vibratome stage rostral side down using cyanoacrylate glue, again with the dorsal surface of the spinal cord facing the cutting blade. Position the edge of the cutting blade immediately distal to where the root enters the spinal cord; this will be the first cut (be sure to have the root out of the way). The next cut will determine the thickness of the slice with the root attached, and should be between 500–600 μm. Lift the root above the blade and then adjust the blade height to obtain the desired thickness. If experiments without an attached root are planned, then slices can be thinner (350–400 μm), and more than one slice can be obtained.

WHOLE-PATCH CLAMP RECORDING FROM ADULT SPINAL CORD SLICES

Direct visualization of neurons in lamina II in the adult spinal cord slice is not feasible due to increases in myelination. However, it is still possible to perform whole cell patch clamp recordings from lamina II neurons using a "blind" approach. Here, a spinal cord slice (with or without the dorsal root) is transferred to a modified plexiglass submersion style chamber where it rests on a nylon mesh and is held in place by a titanium grid while being continuously superfused at 15–30 mL/min with aCSF equilibrated with O_2 / CO_2 (BOX 32.3). The slice is transilluminated from below under a stereomicroscope, and lamina II is clearly visible as a bright translucent band at the outer edge of the dorsal horn. If dorsal root stimulation is used, the free end of the root is positioned in the suction electrode; be sure to keep the root submerged or else it will dry out.

BOX 32.3   A photograph demonstrating an adult spinal cord slice resting on a nylon grid and held in place by a titanium electron microscopy grid supported by a silver wire loop.

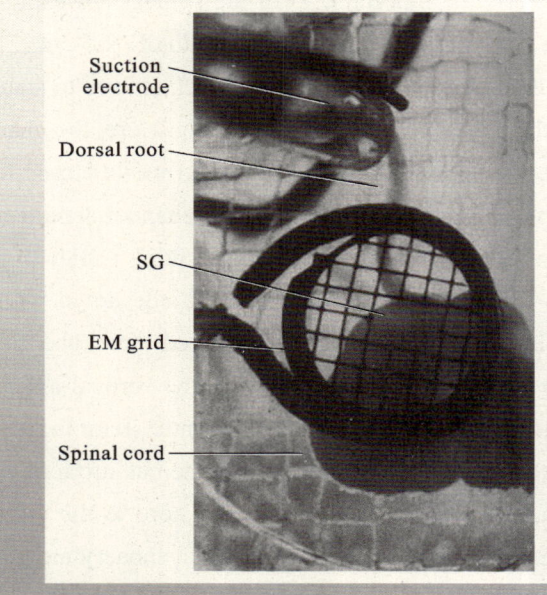

Suction electrode

Dorsal root

SG

EM grid

Spinal cord

The attached dorsal root can be seen in the suction electrode. Lamina II (SG) is the thin translucent band near the outer edge of the slice (from Yoshimura & Nishi, 1993).

The recording electrode is positioned just above the surface of lamina II using a stereomicroscope equipped with 20×to 60×magnification. A small (1–10 mV) square wave pulse is applied to the electrode, and the resistance across the tip of the electrode monitored on either an oscilloscope or computer monitor using the acquisition software. As above, positive pressure is applied to the electrode, which is then slowly and smoothly advanced at a sharp angle (60–75℃) into the spinal cord, and changes in the tip resistance monitored; a 25%–50% increase in resistance suggests that the tip is in contact with a cell membrane. Once contact has been made, positive pressure is released and negative pressure applied to obtain a gigaohm seal as before; the membrane patch is ruptured and whole cell recordings can be obtained.

As indicated above, evoked responses can be obtained in a number of ways. With rat spinal cord slices from juvenile and mature animals with a dorsal root attached, the most informative approach with respect to defined fiber input (Aβ vs. Aδ vs. C) is to stimulate the root using a suction electrode.

THALAMOCORTICAL SLICE PREPARATION

The thalamocortical slice preparation is also valuable for studying synaptic mechanism pertaining to sensory transmission. The ventrobasal (VB) nucleus in the thalamus receives excitatory input via ascending spinothalamic tract fibers as well as from descending corticothalamic fibers arising in the somatosensory cortex. The use of the thalamocortical slice preparation preserves bi-directional connectivity between VB neurons and those in sensory cortex, and whole cell patch clamp recordings in either voltage (BOX 32.4B) or current clamp (BOX 32.4 D–E) configuration can be made from visually identified cortical or thalamic neurons using DIC-IR microscopy as for neonatal spinal cord slices.

BOX 32.4   Recording from cortical and thalamic VB neurons in the thalamocortical slice preparation.

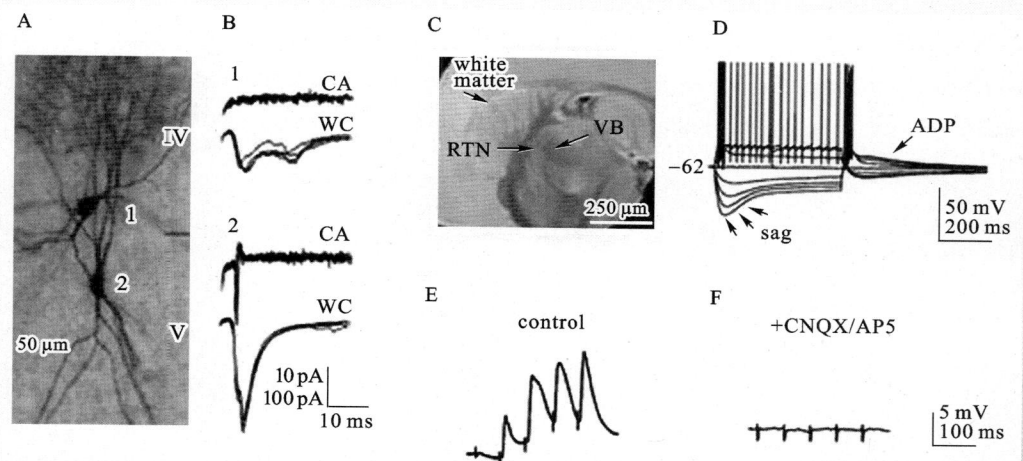

A. Photomicrograph demonstrating two biocytin-filled inhibitory interneurons in the same cortical barrel. B. Four superimposed traces from interneuron 1 (top traces) and 2 (bottom traces) in the cell-attached (CA) and whole cell (WC) modes. Note that despite the close proximity between the two cells, thalamic stimulation elicited spikes only in interneuron 2 (panels A and B from Porter *et al.*, 2001). C. Photomicrograph of a live thalamocortical brain slice containing the ventrobasal (VB) complex, reticular thalamic nucleus, and adjacent connected structures. D. Tonic and rebound burst firing patterns were initiated in a VB neuron with intracellular current pulses (proto- col not shown). A distinct membrane voltage response is characterized by a prominent sag and after-depolarization potential(ADP) in response to hyperpolarizing current steps. The value to the left of the trace indicates membrane potential (in mV). E. Excitatory postsynaptic potentials (EPSPs) showing temporal summation were evoked by extracellular stimulation of corticothalamic fibers in the white matter. F. EPSPs are blocked in the presence of co-applied ionotropic glutamate receptor antagonists (APV 40 μM and CNQX 20 μM) (panels C–F from Ying and Goldstein, 2005).

Thalamocortical slices can be obtained from either mice or rats. Details of slice preparation will vary to some extent, and depend on the nature of the connections to be preserved. Here, we review the methods for preparing thalamocortical brain slices that preserve connections between somatosensory (barrel) cortex and the ventrobasal thalamus in slices prepared from juvenile (P25-55) mice.

Following appropriate guidelines, a mouse is anesthetized and decapitated; the head is immediately submerged in ice-cold carbogenated (95% O_2 / 5% CO_2) sucrose-substituted slicing solution (see above) and the brain is rapidly dissected free. The cerebellum is removed, and the brain anterior to the tectum is placed on a chilled 10° glass ramp, ventral side down (BOX 32.5A). Using a fresh razor blade, a vertical cut is made at a point about one-third of the way back along the anterior-to-posterior axis at an angle of 55° (or 45°) to the right of that axis (BOX 32.5B). The tissue rostral to the cut is discarded and the remaining tissue affixed to a vibratome stage after gently blotting the tissue, cut (rostral) surface down (BOX 32.5C), using cyanoacrylate glue. The pial surface of the brain faces the cutting blade; support to the brain is provided by a 3% agar block that is positioned such that it abuts the brain from the back and is then glued into place.

One the glue has set, the stage is flooded with ice-cold carbogenated slicing solution, and the caudal portion of the brain removed; typically, this is 1600 to 2400 μm worth of tissue (depending on brain size). Once the caudal section is removed, thalamocortical slices (250-500 μm thick) are sectioned, again using very slow forward motion and high oscillation frequency; slicing is terminated once the lateral ventricle (which is tinted pink) is no longer visible. Slices are transferred to an incubation beaker (see above) containing carbogenated aCSF (which contains 124 mMNaCl, 2.5 mMKCl, 2 mMCaCl$_2$, 1.2 mMMgCl$_2$, 26 mMNaHCO$_3$, 1.25 mMNaH$_2$PO$_4$, and 11 mMD-glucose) at 37℃ for 1 h before use.

Whole Cell Patch Recording from Neurons in Thalamocortical Slices

Recordings from visually identified neurons in the barrel cortex and the thalamus are obtained in the same manner as described for recordings from lamina II neurons in neonatal spinal cord slices.

BOX 32.5   Cartoon showing the orientation of the brain for preparing thalamocortical mouse brain slices.

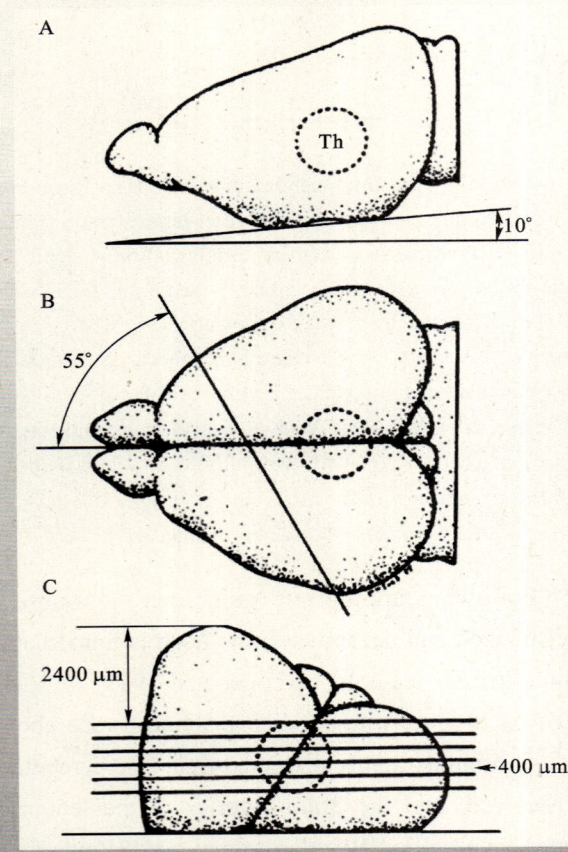

A. The brain is placed on an angled ramp. Th, approximate location of the thalamus. B. Dorsal view showing the angle of the initial cut. C. Brain affixed to vibratome stage. Approximate position of collected slices; typically, two or three slices will retain full thalamocortical connectivity (agmon and Connors, 1991).

GENERAL CITATIONS

Dodt HU, D'Arcangelo G, Zieglgänsberger W. 2000. Infrared Videomicroscopy. In: Yuste R, Lanni F, Konnerth A, eds. *Imaging Neurons*: *A Laboratory Manual*. Cold Spring Harbor: Cold Spring Harbor Press. 7. 1-7.8.

Sakmann B, Stuart G. 1995. Patch-Pipette Recordings from the Soma, Dendrites, and Axon of Neurons in Brain Slices. In: Sakmann B, Neher E, eds. *Single-Channel Recordings*, 2nd Ed. New York: Plenum Press. 199-211.

Steriade M. 2001. *The Intact and Sliced Brain*. Cambridge, MA: The MIT Press.

Yang K, Li Y, Kumamoto E, Furue H, Yoshimura M. 2001. Voltage-clamp recordings of postsynaptic currents in substantia gelatinosa neurons *in vitro* and its applications to assess synaptic transmission. *Brain Res Brain Res Protoc*, 7:235-240.

DISCOVERY CITATATIONS

Agmon A, Connors BW. 1991. Thalamocortical responses of mouse somatosensory (barrel) cortex *in vitro*. *Neuroscience*, 41:365-379.

Alger BE, Dhanjal SS, Dingledine R, Garthwaite J, Henderson G, King GL, Lipton P, North A, Schwartzkroin PA, Sears TA, Segal M, Whittingham TS, Williams J. 1984. Brain Slice Methods. In: Dingledine R, ed. *Brain Slices*. New York: Plenum. 381-437.

Bardoni R, Magherini PC, MacDermott AB. 1998. NMDA EPSCs at glutamatergic synapses in the spinal cord dorsal horn of the postnatal rat. *J Neurosci*, 18:6558-6567.

Bardoni R, Goldstein PA, Lee CJ, Gu JG, MacDermott AB. 1997. ATP P2$_X$ receptors mediate fast synaptic transmission in the dorsal horn of the rat spinal cord. *J Neurosci*, 17:5297-5304.

Blanton MG, Lo Turco JJ, Kriegstein AR. 1989. Whole cell recording from neurons in slices of reptilian and mammalian cerebral cortex. *J Neurosci Methods*, 30:203-210.

Chéry N, de Koninck Y. 1999. Junctional versus extrajunctional glycine and GABA$_A$ receptor-mediated IPSCs in identified lamina I neurons of the adult rat spinal cord. *J Neurosci*, 19:7342-7355.

Chéry N, Yu XH, de Koninck Y. 2000. Visualization of lamina I of the dorsal horn in live adult rat spinal cord slices. *J Neurosci Methods*, 96:133-142.

Edwards FA, Konnerth A. 1992. Patch-clamping cells in sliced tissue preparations. *Methods Enzymol*, 207:208-222.

Kohno T, Kumamoto E, Baba H, Ataka T, Okamoto M, Shimoji K, Yoshimura M. 2000. Actions of midazolam on GABAergic transmission in substantia gelatinosa neurons of adult rat spinal cord slices. *Anesthesiology*, 92:507-515.

Land PW, Kandler K. 2002. Somatotopic organization of rat thalamocortical slices. *J Neurosci Methods*, 119:15-21.

Metherate R, Cruikshank SJ. 1999. Thalamocortical inputs trigger a propagating envelope of g-band activity in auditory cortex *in vitro*. *Exp Brain Res*, 126:160-174.

Nakatsuka T, Park JS, Kumamoto E, Tamaki T, Yoshimura M. 1999. Plastic changes in sensory inputs to rat substantia gelatinosa neurons following peripheral inflammation. *Pain*, 82:39-47.

Okamoto M, Baba H, Goldstein PA, Higashi H, Shimoji K, Yoshimura M. 2001. Functional reorganization of sensory pathways in the rat spinal dorsal horn following peripheral nerve injury. *J Physiol*, 532:241-250.

Park JS, Nakatsuka T, Nagata K, Higashi H, Yoshimura M. 1999. Reorganization of the primary afferent termination in the rat spinal dorsal horn during post-natal development. *Brain Res Dev Brain Res*, 113:29-36.

Porter JT, Johnson CK, Agmon A. 2001. Diverse types of interneurons generate thalamus-evoked feedforward inhibition in the mouse barrel cortex. *J Neurosci*, 21:2699-2710.

Takahashi T. 1990. Membrane currents in visually identified motoneurones of neonatal rat spinal cord. *J Physiol*, 423:27-46.

Turner JP, Salt TE. 1998. Characterization of sensory and corticothalamic excitatory inputs to rat thalamocortical neurones *in vitro*. *J Physiol*, 510 (Pt 3):829-843.

Ying SW, Goldstein PA. 2005. Propofol suppresses synaptic responsiveness of somatosensory relay neurons to excitatory input by potentiating GABA$_A$ receptor chloride channels. *Mol Pain*, 1:2.

Yoshimura M, Jessell TM. 1989. Primary afferent-evoked

synaptic responses and slow potential generation in rat substantia gelatinosa neurons *in vitro*. *J Neurophysiol*, 62:96-108.

Yoshimura M, Jessell T. 1990. Amino acidmediated EPSPs at primary afferent synapses with substantia gelatinosa neu-

rones in the rat spinal cord. *J Physiol*, 430:315-335.

Yoshimura M, Nishi S. 1993. Blind patch-clamp recordings from substantia gelatinosa neurons in adult rat spinal cord slices: pharmacological properties of synaptic currents. *Neuroscience*, 53:519-526.

Whole-cell Patch-clamp Recording *in Vivo*

CHAPTER 33

Megumu Yoshimura[*]

MAJOR CONTRIBUTIONS

1. Furue H, Narikawa K, Kumamoto E, Yoshimura M. 1999. Responsiveness of rat substantia gelatinosa neurons to mechanical but not thermal stimuli revealed by *in vivo* patch-clamp recording. *Journal of Physiology* (*London*), 521:529-535.

2. Sonohata M, Furue H, Katafuchi T, Yasaka T, Doi A, Kumamoto E, Yoshimura M. 2004. Actions of noradrenaline on substantia gelatinosa neurones in the rat spinal cord revealed by *in vivo* patch recording. *Journal of Physiology* 555(2), 515-526.

3. Yoshimura M, Furue H, Nakatsuk T, Matayoshi T, Katafuchi T. 2004. Functional reorganization of the spinal pain pathways in developmental and pathological conditions. *Novartis Foundation Symposium 261, Pathological Pain: From Molecular to Clinical Aspects*, Chadwick DJ, Goode J., eds. John Wiley & Sons, Ltd. 116-131.

4. Kato G, Furue H, Katafuchi T, Yasaka T, Iwamoto Y, Yoshimura M. 2004. Electrophysiological mapping of the nociceptive inputs to the substantia gelatinosa in rat horizontal spinal cord slices. *Journal of Physiology* (*London*), 560(1): 303-315.

5. Yoshimura M, Furue H, Nakatsuka H, Katafuchi T. 2004. Analysis of receptive fields revealed by *in vivo* patch-clamp recordings from dorsal horn neurons and *in situ* intracellular recordings from dorsal root ganglion neurons. The First International Pfizer Science and Research Symposium: Key Topic 2003: Central Mechanism of Neuropathic Pain. Kumazawa T. and Toide K., eds. *Life Sciences*, 74: 2611-2618.

---

* For the introduction of Dr. Yoshimura, please refer to Chapter 7.

MAIN TOPICS

Methods for *in Vivo* patch-clamp recordings

General properties of synaptic responses in SG neurons

    Spontaneous synaptic responses in SG neurons

    Excitatory synaptic responses evoked by mechanical stimuli

    Inhibitory synaptic responses evoked by mechanical stimuli

    Synaptic responses in SG neurons by heat stimulation

Plastic change of spinal nociceptive transmission revealed by *in Vivo* patch-clamp recording methods

In Vivo patch-clamp recording from somatosensory cortex

SUMMARY

In the last two decades, electrophysiological studies for understanding the mechanisms of central sensitization, which have been induced in many cases by overwhelming inputs from the periphery, have been extensively investigated in slice preparations with intracellular or patch-clamp recordings from spinal dorsal horn neurons. The main difficulty in using slice preparations is that there is no information about what modality of afferent fibers elicits a certain response in dorsal horn neurons. To overcome this problem an *in vivo* patch-clamp recording method has been developed. Under the *in vivo* condition, noxious or non-noxious stimuli applied to the skin elicits a barrage of EPSCs in substantia gelatinosa (SG) neurons which have no slow membrane currents, suggesting that the mechanical information is mediated by glutamate through the activation of AMPA type receptors. Unexpectedly, thermal stimuli elicit no response, in spite of the fact that the SG neurons receive abundant inputs from C afferents and express c-FOS in many neurons by thermal stimuli. Further study from deeper laminae shows that the noxious thermal information appears to be transmitted to laminae III - V. However, these responses are mediated by fast EPSCs but not by slow synaptic current. These observations are inconsistent in regard to the assumption that thermal sensation is carried by polymodal afferents, in particular C, which are known to contain various peptides, such as substance P or CGRP. The role of such peptides in sensory transmission is still largely unknown, although it is believed the peptidergic transmission would become obvious under extreme or pathological conditions. In addition to the excitatory responses, an inhibitory response is commonly observed in dorsal horn neurons. The IPSCs have two components: the first being mediated by GABA through GABA$_A$ receptors, the other is glycinergic. GABAergic IPSCs are dominant and have a much longer time course. Intriguingly, the IPSCs are elicited by non-noxious rather than noxious mechanical stimuli in SG neurons. After integration at the spinal cord, sensory information is finally ascended to the primary somatosensory cortex through the thalamus where further sensory processing will be made. Based on the accumulating evidence, pain research is now focusing on clarifying mechanisms of plastic changes in the sensory pathways under pathological conditions.

In this chapter excitatory and inhibitory synaptic responses to physiological stimuli, and plastic changes induced in ovariecotomized rats, which is a model for osteoporosis, are described. Additionally, *in vivo* patch-clamp data from the sensory cortex is shown briefly.

INTRODUCTION

In vivo extracellular and intracellular recordings have been used to analyze a change of excitability in dorsal horn neurons under physiological and pathological conditions. Consequently a large amount of basic knowledge about nociceptive transmission and sensory circuitry in the spinal dorsal horn has been accumulated. However, the extracellular study is confined to analyzing only a firing frequency and not subthreshold synaptic events, similarly the intracellular recording is also limited, only being able to record data from relatively large neurons. To overcome these problems, an *in vivo* patch-clamp recording method has been developed. The original *in vivo* patch-clamp recording which analyzed synaptic responses in the visual cortex of cats was established in 1991. Currently more than 20 labs are examining the sensory processes in the visual, auditory and somatosensory cortices of cats, rats or mice. Unfortunately an *in vivo* patch-clamp recording from spinal dorsal horn neurons was not developed until the original work by Light and Willcockson in 1996. Since then two groups independently developed the same *in vivo* method. However, due to the difficulty in applying this method, at present only two labs continue to use this method for analyzing synaptic transmission in rats and mice. Despite the lack of usage, the *in vivo* patch recording is remarkably stable and lasts for up to 4 hours after establishing the whole cell configuration. This method is also applicable for recordings from deeper neurons, such as lamina III−V and also from the somatosensory cortex in studying how nociceptive information is processed at the higher center. Rats have been, and are commonly used in recording data but now it is also possible to record accurate information from mice. Due to the ability to apply this method to mice it is feasible for analyzing a functional role of a certain molecule that is involved in nociceptive transmission by using knockout mice. A change in synaptic responses studied by *in vivo* examination can be further confirmed by combining this with a slice study. Thus, the *in vivo* patch-clamp recording would be one of the most suitable ways for making a correlation between a change in behavioral and synaptic transmission in slice preparations.

METHODS FOR *IN VIVO* PATCH-CLAMP RECORDINGS

Under anesthesia with urethane or other volatile anesthesia, a lumbo-sacral laminectomy is made and the animal is fixed in a stereotaxic apparatus(Fig.33.1). After opening the dura-mater with scissors, a small window is made with a fine needle in arachnoid and pear mater, then the surface of the spinal cord is perfused with warmed (38±1℃) pre-oxygenated Krebs solution. The known concentrations of drugs are also applied through this line from a three way tap, therefore there is no change in temperature or perfusion rate. Under a binocular microscope, the superficial dorsal grey matter lateral to the dorsal root entry zone is discernible as a relatively translucent band under Lissauer's tract. Recording electrodes having input resistances of 8−12 Ω are inserted through the windor opened in the arachnoid and pear matter, at an angle of 30 degrees from the horizontal line. This approach is suitable for making recordings from SG neurons at a depth of 50−150 μm. Further identification of neurons in the SG are made, in some instances, by the injection of neurobiotin through the recording electrode. After the completion of recordings, recorded neurons are stained and their morphological features

are correlated with synaptic inputs.

Mechanical noxious stimuli are applied to the ipsilateral hind limb by pinching the skin with toothed forceps and a brush or glass rod is used for non-noxious stimuli. Noxious heat stimulation is produced by a halogen lamp focused on the skin and the temperature at the surface is monitored continuously and feedback to control the temperature (Fig.33.2).

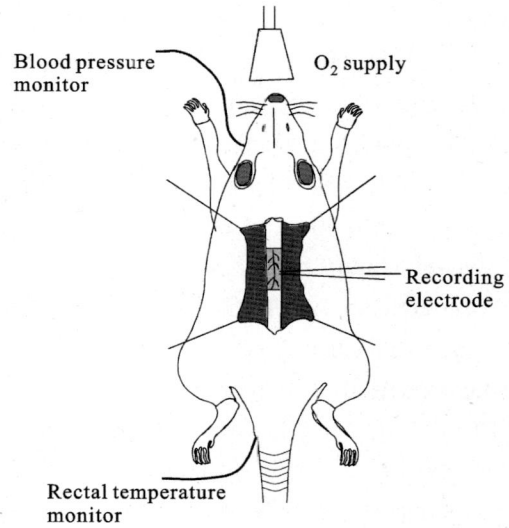

Fig.33.1 Schematic diagram of an *in vivo* patch-clamp recording. After monitoring blood pressure and body temperature, lumbo-sacral laminectomy is performed and a rat is fixed in a stereotaxic apparatus. The surface of the spinal cord is perfused with wormed Krebs solution. Recording electrodes are inserted to substantia gelatinosa neurons.

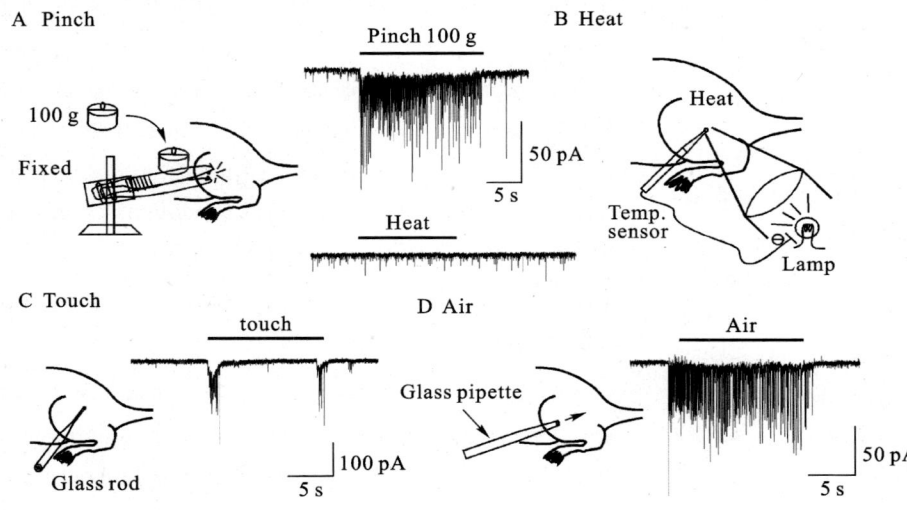

Fig.33.2 Noxious and non-noxious stimulation and evoked synaptic currents. A. Noxious pinch stimulation is applied to the skin by toothed forceps pinching the skin that elicits a barrage of EPSCs. B. Noxious heat stimulation is applied by a halogen lamp focusing on the surface of the skin. No response is elicited by heat stimulation. C. Deformation of the skin with a glass rod produces responses at the beginning and end of the stimulation. D. Air puff application from a glass pipette produces a barrage of EPSCs.

GENERAL PROPERTIES OF SYNAPTIC RESPONSES IN SG NEURONS

Spontaneous Synaptic Responses in SG Neurons

At a holding potential of –70 mV, all SG neurons exhibit spontaneous EPSCs, some of which have a large amplitude, indicating that those are mediated by spontaneous firings of the primary afferent or interneurons. Under the current clamp condition some EPSPs are sufficient to initiate an action potential, but in general SG neurons have relatively higher membrane potentials (about –68mV) and the threshold for action potential is high (–40 to –45mV). Therefore, spontaneous synaptic inputs hardly initiate spikes (Fig.33.3).

The frequency of EPSCs in *in vivo* condition is much higher than that observed in slice preparations and spontaneous IPSCs recorded at a holding potential of 0 mV exhibit a higher frequency than that of spontaneous EPSCs. This difference in the frequencies of spontaneous IPSCs and EPSCs is inconsistent with those in slice preparations. In slice, no significant difference in the frequencies of EPSCs and IPSCs are observed. Spontaneous as well as evoked EPSCs are sensitive to the non-NMDA receptor antagonist, CNQX, and no residual responses are detected, indicating that glutamate is the only transmitter for EPSCs. No slow response is found after the blockade of the fast EPSCs, although a substantial number of C afferents and interneurons are known to contain various peptides and that they are co-released with glutamate. Consistent with the data from slice examinations, spontaneous IPSCs are mediated by either GABA via a GABAA receptor or glycine. GABAergic IPSCs have about a 3 times longer decay time constant than glycinergic IPSCs. Todd *et al.* has reported that some inhibitory interneurons co-release GABA and glycine. Inconsistent with this result, no such IPSCs mediated by both GABA and glycine are detected in adult SG. This discrepancy might be due in part to developmental change, alternatively either

GABA or glycine response is occluded by an unknown mechanism. Chery *et al.* shows that spontaneous IPSCs are mediated by co-released GABA and glycine which is detected only in the presense of benzodiazepine which enhances GABA response.

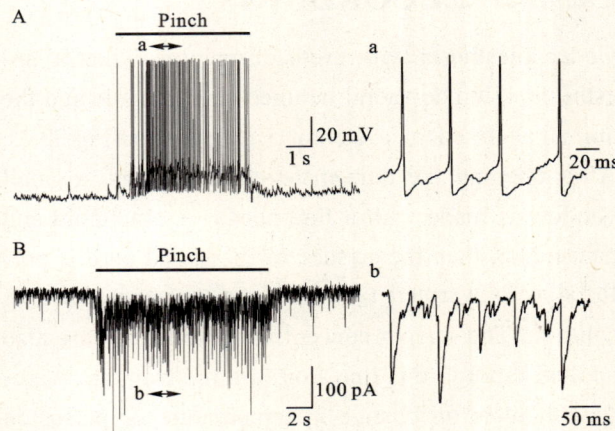

Fig.33.3 Pinch evoked synaptic responses under the current clamp (A) and voltage clamp conditions (B). Note that the pinch stimuli initiate spike firings (a).

Excitatory Synaptic Responses Evoked by Mechanical Stimuli

Noxious or non-noxious stimuli are applied to the ipsilateral hind limb. Noxious as well as non-noxious stimuli elicit a barrage of EPSCs under the voltage-clamp condition, some EPSPs under the current clamp can initiate spikes. Noxious pinch stimuli elicit a continuous barrage of EPSCs, while deformation of the skin with a glass rod produces responses only at the beginning and end of the stimulation, indicating that the receptor responsible for the stimuli shows rapid adaptation. To obtain a continuous barrage of EPSCs, air puff from a glass pipette is applied to the hairy skin or hind paw. The stimulation elicits continuous EPSCs which have similar frequency and amplitude with those evoked by noxious stimuli.

Inhibitory Synaptic Responses Evoked by Mechanical Stimuli

Consistent with the spontaneous IPSCs, non-noxious stimuli elicit a barrage of IPSCs without showing any adaptation when the air puff or brush stimuli are applied to the skin. In contrast, the pinch stimuli evoke

IPSCs at the binning and end of the stimulation. The responses at the beginning and end seem to be mainly due to an activation of non-noxious but not noxious receptor activation, since the pinch stimuli elicits the continuous barrage of EPSCs without any adaptation. This indicates that the noxious stimuli produce continues firings without showing the adaptation of the primary afferent to the spinal cord. These observations suggest that the IPSCs in the majority of SG neurons are elicited only by non-noxious inputs.

Synaptic Responses in SG Neurons by Heat Stimulation

Unexpectedly, no synaptic response is observed in all SG neurons by the heat stimulation, in spite of large synaptic inputs from polymodal C afferents to SG. Intriguingly, capsaicin application on slice preparations significantly increases mEPSCs in all SG neurons, indicating that the SG neurons receive C afferent fibers of which those fiber's terminals are endowed with TRPV1 (previously VR1) receptors. It is believed in general that a receptor expressed at the central end of these terminals is also expressed at the peripheral nerve endings. Therefore, the fibers terminated on SG neurons should but do not respond to

heat stimulation. This clear discrepancy has not been clarified yet. Further study from deeper laminae shows that the noxious thermal information appears to be transmitted to laminae III – V. These responses are, however, mediated by fast EPSCs but not by slow synaptic current (Fig.33.4).

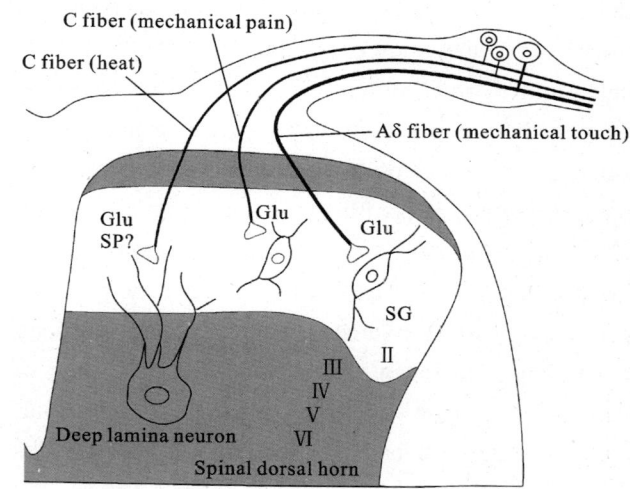

Fig. 33.4 Schematic diagram of the modality dependent synaptic connections between the primary afferents and spinal dorsal horn neurons. Mechanical noxious and non-noxious sensations are terminated on the SG neurons, while the noxious heat information is transmitted to the dendrite of deeper neurons.

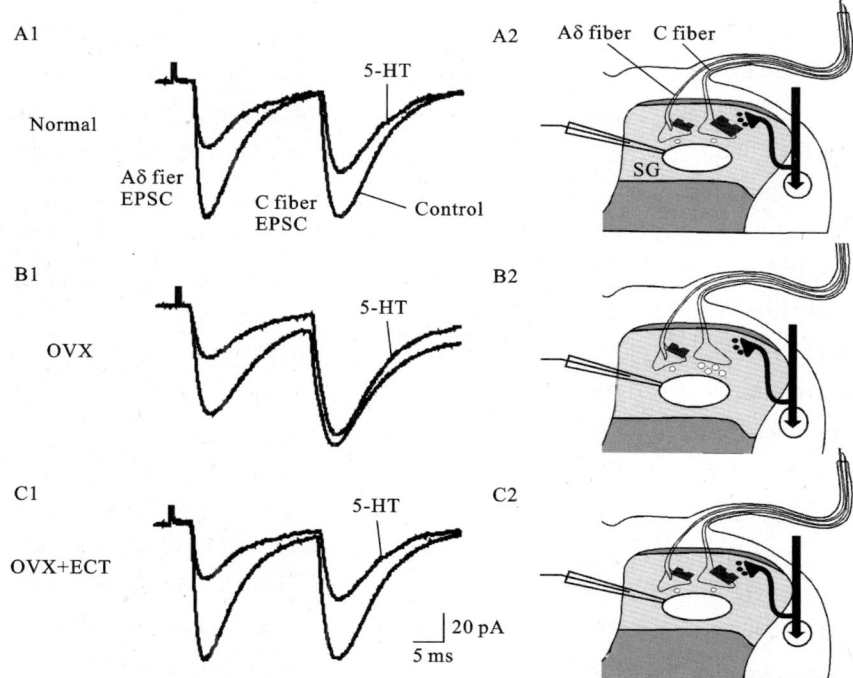

Fig.33.5 Plastic changes induced in the ovariecotmized rats. Left panels show the results obtained from slice experiments and right panels are possible changes in the expression of 5-HT receptor at the C afferent terminals. A. In normal rats, bath applied 5-HT reduces the amplitudes of both Aδ and C afferent evoked EPSCs, indicating that the 5-HT receptors are expressed at the Aδ and C afferent terminals and reduce the release of glutamate. B. In OVX rats, 5-HT depresses only the Aδ afferent evoked EPSCs without affecting the C afferent EPSCs. Based on these results, 5-HT receptors expressed at the C afferent terminals are eliminated by the reduction of estrogen. C. In OVX rats treated with calcitonin, the depressive action of 5-HT on the presynaptic terminals of C afferent is restored. Administration of calcitonin synthesizes 5-HT receptors at the C afferent terminals.

PLASTIC CHANGE OF SPINAL NOCICEPTIVE TRANSMISSION REVEALED BY *IN VIVO* PATCH-CLAMP RECORDING METHODS

It has been demonstrated that ovariectomized (OVX) rat are the commonly used model for osteoporosis. Rats used in the study of osteoporosis exhibit hyperalgesia to thermal stimuli. This hyperalgesia can be alleviated by repeptitive subcutaneous injections of calcitonin, a polypeptide hormone secreted from the parafollicular C cells of the mammalian thyroid gland. Calcitonin is widely used clinically to improve bone mass in osteoporosis and also to relieve the pain accompanying it. Mechanisms for ovariectomy-induced hyperalgesia has been challenged by studies using *in vitro* slices which retain an attached dorsal root, demonstrating that bath applied 5-HT reversibly depresses Aδ and C afferent fiber-evoked EPSCs, by depressing the release of glutamate from the afferent terminals. In OVX rats, 5-HT still depresses the Aδ afferent EPSCs, however, the C afferent EPSCs are not altered. This lack of depressive action of 5-HT is restored, by an administration of calcitonin, suggesting that OVX causes the elimination of 5-HT receptors at the terminals of C afferent fibers and that calcitonin restores the eliminated 5-HT receptors at the C afferent(Fig.33.5). In this slice experiment, identification of afferent fibers responsible for the effects of OVX and calcitonin is available based on the conduction velocities and stimulus intensities. However, it is hard to know what modality of sensory information is modified by OVX. To address this problem, *in vivo* patch-clamp analysis is made to test whether noxious or non-noxious mechanical sensation is modified by OVX.

In normal rats, the frequency and amplitude of EPSCs evoked by noxious and non-noxious stimuli are not significantly different in amplitude and frequency, while the amplitude but not frequency of EPSCs by noxious stimuli in OVX rat SG neurons is greater than that of applied non-noxious stimuli. These findings are consistent with the data obtained from slice studies demonstrating that the release of glutamate from C afferent fibers is not reduced, because of a lack of 5-HT receptors at the terminals. Activation of which causes a reduction of the release of glutamate since bath applied 5-HT depresses both Aδ and C afferent evoked EPSCs, and the C afferent EPSCs are not affected in OVX rats, an effect of 5-HT on a barrage of EPSCs evoked by noxious and non-noxious stimuli is tested in normal and OVX rats. As expected, 5-HT applied to the surface of the spinal cord depresses both noxious and non-noxious responses in normal rats, while only the non-noxious but not noxious response is depressed in OVX rats, consistent with the idea that the noxious sensation is carried by predominantly C afferent fibers. This data further suggests that the 5-HT receptors at the C afferent terminals which convey noxious sensation to the spinal dorsal horn are eliminated in OVX rats. Interestingly pretreatment of OVX rats with calcitonin restore the effect of 5-HT, demonstrating that 5-HT again reduces the amplitude of both noxious and non-noxious responses in SG neurons, suggesting that calcitonin re-expresses the 5-HT receptor at the C afferent terminals. It is still unknown how calcitonin synthesizes 5-HT receptors at the C afferent terminals. As we know, OVX causes a significant reduction of estrogen which is one of steroid hormones known to act through intracellular receptors. Calcitonin might interact with a production of protein regulated by estrogen, however the site of action is unknown and further investigation is clearly required to clarify this.

IN VIVO PATCH-CLAMP RECORDING FROM SOMATOSENSORY CORTEX

Recent imaging studies such as PET and fMRI demonstrate that the sensation of pain is conveyed to the primary sensory cortex through the thalamus and therefore, the primary sensory cortex is one of the targets for the pain research in spite of the fact that stimulation of the region initiates no painful sensation. To address how pain sensation is further processed at the higher center, *in vivo* patch-clamp recording from sensory cortex would be one of the most effective approaches to analyze this. Now more than 20 laboratories are investigating the synaptic transmission in the somatosensory cortex using the *in vivo* patch methods.

The methods used in *in vivo* patch-clamp recording from the somatosensory cortex are similar to that for making an *in vivo* patch-clamp from the spinal cord. Briefly, after an anesthetized rat is fixed in a stereotaxic apparatus, a small recording chamber is fixed on the skull with dental cement. A small hole in the skull on the sensory cortex is drilled and the dura mater is cut with scissors. Following the perfusion of the surface of the brain, a small window is opened on the arachnoid and pear mater with fine scissors to let a patch electrode into the brain. Identification of recorded neurons as pyramidal or non-pyramidal neurons is made by their morphological features by injection of neurobiotin.

More than 95 % of pyramidal and non-pyramidal neurons exhibit bursting activity with a frequency of 0.5 to 4 Hz in urethan anesthetized rats(Fig.33.6). This bursting activity appears to be a summation of excitatory synaptic inputs, since bath applied CNQX 20 μM reversibly depresses it. To exclude the possibility that the bursting activity is due to the movement of the thorax or the pulsation of arteries, ECG and the movement of the thorax are monitored and compared in correlation to the bursting. However, no correlation is found among the bursting, the ECG or the movement of the thorax, indicating that it is not artificial but mediated by synaptic inputs originating from other neurons; possibly from other cortices, ipsilatral, contalateral or more likely the thalamus. The bursting frequency correlates well with the level of anesthesia and is dependent on anesthetics. When a rat is anesthetized with pentobarbital, no bursting activity is observed, suggesting an involvement of GABAergic systems in the generation of the bursting. As expected the bursting frequency correlates well with EEG and interestingly the bursting correlates with both EEG from ipsi- and contra-lateral sides. Due to the presence of this bursting activity, analysis of synaptic responses evoked by noxious or non-noxious stimuli is hampered. In order to analyze the synaptic responses,

pentobarbital or other anesthetics should be used. In fact, some of the somatosensory cortex neurons respond to non-noxious stimuli with a barrage of EPSCs similar to that evoked in spinal dorsal horn neurons. However, only a few cortex neurons respond to noxious stimuli; although the response is analogous to those evoked by non-noxious stimulation. So far no convincing evidence has been reported showing a plastic change in the primary somatosensory cortex induced by pathological conditions. However, as described in Chapter 28 by Min Zhuo, the neuronal circuitry in ACC is a subject of plastic changes induced by chronic pain states.

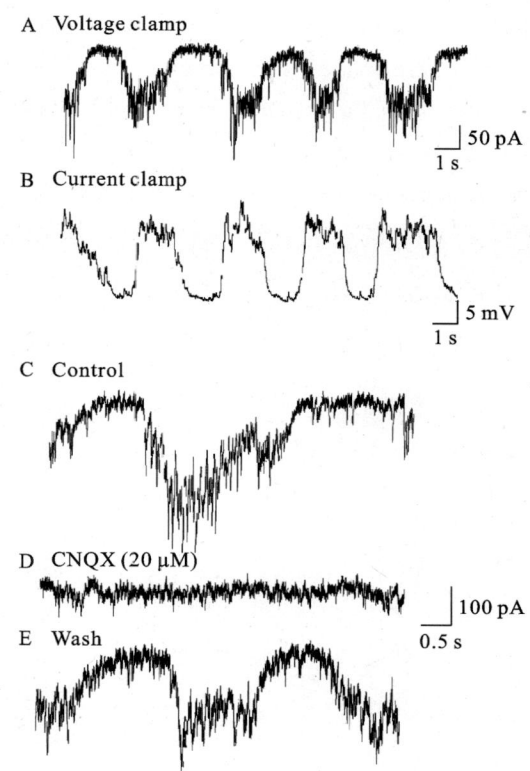

Fig.33.6   Bursting activity of somatosensory neurons recorded in *in vivo* patch-clamp recordings in urethane anesthetized rats. A and B are obtained from the same neuron under the voltage and current clamp condtions. The bursting activities are sensitive to a gultamate receptor antagonist, CNQX (C, D, and E).

CONCLUSION AND FUTURE DIRECTIONS

The *in vivo* patch-clamp recording method is promising

to have fruitful results that would be difficult to obtain with other methods. The great advantage in this method is its ability to analyze responses at the single neuron level in response to physiological stimulation. Although the *in vivo* recording method is feasible for analyzing responses evoked by physiological stimuli applied to the skin or other tissues, there will be confliction, such as when pain related responses are analyzed under the analgesic condition using anesthetics. Ideally it would be quite useful if the *in vivo* recordings were performed under conscious conditions. Recently this method, that being performing *in vivo* recordings under conscious conditions, has been reported to be applicable in rodents. Previously *in vivo* intracellular recordings were made from cortical neurons without any anesthetics using primates. Therefore, beneficial to greater understanding in higher brain functions while it would be possible to make recordings from primate cortical neurons with patch electrodes without any anesthetics, seeing that patch recording is much more stable and applicable to the study of small neurons. This method combined with slice study and imaging analysis may disclose mechanisms of the processing of the sensation of pain in the spinal cord and cortical level. Recently, propagation of neuronal excitation by peripheral stimulation has been assessed by using both voltage sensitive dye and intrinsic fluorescent change methods. The *in vivo* patch-clamp method would be able to combine with either of these methods. Understanding the underlying mechanisms of pain transmission under physiological and pathological conditions should be the first step in providing an idea on how to manage, or on what kind of chemicals are possible in the treatment of patients suffering from a tractable chronic pain.

BOX 33.1   Mechanism for ovariectomy induced hyperalgesia.

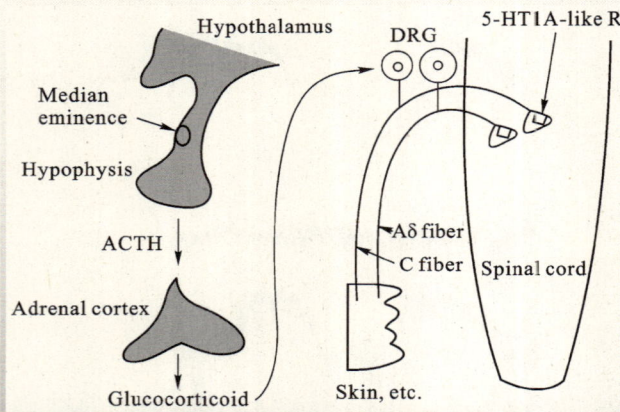

Although the mechanisms of elimination and resumption of 5-HT receptors at the C afferent terminal following ovariecotmy and administration of calcitonin, respectively, are still unknown, one possible explanation for the mechanisms is shown in this figure. It is reported that the elimination of estrogen induced by ovariectomy in rats results in a reduction in corticosterone levels in serum for 3 weeks. It is well established that steroid hormones, such as glucocorticoids, regulate the expression of various genes by forming a complex with their receptors, followed by binding to a particular sequence in the promoter region of gene. Shimizu *et al.* (1997) have demonstrated that a decrease of glucocorticoid levels in OVX rats could be expected to reduce the amount of gene products, including 5-HT receptors. Because it is known in humans that single peripheral injection of calctionin causes a raise in ACTH and subsequently cortisol levels in plasma for >2 h, it may be that repetitive treatment leading to a resumption of synthesis of 5-HT receptors. This hypothesis remains to be verified. In any event, calcitonin may be an exceptional analgesic that acts by altering the density of 5-HT receptors at C fiber terminals innervating SG neurons. Considering that the C fibers convey predominantly diffuse and long-lasting pain sensation, these results indicate that 5-HT receptors may play an important role in controlling pain: identification of the 5-HT receptor subtype may accelerate the development of drugs that potentially affect nociceptive transmission.

GENERAL CITATIONS

Furue H, Narikawa K, Kumamoto E, Yoshimura M. 1999. Responsiveness of rat substantia gelatinosa neurones to mechanical but not thermal stimuli revealed by *in vivo* patch-clamp recording. *J Physiol. (Lond)*, 521(1): 529-535.

Light AR, Willcockson HH. 1999. Spinal laminae I-II neurons in rat recorded *in vivo* in whole cell, tight seal configuration: properties and opioid responses. *J Neurophysiol*, 82: 3316-3326.

Narikawa K, Furue H, Kumamoto E, Yoshimura M. 2000. *In vivo* patch-clamp analysis of IPSCs evoked in rat substantia gelatinosa neurons by cutaneous mechanical stimulation. *J Nurophysiol*, 84: 2171-2174.

Sonohata M, Furue H, Katafuchi T, Yasaka T, Doi A, Kumamoto E, Yoshimura M. 2004. Actions of noradrenaline on substantia gelatinosa neurones in the rat spinal cord revealed by *in vivo* patch recording. *J Physiol*, 555(2): 515-526.

DISCOVERY CITATIONS

Brecht M, Sakmann. 2002. Dynamic representation of whisker deflection by synaptic potentials in spiny stellate and pyramidal cells in the barrels and septa of layer 4 rat somatosensory cortex. *J Physiol* (*Lond*), 4543(1): 49-70.

Caterina MJ, Leffler A, Malmberg AB, Martin WJ, Trafton J, Petersen-Zeitz KR, Koltzenburg M, Basbaum AI, Julius D. 2000. Impaired nociception and pain sensation in mice lacking the capsaicin receptor. *Science*, 288: 306-313.

Chery N, De-Koninck Y. 1999. Junctional versus extrajunctional glycine and GABA(A) receptor-mediated IPSCs in identified lamina I neurons of the adult rat spinal cord. *J Neurosci*, 19(17): 7342-7355

Chung S, Li X, Nelson SB. 2002. Short-term depression at thalamocortical synapses contributes to rapid adaptation of cortical sensory responses *in vivo*. *Neuron*, 34: 437-446.

Graham BA, Brichta AM, Callister RJ. 2004 *In vivo* responses of mouse superficial dorsal horn neurones to both current injection and peripheral cutaneous stimulation. *J Physiol*, 561: 749-763.

Ito A, Kumamoto E, Takeda M, Takeda M, Shibata K, Sagai H, Yoshimura M. 2000. Mechanisms for ovariectomy-induced hyperalgesia and its relief by calcitonin: participation of 5-HT1A-like receptor on C-afferent terminals in substantia gelatinosa of the rat spinal cord. *J Neurosci*, 20: 6302-6308.

Murakami H, Kamatani D, Hishida R, Takao T, Kudoh M, Kawaguchi T, Tanaka R, Shibuki K. 2004. Short-term plasticity visualized with flavoprotein autofluorescence in the somatosensory cortex of anaesthetized rats. *European J Neuro Science*, 19(5):1352-1360.

Orimo H, Morii H, Inoue T, Ymamoto K, Ninaguchi H, Ishii Y, Murota K, Fujimaki E, Watanabe R, Harata S, Honjo H, Fujita T. 1996. Effect of elcatonin on involutional osteoporosis. *J Bone Miner Metab*, 14: 73-78.

Pei X, Volgushev M, Vidyasagar TR, Creutzfeldt OD. 1991. Whole cell recording and conductance measurements in cat visual cortex *in vivo*. *NeuroReport*, 2: 485-488.

Potts Jr JT, Aurbach GD. 1976. Chemistry of the calcitonins. In: Aurbach GD, ed. *Handbook of Physiology*. Vol 7, Washington, DC: American Physiological Society. 423-430.

Shibata K, Takeda M, Ito A, Takeda M, Sagai H. 1998. Ovariecotmy-induced hyperalgesia and antinocieptive effect of calcitonin, a synthetic eel calcitonin. *Pharmacol Biochem Behav*, 60: 371-376.

Shimizu H, Ohtani K, Kato Y, Tanaka Y, Mori M. 1997. Withdrawal of [corrected] estrogen increases hypothalamic neuropeptide Y (NPY) mRNA expression in ovariectomized obese rat . *Neurosci Lett*, 204: 81-84.

Todd AJ, Watt C, Spike RC, Sieghart W. 1996. Colocalization of GABA, glycine, and their receptors at synapses in the rat spinal cord. *J Neurosci*. 16(3): 974-982.

Todd AJ, Spike RC. 1993. The localization of classical transmitters and neuropeptides within neurons in laminae I–III of the mammalian spinal dorsal horn. *Prog Neurobiol*, 41: 609-645.

Vidyasagar TR, Pei X, Volgushev M. 1996. Multiple mechanisms underlying the orientation selectivity of visual cortical neurones. *Trends Neurosci*, 19: 272-277.

Willis Jr. WC, Coggeshall RE. 1991. *Sensory Mechanisms of the Spinal Cord*. New York: Plenum Press.

Yang K, Kumamoto E, Furue H, Yoshimura M. 1998. Capsaicin facilitates excitator but not inhibitory synaptic transmission in substantia gelatinosa of the rat spinal cord. *Nueosci Lett*, 255: 135-138.

Yosimura M, Jessell TM. 1993. Amino acid-mediated EPSPs at primary afferent synapses with substantia gelationsa neurones in the rat spinal cord. *J Physiol*, 430: 315-335.

Yoshimura M, Nishi S. 1995. Primary afferent-evoked glycine- and GABA-mediated IPSPs in substantia gelatinosa neurones in the rat spinal cord *in vitro*. *J Physiol* (*Lond*), 428: 29-38.

Basic Mechanisms of Clinically Used Drugs

CHAPTER 34

Annika B. Malmberg

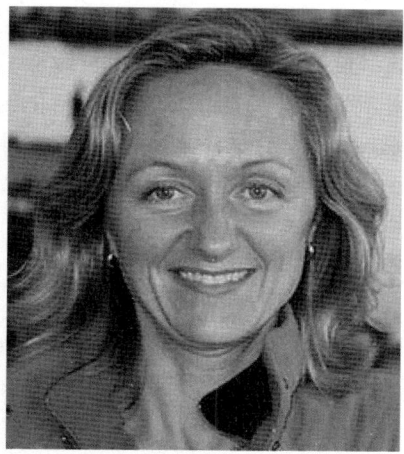

Dr. Malmberg is a Principal Scientist in the Neuroscience group at Amgen in Cambridge, MA, USA. She graduated from University of Uppsala, Sweden, and obtained a MSc in Pharmacy, followed by a PhD in Pharmacology and Physiology at the University of Göteborg, Sweden. She also spent time at the University of California, San Diego during her thesis work and performed postdoctoral training at the University of California, San Francisco, CA.

MAJOR CONTRIBUTIONS

1. Malmberg AB, Yaksh TL. 1992. Hyperalgesia mediated by spinal glutamate or substance P receptor blocked by spinal cyclooxygenase inhibition. *Science*, 257: 1276-1279.
2. Malmberg AB, Yaksh TL. 1995. Cyclooxygenase inhibition and the spinal release of prostaglandin E2 and amino acids evoked by paw formalin injection: A microdialysis study in unanesthetized rats. *J Neurosci*, 15: 2768-2776.
3. Malmberg AB, Chen C, Tonegawa S, Basbaum AI. 1997. Preserved acute pain and reduced neuropathic pain in mice lacking PKC. *Science*, 278: 279-283.
4. Caterina MJ, Leffler A, Malmberg AB, Martin WJ, Trafton J, Petersen-Zeitz KR, Koltzenburg M, Basbaum AI, Julius D. 2000. Impaired nociception and pain sensation in mice lacking the capsaicin receptor. *Science*, 288: 306-313.
5. Malmberg AB, Mizisin A, Calcutt NA, von Stein T, Robbins W, Bley KR, 2004. Reduced heat sensitivity and epidermal nerve fiber immunostaining following single applications of high-concentration capsaicin patches. *Pain*, 111: 360-367.

MAIN TOPICS

Opioids
  Tramadol
Non-opioids/Cyclooxygenase inhibitors
  NSAIDS
  COX-2 inhibitors
  Acetaminophen
  NSAID combinations
Anticonvulsants
  Gabapentin
  Pregabalin
  Phenytoin and carbamazepine
  Lamotrigine
  Topiramate
Tricyclic antidepressants
  Amitriptyline
Spinally delivered agents
  Ziconotide
  Clonidine
Topically applied agents
  Lidocaine
  Capsaicin

SUMMARY

Analgesic drugs represent the most common treatments of pain. Analgesics can be broadly classified into opioid analgesics, non-opioid analgesics and adjuvant or co-analgesics. Opioid analgesics, such as morphine and other opioid receptor agonists, are used to treat moderate to severe pain. Mild to moderate pain is typically relieved with non-opioid drugs, such as nonsteroidal anti-inflammatory drugs (NSAIDs), aspirin and acetaminophen. In addition, certain pain conditions, such as neuropathic pain, are commonly treated with agents that originally were developed for other indications, but have been shown to be effective in some persistent pain conditions. These agents include anticonvulsant drugs, some antidepressants and local anesthetics. This chapter is focusing on the most commonly used analgesics and their proposed mechanisms of action.

INTRODUCTION

Pain is the most common reason for patients seeking medical consultations with their physician and the most used treatment for pain is pharmacological therapies. Pain medications represent one of the largest pharmaceutical markets in the world. Pain therapeutics is typically administered according to severity of the pain; there are different recommendations to treat mild, moderate and severe pain. In addition, severe pain conditions such as neuropathic pain are often treated with additional therapeutics, which originally was developed for other conditions, e.g., epilepsy or CNS disorders. Similarly as there are different types of pain, there are various ways to categorize pharmacological treatments of pain. Broadly, analgesics can be divided into three groups, namely opioid analgesics, non-opioid analgesics and adjuvant or co-analgesics.

Opioid analgesics include morphine and other opioid agonists. These drugs are used to treat moderate to severe pain. Non-opioid analgesics include nonsteroidal anti-inflammatory drugs (NSAIDs), aspirin and acetaminophen. Drugs in this class are most effective for the treatment of mild to moderate pain.

Adjuvant analgesics are a diverse group of drugs, including anticonvulsants, some antidepressants and local anesthetics. These drugs have other primary indications, but are effective in treating some types of pain conditions, particularly neuropathic pain. In addition, there are some newer drugs with specific effects that are not included in the categories above. This chapter is focusing on the most commonly used analgesics and their proposed mechanisms of action.

OPIOIDS

For centuries, pain has been relieved by various preparations of the opium poppy papaver somniferum. It was later discovered that the analgesic effect was produced by the alkaloid morphine. The principal therapeutic action of morphine is analgesia and morphine is essentially effective in all preclinical pain assays. Clinically, morphine is efficacious in treating moderate to severe pain. Other therapeutic effects of morphine include anxiolysis, euphoria and feelings of relaxation. Both adverse and therapeutic effects result from opioid expression in the CNS and gastrointestinal tract. Side effects of morphine and other opioids include sedation, mental clouding or confusion, respiratory depression, nausea, vomiting, constipation, pruritus (itch) and urinary retention.

Morphine and other opioid drugs produce analgesia by binding to opioid receptors expressed in the brain stem, spinal cord and peripheral tissues. Activation of these receptors both account for the analgesic and side effects of opioids. There are three subtypes of opioid receptors, namely the mu-, kappa- and delta-opioid receptors. All three genes encoding the receptors, namely the mu-opioid (MOR), kappa-opioid (KOR) and delta-opioid receptor (DOR) genes have been cloned. Most clinically used opioid drugs mediate their action via activation of the mu receptor. Commonly used mu receptor agonists include morphine, hydromorphone, oxycodone, hydrocodone, fentanyl and meperidine. Some opioids are partial mu agonists, including buprenorphine, profadol and propiram. Butorphanol and nalbuphine are partial kappa agonists.

All of the cloned opioid receptor types belong to the superfamily of G protein-coupled receptors and the subfamily of rhodopsin receptor. All opioid receptors have the putative structure of seven transmembrane domains. It also appears that all opioid receptors couple through G_i/G_o proteins to inhibit adenylate cyclase, activate an inwardly rectifying potassium conductance and to inhibit voltage-gated calcium channels. Additional intracellular responses to opioid receptor stimulation include activation of phospholipase C, phospholipase A2 and mitogen activated protein kinases ERK1 and ERK2. However, differential opioid receptor expression and different intracellular pathways in various cell types is likely to reflect variable effects mediated by the different opioid receptors.

On a systems level, the analgesic effect of opioids is a result of modulation of pain pathways in the CNS; however, peripheral effects are also observed under certain conditions. The potent analgesic effect of opioids is a result of modulation of nociceptive transmission in the CNS, specifically the spinal cord, the brainstem and other supraspinal sites. Opioid receptor expression in the CNS has been determined for several animal species and humans. The expression appears to be restricted to subpopulations of neurons within several brain regions and the cellular expression patterns varies for mu, kappa, and delta opioid receptor. Several studies have indicated that areas such as the periaqueductal grey (PAG) and the rostral ventromedial medulla (RVM) are important anatomical locus for opioid analgesia and opioid activation of descending inhibitory pathways to the spinal cord. At the spinal cord level, mu opioids act presynaptically to inhibit neurotransmitter release and postsynaptically to inhibit firing of transduction neurons. It has been hypothesized that the combination of morphine's actions on both pre- and postsynaptic sites is the reason to morphine's and other opioids potent analgesic effect.

In the periphery, opioids appear to have minimal effect on nociceptive afferent, although opioid receptor expression has been demonstrated in peripheral sensory neurons. However, in models of inflammation, opioid receptor agonists are active in reducing pain. Opioid receptors are expressed on several peripheral cell types, which are involved in pain modulation, including sensory and sympathetic postganglionic nerves, and immune cells. While immune cells may release a number of factors that may enhance pain signaling, opioid agonist efficacy in inflammation appears to be mainly due to an increased number of peripheral opioid receptor on primary afferent neurons following inflammation.

In addition to active opioid receptors by various opioid drugs, an endogenous opioid system regulates pain perception. This system is also modulated by other endogenous neuropeptides, which participate in a homeostatic system tending to reduce the effects of opioids. Understanding these systems may identify new mechanisms for potential therapeutic intervention for the control of opioid functions and alleviating pain, including chronic pain.

Tramadol

Tramadol is usually considered among the opioids, although tramadol possesses weak affinity for the opioid receptor (6 000-fold less than morphine, 10-fold less than codeine and equivalent to dextromethorphan) and exerts unusual actions compared the traditional members of the opioid class. In experimental animal model of pain and clinical studies, he analgesic effect of tramadol is only partially blocked by the opioid antagonist naloxone, suggesting an important nonopioid mechanism.

Tramadol is structurally related to codeine and morphine and consists of two enantiomers, which contribute to analgesic activity via different mechanisms. The (+) entantiomer of tramadol and the metabolite (+)-O-desmethyl-tramadol are agonists of the mu opioid receptor. Furthermore, (+)-tramadol inhibits serotonin reuptake, while (−)-tramadol inhibits norepinephrine reuptake. Tramadol's different mechanisms are likely working in additive or synergistic fashion to improve the analgesic efficacy and tolerability.

NON-OPIOIDS/CYCLOOXYGENASE INHIBITORS

NSAIDS

Mild to moderate pain is typically treated with nonsteroidal anti-inflammatory drugs (NSAIDs), such as ibuprofen and naproxen. NSAIDs are the most widely utilized drugs to treat pain associated with minor surgeries or injuries and disease. In general, these agents act to decreased exaggerated pain signaling (hyperalgesia) associated with tissue injury and inflammation, while having minimal effects on pain signaling per se (e.g., they have limited analgesic effects). Thus, NSAIDs are often highly efficacious to treat the pain following minor trauma or inflammatory conditions. In contrast, severe acute and chronic pain, such neuropathic pain, appears to be less sensitive to these drugs.

The common mechanism shared by all NSAID drugs is inhibition of cyclooxygenase (COX). COX is the rate-limiting enzyme in the production of prostaglandins, which are derived from C-20 unsaturated fatty acids, mainly arachidonic acid (Fig.34.1). Arachidonic acid is formed from membrane phospholipids by activation of phospholipase A2. COX converts arachidonic acid to prostaglandin H2 (PGH2), which is subsequently catalyzed to PGD2, PGE2, PF2a and PGI2 by specific synthases for the different prostaglandins. In addition, COX catalyses the generation of thromboxanes, leukotrienes and lipoxins; together these substances are referred to as eicosanoids. The prostaglandins mediate their action by binding to specific membrane receptors (DP, EP, FP and IP) that are G-protein coupled receptors with seven transmembrane domains.

Two forms of COX, entitled COX-1 and COX-2, have been identified, sequenced and cloned. COX-1 is predominantly constitutively and expressed in most tissues, particularly in platelets, kidneys and stomach. The expression pattern of COX-1 indicates that this enzyme is responsible for production of prostaglandins involved in maintenance of gastric mucosal integrity and platelet function. In contrast, COX-2 is primarily associated with inflammation and is the inducible form localized to inflammatory cells and tissues. However, in the CNS, both constitutive and inducible forms of COX-2 appear to be present.

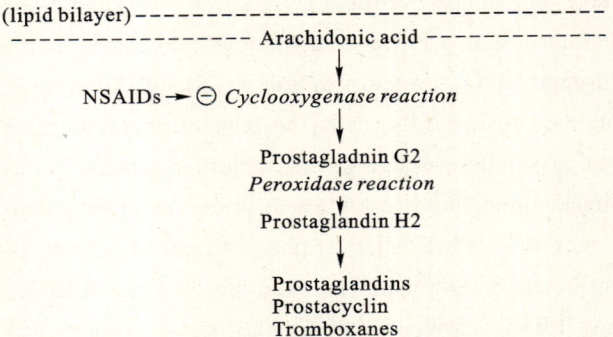

Fig.34.1 Schematic of prostaglandin production and NSAIDs action.

Conventional NSAIDs inhibit both COX-1 and COX-2, with a tendency towards COX-1 preference. Since COX-1 appeared to be responsible for the GI side effects of NSAIDs and COX-2 was mediating the anti-inflammatory effects of NSAIDs, the last 10 years there have been very active efforts by pharmaceutical industry to develop COX-2 selective inhibitors with the goal of generating efficacious anti-inflammatory and analgesic agents without the GI liability. In addition to COX enzyme preference, NSAIDs vary according to the nature of the COX inhibition. For example, aspirin is an irreversible inhibitor of COX-1 and COX-2. Ibuprofen is a reversible and competitive inhibitor of COX-1 and COX-2. Indomethacin is a slow, time-dependent, reversible inhibitor of COX-1 and COX-2. Celecoxib and Rofecoxib are slow, time-dependent, irreversible inhibitors of COX-2.

Table 34.1 Examples of NSAIDs and COX selectivity.	
COX-1 and COX-2 active	**COX-2 selective**
ibuprofen	celecoxib
naproxen	rofecoxib
aspirin	valdecoxib
indomethacin	meloxicam
diclonfenac	
piroxicam	

While the analgesic property of NSAIDs is most likely explained by their COX inhibiting property, several authors have pointed out the dissociation between anti-inflammatory and analgesic potency and proposed additional mechanisms to account for the pain-relieving action. However, rather than additional mechanism, it appears clear that variable CNS penetration could explain at least some of the inconsistency.

Tissue injury and inflammation result in prostanoid production at the site of tissue injury and inflammation. Once released at the site of injury prostaglandins act on prostaglandin receptors on primary afferent terminals to produce sensitization and behavioral hyperalgesia. In addition, tissue injury and inflammation is associated with elevated prostaglandin levels and an induction of COX-2 at the level of the spinal cord. Thus, prostaglandins may not only produce sensitization in the periphery, but also contribute to sensitization mechanisms at the spinal cord level — a phenomenon often referred to as central sensitization. Taken together, these data support the idea that NSAIDs anti-inflammatory action is a result of COX inhibition in peripheral tissues, whereas NSAIDs analgesic effect is mediated via reduction of pro-nociceptive prostaglandins both in the periphery and CNS.

COX-2 Inhibitors

The discovery of COX-2 in the early 1990s resulted in renewed interest in COX / NSAID pharmacology and the development of COX-2 selective drugs. COX-2 inhibitors quickly became established as important anti-inflammatory and pain-relieving therapeutics with potentially fewer side effects. Because of the upregulation of COX-2 after tissue injury and inflammation this enzyme has been thought to be the most important COX enzyme associated with pain and hyperalgesia. While COX-2 inhibitors reduce pain behaviors in rodent models, it is less clear if COX-2 inhibitors are as efficacious as non-selective COX-1/COX-2 inhibitors. Although there is clinical evidence for pain relief, it is not clear if COX-2 inhibitors possess any advantage over traditional NSAIDs for all types of pain. Further research is necessary to clarify the therapeutic potential of COX-2 inhibitors for the treatment of different types of pain.

Recent understanding of cardiovascular liability of COX inhibitors has clouded the excitement about these drugs. An increased relative risk for cardiovascular events, such as heart attack and stroke, was recently shown in large clinical trials for additional indications and this lead to the voluntary action of Merck to withdraw Vioxx (rofecoxib) from the market in the fall of 2004. While originally it was believed that the COX-2 was mainly an inducible enzyme involved in inflammation, studies in more recent years have indicated COX-2 in a number of physiological functions. It is likely that some of these functions are going to support the use of COX-2 inhibitors to prevent disease (certain cancers and CNS disorders), while others are going to define limitations and clinical utility in patients with renal and heart disease.

Acetaminophen

Acetaminophen (paracetamol) is one of the most commonly used drugs for the treatment of pain and fever. The mechanisms by which acetaminophen mediates its action has been highly debated. Acetaminophen does appear to be an inhibitor of COX, but the drug is not active in reducing peripheral inflammation, which is the hallmark activity of traditional NSAIDs. The anti-pyretic and analgesic effects of acetaminophen have been the basis for the suggestion that acetaminophen is particularly active in inhibiting COX enzymes in the CNS.

Two main theories exist for the cellular mechanisms of acetaminophens pharmacological activity. First, it has been proposed that acetaminophen blocks COX activity by interacting with another site than the active site of COX and via this mechanism reduce the active oxidized form of the enzyme to an inactive form. Second, it has been suggested that acetaminophen selectively inhibits another COX enzyme, specifically a splice variant of COX-1 labeled COX-3. However, genomic and kinetic analysis has not supported an interaction between acetaminophen and COX-3. Taken together, most data support that acetaminophen in one way or another mediates its action via an interaction with a COX enzyme at some location, although the cellular mechanism is distinct from NSAIDs.

NSAID Combinations

Inhibition of multiple pain pathways by combining analgesics with different mechanisms may provide more effective pain relief for a broader spectrum of pain. In addition, combinations may be associated with lower incidence of adverse drug reactions. Particularly, combining NSAIDs or acetaminophen with an analgesic that acts via a different mechanism, such as an opioid, may be beneficial and is often employed. While COX inhibitors represents the first step in the World Health Organizations scheme for the treatment of chronic (cancer) pain, mild opioids, such as codeine or oxycodone combined with an NSAIDs or acetaminophen, is recommended for the treatment of moderate pain. The rationale for the combination is not only to achieve potential benefits from using agents that act at different sites, peripheral and central, but also interaction between different pain pathways within the CNS. Experimental studies in animals have indicated a synergistic interaction between opioids and NSAIDs in the CNS.

ANTICONVULSANTS

The group of compounds referred to as anticonvulsant or antiepileptic drugs are also being used to treat pain, particularly neuropathic pain. Most of this use is off label. All these drugs were initially developed to treat epilepsy and were introduced on the market as antiepileptics. However, subsequently, preclinical and clinical studies have demonstrated that several of these agents are also valuable for the treatment of pain associated with nerve disorders. The first drugs to be shown to possess pain-relieving actions were the older anticonvulsants, carbamazepine and phenytoin. Recently, several newer anticonvulsants have been investigated in clinical trials and shown to be effective in treating neuropathic pain. Examples of anticonvulsants with pain-relieving effects in clinical and preclinical studies are presented in Table 34.2.

Table 34.2 Mechanisms of antinociceptive action of anticonvulsant drugs.	
Drug	Mechanisms
Carbamazepine	sodium channel inhibition
Felbamate	sodium channel block, decreased GABA inhibition and increased glutamate excitation
Gabapentin	calcium channel modulation, increased GABA turnover, GABAB receptor modulation
Lamotrigine	sodium and calcium channel blockade and inhibition of glutamate release
Lidocaine	sodium channel inhibition
Phenytoin	sodium and calcium channel inhibition
Pregabalin	calcium channel modulation and GABAB receptor modulation
Tiagabine	inhibition of GABA uptake by blockade of GAT1 GABA transporter
Topiramate	sodium/calcium channel and glutamate receptor modulation, increased GABA inhibition
Valproic acid	Sodium channel modulation, increased GABA turnover
Zonisamide	sodium and calcium (T-type) channel inhibition

The anticonvulsants represent a group of compounds with diverse chemical structures and different mechanisms of action. Several anticonvulsants are potent blockers of voltage-gated sodium channels, including carbamazepine, phenytoin, lamotrigine, topiramate and felbamate. Gabapentin is the only anticonvulsant approved for the treatment of neuropathic pain (postherpetic neuralgia) and its activity is thought to be a result of inhibition of voltage-sensitive calcium channels (via binding to the alpha2delta subunit) and modulation of the GABA system. Valproic acid appears to mediate its effect via several mechanisms, including modulation of sodium channels, calcium channels and GABA synthesis and turnover, while vigabatin is an irreversible inhibitor of GABA transaminase, which is an enzyme involved in GABA degradation. Some of the anticonvulsant agents that have been shown to reduce neuropathic pain are discussed below and the mechanisms of several anticonvulsants are summarized in Table 34.2.

Gabapentin

Gabapentin (1-(aminomethyl)cyclohexaneacetic acid, Neurontin®) is a lipophilic analog of GABA that initially was developed as an anticonvulsant and approved for certain types of epilepsy treatment in 1994. Clinical trials and experience with gabapentin indicated that the drug possessed additional therapeutic advantages. To date, a number of clinical studies have demonstrated pain-relieving effect of gabapentin, specifically against neuropathic pain. In randomized controlled clinical trials, gabapentin has shown significant pain relief against painful diabetic neuropathy and postherpetic neuralgia. In the US, Neurontin® (gabapentin) is indicated for the management of postherpetic neuralgia in adults, in addition to epilepsy (as adjunctive therapy in the treatment of partial seizures).

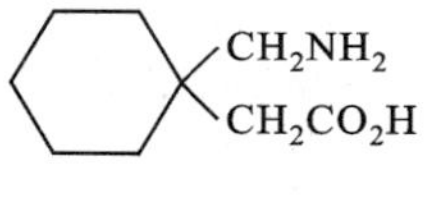

Fig.34.2   Structure of Gabapentin.

While gabapentin's effectiveness in treating neuropathic pain has been proved in several clinical trials, the mechanisms of action are still debated. Several reviews of gabapentin's pharmacology and mechanisms of action have been published. The hypotheses that have been proposed to explain gabapentin's pharmacological activity include modulation of calcium channels, reduction of neurotransmitter release, increase of GABA synthesis and release, and GABAB receptor actions (Table 34.2).

Gabapentin interacts with a high affinity binding site in brain membranes that has been identified as an accessory alpha2delta subunit of voltage-gated calcium channels. Functional effects of gabapentin binding to the alpha2delta subunit include inhibitory actions of gabapentin on voltage-gated calcium channels and inhibition of calcium influx into synaptosomes. Furthermore, nerve injury-evoked changes in alpha2delta subunit expression in the spinal cord and DRG of rats corresponds to pain-related behaviors and efficacy of gabapentin.

Gabapentin also appears to activate, directly or indirectly, GABAB receptors, although others refute this finding. Specifically, gabapentin-evoked suppression of potassium-evoked calcium influx via voltage-dependent calcium channels was shown to be selectively inhibited by GABAB antagonism and dependent on functional GABAB gb1a-gb2 receptors. In another study, gabapentin was shown to act as a selective agonist at the gb1a-gb2 heterodimer and postsynaptic GABAB receptors, which couple to inwardly rectifying potassium channels.

Several studies have demonstrated an effect of gabapentin on neurotransmitter release. Gabapentin reduced the release of noradrenaline, dopamine and glutamate from various brain slice preparations. In addition, gabapentin was shown to inhibit glutamate release from rat brainstem slice preparations containing the spinal trigeminal caudal subnucleus. Gabapentin had no effect on baseline levels of potassium-evoked release of glutamate, while subtance P or CGRP-evoked facilitation of glutamate release via activation of PKC or adenylyl cyclase was inhibited by gabapentin.

While gabapentin clearly reduces facilitated neuronal signaling, it has minimal effect on physiological synaptic transmission. This is also consistent with the effect of gabapentin in animal models. A significant literature shows that gabapentin prevents exaggerated pain behaviors (allodynia and hyperalgesia) in several models of neuropathic pain in rats or mice (e.g. spinal nerve ligation models, streptozocin-induced diabetes model, spinal cord injury model, acute herpes zoster infection model). Gabapentin also decreases pain-like behavioral responses after peripheral inflammation (carrageenan or CFA-evoked inflammation, and 2nd phase formalin test). In contrast, gabapentin has little effects in acute models of pain.

Pregabalin

Pregabalin (Lyrica™) is a gabapentin-related compound that has a similar pharmacological profile to that of its developmental predecessor and binds the alpha2delta subunit of voltage-gated calcium channels with high affinity. Pregabalin exhibits robust effect in preclinical assays indicative of antiepileptic, anxiolytic, and antinociceptive efficacy. Developed by Pfizer, pregabalin received approval from the U.S. Food and Drug Administration (FDA) in January (2005) to market Lyrica™ for the management of neuropathic pain associated with diabetic peripheral neuropathy and postherpetic neuralgia.

Phenytoin And Carbamazepine

Phenytoin was the first anticonvulsant drug to be used to threat neuropathic pain. However, clinical studies show conflicting results regarding the efficacy of the drug. Carbamezepine is another anticonvulsant that in early clinical studies showed beneficial effect in the treatment of neuropathic pain. Initial evidence was demonstrated in patients with trigeminal neuralgia. Since then, several placebo controlled clinical trials have proved the usefulness of carbamazepine in treating neuropathic pain, including diabetic neuropathy, postherpetic neuralgia and trigeminal neuralgia. The main drawback with these older anticonvulsants the side effects, such as hepatic enzyme induction for both compounds, gingival hyperplasia for phenytoin and altered lipid levels, sex hormone and serum sodium concentrations for carbamazepine. Regarding mechanism of action, both phenytoin and carbamazepine most likely mediate their pain relieving effects via blockade of voltage-sensitive sodium channels.

Lamotrigine

Lamotrigine was introduced 1994 in the US as a treatment for epilepsy. Since then the drug has seen progressively greater application, including the treatment of pain, specifically neuropathic pain and psychiatric diseases, particularly the treatment of bipolar disorder. There is both preclinical and clinical evidence that lamotrigine is effective in treating neuropathic pain. Clinical efficacy of lamotrigine has been reported in patients with diabetic neuropathy, HIV-associated peripheral neuropathy, trigeminal neuralgia and some other neuropathic pain states. While lamotrigine is better tolerated compared to older anticonvulsants, the compound may induce a serious rash, however, decreasing the rate of dose escalation may decrease the incidence of side effects. The therapeutic effect of lamotrigine is mediated by inhibition of voltage-sensitive sodium and calcium channels, while the rash side effect is not thought to be target dependent.

Topiramate

Clinical studies have demonstrated that topiramate is effective in the treatment of neuropathic pain. In particular there is evidence for benefits treating pain associated with diabetic neuropathy, although some placebo-controlled studies have shown inconsistent effects. Experimental studies have showed that topiramate reduce pain-like behaviors in animals following nerve injury, although there is little evidence for neruroprotective effects of the agent. Topiramate's effect on neuropathic pain may be mediated via blocking action on voltage-sensitive sodium channels, but other mechanisms may contribute as well. In addition, topiramate appears to potentiate the inhibitory actions of GABA and modulate the activity of several ligand and voltage-sensitive ion channels, including voltage-sensitive Ca^{2+} channels, at least one type of K^+ channel and AMPA and kainate subtypes of glutamate receptors.

TRICYCLIC ANTIDEPRESSANTS

In addition to its effects on mood disorders, tricyclic antidepressant drugs (TCAs) may be effective in treating painful conditions such as neuropathic pain.

Clinical trials have shown superior pain relieving effects of TCAs compared to placebo or other antidepressants in patients with diabetic neuropathy and postherpetic neuralgia, but less efficacious in HIV-induced neuropathy. Additionally, TCAs have been shown to reduce other types of pain, including pain associated with arthritis, back pain and fibromyalgia. The efficacy of TCAs in neuropathic pain appears to be independent of the effect on depression.

Several mechanisms may contribute to the pain-relieving effects of TCAs. These include reuptake inhibition of noradrenaline and serotonin, blockade of ion channels and inhibition of NMDA adrenergic and cholinergic receptors. Particularly, TCAs that inhibit serotonin and/or noradrenaline uptake, such as amitriptyline and desipramine, have been used clinically to treat neuropathic pain. In contrast, selective serotonin reuptake inhibitors (SSRIs) appear to be less effective. The reason for TCAs effect in reducing neuropathic pain may be related to complex changes that occur in both ascending and descending pain pathways in the brain and spinal cord in persistent pain conditions. Serotonin and noradrenaline have been implicated in descending inhibitory pain pathways. In addition, several TCAs possess additional activities, specifically sodium channel blockade and NMDA receptor antagonism, which are mechanisms likely to significantly contribute to the analgesic effect TCAs in neuropathic pain states.

Amitriptyline

The TCA amitriptyline is widely used in treating chronic pain. Amitriptyline has been shown to reduce pain behaviors in number of preclinical pain models and several clinical trials have proven the drug efficacious in treating neuropathic pain, inflammatory pain and possibly some other pain conditions. While the antidepressive effect of amitriptyline is most likely related to its inhibitory action on monoamine re-uptake, the pain-relieving action may be related to a different mechanism. Amitriptyline is a potent inhibitor of voltage-sensitive sodium channels and its effect on pain may well be explained by this mechanism of ac-

tion. Thus, TCAs such as amitriptyline may be efficacious in reducing pain, specifically neuropathic pain, via a mechanism that is similar to that of many anticonvulsants, that is, inhibition of voltage-sensitive (sodium) ion channels.

SPINALLY DELIVERED AGENTS

Ziconotide

Ziconotide (Prialt®) was recently approved by the FDA for the management of severe chronic pain in patients or whom intrathecal therapy is warranted and who are intolerant or refractory to other treatment. Ziconotide is a synthetic version of the naturally occurring omega-conotoxin MVIIA. The mechanism of action underlying ziconotide's therapeutic effect derives from selective, potent and reversible inhibition of neuronal N-type voltage-sensitive calcium channels. N-type calcium channels are found throughout the nervous system. N-type calcium channels are the predominant calcium channels expressed on peptide containing small diameter nociceptive afferents and inhibition of pre-synaptic N-type calcium channels by ziconotide may regulate noxious-evoked neurotransmitter release in the spinal cord. In addition, post-synaptic N-type calcium channels located on cell bodies, dendritic spines shafts and spines may modulate neuronal excitability and plasticity.

Clonidine

Clonidine was originally used for the treatment of hypertension and migraine. A large number of preclinical studies have demonstrated analgesic efficacy of clonidine, in a wide range of animal models, particular following spinal administration. However, cardiovascular side effects limit its use. Clinical studies have shown that epidural clonidine is an effective pain treatment and has been approved of neuropathic cancer pain. The analgesic action of spinally delivered clonidine is most likely related to activation of alpha-2 adrenergic receptors.

Three different alpha-2 adrenergic receptor subtypes, alpha-2A, alpha-2B and alpha-2C, have been identified and all three subtypes are located in regions associated with the processing of nociceptive information, including the dorsal root ganglia and the superficial layers of the spinal cord dorsal horn. Experimental studies using mice with either a point mutation or a null mutation in the different alpha2 adrenergic receptors indicate that the analgesic effect of alpha-2 adrenergic agonists is mediated via an activation of alpha-2A adrenergic receptors. Unfortunately, systemic side effects produced by alpha-2 adrenergic agonists, such as sedation and hypothermia, is also mediated by the alpha-2A adrenergic receptor subtype. Since the majority of alpha-2A adrenergic receptors in the spinal cord are located on peptide containing primary afferents neurons that terminate in the dorsal horn, alpha-2 adrenergic-induced analgesia may involve inhibition of peptide release at these terminals, possibly via an action on N-type calcium channels. In addition, alpha-2 adrenergic agonists may mediate analgesia by postsynaptic inhibitory mechanisms, via alpha-2 adrenergic receptors expressed on pain projection neurons.

TOPICALLY APPLIED AGENTS

Lidocaine

The lidocaine patch (Lidoderm®) is a topical treatment that was approved ~5 years ago for the treatment of postherpetic neuralgia. While systemic doses of lidocaine may produce cardiovascular effects, the 5% lidocaine patch is a transdermal treatment that results in insignificant serum levels even with chronic use. Clinical studies have supported the use of the lidocaine patch for additional chronic neuropathic pain conditions other than postherpetic neuralgia.

Lidocaine is an amide-type local anesthetic that mediates its effect by blocking sodium channels expressed on peripheral neurons, which results in decreased excitability in peripheral nociceptors. The structure of lidocaine is presented in Fig.34.3. Sodium channels are fundamentally involved in sensory neuron physiology and pathophysiology, including normal and abnormal pain signaling. The lidocaine patch

typically reduces pain associated with hypersensitivity of primary afferents, that is, when the pain results from a peripheral problem. In contrast, patients in which the pain is a result of small fiber deafferentation and a more centrally located underlying mechanisms, the pain may be more resistant to peripheral treatments, including topical lidocaine.

One of the mechanisms underlying neuropathic pain appears to be nerve injury-induced abnormal sodium channel expression and function followed by hyperexcitability in primary afferents neurons. While lidocaine non-selectively inhibit sodium channels and affect normal sensitivity as well as pain, academic and industry research over the last decade have focused on characterizing the sodium channels that are involved in abnormal neuronal excitability and firing after nerve injury. The ultimate goal is to develop novel therapeutics for the treatment of pain, while leaving normal sensation intact.

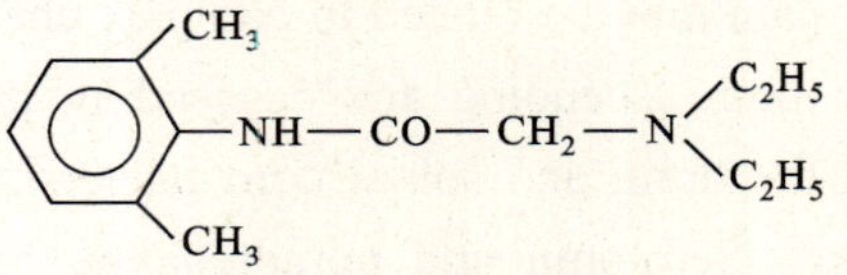

Fig.34.3   Structure of Lidocaine

Capsaicin

Capsaicin has been used as topical treatment of a variety of pain conditions for over a century. Several capsaicin-containing creams, lotions and patches are sold without prescription. These products typically contain 0.025%–0.09% capsaicin or mixtures of capsaicin and capsaicin-related compounds such as dihydrocapsaicin and homohydrocapsaicin. Clinical studies have shown that topical applications of capsaicin creams three to four times daily for two to six weeks produce pain relief, particularly for conditions such as postherpetic neuralgia, diabetic neuropathy and osteoarthritis. However, a recent meta analysis concluded that topically applied capsaicin has moderate to poor efficacy in the treatment of chronic musculoskeletal or neuropathic pain but may be useful in patients who do not respond to or tolerate other treatments.

Capsaicin mediates its effect by activating the

transient receptor potential type 1 (TRPV1) receptor, a ligand-gated, non-selective, cation channel preferentially expressed in small-diameter, primary afferent neurons. The initial effect of topical capsaicin application is activation of cutaneous nociceptive afferent fibers, resulting in a burning sensation, hyperalgesia, allodynia, and erythema. The induction of edema is due to the release of vasoactive neuropeptides, such as GCRP or substance P, from small-diameter primary afferents, and this effect is commonly referred to as neurogenic inflammation. After prolonged exposure to capsaicin, there is not only a loss of sensitivity to capsaicin, but also loss of responsiveness to heat and noxious stimulation. These effects of persistent capsaicin treatment are frequently referred to as "desensitization", although this terminology has been used to both describe the cellular effects (e.g., tachyphylaxis of the TRPV1 receptor) and psychophysical reports of reduced pain sensitivity in humans following prolonged capsaicin exposure.

The mechanisms underlying pain relief following repeated application of capsaicin cream appears to be a result of alterations in the peripheral nerve ending in the skin. An experimental study in human subjects demonstrated that the onset of analgesic effect of repeated applications of capsaicin cream correlates with loss of immunocytochemical markers for the peripheral endings of small-diameter afferent nerves that are found in the epidermis. The authors also showed that discontinuation of the capsaicin treatment resulted in apparent re-innervation of the epidermis and a return of the ability to detect noxious sensations. While topical capsaicin alters peripheral primary afferent nerve endings, the cell bodies in DRG and the majority of the neuron remains intact.

Since topical application of capsaicin produces a burning sensation and burning may be a particular problem in those patients with intact primary afferent a main problem with topical capsaicin treatment is compliance. This is unfortunately since these patients may benefit the most from capsaicin treatment. Recently, it has been indicated that long lasting pain relief may be obtained by using higher doses of capsai-

cin applied for shorter periods.

Since topical application of capsaicin produces a burning sensation a main problem with capsaicin treatment is compliance. It is particularly unfortunate that those patients who may benefit the most from the capsaicin treatment may experience the most burning. Recently, it has been indicated that long lasting pain relief may be obtained by using higher doses of capsaicin applied for shorter periods.

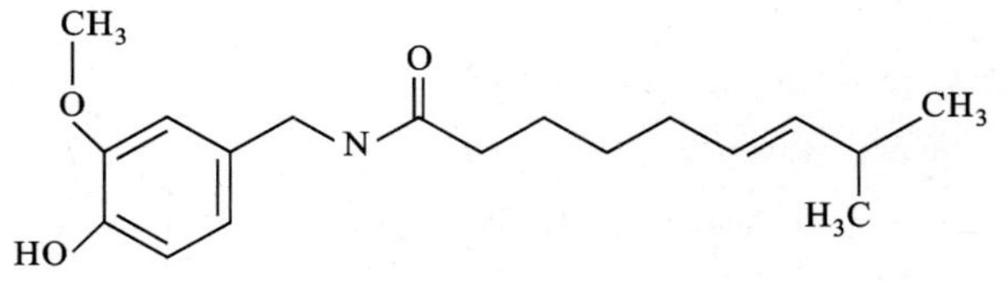

Fig.34.4   Structure of Capsaicin.

CONCLUSIONS

Limitations of pharmacological treatments for persistent pain conditions continue to be a major clinical problem. Several of the traditional treatments are limited by efficacy, tolerability and abuse/diversion liability. The most commonly used pain drugs were discovered a long time ago and very few new therapies have recently entered the market. Furthermore, pharmacological agents that are currently used to treat for neuropathic pain conditions were originally developed for other CNS disorders, such as epilepsy and depression. Although these drugs have contributed to the understanding of mechanisms underlying neuropathic pain, improved therapies for neuropathic pain are necessary. Current research focuses on trying to understand the mechanisms involved in pain transmission and changes that occur in pain pathways after injury in order to identify improved targets to treat chronic pain conditions. Clearly experience from both clinical practice and basic research is critical for both better utility of current pain drugs and the development of new therapies.

GENERAL CITATIONS

Backonja M. 2004. Neuromodulating drugs for the symptomatic treatment of neuropathic pain. *Curr Pain Headache*

Rep, 8(3):212-216.

Graham GG, Scott KF. 2005. Mechanism of action of paracetamol. *Am J Ther*, 12(1):46-55.

Hinz B, Brune K. 2002. Cyclooxygenase-2—10 years later. *J Pharmacol Exp Ther*, 300(2):367-375.

Martin TJ, Eisenach JC. 2001. Pharmacology of opioid and nonopioid analgesics in chronic pain states. *J Pharmacol Exp Ther*, 299(3):811-817.

McCleane G. 2003. Pharmacological management of neuropathic pain. *CNS Drugs*, 17(14):1031-1043.

McCormack K, Brune K. 1991. Dissociation between the antinociceptive and anti-inflammatory effects of the nonsteroidal anti-inflammatory drugs: a survey of their analgesic efficacy. *Drugs*, 41(4):533-547.

Miljanich GP. 2004. Ziconotide: neuronal calcium channel blocker for treating severe chronic pain. *Curr Med Chem*, 11(23):3029-3040.

Priestley T. 2004. Voltage-gated sodium channels and pain. *Curr Drug Targets CNS Neurol Disord*, 3(6):441-456.

Rogawski MA, Loscher W. 2004. The neurobiology of antiepileptic drugs for the treatment of nonepileptic conditions. *Nat Med*, 10(7):685-692.

Rogawski MA, Loscher W. 2004. The neurobiology of antiepileptic drugs. *Nat Rev Neurosci*, 5(7):553-564.

Sindrup SH, Jensen TS. 1993. Efficacy of pharmacological treatments of neuropathic pain: an update and effect related to mechanism of drug action. *Pain*, 83(3):389-400.

Stein C, Machelska H, Binder W, Schafer M. 2001. Peripheral opioid analgesia. *Curr Opin Pharmacol*, 1(1):62-65.

Szallasi A, Blumberg PM. 1999. Vanilloid (capsaicin) receptors and mechanisms. *Pharmacol Rev*, 51:159-211.

Taylor CP. 1997. Mechanisms of action of gabapentin. *Rev Neurol (Paris)*, 153 (Suppl 1):S39-45.

Vane JR, Bakhle YS, Botting RM. 1998. Cyclooxygenases 1 and 2. *Annu Rev Pharmacol Toxicol*, 38:97-120.

Wood JN, Boorman JP, Okuse K, Baker MD. 2004. Voltage-gated sodium channels and pain pathways. *J Neurobiol*, 61(1):55-71.

DISCOVERY CITATIONS

Argoff CE. 2000. New analgesics for neuropathic pain: the lidocaine patch. *Clin J Pain*, 16(2 Suppl): S62-66.

Caterina MJ, Schumacher MA, Tominaga M, Rosen TA, Levine JD, Julius D. 1997. The capsaicin receptor: a heat-activated ion channel in the pain pathway. *Nature*, 389(6653):816-824.

Hunter JC, Fontana DJ, Hedley LR, Jasper JR, Lewis R, Link RE, Secchi R, Sutton J, Eglen RM. 1997. Assessment of the role of alpha2-adrenoceptor subtypes in the antinociceptive, sedative and hypothermic action of dexmedetomidine in transgenic mice. *Br J Pharmacol*, 122(7): 1339-1344.

Hunter JC, Gogas KR, Hedley LR, Jacobson LO, Kassotakis L, Thompson J, Fontana DJ. 1997. The effect of novel anti-epileptic drugs in rat experimental models of acute and chronic pain. *Eur J Pharmacol*, 324(2-3):153-160.

Kieffer BL, Gaveriaux-Ruff C. 2002. Exploring the opioid system by gene knockout. *Prog Neurobiol*, 66(5):285-306.

Kuo CC. 1998. A common anticonvulsant binding site for phenytoin, carbamazepine, and lamotrigine in neuronal Na^+ channels. *Mol Pharmacol*, 54(4): 712-721.

Law PY, Wong YH, Loh HH. 2000. Molecular mechanisms and regulation of opioid receptor signaling. *Annu Rev Pharmacol Toxicol*, 40: 389-430.

Lucas R, Warner TD, Vojnovic I, Mitchell JA. 2005. Cellular mechanisms of acetaminophen: role of cyclo-oxygenase. *FASEB J*, 19(6):635-637.

Luo ZD, Calcutt NA, Higuera ES, Valder CR, Song YH, Svensson CI, Myers RR. 2002. Injury type- specific calcium channel alpha 2 delta-1 subunit up-regulation in rat neuropathic pain models correlates with antiallodynic effects of gabapentin. *J Pharmacol Exp Ther*, 303(3): 1199-1205.

Nolano M, Simone DA, Wendelschafer-Crabb G, Johnson T, Hazen E, Kennedy WR. 1999. Topical capsaicin in humans: parallel loss of epidermal nerve fibers and pain sensation. *Pain*, 81: 135-145.

Shank RP, Gardocki JF, Streeter AJ, Maryanoff BE. 2004. An overview of the preclinical aspects of topiramate: pharmacology, pharmacokinetics, and mechanism of action. *Epilepsia*, 41 (Suppl 1):S3-9.

Wang GK, Russell C, Wang SY. 2004. State-dependent block of voltage-gated Na^+ channels by amitriptyline via the local anesthetic receptor and its implication for neuropathic pain. *Pain*, 110(1-2):166-174.

Selected References

1. Casey KL. 1971. Somatosensory responses of bulboreticular units in awake cat: relation to escape-producing stimuli. *Science*, 173: 77-80.

2. Yaksh TL and Rudy TA. 1976. Analgesia mediated by a direct spinal action of narcotics. *Science*, 192: 1357-1358.

3. Hosobuchi Y, Rossier J, Bloom FE, Guillemin R. 1979. Stimulation of human periaqueductal gray for pain relief increases immunoreactive beta-endorphin in ventricular fluid. *Science*, 203: 279-281.

4. Lewis JW, Cannon JT, Liebeskind JC. 1980. Opioid and nonopioid mechanisms of stress analgesia. *Science*, 208: 623-625.

5. Yaksh TL, Jessell TM, Gamse R, Mudge AW, Leeman SE. 1980. Intrathecal morphine inhibits substance P release from mammalian spinal cord *in vivo*. *Nature*, 286: 155-157.

6. Meyer RA and Campbell JN. 1981. Myelinated nociceptive afferents account for the hyperalgesia that follows a burn to the hand. *Science*, 213: 1527-1529.

7. Woolf CJ. 1983. Evidence for a central component of post-injury pain hypersensitivity. *Nature*, 306: 686-688.

8. Yoshimura M and North RA. 1983. Substantia gelatinosa neurones hyperpolarized *in vitro* by enkephalin. *Nature*, 305: 529-530.

9. Sato J and Perl ER. 1991. Adrenergic excitation of cutaneous pain receptors induced by peripheral nerve injury. *Science*, 251: 1608-1610.

10. Talbot JD, Marrett S, Evans AC, Meyer E, Bushnell MC, Duncan GH. 1991. Multiple representations of pain in human cerebral cortex. *Science*, 251: 1355-1358.

11. Trujillo KA and Akil H. 1991. Inhibition of morphine tolerance and dependence by the NMDA receptor antagonist MK-801. *Science*, 251: 85-87.

12. Malmberg AB and Yaksh TL. 1992. Hyperalgesia mediated by spinal glutamate or substance P receptor blocked by spinal cyclooxygenase inhibition. *Science*, 257: 1276-1279.

13. Ingram SL and Williams JT. 1994. Opioid inhibition of Ih via adenylyl cyclase. *Neuron*, 13: 179-186.

14. Taddese A, Nah SY, McCleskey EW. 1995. Selective opioid inhibition of small nociceptive neurons. *Science*, 270: 1366-1369.

15. Flor H, Elbert T, Knecht S, Wienbruch C, Pantev C, Birbaumer N, Larbig W, Taub E. 1995. Phantom-limb pain as a perceptual correlate of cortical reorganization following arm amputation. *Nature*, 375: 482-484.

16. Strassman AM, Raymond SA, Burstein R. 1996. Sensitization of meningeal sensory neurons and the origin of headaches. *Nature*, 384: 560-564.

17. Craig AD, Reiman EM, Evans A, Bushnell MC. 1996. Functional imaging of an illusion of pain. *Nature* 384: 258-260.

18. Rainville P, Duncan GH, Price DD, Carrier B, Bushnell MC. 1997. Pain affect encoded in human anterior cingulate but not somatosensory cortex. *Science*, 277: 968-971.

19. Caterina MJ, Schumacher MA, Tominaga M, Rosen TA, Levine JD, Julius D. 1997. The capsaicin receptor: a heat-activated ion channel in the pain pathway. *Nature*, 389: 816-824.

20. Gu JG and MacDermott AB. 1997. Activation of ATP P2X receptors elicits glutamate release from sensory neuron synapses. *Nature*, 389: 749-753.

21. Pan ZZ, Tershner SA, Fields HL. 1997. Cellular mechanism for anti-analgesic action of agonists of the kappa-opioid receptor. *Nature*, 389: 382-385.

22. Tominaga M, Caterina MJ, Malmberg AB, Rosen TA, Gilbert H, Skinner K, Raumann BE, Basbaum AI, Julius D. 1998. The cloned capsaicin receptor integrates multiple

482   Selected References

pain-producing stimuli. *Neuron*, 21: 531-543.

23. Meng ID, Manning BH, Martin WJ, Fields HL. 1998. An analgesia circuit activated by cannabinoids. *Nature*, 395: 381-383.

24. Li P and Zhuo M. 1998. Silent glutamatergic synapses and nociception in mammalian spinal cord. *Nature*, 393: 695-698.

25. De Felipe C, Herrero JF, O'Brien JA, Palmer JA, Doyle CA, Smith AJ, Laird JM, Belmonte C, Cervero F, Hunt SP. 1998. Altered nociception, analgesia and aggression in mice lacking the receptor for substance P. *Nature*, 392: 394-397.

26. Ji RR, Baba H, Brenner GJ, Woolf CJ. 1999. Nociceptive-specific activation of ERK in spinal neurons contributes to pain hypersensitivity. *Nat Neurosci*, 2: 1114-1119.

27. Li P, Kerchner GA, Sala C, Wei F, Huettner JE, Sheng M, Zhuo M. 1999a. AMPA receptor-PDZ interactions in facilitation of spinal sensory synapses. *Nat Neurosci*, 2: 972-977.

28. Hutchison WD, Davis KD, Lozano AM, Tasker RR, Dostrovsky JO. 1999. Pain-related neurons in the human cingulate cortex. *Nat Neurosci*, 2: 403-405.

29. Lewin MR and Walters ET. 1999. Cyclic GMP pathway is critical for inducing long-term sensitization of nociceptive sensory neurons. *Nat Neurosci* 2: 18-23.

30. Caterina MJ, Rosen TA, Tominaga M, Brake AJ, Julius D. 1999. A capsaicin-receptor homologue with a high threshold for noxious heat. *Nature*, 398: 436-441.

31. Li P, Wilding TJ, Kim SJ, Calejesan AA, Huettner JE, Zhuo M. 1999b. Kainate-receptor-mediated sensory synaptic transmission in mammalian spinal cord. *Nature*, 397: 161-164.

32. Caterina MJ, Leffler A, Malmberg AB, Martin WJ, Trafton J, Petersen-Zeitz KR, Koltzenburg M, Basbaum AI, Julius D. 2000. Impaired nociception and pain sensation in mice lacking the capsaicin receptor. *Science*, 288: 306-313.

33. Craig AD, Chen K, Bandy D, Reiman EM. 2000. Thermosensory activation of insular cortex. *Nat Neurosci*, 3: 184-190.

34. Pan Z, Hirakawa N, Fields HL. 2000. A cellular mechanism for the bidirectional pain-modulating actions of orphanin FQ/nociceptin. *Neuron*, 26: 515-522.

35. Souslova V, Cesare P, Ding Y, Akopian AN, Stanfa L, Suzuki R, Carpenter K, Dickenson A, Boyce S, Hill R, *et al.* 2000. Warm-coding deficits and aberrant inflammatory pain in mice lacking P2X3 receptors. *Nature*, 407: 1015-1017.

36. Cockayne DA, Hamilton SG, Zhu QM, Dunn PM, Zhong Y, Novakovic S, Malmberg AB, Cain G, Berson A, Kasso-takis L, *et al.* 2000. Urinary bladder hyporeflexia and reduced pain-related behaviour in P2X3-deficient mice. *Nature*, 407: 1011-1015.

37. Bhave G, Karim F, Carlton SM, Gereau RWT. 2001. Peripheral group I metabotropic glutamate receptors modulate nociception in mice. *Nat Neurosci*, 4: 417-423.

38. Wei F, Wang GD, Kerchner GA, Kim SJ, Xu HM, Chen ZF, Zhuo M. 2001. Genetic enhancement of inflammatory pain by forebrain NR2B overexpression. *Nat Neurosci*, 4: 164-169.

39. Becerra L, Breiter HC, Wise R, Gonzalez RG, Borsook D. 2001. Reward circuitry activation by noxious thermal stimuli. *Neuron*, 32: 927-946.

40. Wei F, Qiu CS, Liauw J, Robinson DA, Ho N, Chatila T, Zhuo M. 2002a. Calcium calmodulin-dependent protein kinase IV is required for fear memory. *Nat Neurosci*, 5: 573-579.

41. Viana F, de la Pena E, Belmonte C. 2002. Specificity of cold thermotransduction is determined by differential ionic channel expression. *Nat Neurosci*, 5: 254-260.

42. Wei F, Qiu CS, Kim SJ, Muglia L, Maas JW, Pineda VV, Xu HM, Chen ZF, Storm DR, Muglia L J, Zhuo M. 2002b. Genetic elimination of behavioral sensitization in mice lacking calmodulin-stimulated adenylyl cyclases. *Neuron*, 36: 713-726.

43. Bhave G, Zhu W, Wang H, Brasier DJ, Oxford GS, Gereau RWT. 2002. cAMP-dependent protein kinase regulates desensitization of the capsaicin receptor (VR1) by direct phosphorylation. *Neuron*, 35: 721-731.

44. Lorenz J, Cross D, Minoshima S, Morrow T, Paulson P, Casey K. 2002. A unique representation of heat allodynia in the human brain. *Neuron*, 35: 383-393.

45. Ikeda H, Heinke B, Ruscheweyh R, Sandkuhler J. 2003. Synaptic plasticity in spinal lamina I projection neurons that mediate hyperalgesia. *Science*, 299: 1237-1240.

46. Dina OA, McCarter GC, de Coupade C, Levine JD. 2003. Role of the sensory neuron cytoskeleton in second messenger signaling for inflammatory pain. *Neuron*, 39: 613-624.

47. Bao L, Jin SX, Zhang C, Wang LH, Xu ZZ, Zhang FX, Wang LC, Ning FS, Cai HJ, Guan JS, *et al.* 2003. Activation of delta opioid receptors induces receptor insertion and neuropeptide secretion. *Neuron*, 37: 121-133.

48. Immke DC and McCleskey EW. 2003. Protons open acid-sensing ion channels by catalyzing relief of Ca^{2+} blockade. *Neuron*, 37: 75-84.

49. Coull JA, Boudreau D, Bachand K, Prescott SA, Nault F, Sik A, de Koninck P, de Koninck Y. 2003. Trans-synaptic

shift in anion gradient in spinal lamina I neurons as a mechanism of neuropathic pain. *Nature*, 424: 938-942.

50. Tsuda M, Shigemoto-Mogami Y, Koizumi S, Mizokoshi A, Kohsaka S, Salter MW, Inoue K. 2003. P2X4 receptors induced in spinal microglia gate tactile allodynia after nerve injury. *Nature*, 424: 778-783.

51. Johansen JP and Fields HL. 2004. Glutamatergic activation of anterior cingulate cortex produces an aversive teaching signal. *Nat Neurosci*, 7: 398-403.

52. Hartmann B, Ahmadi S, Heppenstall PA, Lewin GR, Schott C, Borchardt T, Seeburg PH, Zeilhofer HU, Sprengel R, Kuner R. 2004. The AMPA receptor subunits GluR-A and GluR-B reciprocally modulate spinal synaptic plasticity and inflammatory pain. *Neuron*, 44: 637-650.

53. Hofstetter CP, Holmstrom NA, Lilja JA, Schweinhardt P, Hao J, Spenger C, Wiesenfeld-Hallin Z, Kurpad SN, Frisen J, Olson L. 2005. Allodynia limits the usefulness of intra-spinal neural stem cell grafts; directed differentiation improves outcome. *Nat Neurosci*, 8: 346-353.

Units in Pain Research

Pharmacology			
half effective dose	EC_{50}	$mol \cdot kg^{-1}$	molar(effective) concentration producing 50% of the maximum possible response
gram	G	g	1 gram is equal to one-thousandth (10^{-3}) of a kilogram
half inhibitory dose	IC_{50}	$mol \cdot kg^{-1}$	molar inhibitor dose reducing a control response by 50%
half lethal dose	LD_{50}	$mol \cdot kg^{-1}$	1 LD_{50} is equal to molar dose producing 50 % of lethal response
molar	M	$mol \cdot L^{-1}$	1 molar is equal to one mole of solute per liter of solution
		$mg \cdot kg^{-1}$	to inject an amount of drug (mg) per kilogram of body weight
microliter		μL	one million microliters makes one liter

Electrophysiology			
Ampere	A		1 ampere of current is defined as movement of 1 Coulomb of charge per second
Coulomb	C	$s \cdot A$	1 Coulomb is equal to the charge transferred in one second by a steady current of one Ampere
Farad	F	$m^{-2} \cdot kg^{-1} \cdot s^{4} \cdot A^{2}$	1 Farad is equal to the capacitance of a capacitor having an equal and opposite charge of 1 Coulomb on each plate and a potential difference of 1 Volt between the plates
Hertz	Hz	s^{-1}	1 Hertz equals to one cycle per second
Siemens	S	$m^{-2} \cdot kg^{-1} \cdot s^{3} \cdot A^{2}$	1 Seimens equals to the conductance of a conductor if an electrical potential difference of 1 Volt produces a 1 Ampere current in it
Volt	V	$m^{2} \cdot kg \cdot s^{-3} \cdot A^{-1}$	1 Volt is defined as the energy required to move 1 Coulomb a distance of 1 meter against a force of 1 Newton
Ohm	Ω	$m^{2} \cdot kg \cdot s^{-3} \cdot A^{-2}$	1 Ohm equals to the resistance of a conductor in which a current of one Ampere is produced by a potential of one Volt across its terminals

Molecular Biology			
base pair		bp	two nucleotides on opposite complementary DNA or RNA strands that are connected
kilobase		kb	1 kilo base =1000 base pairs
molecular weight	MW		the mass of one molecule of that substance, relative to the unified atomic mass unit
melting temperature	T_m		The temperature where 50% of the DNA is in a duplex form, 50% of the DNA has been denatured into single strands

Behavior			
centimeter	cm		Distance moved is measured in centimeters. One hundred centimeters make one meter
intraperitoneal injection	i.p.		injections that are made within the peritoneal cavity, an area that contains the abdominal organs
subcutaneous	s.c.		An injection made into the fatty layer of tissue just under the skin
seconds		s	Latency to a response is measured in seconds Sixty seconds make up one minute
% freezing		%	The percentage of time during a given period spent in freezing behavior, "freezing" is defined as a lack of any movement aside from respiration

Useful Websites for the Study of Pain

Society for Neuroscience

http://web.sfn.org/

FENS, the Federation of European Neuro-science Societies

http://fens.mdc-berlin.de/

International Association for the Study of Pain® (IASP)

http://www.iasp-pain.org/meetopen.html

American Pain Society

http://www.ampainsoc.org/

APS: The American Physical Society

http://www.aps.org/

National Institute of Neurological Disorders and Stroke

Chronic Pain: Hope Through Research

http://www.healthieryou.com/chronpn.html

Pain—Learn more from MedlinePlus

http://www.ninds.nih.gov/disorders/chronic_pain/chronic_pain.htm

List of Scientific Journals Publishing Studies in Pain

 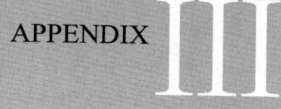

Nature
http://www.nature.com/index.html

Science
http://www.sciencemag.org/

Neuron
http://www.neuron.org/

Nature Neuroscience
http://www.nature.com/neuro/index.html

J Neuroscience
http://www.jneurosci.org/

European Journal of Neuroscience
http://www.blackwell-synergy.com/servlet/useragent?
func=showIssues&code=ejn

J Neurophysiology
http://jn.physiology.org/

J Physiology
http://jp.physoc.org/

JBC
http://www.jbc.org/

Journal of Pain
http://journals.elsevierhealth.com/periodicals/yjpai

Molecular Pain (first free online access journal)
http://www.molecularpain.com/articles/top/browse.asp

Pain
http://www.sciencedirect.com/science/journal/03043959

European J Pain
http://www.sciencedirect.com/science/journal/10903801

Neuroscience
http://www.sciencedirect.com/science/journal/03064522

Brain Research
http://www.sciencedirect.com/science/journal/00068993

Fundamental and Innovative Contribution to Understanding of Basic Mechanism of Pain, Analgesia and Persistent Pain

1965–1970

1965   Publication of the "gate control theory"

1970–1980

1971   Somatosensory responses of bulboreticular units in awake cat: relation to escape-producing stimuli

1973   Opiate binding sites in the brain are identified

1975   Anaesthetisation of prefrontal cortex and response to noxious stimulation

1976   Sensitization of nociceptors and discovers peripheral sensitization

1979   Descending inhibitory modulation of spinal nociception

1980–1990

1983   Morphine and enkephalin produced postsynaptic inhibitory effects in spinal cord dorsal horn neurons

1983   Central sensitization of dorsal horn neurons is shown to contribute to pain hypersensitivity, representing a major target for analgesic intervention

1987   C-fiber stimulation trigger dynamic receptive field plasticity in rat spinal cord dorsal horn

1990–2000

1990   Descending facilitatory system from the brainstem on spinal nociceptive transmission

1991   Multiple presentations of pain in human cerebral cortex

1994   Thermal grill illusion: unmasking the burn of cold pain

1995   Phantom-limb pain and cortical reorganization following arm amputation

1995   Selective opioid inhibition of small nociceptive neurons

1996   Sensitization of meningeal sensory neurons and the origin of headaches

1996   Kappa-opioids produce significantly greater analgesia in woman than in man, raising the sex-differences in analgesia in humans

1997   Cloning of the capsaicin receptor TRPV1

1997   Presynaptic ATP P2x receptor activation trigger glutamate release, making presynaptic P2X receptors as a possible target for pain therapy

1997   Pain affect is encoded in human ACC but not somatosensory cortex

1998   Silent glutamatergic synapses in spinal cord dorsal horn

1998 Phantom sensations generated by thalamic microstimulation

1999 Kainate receptor mediated nociceptive synapses transmission and modulation

1999 Pain responsive neurons in human ACC using electrophysiological recordings from humans

2000–present

2000 Warm-coding deficits and aberrant inflammatory pain in mice lacking P2X3 receptors

2001 Smart mice Doogie suffer more chronic pain, suggesting that NMDA NR2B receptors in the forebrain may serve as a target for treating chronic pain

2001 Reward circuitry activation by noxious thermal stimuli

2001 LTP in the ACC induced by a single digit amputation

2002 Calcium-stimulated AC1 and AC8 are required for neuropathic and inflammatory pain

2003 LTP in spinal lamina I projection neurons that mediate hyperalgesia

2003 Cytoskeleton as a critical regulator for pain plasticity

2003 Trans-synaptic shift in anion gradient contribute to neuropathic pain

2003 Spinal microglia was reported to be involved in nerve injury related allodynia

2003 Analgesia and hyperalgesia from GABA-mediated modulation of the cerebral cortex

2004 Glutamatergic activation of ACC produced an aversive teaching signal

2005 Stimulation in the ACC generated "fearful" memory in freely moving mice and inhibition of NMDA NR2B receptor attenuated the formation of fear

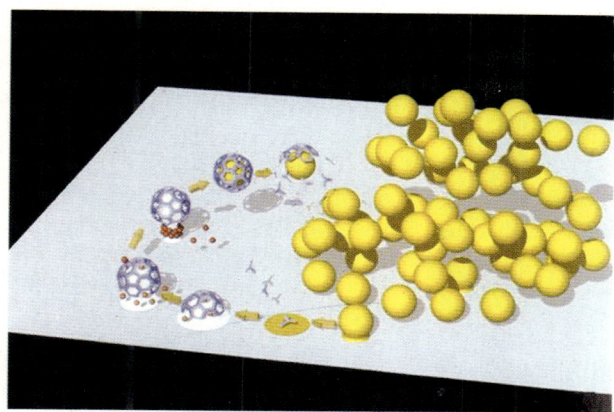

Fig.3.4 The model of clathrin-mediated endocytosis.

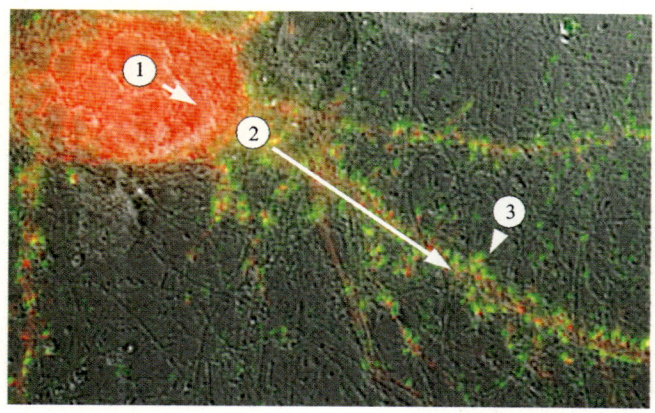

① Synthesis, Modification & Sorting   ② Trafficking   ③ Complex assembly, Specification of synaptic structure & function

Fig.6.2 The construction of excitatory synapses is thought to involve three successive processes.

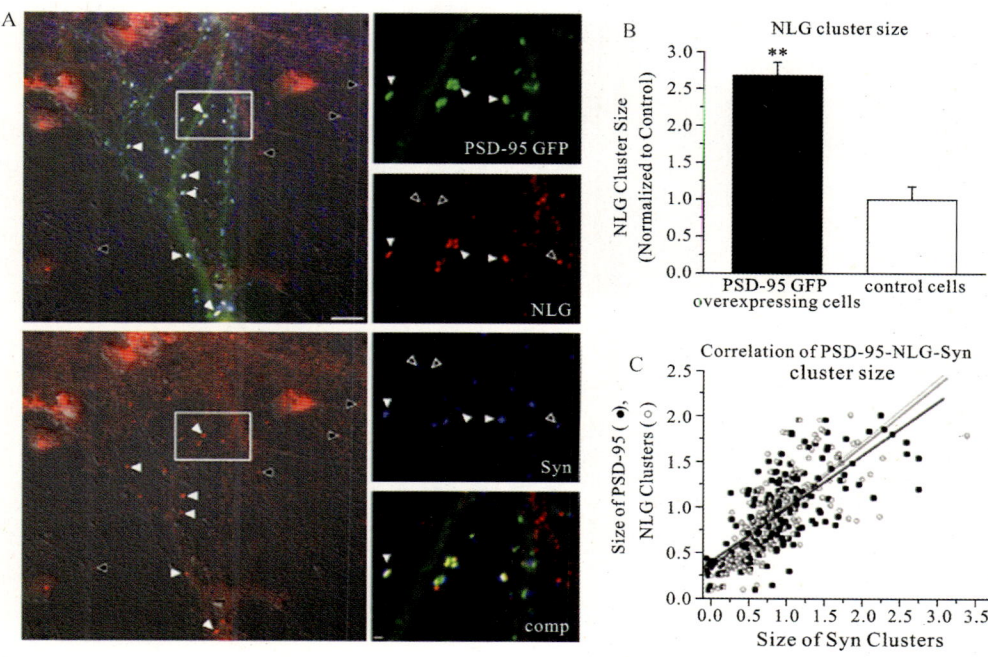

Fig.6.4 PSD-95 recruits neuroligins to the synapse and regulates presynaptic maturation.

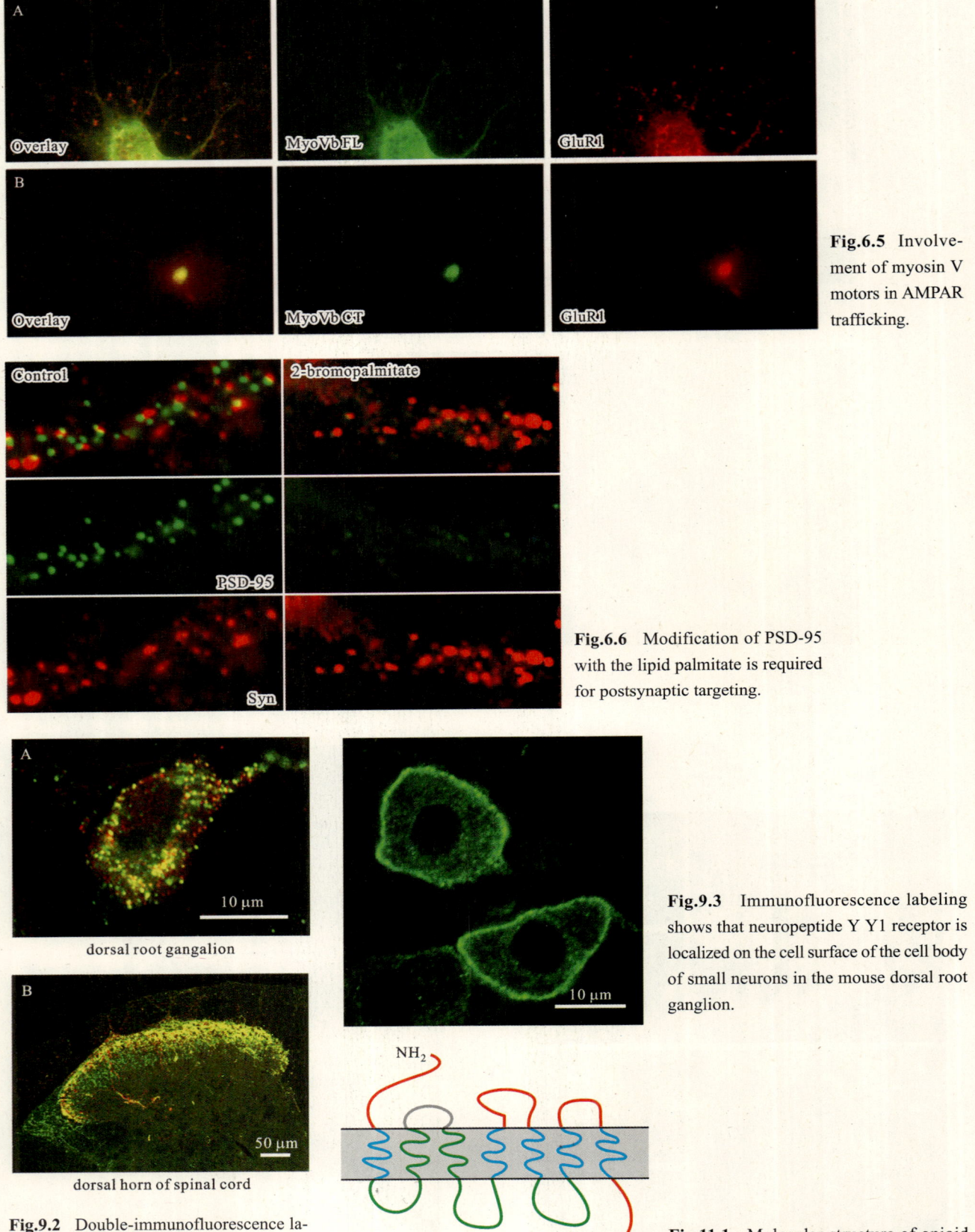

Fig.6.5 Involvement of myosin V motors in AMPAR trafficking.

Fig.6.6 Modification of PSD-95 with the lipid palmitate is required for postsynaptic targeting.

Fig.9.3 Immunofluorescence labeling shows that neuropeptide Y Y1 receptor is localized on the cell surface of the cell body of small neurons in the mouse dorsal root ganglion.

Fig.9.2 Double-immunofluorescence labeling shows colocalization of δ-opioid receptor.

Fig.11.1 Molecular structure of opioid receptors.

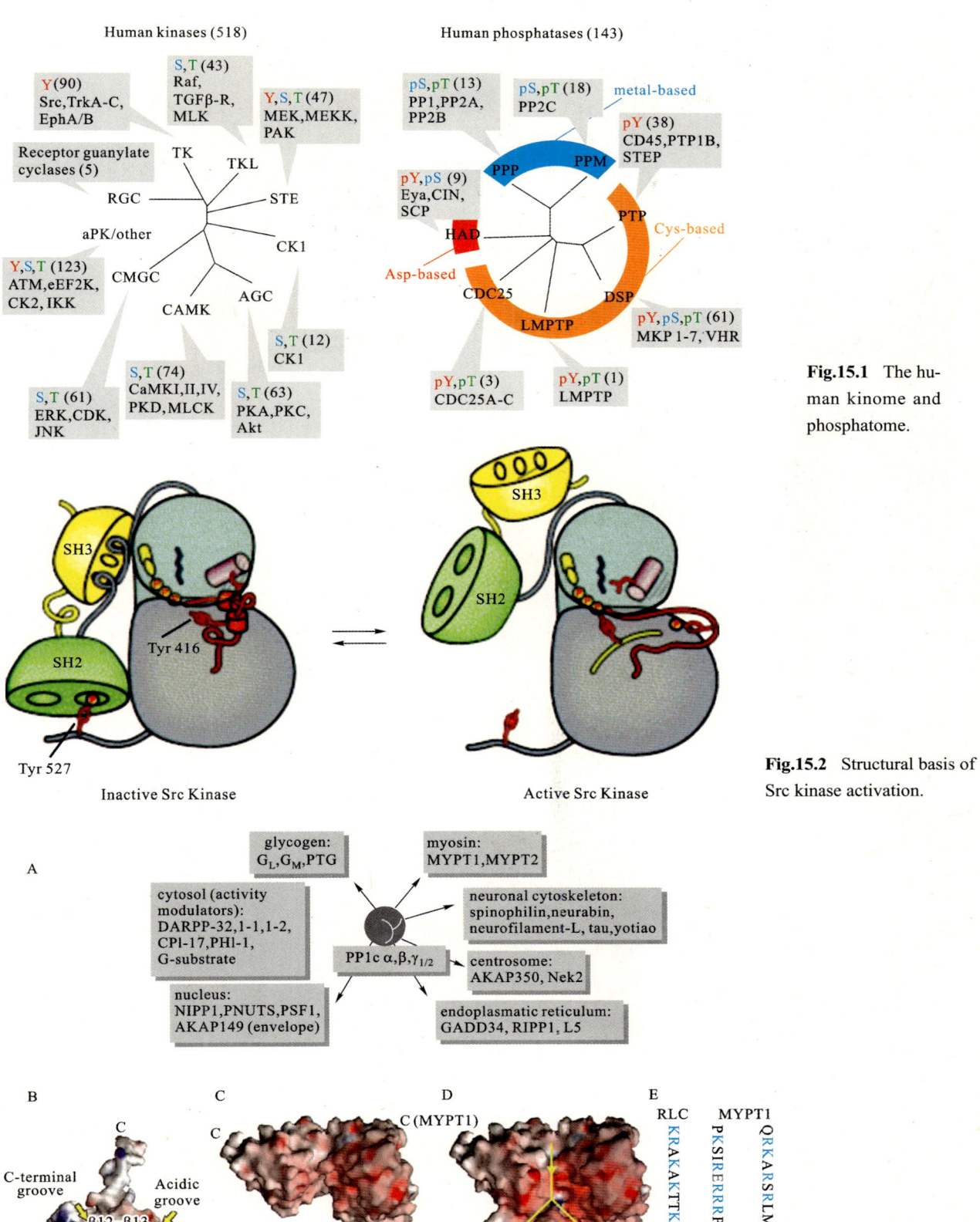

Fig.15.1 The human kinome and phosphatome.

Fig.15.2 Structural basis of Src kinase activation.

BOX 15.1 Structural basis of PP1 substrate specificity.

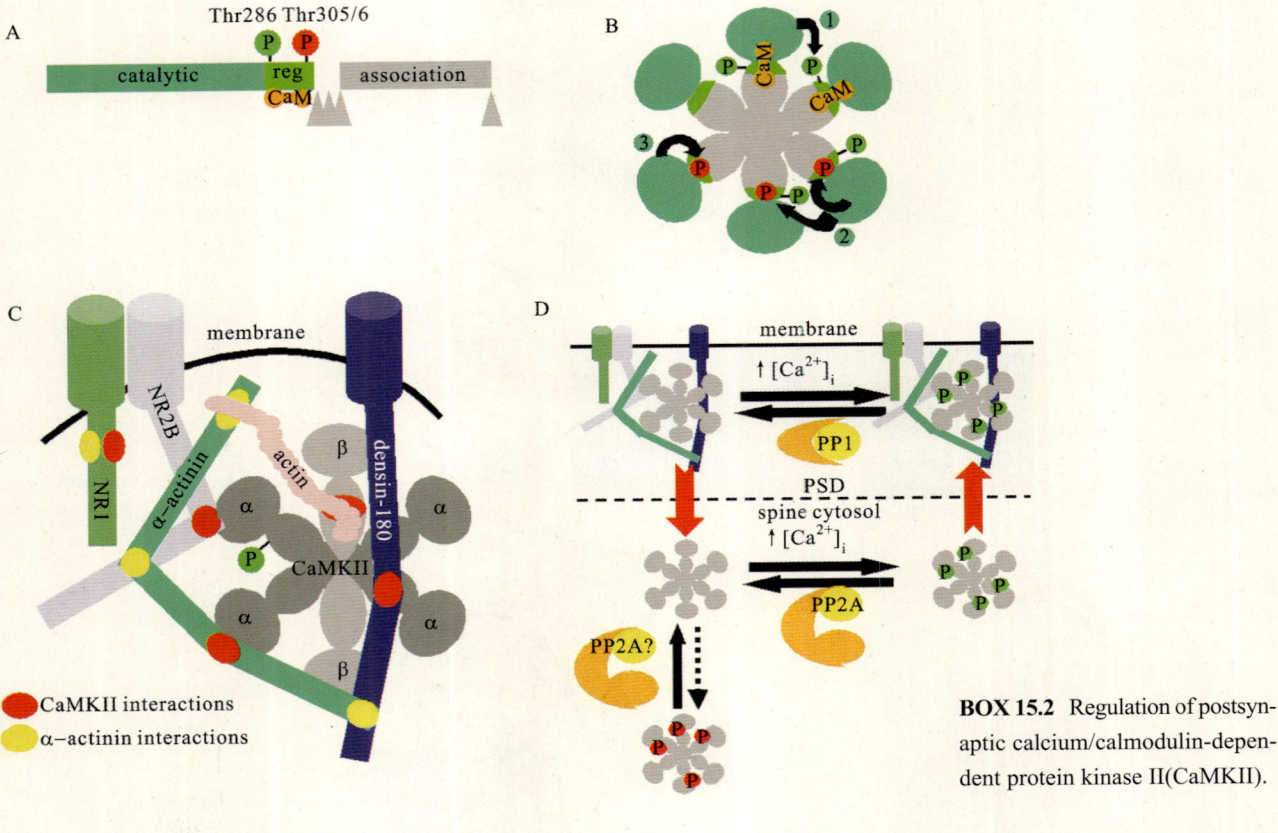

BOX 15.2 Regulation of postsynaptic calcium/calmodulin-dependent protein kinase II(CaMKII).

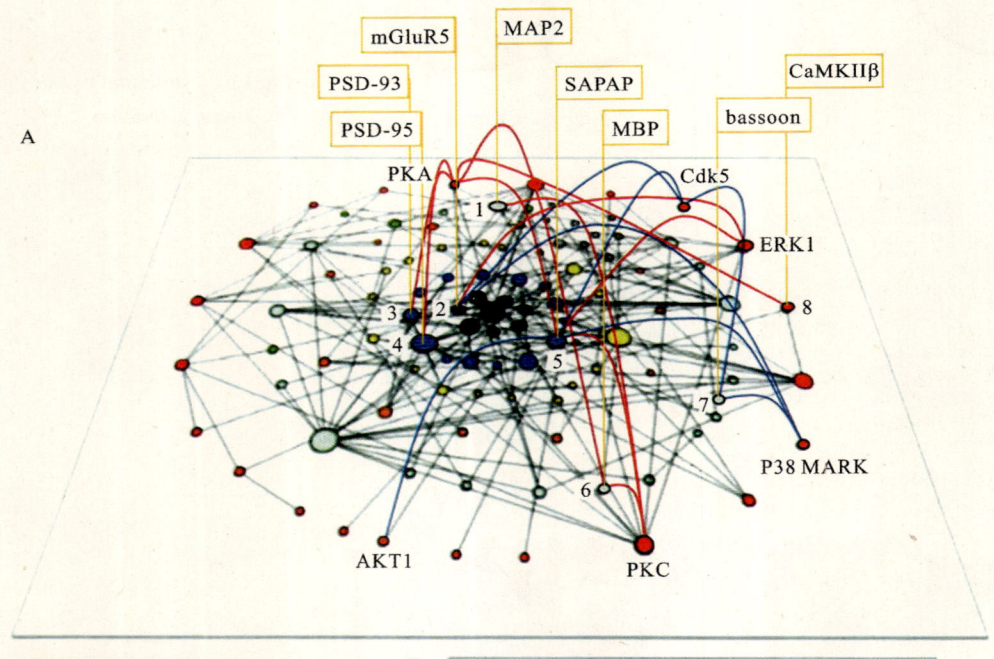

BOX 15.5 A protein-protein interaction and phosphorylation network centered on the NMDA-type glutamate receptor.

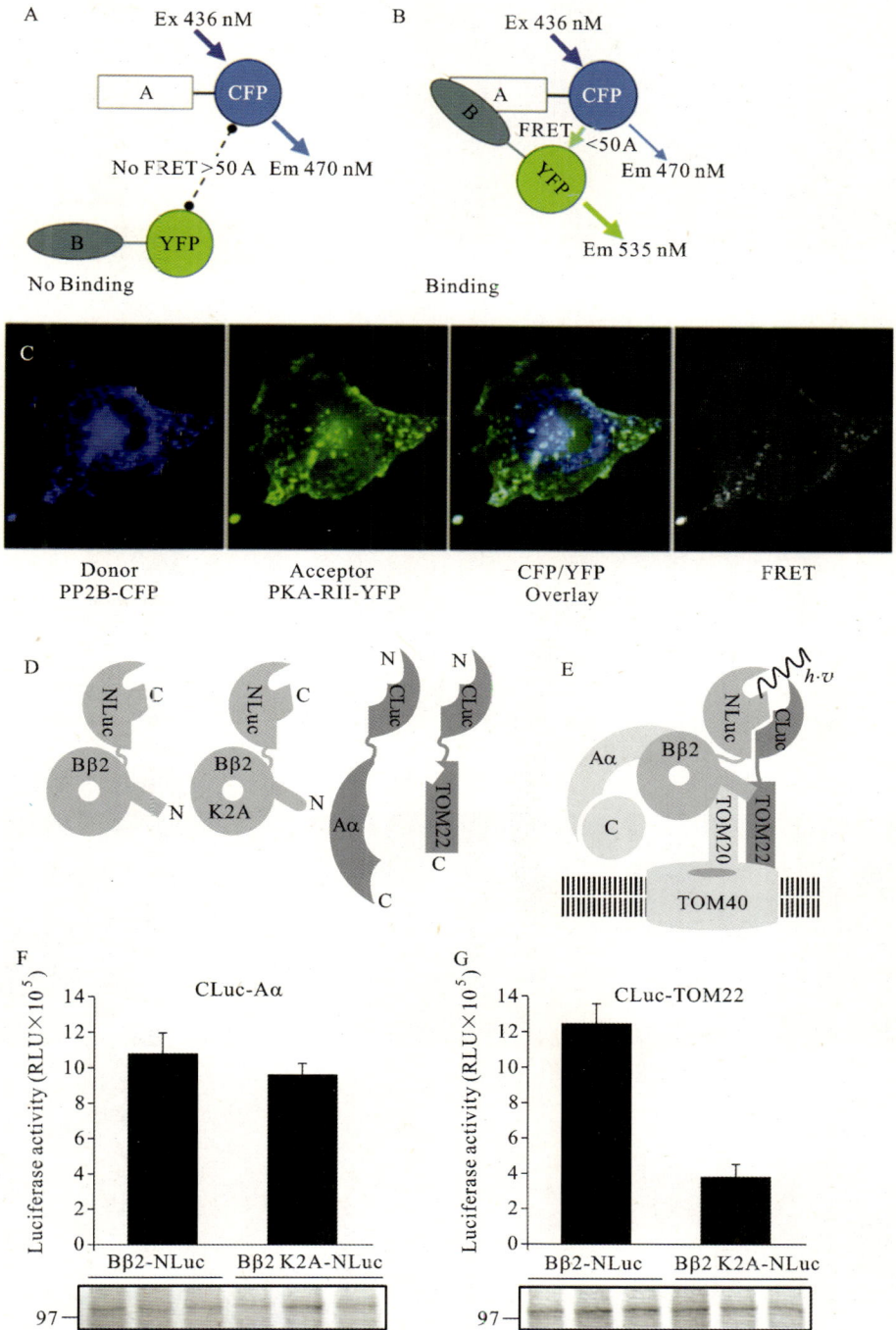

BOX 15.3 Detecting kinase/phosphatase complexes in living cells.

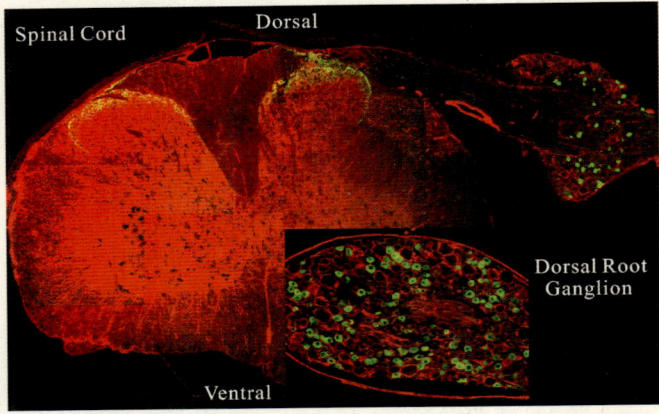

Fig.19.3 Expression of TRPV1 proteins in rat lumbar spinal cord (indicated in green) detected by anti-TRPV1 antibody.

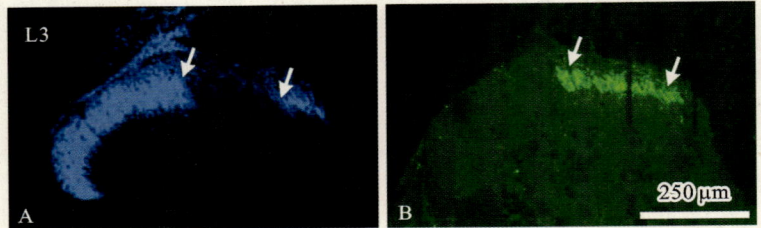

Fig.23.2 Alterations to C fibres after peripheral axotomy.

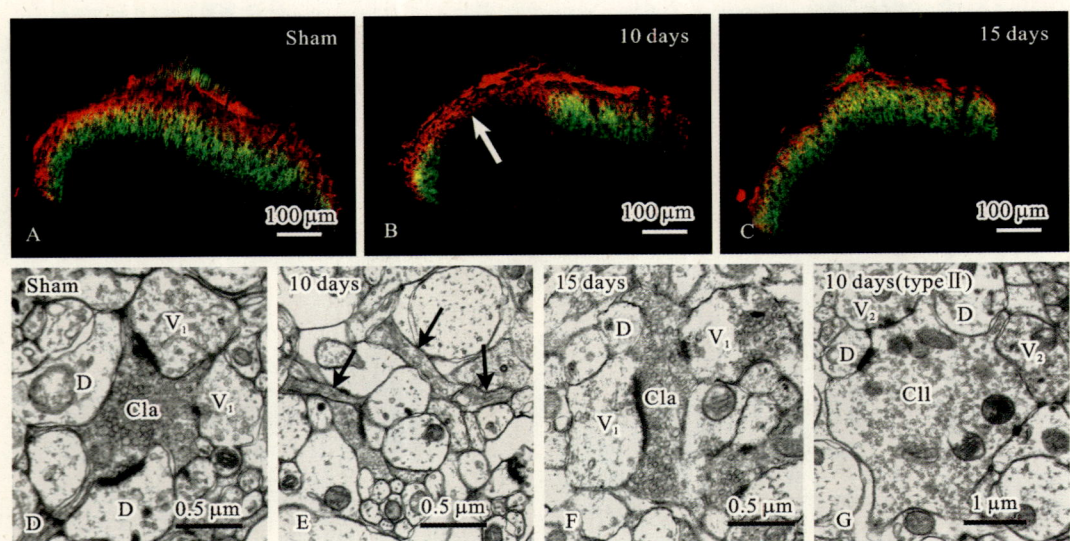

Fig.23.3 Transient loss of non-peptidergic nociceptive C afferents following the application of a polyethylene cuff to the sciatic nerve of the rat.

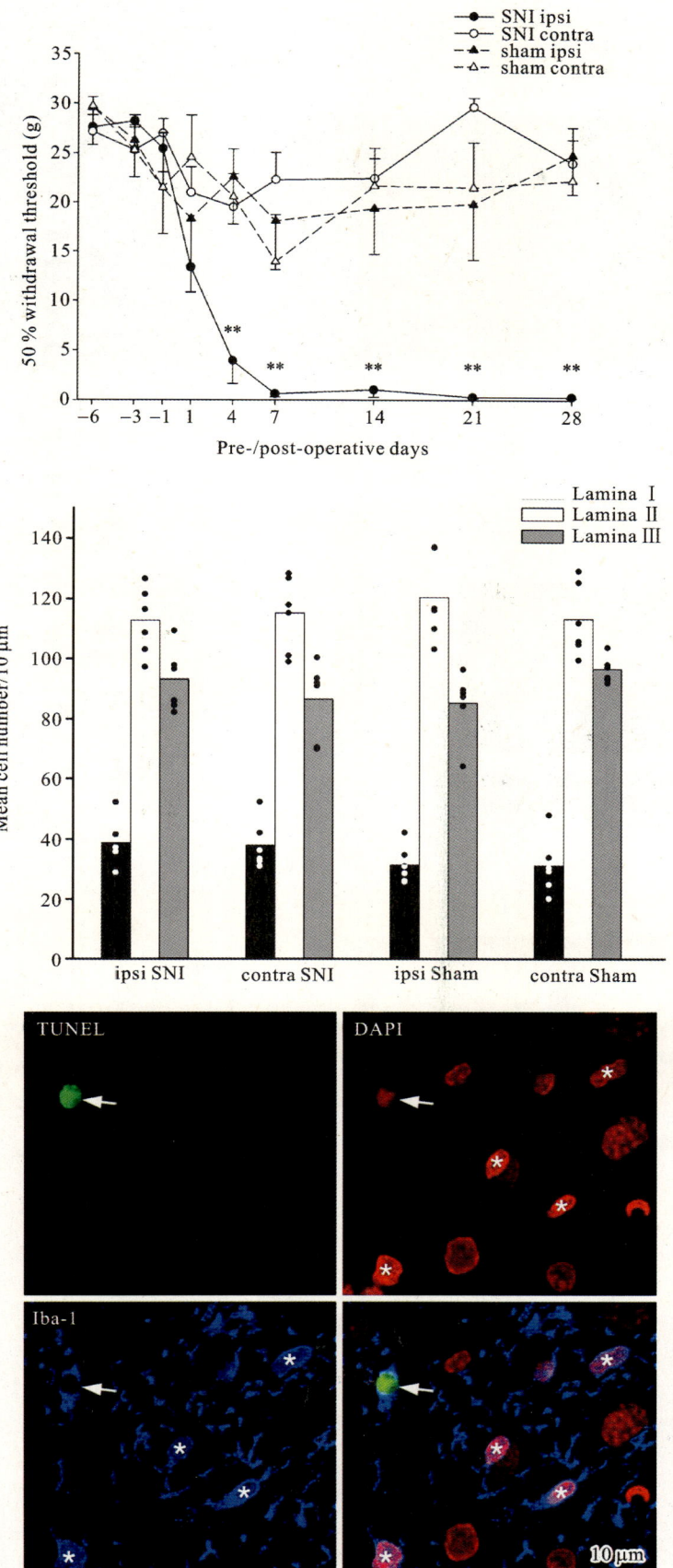

Fig.23.4 Evidence that loss of neurons from the superficial dorsal horn is not required for development of tactile allodynia in the spared nerve injury (SNI) model.

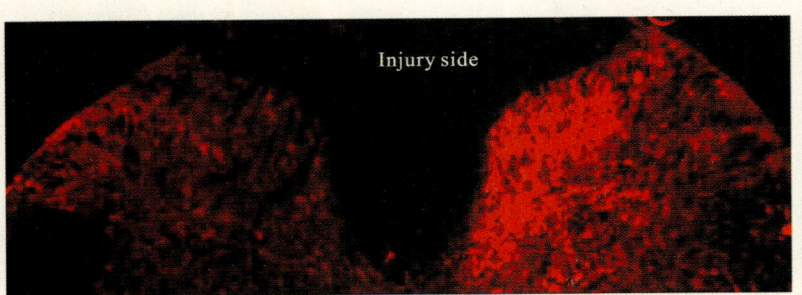

Fig.24.2 Activation of microglia in the spinal cord ipsilateral to the side of peripheral nerve injury.

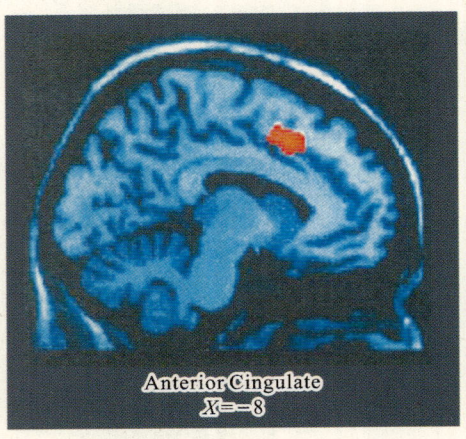

Fig.25.1 Activation of the ACC is related to pain unpleasantness.

A

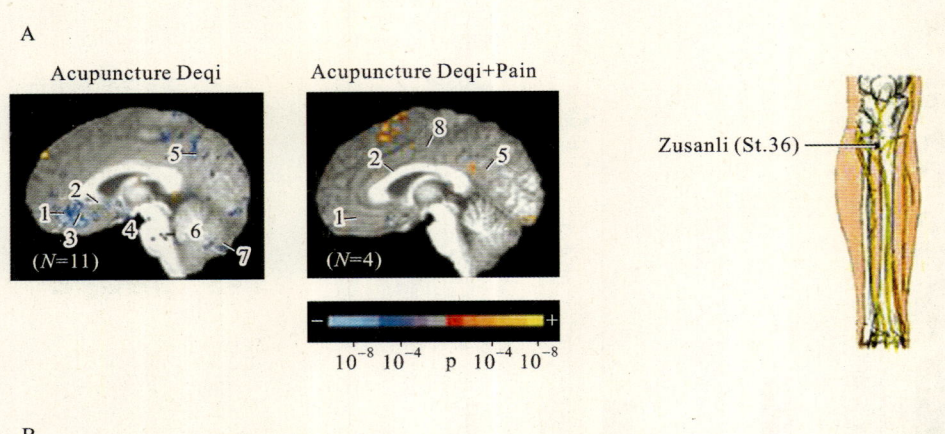

Acupuncture Deqi

Acupuncture Deqi+Pain

B

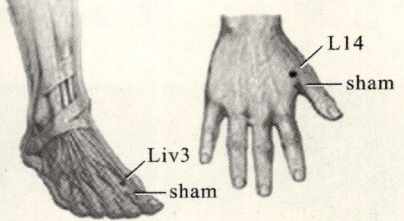

Zusanli (St.36)

Fig.29.5 Acupucture-induced change in brain neuroimage.

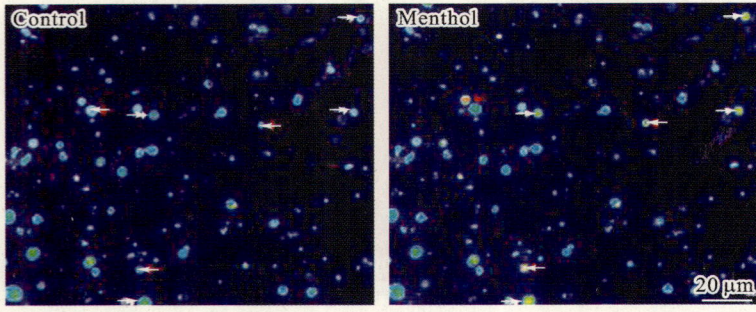

Fig.32.3 Identification of menthol-sensitive neurons.

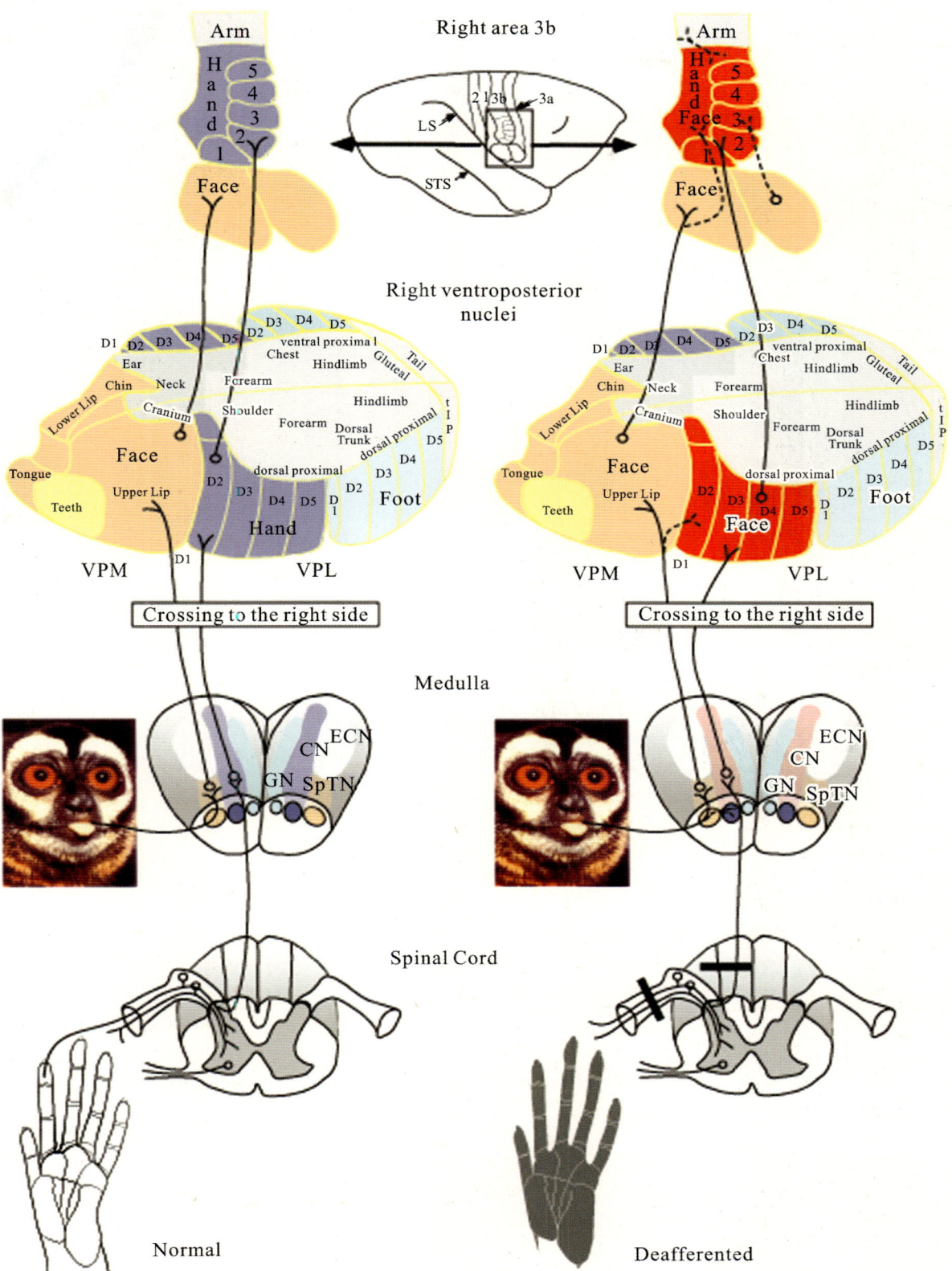

Fig. 26.2 The relay of sensory information from the skin to somatosensory cortex in a normal monkey (left) and a monkey (right) with the loss of inputs from the hand by peripheral nerve injury (bar on dorsal root of nerve) or dorsal column pathway section (bar on spinal cord).